Principles and
Practice of Equine
Sports Medicine

THE
ATHLETIC
HORSE

Principles and Practice of Equine Sports Medicine

THE ATHLETIC HORSE

David R. Hodgson

BVSc, PhD, FACSM, Diplomate, ACVIM

Superintendent, Rural Veterinary Centre
Department of Animal Health
University of Sydney
Camdem, Australia

formerly Associate Professor
Department of Veterinary Clinical Medicine and Surgery
Washington State University
Pullman, Washington

Reuben J. Rose

DVSc, PhD, FRCVS, DipVetAn, MACVSc

Professor of Veterinary Clinical Studies
Department of Veterinary Clinical Sciences
University of Sydney, Sydney, Australia

formerly Appleton Professor of Equine Surgery
College of Veterinary Medicine
University of Florida, Gainesville, Florida

W.B. SAUNDERS COMPANY

A Division of Harcourt Brace & Company

Philadelphia • London • Toronto • Montreal • Sydney • Tokyo

W. B. SAUNDERS COMPANY
A Division of Harcourt Brace Company

The Curtis Center
Independence Square West
Philadelphia, PA 19106

Library of Congress Cataloging-in-Publication Data

The Athletic horse : principles and practice of equine sports medicine
/ [edited by] David R. Hodgson, Reuben J. Rose. — 1st ed.
     p.   cm.
  ISBN 0-7216-3759-0
  1. Equine sports medicine.   2. Horses—Exercise—Physiological
effects.   I. Hodgson, David R.   II. Rose, R. J. (Reuben J.)
SF956.A88   1994
636.1'08971027—dc20   94-7652

THE ATHLETIC HORSE: Principles and Practice of Equine Medicine   ISBN   0–7216–3759–0

Printed in the United States of America

Last digit is the print number: 9   8   7   6   5   4   3   2   1

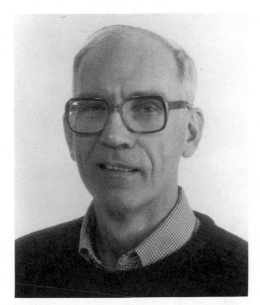

In memory of Dr. Philip D. Gollnick—eminent scientist, mentor, and friend
1936–1991

Contributors

TATIANA ART, D.V.M., Ph.D.

Assistant Professor, Head Equine Sports Medicine Unit, Faculty of Veterinary Medicine, University of Liege, Belgium.

The Respiratory System: Anatomy, Physiology, and Adaptations to Exercise and Training

HILARY M. CLAYTON, B.V.M.S, Ph.D., M.R.C.V.S.

Professor and Head, Department of Veterinary Anatomy, Western College of Veterinary Medicine, University of Saskatchewan, Saskatoon, Saskatchewan, Canada.

Training Show Jumpers

GORAN DALIN, D.V.M., Ph.D.

Associate Professor, Department of Anatomy and Histology, Faculty of Veterinary Medicine, Swedish University of Agricultural Sciences, Uppsala, Sweden; State Veterinarian, Equine Unit, Natimal Veterinary Institute, Uppsala, Sweden.

Biomechanics, Gait, and Conformation

KEVIN D. DERMAN, B.Sc.(Med.)

Researcher, Bioenergetics of Exercise Research Unit, University of Cape Town Medical School, South Africa.

Comparative Aspects of Exercise Physiology

SUE J. DYSON, B.A., Vet. M.B., D.E.O., F.R.C.V.S.

Head, Equine Clinical Services, Animal Health Trust, Newmarket, Suffolk, England.

Training the Event Horse

MICHAEL D. EATON, B.V.Sc.

Research Fellow, Equine Exercise Physiology, Equine Performance Laboratory, University of Sydney, NSW, Australia.

Energetics and Performance

DAVID L. EVANS, B.V.Sc., Ph.D.

Senior Lecturer, Department of Animal Science, The University of Sydney, NSW, Australia. Associate Director, Equine Performance Laboratory, University of Sydney, NSW, Australia.

The Cardiovascular System: Anatomy, Physiology, and Adaptations to Exercise and Training; Training Regimens: Overview; Training Thoroughbred Racehorses

KEN W. HINCHCLIFF, B.V.Sc., Ph.D., Diplomate A.C.V.I.M.

Assistant Professor, Department of Veterinary Clinical Sciences, College of Veterinary Medicine, The Ohio State University, Columbus, Ohio.

Drugs and Performance

DAVID R. HODGSON, B.V.Sc., Ph.D., Diplomate A.C.V.I.M., F.A.C.S.M.

Superintendent, Rural Veterinary Centre, University of Sydney, Camden, NSW; Associate Director, Equine Performance Laboratory, University of Sydney, NSW, Australia.

An Overview of Performance and Sports Medicine, Hematology and Biochemistry, Evaluation of Performance Potential, Clinical Exercise Testing, Investigation of Poor Performance, Training Regimens: Physiologic Adaptations to Training

LEO B. JEFFCOTT, B.V.Sc., Ph.D., F.R.C.V.S., D.V.Sc.

Dean, Veterinary School, Professor of Veterinary Clinical Studies, Department of Veterinary Medicine, University of Cambridge, Cambridge, England.

Biomechanics, Gait, and Conformation

LAURIE LAWRENCE, M.S., Ph.D.

Associate Professor, Department of Animal Sciences, University of Kentucky, Lexington, Kentucky.

Nutrition and the Athletic Horse

DESMOND P. LEADON, M.V.B., M.A., M.Sc., F.R.C.V.S.

Head, Clinical Pathology Unit, Irish Equine Centre, Johnstown, Naas, Co., Kildare, Ireland.

Transport Stress

PIERRE LEKEUX, D.V.M., Ph.D.

Professor and Head, Department of Physiology, Faculty of Veterinary Medicine, University of Liege, Belgium.

The Respiratory System: Anatomy, Physiology, and Adaptations to Exercise and Training

DAVID K. LOVELL, B.V.Sc.

Private Practitioner, 433 Boundary Rd., Thornlands, Qld, Australia.

Training Standardbred Trotters and Pacers

FINOLA McCONAGHY, B.V.Sc., Dip. Vet. Clin. Stud.

Graduate Student, Department of Animal Health, Rural Veterinary Centre, University of Sydney, Australia.

Thermoregulation

TIMOTHY D. NOAKES, M.B., Ch.B., M.D., F.A.C.S.M.

Liberty Life Chair of Exercise and Sports Science, University of Cape Town Medical School, Director, Medical Research Council, University of Cape Town Bioenergetics Exercise Research Unit, Cape Town, South Africa.

Comparative Aspects of Exercise Physiology

KERRY J. RIDGWAY, D.V.M.

Private Practitioner, Garden Valley, California.

Training Endurance Horses

REUBEN J. ROSE, D.V.Sc., Ph.D., F.R.C.V.S., M.A.C.V.Sc.

Professor, Veterinary Clinical Studies, Director, Equine Performance Laboratory, University of Sydney, NSW, Australia.

An Overview of Performance and Sports Medicine, Hematology and Biochemistry, Evaluation of Performance Potential, Clinical Exercise Testing, Investigation of Poor Performance, Training Regimens: Physiologic Adaptations to Training

RICHARD A. SAMS, Ph.D.

Department of Veterinary Clinical Sciences, College of Veterinary Medicine, The Ohio State University, Columbus, Ohio.

Drugs and Performance

MICHAEL C.A. SCHRAMME, D.V.M., Cert. E.O., M.R.C.V.S.

Lecturer in Equine Surgery, Department of Large Animal Medicine and Surgery, Royal Veterinary College, University of London, England.

Diagnostic Imaging in the Athletic Horse: Scintigraphy

ROGER K.W. SMITH, M.A., Vet. M.B., Cert. E.O., M.R.C.V.S.

Department of Large Animal Medicine and Surgery, Royal Veterinary College, University of London, England.

Diagnostic Imaging in the Athletic Horse: Radiology; Diagnostic Imaging in the Athletic Horse: Musculoskeletal Ultrasonography; Diagnostic Imaging in the Athletic Horse: Scintigraphy

DAVID H. SNOW, D.V.Sc., B.Sc (Vet.)., Ph.D., M.R.C.V.S.

Consultant Clinical Pathologist, Macquarie Vetnostic Services; Consultant Equisci International, Sydney, NSW, Australia.

Muscle Anatomy, Physiology, and Adaptations to Exercise and Training

VICTOR C. SPEIRS, B.V.Sc., Dr. Med. Vet., Ph.D., F.A.C.V.Sc, Diplomate A.C.V.S

Professor and Head, Equine Surgery, University of Bern, Bern, Switzerland.

Lameness: Approaches to Therapy and Rehabilitation

STEPHANIE VALBERG, D.V.M., Ph.D., Diplomate A.C.V.I.M.

Assistant Professor, Department of Clinical and Population Sciences, College of Veterinary Medicine, University of Minnesota, St. Paul, Minnesota; Large Animal Clinic, Department of Clinical and Population Sciences, College of Veterinary Medicine, University of Minnesota, St. Paul, Minnesota.

Muscle Anatomy, Physiology, and Adaptations to Exercise and Training

PETER WEBBON, B. Vet. Med, Ph.D., D.V.R.

Senior Lecturer, Equine Medicine, Department of Large Animal Medicine and Surgery, Royal Veterinary College, University of London, England.

Diagnostic Imaging in the Athletic Horse: Radiology; Diagnostic Imaging in the Athletic Horse: Musculoskeletal Ultransonography; Diagnostic Imaging in the Athletic Horse: Scintigraphy

Preface

Over the past 10 years, there has been considerable interest in equine exercise physiology in all parts of the world. Much has been written of the lack of improvement in racetrack times over the last 100 years, in contrast with human athletic performance. Assumptions have been made that similar improvements should be possible in equine performance, but so far there is no evidence to substantiate these claims. The athletic horse is not just a big version of a human athlete but rather an animal with unique physiology and limitations to its exercise capacity. Some of these unique features have not been understood by writers of various popular books on fitness and training methods in horses. An understanding of the major body systems involved in exercise, together with interpretation of the results of various research papers, provides a useful starting point in production of fitter athletic horses who have a lower incidence of musculoskeletal injuries.

The contributors to this book have done an outstanding job in providing an overview of performance in the athletic horse. The international representation of the authors indicates worldwide interest in the athletic horse. We thank all contributors for their care in preparation of their manuscripts and for meeting the deadlines so that timely production of the book was possible. The book is arranged in two major sections: Section 1 covers basic structure and function with details of anatomy, physiology, and biochemistry of the major body systems involved in performance. Section 2 covers more practical aspects of exercise science with material on nutrition, poor performance, exercise testing, training, and drugs. We hope that this book will be useful at a wide range of levels. It should be a valuable text for students of animal science and veterinary medicine as well as veterinarians involved with athletic horses, horse owners, and trainers.

We thank our wives Jennifer and Suzette for their forbearance during the production of this book. Ray Kersey and Linda Mills, Senior Medical Editors at Saunders, played vital roles in bringing this book to fruition, and we are grateful for their assistance. John Fitzpatrick provided expert editorial assistance and we thank him for his care and attention to detail. Our thanks also to Bozena Jantulik for her outstanding drawings, and to Shirley Ray, Louise Southwood, Jennifer Wright, and Ruth Davis for editing and research assistance. We also thank our colleagues and research students in the Equine Performance Laboratory at the University of Sydney: David Evans, Michael Eaton, David Lloyd, Finola McConaghy, Allan Davie, Christine King, Joanne Rainger, Shaun McKane, Leopoldo Sosa Leon, Cathy Tyler, Lorraine Golland, Robert Christley, and Chris Whitton. Finally, we acknowledge the support of the Australian Equine Research Foundation, the New South Wales Racing Research Fund, the Australian Research Council, Vetsearch International, and the University of Sydney for financial support over the last 15 years for studies into equine exercise physiology.

D.R. HODGSON AND R.J. ROSE
JUNE, 1994

Contents

I

Structural Considerations in Equine Sports Medicine

1

An Overview of Performance and Sports Medicine

R. J. ROSE AND D. R. HODGSON

Introduction

The study of equine sports medicine, while now out of its infancy, can only be said to be in its adolescence compared with investigations into human exercise and sports science, which appear to have reached maturity. Early studies of equine exercise physiology at the end of the 19th century[1] through until the mid-1930s[2] focused on energy metabolism, with particular relevance to the work horse. While the work horse is still used in some parts of the world, increasing mechanization in Western countries has resulted in the horse being used mainly for recreational purposes. Revenue from gambling has been an important driving force for a thriving racing industry in most developed countries.

In the 1950s and 1960s, there was an upsurge in interest in the physiology of the athletic horse,[3–8] and over the last 10 years, there has been a dramatic acceleration in information that is available from a range of research studies performed around the world. The real pioneer of equine exercise science is Professor Sune Persson, who commenced his studies of the Swedish trotter in the early 1960s. Persson was the first person to utilize the treadmill to study the physiology of exercise, and the treadmill has now become widely used for research as well as commercial training. Persson's work has stimulated a wide range of studies throughout the world examining the science of equine exercise. The widespread interest in the physiology of the athletic horse can be gauged by the response to three international conferences on equine exercise physiology held in Oxford, U.K., San Diego, U.S.A., and Uppsala, Sweden, between 1982 and 1990 involving the publication of 200 original papers.[9–11] Clearly, there is both scientific and commercial interest in factors that contribute to successful athletic performance.

Equine Sports Medicine and the Athletic Horse

In contrast to earlier investigations into exercise that were stimulated by the horse's role in agriculture, today the horse is largely used for recreation, and the range of activities has become increasingly diversified. A variety of breeds are involved in an assortment of athletic endeavors, including thoroughbred, standardbred, and quarter horse racing, endurance riding, show jumping, 3-day eventing, driving events, and vaulting. Added to this are activities such as dressage, western pleasure, rodeo, barrel racing, and polo. Riders, drivers, trainers, and veterinarians are better informed, and there is acknowledgment that traditional training and feeding methods require investigation. Appropriate changes could be made to such areas as training strategies in light of new information from research studies. However, it must be acknowledged that there is some disillusionment with equine sports medicine because of expectations that the principles used in human exercise science could be transposed easily to training the athletic horse. Several popular books[12,13] proposed simple recipes for success in training horses, but these regimens had not received scientific investigation, and many methods proposed were time-consuming and ultimately produced no improvement in athletic performance. There are no easy methods for producing athletic success in horses. However, the extensive information that is now available from various research studies does provide the opportunity for some guidelines for horse owners, trainers, and veterinarians. Superior athletic performance is multifaceted and is the result of integration of the major body systems involved in delivering energy, as well as biomechanical factors (Fig. 1–1). Aerobic energy delivery, a function of heart rate, stroke volume, and oxygen

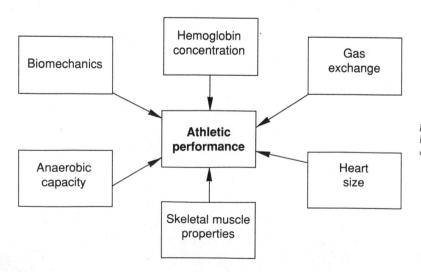

Figure 1-1. Some of the major physiological factors contributing to superior athletic performance in horses.

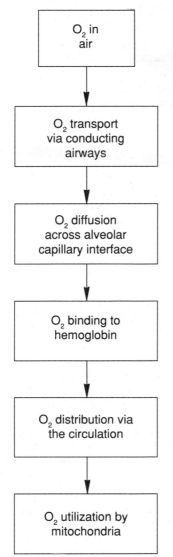

Figure 1-2. *The oxygen transport chain showing the various steps in transport from the air breathed in to final utilization by the mitochondria.*

extraction by muscle, is the result of a complex chain of events involving the oxygen transport chain (Fig. 1–2). In contrast, anaerobic energy delivery is more direct and predominates in the rapid delivery of energy for brief periods of intense exercise (Fig. 1–3). While it is clear that physiologic capacity is closely related to athletic performance, it appears almost impossible to define what contributes to that elusive "will to win" that distinguishes the champion horse within an elite group.

Energy Demands of Exercise and Implications for Training

If one compares events as diverse as endurance riding (160 km) and racing (up to 3200 m), it is clear that there are great differences in energy demands, biomechanical function, thermoregulation, and training strategies. Other athletic activities such as dressage and show jumping focus on biomechanical skills rather than energy availability. However, in all these activities, an important consideration is the provision of energy from the available reserves, which are chiefly glycogen in liver and skeletal muscle and fat in the various fat depots. A detailed consideration of energy utilization during exercise is provided in Chapter 4. Knowledge of the patterns of energy use in different competitive events allows specific training strategies to be adopted to maximize the adaptations in various body systems. While both aerobic and anaerobic energy supplies coexist in all events, aerobic energy production predominates in the majority of equine competitive activities. This has important implications for training strategies because an emphasis on aerobic training appears to be an important foundation for all events. However, much more information is required for assessing different training schemes and experimental methods to determine factors such as

- The optimal age to commence training
- Specificity of training for speed rather than stamina
- The time course of adaptations of bone and supporting structures to training exercise
- The selection of horses for specific events prior to the onset of training
- The rate of decrease in fitness following cessation of training

Many of these questions can be answered by specific experiments, but it is doubtful whether sufficient resources are available to determine whether physiologic measurements may be used to forecast future athletic performance accurately.

Training and Musculoskeletal Injuries

The major problem in training horses for athletic activities is to keep them free of injury. Studies examining racehorses in training have shown that by far the most common reason for wastage is musculoskeletal injury.[14,15] While a variety of factors are obviously involved, including the conformation, training surface, age of the horse, and stage of training, there have been few studies that have examined the role of training in maximizing the strength of soft tissue and bone. Most racehorses commence training when they are 18 to 20 months of age, which is long before the attainment of bone maturity. In growing horses there is little change in bone mineral density, whereas bone mineral content increases from weaning to the onset of training.[16] With training, noninvasive methods for assessment of bone quality have shown no changes in bone mineral content or bone mineral density.[17] However, studies by Jeffcott and colleagues[17,18] demonstrated an increase in apparent ultrasound velocity, indicating an increase in bone strength due to reduced bone porosity. These studies have shown the importance of adaptations of bone to training, but there is little or no information on adapta-

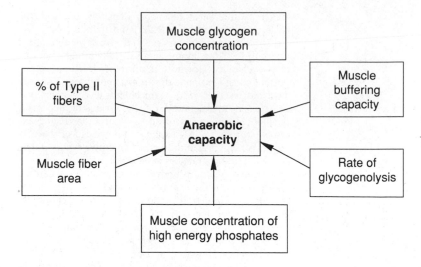

Figure 1-3. *A summary of important factors contributing to anaerobic capacity.*

tions of important soft-tissue structures such as ligaments and tendons. Recently, there has been evidence of a decrease in density and increase in area of the superficial flexor tendon during training.[19] Further experiments are necessary to determine the optimal training regimens for strengthening of bone and soft tissues in horses of different ages involved in the variety of equine athletic endeavors.

Limitations to Performance

Fatigue is a complex chain of events, with central as well as peripheral contributions. Short-duration, high-intensity exercise such as is performed in thoroughbred, quarter horse, and standardbred racing is not limited by availability of substrates but, more likely, by failure of energy production associated with an increase in protons and a decrease in [ATP].[20] In contrast, longer-duration exercise such as endurance riding results in substantial muscle glycogen depletion, which eventually may limit the horse's capacity to continue exercise.[21,22] In addition, long-distance exercise also imposes substantial thermoregulatory demands, with evaporative cooling from sweat production as the major mechanism for heat dissipation. Some of the factors involved in fatigue and poor performance are discussed in detail in Chapter 13, while thermoregulation is reviewed in Chapter 9.

New Technology

Along with the increase in scientific studies on the athletic horse over the last 10 years has come a range of technology to aid in training, evaluation of fitness, and assessment of response to exercise. Formerly, the complete blood count and plasma or serum biochemical "profile" were the main diagnostic aids used by veterinarians to assess clinical and subclinical disease in performance horses. However, a range of equipment is now available to assist veterinarians and trainers in determining exercise capacity and fitness, including treadmills, heart rate meters, and rapid lactate analyzers.

TREADMILLS

Until the mid-1980s, studies utilizing a high-speed treadmill were confined to those conducted at the Swedish University of Agricultural Sciences in Uppsala, Sweden.[8,23–25] However, it is interesting to note that in April of 1891, mechanical treadmills were used in the theater to simulate horse races (Fig. 1–4). A report in *Scientific American* noted, "One of the 'hits' of Messrs. Montreal and Blondeau's 'Paris Port de Mer,' played at the Varieties Theater, is a horse race. The horses are free from all restraint, and really gallop, but the ground disappears under their feet, moving in a direction opposite that of their running, and the landscape as well as the fences also fly in a direction contrary to the forward motion of the horses."[26] During the last 8 to 10 years, high-speed treadmills (Fig. 1–5) have been installed in a large number of veterinary schools as well as being utilized by thoroughbred and standardbred horse trainers to aid in the training of racehorses. Additionally, many stud farms use lower-speed treadmills to walk and trot yearlings for conditioning prior to annual sales. Two main companies are involved in treadmill manufacture: Kagra AG, a Swiss company that manufactures the Mustang treadmill (Kagra AG, Fahrwangen, Switzerland), and Säto, a Swedish company whose treadmills are now distributed in the United States (Säto, Kansas City, MO). Both these companies make a lower-cost treadmill that is suited to training establishments and veterinary practices, as well as a more sophisticated machine used by institutions.

Much of our current knowledge concerning the physiologic responses to exercise is the result of a variety of treadmill studies examining cardiovascular, respiratory, metabolic, thermoregulatory, hematologic, and hormonal changes in horses exercising over different distances and intensities. However, it should be remem-

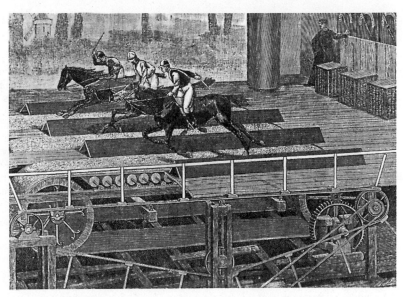

Figure 1-4. Simulated horse race with horses "running in place" on treadmills. This simulated race took place at the Varieties Theater and was reported in the Scientific American in April of 1981. (Illustration courtesy of Scientific American, with permission.)

bered that treadmill exercise is an artificial method for exercising horses that cannot duplicate the effects of air movement, ground surface, and the impact of a rider when horses are exercised on grass or dirt. Horses exercising on a treadmill have no momentum because the motorized treadmill provides the driving force. Thus the actual work performed by horses during treadmill exercise is quantitatively different from track work. Care must be taken when extrapolating treadmill exercise to the competitive event. Nonetheless, training horses utilizing a treadmill has a number of advantages over track training. Treadmill training provides a consistent exercise surface, permits exercise during inclement weather, allows precise control over the training intensity, and permits monitoring of the level of fitness using standardized exercise tests. Simple measurements such as plasma or blood lactate concentrations at various submaximal treadmill speeds, as well as alterations in heart

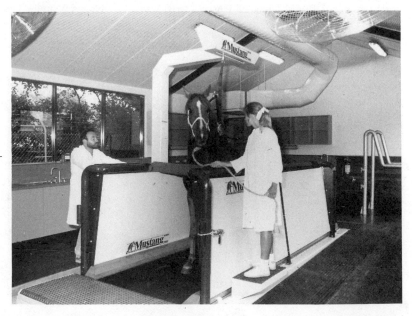

Figure 1-5. A Mustang (Kagra AG, Switzerland) treadmill used at the University of Sydney Equine Performance Laboratory.

rate, can assist in determining responses to the training level. Further aspects of the use of treadmills for exercise testing and as a training aid are discussed in Chapters 12 and 17.

To reduce the speed at which horses exercise, most research workers and horse trainers use treadmills inclined at slopes varying from 5 to 19 (2 to 11 degrees) percent so that a high workload can be maintained at a lower overall speed. The major advantage of this is lessening of the chance of musculoskeletal injury because speeds above 12 to 13 m/s are unnecessary. Our studies have shown that inclining the treadmill at a slope of 10 percent (6 degrees) results in most horses reaching their maximum oxygen uptake at speeds in the range 10 to 12 m/s compared with 14 to 15 m/s on the flat. Most treadmills can have the incline changed from the flat up to +10 percent slope, while speeds may be varied from 0 to 15 m/s. Some less expensive treadmills that permit only speeds up to 6 m/s have a fixed incline in excess of 10 percent. These treadmills are appropriate for mild to moderate exercise, but the steep treadmill incline may have adverse effects on biomechanical function.

HEART RATE METERS

Heart rate meters (Fig. 1–6) have been available for the past 10 to 12 years and have been used widely by sections of the thoroughbred and standardbred racing industries, as well as riders involved in endurance and 3-day events. The majority of heart rate meters are accurate[27,28] and relatively easy to use. The two major heart rate meters that we have worked with are the Equistat HR7 (EQB, Unionville, PA) and the Hippocard (Ingenieurburo Isler, Zurich, Switzerland), and both have storage mechanisms for replaying the heart rate after the exercise bout. The EQB heart rate meter has been designed principally for use in riding horses, whereas the Hippocard functions by telemetry, transmitting the heart rate signal for a distance of 1 m to a wrist watch

receiver. In both these heart rate meters, electrodes are placed over the wither region and the ventral midline, being maintained in position using a saddle or girth strap. Accurate heart rate values can be achieved only by good electrode contact with the skin, and this is often difficult in the galloping horse. Electrode gel or a concentrated saltwater solution is useful for enhancing electrode-skin contact.

Heart rate meters may be used to monitor the intensity of an exercise bout on the basis that there is a linear relationship between heart rate and exercise intensity (Fig. 1–7) in the range 120 to 210 beats per minute.[29] Factors affecting the heart rate response to exercise and training are discussed in Chapter 7.

RAPID LACTATE ANALYZERS

Measurement of blood or plasma lactate, during or after exercise, is one of the simplest and most useful methods for monitoring the relative intensity of an exercise bout and the response to training. Lactate values in plasma are between 30 and 50 percent higher than whole-blood lactate, but because there is no consistent relationship between values in plasma and blood, one or the other should be used consistently. Lactate increases exponentially with increasing workload (Fig. 1–8), and values during submaximal exercise decrease with increasing fitness (see Chap. 17). The availability of rapid lactate analyzers (Yellow Springs Instruments, Columbus, OH) has allowed lactate measurements to be performed, if necessary, at the trackside. Machines are available for less than $5000, are simple to operate, and require minimum maintenance.

MUSCLE BIOPSY

Sampling of skeletal muscle using the technique of needle biopsy was introduced into equine exercise physiology by Lindholm and Piehl.[30] Over the past 20 years,

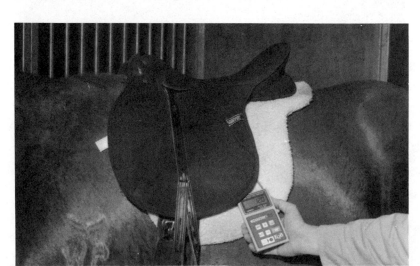

Figure 1-6. An EQB (Unionville, PA) heart rate meter used for monitoring the heart rate during exercise and recovery from exercise.

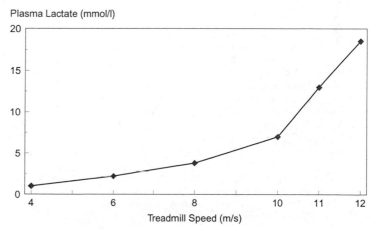

Heart Rate (beats/min)

Figure 1-7. Normal heart rate response to exercise in a 3-year-old thoroughbred horse during an incremental exercise test on a treadmill inclined at a slope of 6 degrees (10 percent).

Treadmill Speed (m/s)

a wide range of research investigations have been performed to determine response of muscle to exercise and training (see Chap. 8). While early studies indicated that there was a relationship between muscle fiber type and competitive activity for which the horse was used,[31,32] more recent research has indicated that there is too much variation for the needle biopsy technique to be used to predict performance.[22,33] Thus muscle biopsy is unlikely to become an important practical tool within veterinary practice. However, muscle biopsy remains an important method for scientific investigations into the responses to exercise and training because some of the major adaptations occur in skeletal muscle.

DIAGNOSTIC EQUIPMENT

The high incidence of musculoskeletal injuries among athletic horses has given rise to various pieces of equipment that can be used to assist in the early diagnosis and prognosis of injuries.

Thermography. Thermography has been used for detecting areas of inflammation by determination of changes in skin surface temperature.[34,35] Thermography equipment has been available for many years, and newer equipment permits a hard-copy printout of the color image. While the equipment is useful for comparing skin temperature differences between the forelegs or hindlegs, thermography is probably useful only for detecting acute injuries.

Ultrasound. Now widely used diagnostically to assess tendon and ligament injuries (see Chap. 14), ultrasound permits better approaches to rehabilitation. Ultrasound also has been used to evaluate changes in bone quality during training[17] by assessing changes in ultrasound velocity. A study by Jeffcott and colleagues[17] demonstrated that there was a decrease in ultrasound velocity prior to development of signs of metacarpal periostitis ("bucked shins"). This information could be applied within a commercial training context to detect subtle subclinical bone disease prior to signs of lameness becoming evident.

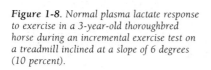

Plasma Lactate (mmol/l)

Figure 1-8. Normal plasma lactate response to exercise in a 3-year-old thoroughbred horse during an incremental exercise test on a treadmill inclined at a slope of 6 degrees (10 percent).

Treadmill Speed (m/s)

Nuclear Scintigraphy. This is a technique used for diagnosis of lameness due to problems such as fissure fractures involving the metacarpal bones, tibia, and humerus. It is used by specialist institutions and university veterinary clinics because of the cost of the equipment and the need for radiation-control measures. However, hand-held gamma cameras are now available together with a computer software package that permits analysis of the results, for about $7500 (Oakfield Instruments, Ltd, Eynsham, England). This may result in more widespread use of scintigraphy by clinics that specialize in sports medicine injuries. Scintigraphy is not a technique that can be used as a screening procedure for lameness because of the cost of ^{99m}Tc-MDP and the need to keep horses isolated for several days after injection of the ^{99m}Tc.

The Future for Equine Sports Medicine

For generations, the care and training of athletic horses have been based on tradition. This accent on horse husbandry continues to be a key to successful athletic performance, but some of the principles of exercise physiology will find their way into commercial training programs, as well as being available for use by specialized veterinary practices. Training of research students in exercise science will provide the knowledge base and expertise for wide areas of the equine industry.

Much of the basic knowledge of the physiology and biochemistry of equine exercise is now known. However, a great deal of the available information is purely descriptive, and therefore, considerable further research is required before specific recommendations can be made about optimal training methods or selection for performance potential. The high expectations for improved performance in athletic horses as a result of the use of human athletic training principles have given way to more modest hopes. Application of the principles of exercise physiology should enable improved fitness of athletic horses and a reduction in the high incidence of limb injuries. Better measurements of fitness are necessary for evaluating training programs so that it is possible to determine when horses are ready for competition. Such indices may come from objective measurements of improvements in oxygen transport, such as maximal oxygen uptake ($\dot{V}_{O_2max}$) or a standardized test that allows calculation of measurements such as the speed at which a plasma lactate of 4 mmol/liter (V_{LA4}) is reached. These tests require treadmills, but it may be possible to develop further track or field tests to aid in fitness evaluation. Much more laboratory work is necessary to allow decisions on training strategies to be based on objective indicators of improvements in fitness rather than the current subjective impressions. These data should become available as further studies are performed by various research groups around the world.

Selection of the horse with outstanding physiologic potential for the particular competitive event prior to commencement of training is one of the unrealized dreams of those involved in equine exercise physiology. While the various factors associated with superior performance are well known (see Fig. 1–1), the weighting of these and the potential for forecasting athletic success from physiologic indices are unknown. To undertake a project to examine predictors of performance, a huge range of resources is required so that a large number of weanlings and yearlings could be assessed and evaluated against some objective indices of performance. This has such obvious commercial ramifications that it seems likely that the project will eventually be undertaken, although the results may never be published.

Conclusions

The athletic horse is a remarkable animal, with both grace and stamina. A high heart weight to body weight ratio, large mass-specific cardiac output, and substantial capacity for oxygen carriage resulting from splenic erythrocyte release during exercise all contribute to the potential of the athletic horse to run at speeds up to 10 to 12 m/s for long distances and reach peak speeds of 17.5 to 18 m/s.[36,37] We need to further understand the limitations to equine performance as well as the adaptations that are possible for the wide range of equine competitive activities.

References

1. Zuntz N, Hagemann O: Untersuchungen uber den Stoffwechsel des pferdes bei ruhe und arbeit. Landw Jahrb 1898; 27:1.
2. Procter RC, Brody S, Jones MM, et al: Growth and development with special reference to domestic animals: XXXIII. Efficiency of work in horses of different ages and body weights. Univ Missouri Agr Exp Stat Res Bull 1934; 209:1.
3. Irvine CHG: The blood picture in the racehorse: I. The normal erythrocyte and hemoglobin status: a dynamic concept. J Am Vet Med Assoc 1958; 133:97.
4. Steel JD, Whitlock L: Observations on the haematology of thoroughbred and standardbred horses in training and racing. Aust Vet J 1960; 36:136.
5. Steel JD: Studies on the Electrocardiogram of the Racehorse. Sydney, Australia, Australasian Medical Publishing Company, 1963.
6. Karlsen GG, Nadaljak EA: Gas and energy exchange in breathing of trotters during exercise (title translated from Russian). Konevodstovo 1964; 11:21.
7. Holmes JR, Alps BJ, Darke PGG: A method of radiotelemetry in equine electrocardiography. Vet Rec 1966; 79:90.
8. Persson SGB: On blood volume and working capacity in horses. Acta Physiol Scand 1967; (suppl 19):1.
9. Snow DH, Persson SGB, Rose RJ (eds): Equine Exercise Physiology. Cambridge, Granta Editions, 1983.
10. Gillespie JR, Robinson NE (eds): Equine Exercise Physiology 2. Davis, CA, ICEEP Publications, 1987.
11. Persson SGB, Lindholm A, Jeffcott LB (eds): Equine Exercise Physiology 3. Davis, CA, ICEEP Publications, 1991.
12. Ivers T: The Fit Racehorse. Cincinnati, OH, Esprit Racing Team, Ltd, 1983.
13. Swan P: Racehorse Training and Feeding. Victoria, Australia, Racehorse Sportsmedicine and Scientific Conditioning, 1984.
14. Jeffcott LB, Rossdale PD, Freestone J, et al: An assessment of wastage in thoroughbred racing from conception to 4 years of age. Equine Vet J 1982; 14:185.
15. Rossdale PD, Hopes R, Oxford K, et al: Epidemiological study of wastage among racehorses 1982 and 1983. Vet Rec 1985; 116:66.
16. Buckingham SHW, Jeffcott LB: Changes in bone strength and density in standardbreds from weaning to onset of training. In Gillespie JR, Robinson NE (eds): Equine Exercise Physiology 2. Davis, CA, ICEEP Publications, 1987, p 631.

17. Jeffcott LB, Buckingham SHW, McCartney RN. Noninvasive measurements of bone quality in horses and changes associated with exercise. *In* Gillespie JR, Robinson NE (eds): Equine Exercise Physiology 2. Davis, CA, ICEEP Publications, 1987, p 615.

18. McCarthy RN, Jeffcott LB: Treadmill exercise intensity and its effects on cortical bone in horses of various ages. *In* Persson SGB, Lindholm A, Jeffcott LB (eds): Equine Exercise Physiology 3. Davis, CA, ICEEP Publications, 1991, p 419.

19. Gillis C: A comparison of clinical, ultrasonographic and histologic analyses of the response of equine superficial flexor tendons to race training. *In* American Association of Equine Practice 38th Convention, Summaries, 1992, p 130.

20. Snow DH, Harris RC, Gash SP: Metabolic response of equine muscle to intermittent maximal exercise. J Appl Physiol 1985; 58:1689.

21. Snow DH, Baxter P, Rose RJ: Muscle fibre composition and glycogen depletion in horses competing in an endurance ride. Vet Rec 1981; 108:374.

22. Hodgson DR, Rose RJ, Allen JR: Muscle glycogen depletion and repletion patterns in horses performing various distances of endurance exercise. *In* Snow DH, Persson SGB, Rose RJ (eds): Equine Exercise Physiology. Cambridge, Granta Editions, 1983, p 229.

23. Lindholm A, Bjerneld A, Saltin B: Glycogen depletion pattern in muscle fibers of trotting horses. Acta Physiol Scand 1974; 90:475.

24. Persson SGB, Essen B, Lindholm A: Oxygen uptake, red cell volume, and pulse/work relationship in different states of training in trotters. *In* Proceedings of the 5th Meeting of the Academic Society of Large Animal Veterinary Medicine, 1980, p 34.

25. Fredericson I, Drevemo S, Dalin G, et al: The application of high-speed cinematography for quantitative analysis of equine locomotion. Equine Vet J 1980; 12:54.

26. The horse race on stage. Sci Am 1891; 64:263.

27. Evans DL, Rose RJ: Method of investigation of the accuracy of four digitally-displayed heart rate meters suitable for use in the exercising horse. Equine Vet J 1986; 18.129.

28. Physick-Sheard PW, Harman JC, Snow DH, et al: Evaluation of factors influencing the performance of four equine heart rate meters. *In* Gillespie JR, Robinson NE (eds): Equine Exercise Physiology 2. Davis, CA, ICEEP Publications, 1987, p 103.

29. Persson SGB: Evaluation of exercise tolerance and fitness in the performance horse. *In* Snow DH, SGB Persson, Rose RJ (eds): Equine Exercise Physiology. Cambridge, Granta Editions, 1983, p 441.

30. Lindholm A, Piehl K: Fiber composition, enzyme activities and concentrations of metabolites and electrolytes in muscles of standardbred horses. Acta Vet Scand 1974; 15:287.

31. Snow DH, Guy PS: Fiber type and enzyme activities of the gluteus medius in different breeds of horse. *In* Poortmans J, Niset G (eds): Biochemistry of Exercise IV-B. Baltimore, University Park Press, 1981, p 275.

32. Snow DH, Guy PS: Muscle fiber type composition of a number of limb muscles in different types of horse. Res Vet Sci 1980; 28:137.

33. Kline KH, Lawrence LM, Novakofski J, et al: Changes in muscle fiber type variation within the middle gluteal of young and mature horses as a function of sampling depth. *In* Gillespie JR, Robinson NE (eds): Equine Exercise Physiology 2. Davis, CA, ICEEP Publications, 1987, p 271.

34. Turner TA, Purohit RC, Fessler JF: Thermography: A review in equine medicine. Compend Contin Educ Pract Vet 1986; 8:855.

35. Turner TA, Wolfsdorf K, Jourdenais J: Effects of heat, cold, biomagnets, and ultrasound on skin circulation in the horse. *In* Proceedings of the Annual Convention of the American Association of Equine Practice, 1991, vol 36, p 249.

36. Evans DL, Rose RJ: Cardiovascular and respiratory responses in thoroughbred horses during treadmill exercise. J Exp Biol 1988; 134:397.

37. Rose RJ, Hodgson DR, Kelso TB, et al: Maximum O_2 uptake, O_2 debt and deficit, and muscle metabolites in thoroughbred horses. J Appl Physiol 1988; 64:781.

2

Comparative Aspects
of Exercise Physiology

K. D. DERMAN AND T. D. NOAKES

Introduction

Besides appreciating their own athletic ability, humans have, uniquely, also trained other animals to compete in athletic events, thereby stimulating scientific investigation of the athletic capabilities of many other species, including the racehorse. This chapter examines some different animal species involved in athletic sports; it briefly considers historical aspects of that involvement, the physiologic factors that might explain differences in athletic ability between different species, and the nature of the improvements in the athletic achievements of these different species over the last century. This information provides insight into those possible factors whose modification might enhance the efficiency and success of training thoroughbred racehorses.

Historical Overview of the Application of Sports Medicine and Exercise Science in the Different Athletic Species

Interest in the physiologic changes that occur during exercise in humans began at the end of the last century. By the early 1920s, scientists began to address practical questions, including the possible biochemical and physiologic causes of the fatigue that develops during exercise.[1,2] However, it was only from the late 1960s that research in sports medicine and the exercise sciences began to develop as a reputable academic discipline. Perhaps two of the principal reasons stimulating this development were an international trend toward an increased interest in health and the growing dominance of international sport by athletes from eastern European countries, especially the former German Democratic Republic (East Germany). The success of athletes from socialist countries posed a challenge to the Western nations, especially the United States, who were anxious that the perceived superiority of the capitalist system in all spheres of human endeavor should not be undermined. Thus financial and political support for sports-related research increased in most Western countries, stimulating the rebirth of these disciplines on a global scale.

In contrast, the exercise sciences have received little financial and intellectual support in the horse racing community. In his book, *The Fit Racehorse,* Tom Ivers[3] has written that " . . . [the racehorse] industry honors the past more ferociously than it defends its own existence." It is very apparent that the principal focus of the horse racing industry is in its past, i.e., in examining the breeding history of the species, especially of its champions. Little, if any, attention is paid to its future, which should involve the application of scientific knowledge and techniques to the study of horses and horse racing. As a direct result, progress in equine exercise science research lags behind its human counterpart by decades.

Perhaps there are two major reasons for the general lack of interest that the horse racing community has for the application of science to its industry. First, any new development, be it a training technique, nutritional advance, apparatus, or drug treatment, that may aid performance is seldom, if ever, adequately evaluated in a scientifically valid manner. In part, this may be because of financial pressures that induce artificial time constraints. In their perpetual search for a "quick fix," owners and trainers eschew the protracted process necessary for adequate scientific evaluation of these interventions. As a result, no distinction can be made between quackery and interventions that may be of real long-term value to the industry. This is clearly to the ultimate detriment of the horse racing industry.

A second possible explanation is that in the majority of races, the winning time is unimportant because there are no additional financial rewards for record performances. Patrick Cunningham[4] wrote that "nobody is much interested in improving the average racing times. . . . what does it matter if all horses race 10 percent faster?" Hence there is no incentive to improve the performances of all racehorses progressively and in a systematic manner.

However, the clever application of science to horse racing will achieve much more than faster racing times. The benefits range from fewer injuries to fewer working hours spent in training if the most effective training methods were identified. The long-term financial benefits for owners and trainers are likely to be substantial. Indeed, the involvement of science in the horse racing industry should be encouraged as a matter of priority if the existence of the industry is to be secured for the future.

The Aim of Scientific Investigation

The aim of science is to test hypotheses through objective measurement. Much that is written or spoken about horses represents little more than qualitative opinions. For example, the horse's appearance often is assessed by observation. Muscles are described as "looking firm," or the jockey "feels" that the horse is running better. In contrast, science deals with measurable numbers: How many grams of carbohydrate and how much oxygen were consumed in a 2000-m race? What percentage of an individual horse's muscle fibers comprise slow-twitch fibers?

The scientist tests the validity of any hypothesis by applying statistics to the numbers that have been collected. This allows an assessment of whether the intervention under study produced an effect and whether that effect could be ascribed to chance alone or resulted directly from the specific intervention.

It is our contention that research studies of a quantitative nature are urgently needed in the horse racing industry. Questions that are open to scientific investigation and which would seem worthy of analysis include

- What physiologic factors determine athletic success in racing horses?
- What is the nature of the fatigue experienced by racing horses?
- How can race horses be better prepared to resist the onset of fatigue, i.e., what are the optimal training methods?

• How can we ensure fewer injuries during training and racing?

We will next examine and compare the physiologic attributes of the main athletic species and describe the tests used commonly by exercise physiologists that allow some of these questions to be answered.

THE MAIN ATHLETIC SPECIES

Of all the athletic species in the world, the physiology of four have been studied to varying degrees. These are the athletic human, the racehorse, the greyhound, and the racing camel (Fig. 2–1). Of these species, the human athlete has received the most attention; the greyhound and the camel, the least. The racehorse occupies an intermediate position.

The Human Athlete
Competitive racing for humans and horses shares a common origin—the use of these species for transport. The Greeks and Romans used runners to deliver messages by foot, often over long distances. This tradition continued in Britain in the 10th century A.D.[5] However, only from the 17th century onward was running established as a competitive sport, originating mainly in Britain.[5]

Distances. The very earliest human footraces were usually over extremely long distances. It is recorded that a race of 237 km took place in Rome during the Roman Empire.[5] Recognized distances for modern footraces range from sprints of 100 m to ultramarathon races of 1000 km or more, lasting many days. The top speeds achieved by human sprinters exceed 36 km/h (22 miles/h), whereas speeds of around 16 km/h (10 miles/h) are more common in ultramarathon races of up to 100 km and of 6 to 8 km/h (4 to 5 miles/h) in races of 1000 km or more.

The Equine Athlete
Horse racing originated with the Bedouins of the Middle East, who dehydrated their horses and trained them to race to the nearest water hole.[6] However, it was only in the late 17th century (circa 1665) that organized horse racing first took place in New York and in Newmarket, England.[6]

Distances. The earliest horse races were run over distances of 6 miles. However, the distances of modern track races for thoroughbreds vary from 1000 m for "sprinters" to the longer 3000-m races for "stayers." Endurance races of 80 to 160 km (50 to 100 miles) and longer are also held over all types of terrain.[6] Quarter horses race over 400-m tracks, attaining top speeds of up to 70 km/h (44 miles/h).

The Racing Camel
The camel is known for its endurance ability in hot, dry environments. In the Middle East, specially bred camels are raced over distances of 4 to 10 km and achieve speeds of approximately 36 km/h (22 miles/h).[7]

Racing Dogs
The Greyhound. From as early as 1835, greyhounds were raced against each other, sometimes in races involving as many as 64 participants.[8] In 1858, the sport was officially organized with the formation of a governing body, the National Coursing Club, in Britain.

DISTANCES. The length of greyhound races varies from 250-m sprints to "long-distance races" of 600 to 1000 m. Dogs can reach speeds of up to 60 km/h (37 miles/h) during races of up to 500 m.

The Husky. The endurance ability and resistance to cold temperatures of the husky and related species have long been recognized. These dogs are the principal means of transport for polar travel. The first races were held in Alaska in 1907 over 600 km (400 miles).[9] The most famous modern race is the Iditarod, in which dogs race from Fairbanks to Nome in Alaska over 1710 km (1049 miles). This race takes 12 to 14 days to complete.[10]

TECHNIQUES AND INSTRUMENTATION NEEDED FOR LABORATORY RESEARCH OF THE ATHLETIC SPECIES

Animals are substantially more difficult to study than are humans. Apart from the inability to obtain their un-

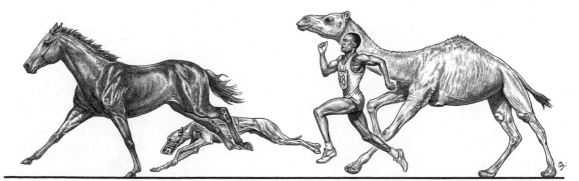

Figure 2-1. *The four main athletic species showing the relative maximum speeds during exercise. Maximum speeds in the different species are 19 m/s (thoroughbred horse), 16.6 m/s (greyhound), and 10 to 11 m/s (human athlete and racing camel).*

divided cooperation, extreme precautions must be taken to ensure their safety, especially of large animals such as the horse.[11]

The Treadmill

The treadmill allows the investigator to study the athlete during any intensity of exercise, as well as at rest before or after exercise. Tests more specific to horses that can be performed on a treadmill include dynamic hoof balancing, gait analysis, endoscopic evaluation of upper airway function, and tests of exercise performance.[12] It is the latter test that has the widest potential use for, among others, determining superior athletic ability or, alternatively, explaining poor racing performance in individual horses; identification of possible physiologic factors that may alter with training; and studying the biochemical and physiologic nature of fatigue during exercise.

Respiratory Gas Analysis

In both humans and horses, air expired during exercise can be measured for its oxygen and carbon dioxide content, thereby allowing the calculation of the rate of oxygen consumption during exercise of different intensities. Measurement of oxygen consumption allows calculation of energy expenditure at any specific workload or running speed and gives an idea of an individual horse's efficiency or "economy of movement." The respiratory exchange ratio (RER), which is calculated as the ratio of carbon dioxide (CO_2) production to oxygen (O_2) consumption, provides an indication of the relative proportions of the metabolic fuels that are used at a specific exercise intensity (see Chap. 4). This information allows for calculation of the dietary requirements of animals with different levels of habitual activity.

Maximal oxygen consumption ($\dot{V}_{O_2max}$) is the maximal amount of oxygen used by the athlete during maximal exercise to exhaustion. It is determined by increasing the workload or speed of the treadmill in a stepwise manner with continuous monitoring of the rate of oxygen consumption. $\dot{V}_{O_2max}$ is sometimes termed the *peak aerobic power.*

In humans, there is a trend for the best athletes to have the highest $\dot{V}_{O_2max}$ values.[5] Elite human athletes have $\dot{V}_{O_2max}$ values ranging between 69 and 85 ml O_2/kg/min, whereas thoroughbred racehorses have $\dot{V}_{O_2max}$ values twice as high, about 160 ml O_2/kg/min.[13–15] The higher $\dot{V}_{O_2max}$ values of the racehorse are best understood in terms of the physiologic factors that determine how rapidly oxygen can be transferred from the air to the active muscles where it is used.

The rate of oxygen consumption can be calculated as the product of the cardiac output multiplied by the difference in the oxygen (O_2) content of the arterial blood traveling to the muscles and the venous blood returning to the heart, having delivered much of its oxygen to the active muscles. The difference in the oxygen content of the arterial and venous blood is known as the *arteriovenous O_2 difference* [(a-v)D_{O_2}].

Cardiac output is the volume of blood pumped by the heart each minute. It is the product of the heart rate and the stroke volume, which is the amount of blood ejected from the heart with each contraction. Cardiac output increases during exercise as a result of an increase in both heart rate and stroke volume. During exercise, both these responses occur to a greater extent in horses than in humans.

Resting heart rates are in the low twenties in fit horses,[10,16] whereas values of 40 to 60 are more usual in athletic humans under the same conditions.[5] During exercise, maximal heart rates of between 240 and 250 beats per minute have been recorded in racehorses,[17] whereas maximal values in the range of 180 to 200 beats per minute are more common in athletic humans.[5]

Thus the thoroughbred racehorse has the ability to increase its heart rate almost tenfold from rest to maximal exercise, whereas in humans this range is of the order of three- to fourfold.[16] This difference contributes in large measure to the greater $\dot{V}_{O_2max}$ of the thoroughbred racehorse compared with the elite human athlete.

The resting stroke index (stroke volume divided by body weight) for horses is between 1.3 and 2.3 ml/kg, increasing to 2.5 to 2.7 ml/kg during maximal exercise,[17] similar to the human resting value of 1.1 to 1.4 ml/kg, which increases to around 1.5 ml/kg during maximal exercise.[18] Although the stroke index increases in both humans and horses, the increase is, at most, of the order of one- to twofold. Hence it is the much larger (four- to tenfold) increase in heart rate that is the main contributor to the increase in cardiac output during exercise in both racehorses and human athletes.[13,17,19]

The arteriovenous oxygen difference represents the difference in the (high) oxygen content of the blood in the arteries and the (much lower) oxygen content of the venous blood returning to the heart. The amount of oxygen carried in the arterial blood is dependent on the concentration of red blood cells in the circulation and their hemoglobin content. Another measure of the number of circulating red blood cells is the hematocrit, which is the percentage of the total blood volume occupied by red blood cells.

The human athlete maintains this hematocrit value at between 40 and 50 percent.[19] During exercise in humans the hematocrit tends to rise slightly as a result of a fall in the amount of fluid, the plasma volume, in which the red blood cells circulate. The total number of red blood cells contained in that volume may increase only slightly during exercise in humans.[19]

In contrast, the horse has the unique ability, specifically during exercise, to release a large number of red blood cells from their storage site in an intra-abdominal organ, the spleen. As a result, the hematocrit of the horse can increase from around 32 to 46 percent to 60 to 70 percent during maximal exercise.[16] This ability dramatically increases the oxygen-carrying capacity of the horse's blood during exercise.

Some human athletes have attempted to mimic this physiologic response by using an illegal technique known as "blood doping." In this procedure, red blood cells are withdrawn from the athlete and stored frozen. At some point in time, usually hours before competition, the red blood cells are reinjected, thereby increasing the oxygen-carrying capacity of the blood and potentially aiding performance.[20]

The maximum $(a-v)D_{O_2}$ measured in the horse during maximal exercise is only very slightly greater than values measured in elite human athletes under similar conditions.[17] Thus a larger $(a-v)D_{O_2}$ accounts for only about 23 percent of the greater $\dot{V}_{O_2max}$ of the racehorse compared with the elite human athlete; the much greater cardiac output and oxygen-carrying capacity of the blood accounts for the other 77 percent.[17]

Thus the greater capacity for oxygen transport in the racehorse is the result of a larger capacity to increase cardiac output, with heart rate as the main contributor; the greater oxygen-carrying capacity of the blood during exercise; and finally, a small increase in the capacity to extract oxygen in the active muscles, measured as a greater $(a-v)D_{O_2}$.[21]

With regard to the other athletic species, the greyhound has a maximal heart rate of about 300 beats per minute, only a threefold increase from resting values.[10] $\dot{V}_{O_2max}$ in this species is in excess of 100 ml O_2/kg/min.[10] Greyhounds have high resting hematocrit levels of about 54 percent; these increase to around 64 percent during maximal exercise.[22] It is not known whether this is due to the release of red blood cells from the splenic reserve or results from a decrease in plasma volume causing an increase in the concentration of red blood cells.[22]

The camel, on the other hand, has the lowest $\dot{V}_{O_2max}$ value (51 ml/kg/min) of the four common athletic species, the horse, greyhound, camel, and human[7] (Table 2–1). The racing camel can increase heart rate fourfold from a resting rate of about 33 beats per minute to about 150 beats per minute during maximal exercise.[7] The hematocrit of the racing camel increased from 33 percent at rest to 36 percent at maximal exercise.[7] Of the four athletic species, the camel therefore has the lowest concentration of red blood cells. This together with a rela-

tively low maximum heart rate might explain the relatively low $\dot{V}_{O_2max}$ of this species.

$\dot{V}_{O_2max}$ as a Predictor of Athletic Ability

Although $\dot{V}_{O_2max}$ is generally considered to be the best predictor of athletic potential, there is evidence to dispute this belief.[23] For example, although elite human athletes do have high $\dot{V}_{O_2max}$ values, so too do many less conditioned athletes. Athletes with similar athletic abilities may have quite different $\dot{V}_{O_2max}$ values.[5]

The same relationship is found in racehorses, in which there is no significant difference between the $\dot{V}_{O_2max}$ values of standardbred (165 ml/kg/min) and thoroughbred, (164 ml/kg/min) horses.[12] Clearly, if $\dot{V}_{O_2max}$ was the sole predictor of athletic ability, the value should be much higher in thoroughbred than in standardbred horses. Hence factors other than $\dot{V}_{O_2max}$ must be important in determining the superior athletic ability of the thoroughbred racehorse.

Two important factors are locomotive efficiency, which is the oxygen cost per kilogram per kilometer traveled, and he percentage of $\dot{V}_{O_2max}$ that can be sustained during prolonged exercise.[5,24,25] Subjects able to run at a higher percentage of their $\dot{V}_{O_2max}$ for longer periods might be said to exhibit superior fatigue resistance.[25] For example, the $\dot{V}_{O_2max}$ of the thoroughbred racehorse is about three times greater than that of the racing camel, which is of similar mass[26] (see Table 2–1). Yet the camel can exercise at a very high intensity (100 percent $\dot{V}_{O_2max}$) for a much longer period than can the horse (18 versus 3 to 5 min).[26] Thus the performance of the camel in races lasting more than 10 to 15 minutes is likely to be more similar to that of the racehorse because of the former's ability to exercise at a much higher percentage of $\dot{V}_{O_2max}$ for much longer despite a substantially lower $\dot{V}_{O_2max}$. Hence in the assessment of an athlete's potential it is necessary to consider not only the $\dot{V}_{O_2max}$ but

Table 2-1. Comparitive Table for $\dot{V}_{O_2max}$, Heart Rate, Peak Blood Lactate, Hematocrit, Stroke Index, and Muscle Fiber Composition

	Human athlete[a]	Thoroughbred racehorse	Greyhound dog[b]	Racing camel[c]
$\dot{V}_{O_2max}$ (ml O_2/kg/min)	69–85	160[d]	100	51
Resting HR (bpm)	40–60	20–30[e]	100	33
Max exercise HR (bpm)	190	240[f]	300	147
Resting stroke index (ml/kg)	1.1–1.4[g]	1.3–2.3[f]	—	—
Max stroke index (ml/kg)	1.5[g]	2.5–2.7[f]	—	—
Resting hematocrit (%)	40–50	32–46	54[h]	33[i]
Max hematocrit (%)	40–50	60–70	64[h]	36[i]
Peak lactate (mmol/liter)	15	30[j]	20	12
Muscle fiber composition	Sprinters type II > 75 %	Sprinters type II[e] > 80 %	Type II > 75 %	Type I > 70 %
	Endurance type I > 75 %	Endurance type I[k] ~30 %	—	—

Sources: Data from [a]Noakes[5]; [b]Snow[10]; [c]Rose and colleagues[26]; [d]Rose and colleagues[14]; [e]Snow and Vogel[16]; [f]Physick-Sheard[17]; [g]Ganong[18]; [h]Snow and colleagues[22]; [i]Evans and colleagues[7]; [j]McMiken; [k]Rose.[43]

also the percentage of $\dot{V}_{O_2max}$ that can be sustained during prolonged exercise.

Factors relating to running economy that are of importance in determining success in human runners[5] and cyclists,[27] in particular a lower than average oxygen cost at any running speed, have yet to be evaluated in racehorses and the other athletic species. However, when comparing the oxygen cost of exercise in camels and horses, it is clear that the oxygen cost per kilometer traveled in camels is much less than in the horse, indicating superior economy of locomotion.

Heart Rate

Specific heart rates are seldom used as a predictor of athletic performance in humans. However, equine physiologists use a measure termed the V_{200}, which is the velocity a horse achieves at a heart rate of 200 beats per minute. The V_{200}, which is said to approximate the maximal aerobic power achieved by the horse,[17] is calculated from heart rates measured during a series of runs at different speeds on a treadmill or on the racetrack. The V_{200} can be used as a simple, yet effective measurement to monitor training adaptations during and at the completion of a training program. Increases in the V_{200} would be interpreted to indicate a favorable training adaptation, whereas the reverse would apply if the V_{200} fell.

In addition, measurement of heart rate can be a most valuable training aid because it allows for accurate control of the intensity of any exercise training session.[28] In general, it is now believed that intensity is the most important variable in the training program, since the extent of the training adaptation is determined by the intensity rather than the volume of training.[5] However, if training intensity is excessive, injury and overtraining are the likely results. Furthermore, abnormal elevations of heart rate at rest and during exercise are an excellent marker of chronic fatigue and overtraining.[5] These elevations would indicate the need for rest rather than more training.

Blood Samples

Blood samples are taken routinely during exercise tests. In humans and horses, the most common blood biochemical measured is the *blood lactate concentration*. During exercise of progressively increasing intensity, the lactate concentration rises progressively from the resting concentration of about 1 mmol/liter. The exercise intensity at which lactate concentrations rise more steeply is often termed the *lactate threshold* (Fig. 2–2). This threshold has been used as a measure of both fitness and athletic ability in humans and horses. In general, less fit horses show a rise in blood lactate concentration at lower exercise intensities or running speeds, and hence they exhibit an earlier lactate threshold than fit horses.[12] The same relationship is seen in better-performing human athletes[5] (see Fig. 2–2). Other studies have shown that blood lactate concentrations after maximal exercise are higher in better-performing horses.[29] McMiken[30] suggests that training increases the capacity of the horse to break down muscle glycogen to pyruvate in the glyco-

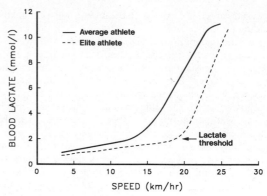

Figure 2-2. *The lactate curve with increasing speed for an average and elite human athlete.*

lytic pathway, thus causing the higher blood lactate concentrations in the better-trained horses.

It is believed that increasing acidity, shown as a fall of the pH in active muscles, is a potent cause of fatigue[19] during exercise of very high intensity and short duration, as typified by horse races of 1000 to 3000 m. Muscles with an increased buffering capacity are more resistant to changes in pH and thus have a greater capacity to continue contracting during high-intensity exercise.

Both the horse and dog are able to produce higher peak blood lactate concentrations after maximal exercise than are humans[10,14] (see Table 2–1). However, the correlation between muscle lactate and pyruvate concentrations and the muscle pH is similar in humans and horses, indicating a similar buffering capacity.[31] Also, respiratory compensation for this metabolic acidosis increases 16-fold in both the horse (100 to 1600 liters/min) and the human athlete (6 to 100 liters/min).[16,18] Thus the higher peak lactate concentrations after maximal exercise in the horse are associated with lower muscle pH levels than in human athletes (6.2 versus 6.6).[32–34]

Blood Glucose and Insulin Concentrations

Premature fatigue during prolonged exercise lasting more than 1 to 2 hours can be caused by hypoglycemia (low blood glucose concentration).[35] Monitoring of the blood concentrations of glucose and insulin, the hormone that regulates the blood glucose concentration, can identify if hypoglycemia is the cause of fatigue during this type of exercise.

Blood Enzyme Assays

The condition of rhabdomyolysis, or the "tying-up syndrome," can be diagnosed by measuring the activity in the blood of certain enzymes released from damaged muscles. The condition is brought on by exercise and presents as an inability to move without pain. As a result of the muscle damage that causes the condition, the activities of the muscle enzymes creatine kinase (CK), aspartate aminotransferase (AST), and lactate dehydrogenase (LDH) increase in the bloodstream. The activities of these enzymes peak within 6 to 12 hours after exercise.

This condition is not unique to horses. Humans can experience a similar condition known as *delayed-onset muscle soreness* (DOMS). A number of theories have been offered to explain this phenomenon, but the exact etiology is unclear.[36–38] However, it is certain that eccentric muscle contractions, in which the muscle lengthens while under tension, as occurs in the quadriceps muscle during downhill running, increase the frequency and severity of DOMS.[39,40]

Eccentric muscle contractions occur especially in the racehorse after crossing the finishing line as the horse is "pulled up" and decelerates. Therefore, it is likely that the damage caused to the muscle in horse racing occurs not only during the race but also at the end of a sprint as the horse decelerates. Most trainers advocate that in order to prevent any further muscle damage, training should cease until muscle enzyme activities have returned to normal.[16] However, human studies have shown that the elevated plasma CK activity is dissociated from both the extent of the pain and the impairment of muscle function.[38] Human athletes who continued to train at low intensity after developing DOMS did not show a delayed rate of recovery compared with those who stopped training altogether.[41] It is unknown if the same response would occur in horses; however, low-intensity exercise should be possible if the horse is pain-free.

The Muscle Biopsy
In this procedure, a small sample of muscle is removed via insertion of a hollow cutting needle through a small cut in the skin.[42] Muscle samples are commonly tested for carbohydrate (glycogen) content, muscle enzyme activities, and muscle fiber typing.

There are two main muscle fiber types, classified as type I (slow twitch, or ST) and type II (fast twitch, or FT) (see Chap. 8). The type II fibers are further subdivided into type IIa and type IIb fibers.[30] The ratio of type I to type II fibers is genetically determined. What is more, the muscle fiber type present in any individual may predispose that individual to success in specific athletic activities.[42] Human sprinters have a majority (>75 percent) of type II fibers, while endurance athletes have a predominance (>75 percent) of type I fibers.[5]

The muscle fiber composition of horses also varies according to their athletic abilities. Endurance horses have a larger percentage of type I fibers than do sprint horses. However, as a species, the horse has a low percentage of type I fibers, with a maximum of around 40 percent for endurance horses, compared with human endurance athletes, who usually have more than 75 percent type I fibers.[5,16,43]

Although the proportion of muscle fibers is strongly genetically controlled, training can alter the relative proportions, at least to a limited extent. Especially a transition of type IIB to type IIA fibers and vice versa might occur, depending on the training regimen.[16,44,45]

The racing camel has a large percentage of type I fibers (70 percent), with the remainder being type IIa, with few or no type IIb muscle fibers.[26] Thus the camel is well suited to low-intensity endurance activities. In contrast to the camel and the racehorse, the greyhound has an almost complete dominance of type II muscle fibers.[10]

THE RELEVANCE OF PHYSIOLOGIC TESTING

The main reasons for the physiologic testing of racehorses is to predict their athletic capacity, to monitor improvements with training, and to determine the likely causes for impaired exercise performance. It is therefore important to ensure that the variables being tested in the laboratory will give information that is of relevance to the clinical setting. For example, the human runner has minimal external interference to his or her performance. The same equipment is utilized on the track and on the laboratory treadmill. In contrast, during competition but not during laboratory testing, the horse needs a jockey to control positioning and speed. In addition, there is the racing tack, including the bridle and saddle, necessary for competition. This introduces variables into the laboratory testing that need to be considered. Hence care must be taken when predictions of track racing performance are made on the basis of laboratory measurements of physiologic function during treadmill exercise in racehorses.

For example, studies have determined that oxygen consumption measured in humans during treadmill running in the laboratory is not significantly different from values measured in the field.[46] Because of the weight of the jockey, the equipment, and the track conditions, it is not known whether the same is true for horses. Thus studies must be performed to identify all the possible variables that might influence the interpretation of laboratory test results in racehorses.

The History of Improvement in Racing Times in the Different Species

THE IMPROVEMENT IN RACING TIMES IN HORSES, DOGS, AND HUMANS

Records in all athletic activities improve with time. However, some limiting speed or distance must ultimately be reached beyond which no further improvement is possible. This stage has yet to be reached in any human athletic event.[5] Rather, world records for all events continue to improve. However, the rate of improvement of these records differs in different sports and between the different athletic species. To illustrate this difference, we analyzed the records of three famous athletic events contested by the three different species. All these races are run at roughly the same exercise intensity (90 to 100 percent $\dot{V}_{O_2max}$). These races are the 1-mile (1609-m) foot race for humans, the Kentucky Derby (1.25 miles, 2018 m) for thoroughbreds, and the Puppy Derby (460 m) for greyhounds (Fig. 2–3). The slope of the regression lines in Figure 2–3 represent the rate of improvement with time of the winning times in the different events. The rate of progression of the winning

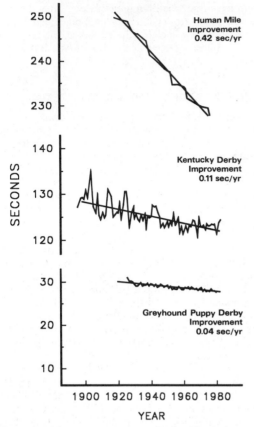

Figure 2-3. *The winning times over the years for the human mile, Kentucky Derby, and the greyhound Puppy Derby.*

time in the human foot race (0.42 s/yr) is 4 times greater than in the Kentucky Derby (0.11 s/yr) and 11 times greater than in the Puppy Derby (0.038 s/yr). Expressed as a percentage of the record times in 1935, the rates of improvement per year for the different species in the different events are 0.17, 0.09, and 0.13 percent for the three species, respectively.

This comparison invites the question, Why should the rate of improvement of human athletic records be superior to that of thoroughbreds and somewhat better than that of greyhounds? To answer this question, we need first to consider the factors that determine racing performance and how these may be influenced by different factors in the different species.

Factors Determining Athletic Ability in Any Species

Athletic ability, regardless of sport or species, is determined by three main factors: genetics, environment, and training.

GENETICS

It has been said that the most effective way to become a champion athlete is to be selective when choosing one's parents.[19] A measure of this genetic contribution to athletic ability is provided by studies of groups of identical twins, whose $\dot{V}_{O_2max}$ values are almost identical ($R = 0.92$).[47,48] Further, the endurance capacity of identical twins during prolonged exercise is quite similar and is more similar than is the endurance capacity of nonidentical twins, whose performance is also more similar than that of brothers.[47] This indicates a strong genetic component for athletic performance, estimated to be between 40 and 60 percent for $\dot{V}_{O_2max}$ and endurance capacity, respectively.[47,48]

Although genetic factors determine the ultimate limit of each athlete's performance, environmental and training factors determine how closely each athlete approaches that limit. Paradoxically, unlike the human athlete, the thoroughbred racehorse has been bred with one objective—to run faster than any other horse. The evidence provided in Figure 2–3, however, suggests that careful breeding has failed to produce the desired result.

Thoroughbred breeding records have been kept since 1791, when James Weatherby established the *Stud Book*. Since then, the breeding of horses has been recorded in elaborate detail. Weatherby's book indicates that just over 50 percent of all the genes in the present thoroughbred population come from only 10 horses[4] and 80 percent from 31 horses.[49] Thus a very small genetic pool exists in the racing breed.

The first book recording the breeding records of greyhounds was published in 1882.[8] Controlled breeding of greyhounds therefore began much later than that of thoroughbred horses. Again, the question must be asked, if genetic factors are such important determinants of athletic performance, especially in thoroughbred racehorses, why then has the breed with the longest history of controlled breeding not made the greatest improvements in racing performances? One explanation for the slow improvement in the winning times of thoroughbred racehorses contends that inbreeding has led to a limited gene pool, leaving little room for further improvement. Support for this contention is the finding that between 1804 and 1910 the winning times for certain thoroughbred races improved more rapidly than in subsequent years. The assumption is that as the thoroughbred breed has become progressively more inbred, the potential for further improvement has decreased.[4] However, Gaffney and Cunningham[49] do not believe that the slow rate of improvement in modern thoroughbred racing performances is due to insufficient genetic variance in the breed as a whole.

To examine the effect of controlled breeding, Cunningham[4] used the Timeform ratings as a measure of racing performance in 31,263 three-year-old thoroughbred racehorses. He compared the Timeform ratings of half-brothers and sisters with those of randomly selected groups and of parents and their offspring compared with random pairings from two consecutive generations. He concluded that only 35 percent of the variance in ability is explained by hereditary factors; the remaining 65 percent is due to environmental factors, such as training and nutrition.[4]

If genetic factors explain only 35 percent of the variance in athletic performance in thoroughbreds, is it therefore appropriate to expend so much time, money, and effort on selective breeding? The answer is both yes and no. According to Gaffney and Cunningham,[49] selective breeding contributes to an increase in the Timeform ratings of about 1 percent per annum. Other research in the quarter horse also suggests that selective breeding will continue to improve racing performances in future generations.[50] But perhaps the most important practical point is that since genetic factors explain less than 40 percent of a thoroughbred's racing potential, and since that contribution is fixed at birth in any individual horse, it follows that more attention should be paid to those environmental and training factors which determine performance and which can be actively and successfully modified.

ENVIRONMENT

Environmental factors that influence athletic performance include all the equipment necessary to participate in the sport, the surface upon which the sport is performed, and the nutrition of the athlete. The jockey adds an additional environmental component that must be considered in the racehorse.

Athletic Nutrition
The aim of athletic nutrition is to meet the athlete's energy and nutrient requirements. Athletes consume 50 to 75 percent more energy than nonathletes.[51] Carbohydrate, fat, and protein form the three primary nutritional fuels (see Chap. 10). All ingested foods are either used directly by the body or converted and stored for later use. As a completely herbivorous animal, the horse has developed a digestive system to break down vegetable cellulose (see Chap. 10). Thus the equine athlete's nutritional processes and demands are far more complex than those of the human. The horse's digestive system, like that of all herbivores, operates with an intake limitation, functioning optimally only at a certain fullness.[52]

Therefore, in order to meet the energy demands of the racehorse undergoing athletic training, the trainer must increase the frequency of feeds instead of increasing only the amount of food.[52] Also, the energy density of the diet can be increased.[53] While moderate exercise has been shown to increase appetite in horses, intense exercise does the opposite.[52] Both humans and horses utilize nonesterified fatty acids (NEFA) as the main fuel for the muscles during rest or walking at a slow pace.[30] This is shown by an RER less than 0.8, indicating fat utilization. As the exercise intensity increases, fats can no longer supply the high rate of energy demands, and carbohydrates become progressively more important as the energy source (RER = 0.8 to 1.0). Carbohydrates are derived from muscle glycogen or glucose transported in the bloodstream.

In the early 1920s, scientists realized that low blood glucose concentrations were associated with fatigue in human athletes[54,55] and that carbohydrate ingestion could rapidly reverse this fatigue.[56] These findings suggested that human athletes should eat a high-carbohydrate diet in the 24 hours prior to a race and consume carbohydrates during long-distance races.[2] Modern research has confirmed these findings.[35,57] Horses involved in endurance races also ingest high-carbohydrate diets when given free access to grain and roughage during prolonged exercise.[53]

The timing of precompetition meals may be of importance to both humans and horses. Studies performed in human athletes who ingested carbohydrate 45 minutes prior to exercise showed that their blood glucose concentrations fell as a result of increased serum insulin concentrations.[58] A similar study in horses that exercised 2 hours after a feed also showed that blood glucose concentrations fell during subsequent exercise.[59] Whether or not this fall in blood glucose concentration impairs exercise performance remains to be clearly established.

The National Research Council of North America (NRC) recommends that the dietary intake of horses in heavy athletic training should contain 33 percent roughage and 67 percent concentrate.[53] The main source of carbohydrate is obtained from the cereals and hay, which also provide the roughage. Horses in heavy training are sometimes fed fats, in the form of soya bean or maize oils, as a potential high source of energy. Concentrations of fat of up to 20 percent (in terms of calories consumed) of the diet have been found to be tolerated by horses.[16] Even though the regular training diet contains only 1 to 2 percent fat. Human athletes are advised to eat diets composed of 50 to 65 percent carbohydrate, 12 to 15 percent protein, and 20 to 30 percent fat.[60]

Track Surfaces
Running surfaces often can contribute to injuries in both equine and human athletes. Advances in the design of track surfaces for racehorses have trailed behind advances made in human athletics. For example, a "sprung" track tuned to the specific biomechanical characteristics of the human body has been developed and may reduce injury risk in human athletes.[61]

Equine tracks traditionally have been either turf or dirt. Each has its own drawbacks. Turf can withstand only limited use, whereas dirt tracks rely on the soil type and moisture level for optimal performance.[62] However, new advances in hydrophobic (water-repelling) polymers have enabled coating of the sand particles. This innovation is preparing the way for new equine racetracks which may combine the benefits of both turf and dirt tracks. Clearly, more needs to be done to develop surfaces that reduce injury risk. This is critically important given the large number of training injuries in thoroughbred racehorses.

Shoes
Advances in human sporting achievements have always relied on equivalent technological advances in sporting equipment. From lighter and more aerodynamic bicycle designs, exemplified most recently by the Lotus bicycle raced to victory by Chris Boardman in the 1992 Barcelona Olympic Games, to the aerodynamically designed javelin that could be thrown so far that the safety of the spectators was threatened, humans have always searched for unique ways to improve their sporting achievements. Perhaps the most visible modern development has been the design of running shoes for humans. Running shoes

have become so sophisticated that there are now over 150 different shoe types from which to choose. Since no man or woman is anatomically identical, running shoe companies have manufactured shoes to deal with this wide variety of anatomic imperfections.

On the other hand, the horse shoe has changed little during the last century, yet lameness accounts for 70 percent of lost training days in racehorses, with 80 percent of injuries occurring in the front legs.[63] This is due to the some 5000-kg of force that is transferred through the horse's front legs when racing.[63] Thus some horses may require novel innovations to soften impact loading during training and racing. However, this possibility has not been addressed until recently, with greater attention being paid to the optimal training surfaces and with introduction of a range of "shock-absorbing" horse shoes, which have had some success in rehabilitating lame horses.[64] These shoes are made either from an acetal resin or from polyurethane in place of the usual hard metal and are lighter than metal shoes. This is of importance, since weight added to the hoof has been found to affect the stride length of the horse.[16] Aluminum horse shoes were developed to decrease the weight of the shoe; however, the durability of the shoe is inferior due to the light-weight material now used.

Thus some progress has been made in the development of more advanced shoes for horses. However, there is a need to increase this research effort so that horses may be at a lesser risk of disabling injuries during both training and racing.

The Jockey

Unlike humans, the equine athlete's positioning, speed, and racing strategy are determined by the jockey. The jockey's weight, positioning, and experience play an integral part in the sport. In order to succeed, the jockey must be an expert judge of pace and of the horse's capabilities.

The jockey represents not only added weight for the horse but also additional surface area, which increases overall aerodynamic drag. It is in this area that the jockey can learn from competitors in other high-speed sports, including cycling and downhill ski racing. Competitors in these events have discovered the value of wearing clothing and equipment designed to reduce the aerodynamic drag. It is estimated that 25 percent of the horse's energy expenditure is used to overcome air resistance at high speeds. Improvements in aerodynamic profiling of the jockey by attention to the riding position, equipment, and clothing would likely reduce this percentage and could conceivably influence the outcome of closely contested races.[62] We should therefore expect more attention to be paid to this area in the future.

TRAINING

After genetics, training is the single most important variable determining athletic success. An essential advantage enjoyed by the coach of human athletes is that the athlete can communicate ideas and especially sensations to the trainer. Unfortunately, the equine trainer lacks the benefit of direct feedback from the horse.

Hence it is less likely that training programs are ever absolutely specific to the unique needs of individual horses. However, since the elite athlete, whether human or horse, always treads a fine line between peak condition and overtraining, the absence of this feedback complicates the task of training immeasurably. Nevertheless, exercise scientists have developed techniques to monitor the effects of training, including monitoring of the heart rate and performance during specific workouts. It is vital that trainers and exercise physiologists work together so that this information from the human experience can be transferred, with benefit, to the training of horses.

With the wise application of scientific principles established in human athletes,[5] the trainer and exercise physiologist working together can bridge the "communication gap" and develop specific training programs for individual horses that will ensure that each achieves its optimal performance relative to genetic abilities.

Training Methodology

With the advances that have been made in the human exercise sciences, an ever-increasing interest has centered on improving training methods by scientifically evaluating the real (as apposed to surmised, but untested) effects of different training methods. Unfortunately, many trainers of either horses or humans continue to use training methods that have been handed down from generation to generation without ever undergoing scientific validation. Worse, many trainers are reluctant to innovate.

A traditional training method for thoroughbred racehorses consists of a single exercise session with one single bout of exercise, e.g., a run of 800 m. The intensity and duration may vary from day to day, with an occasional hard gallop or "breeze" at about racing speed. The distance covered is usually shorter than the racing distance.[65] But the publication of Tom Ivers book[3] prompted many to change their interest to the potential value of interval training.

Interval training is a training method in which a single exercise bout is divided into segments which vary according to intensity, duration, and frequency. Interval training was developed by the German athletics coach Woldemar Gerschler in the 1930s.[19] It is claimed that training of this type will delay the onset of fatigue and strengthen the weight-bearing structures, thereby reducing the risk of injury.[3] A few horse trainers have introduced some of these techniques but, due to an inappropriately sudden transition to a high-intensity training program in horses unprepared for the change, have experienced problems, particularly lameness. This invites the question of whether horses can really be trained according to the principles used by human athletes.

Trainers of both humans and horses use a variety of different training methods. However, most use a variation on a basic model that incorporates three phases, including some form of interval training in the final, precompetition phase. The three phases are (1) a foundation phase, (2) a cardiovascular or aerobic interval phase, and (3) an anaerobic interval phase.[66]

The foundation phase is probably the most important, since it is in this phase that the bones, tendons, and muscular system are strengthened; in equine terminology, this is referred to as *continuous* or *endurance training*. During this phase, a great deal of patience is required. Should the phase not be completed properly for any reasons, injuries are likely to develop subsequently. It is important that the training load be increased gradually to prevent any sudden unusually large demands on the horse.[66] No competitive racing should be undertaken during the foundation phase.

A recent study of interval training in horses found that the time required to complete the first phase varied from 14 to 20 weeks.[67] At the end of phase I, all horses could complete a 9600-m gallop at 460 m/s.

In phase II, the aerobic interval phase, the training volume is maintained, but sessions of higher-quality, more-intensive training are included. In these sessions, repeated runs at a faster pace with brief rest intervals introduce the horse to more intensive training[66] (Fig. 2–4). Ivers[3] advised rest intervals of 5 to 10 minutes.[3] This allows the heart rate to recover fully during the rest phase. There is debate about the optimal length of the recovery phase. Costill[66] suggests that brief rest periods of as little as 5 to 15 seconds should be used in human athletes. Phase II takes between 10 to 12 weeks in the horse.[67]

Phase III, the anaerobic interval stage, is used to develop the strength required for racing at top speed and to optimize the development of coordinated neuromuscular functioning. High-intensity work over short distances is performed. The rest periods between exercise bouts must be of sufficient length to facilitate heart rate recovery to about 60 to 70 percent of the maximum heart rate (Fig. 2–5). This phase is suggested to last for about 6 weeks for horses.[67] However it should be used as a continual method for maintaining fitness and racing condition throughout the competitive racing season.

Scientifically valid training studies are extremely difficult to complete. However, some studies of interval training in horses have been reported. Lindholm and Saltin[68] and Thorton and colleagues[69] have shown that interval training of repeated bouts of 700 to 1000 m at near-maximal speed (11.4 to 12.5 m/s) produced heart rates and blood lactate concentrations similar to those found during racing. Similar findings also have been

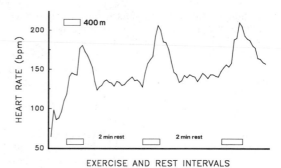

Figure 2-5. Anaerobic interval training and the heart rate response in the thoroughbred horse.

shown with intervals of four times 620-m gallops in thoroughbred horses.[32]

However, to date, only one study has examined the effect of an interval training program in thoroughbred racehorses. Hawkins and colleagues[67] showed that thoroughbred horses trained with an adaptation of the Ivers[3] three-phase interval training program for a period of 7 months improved their anaerobic capacity. This was indicated by an increased slope for lactate recovery, which is due to an increased lactate clearance rather than a reduction in the rate of lactate production.[70] Tests of longer duration would be necessary to test the effect of training on the ability to maintain racing speed. However, the interval trained group did show a trend to an increased peak speed (989 versus 966 m/min), which was averaged for each 200-m segment, compared with the conventionally trained group.[67]

Interval training would seem to be of benefit to human and equine athletes. However, more studies of the specific design of training programs need to be completed so as to establish methods that achieve the maximum training benefits with minimal injuries. Studies also must be done to examine the effect of interval training and a more gradual and delayed introduction to racing at an older age on the competitive longevity of the horse. It must be stressed that there is no substitute for a solid training foundation, especially when initiating an interval training program.

Swimming training or running in water have long been used by horse trainers as additional methods of training. Human athletes also have utilized these methods, although mainly for injury rehabilitation.[71] A specially designed buoyant vest has been developed to enable human athletes to run in water. To achieve the same effect, horses have either swum in a circular pool or have run on a submersed treadmill.[16,71] The heart rates of both humans and horses are lower when exercising in water compared with when running at a similar intensity on land. However, increased blood lactate concentrations have been measured in humans running in water compared with over land. One possible explanation is a lower leg muscle blood flow when exercising in water.[71] Perceived exertion also was higher in humans running in water than over land.[71]

It would seem that the main use of swimming and running in water is for the purposes of rehabilitation

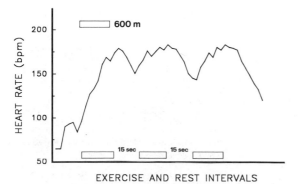

Figure 2-4. Aerobic or cardiovascular interval training and heart rate response in the thoroughbred horse.

from injury, training young horses, since the buoyancy properties of water decrease the concussive forces on the bones and joints, and to add variety to training programs.[16] As Snow[16] states, the use of large amounts of swimming training for horses would only be beneficial if horses also competed in swimming races.

Conclusion

Apart from being the fastest competitive athletic species, the thoroughbred racehorse shows some rather unique physiologic adaptations to exercise. This makes it difficult to apply findings from human physiologic studies directly to the horse. Hence there is a real need to develop a body of scientific knowledge specific to the racing horse.

The need for this information is perhaps best shown by the finding that despite the longest history of selective breeding for athletic success, the improvement in winning race times is much less in thoroughbreds than in humans. It is unlikely that this is due a small genetic pool that limits further improvement, and therefore, other possible factors should be considered.

A more scientific approach to the application of training methods shown to be effective in humans might both improve the athletic ability of the thoroughbred horse and also reduce their high incidence of injury. Indeed, human athletes benefit from the input of a team of advisers, including coaches, trainers, exercise physiologists, and medical doctors. In the sport of horse racing, in which communication with the athlete is of importance but virtually impossible, it would seem that the assistance of a qualified team would be even more important. The probable result of this team approach would likely be improved racing times, fewer injuries, stronger and healthier racehorses, and a more prosperous horse racing industry.

References

1. Hill AV, Lupton H: Muscular exercise, lactic acid and the supply and utilization of oxygen. Q J Med 1923; 16:135.
2. Gordon B, Kohn LA, Levine SA, et al: Sugar content of the blood in runners following a marathon race. JAMA 1925; 185:508.
3. Ivers T: The Fit Racehorse. Cincinnati, Ohio, Esprit Racing Team, Ltd, 1983, pp 4 and 77.
4. Cunningham P: The genetics of thoroughbred horses. Sci Am 1991; 264:56.
5. Noakes TD: Lore of Running. Cape Town, Oxford University Press, 1992, pp 186, 33, 312, 162, 38, 147, 88, 26, 398.
6. Kidd J: The Complete Horse Encyclopedia. London, Salamander Books, 1976, p 126.
7. Evans DL, Rose RJ, Knight PK, et al: Physiological responses during an incremental treadmill exercise test in the camel. *In* Proceedings of the 1st International Camel Conference. Newmarket, R and W Publications, 1992, p 223.
8. Genders R: The NGRC Book of Greyhound Racing. London, Pelham Books, 1990, pp 43 and 228.
9. Sayer A: The Complete Dog. New York, Prion Books, 1989, p 105.
10. Snow DH: The horse and dog, elite athletes: Why and how? Proc Nutr Soc 1985; 44:267.
11. Seeherman HJ: Treadmill exercise testing: Treadmill installation and training protocols used for clinical evaluations of equine athletes. Vet Clin North Am Equine Pract 1991; 7:259.
12. Morris E: Application of clinical exercise testing for identification of respiratory fitness and disease in the equine athlete. Vet Clin North Am Equine Pract 1991; 7:383.
13. Weber J, Dobson GP, Parkhouse WS, et al: Cardiac output and oxygen consumption in exercising thoroughbred horses. Am J Physiol 1987; 253:R890.
14. Rose RJ, Hodgson DR, Kelso B, et al: Maximum O_2 uptake, O_2 debt and deficit, and muscle metabolites in thoroughbred horses. Am J Physiol 1988; 64:781.
15. Hilldridge CJ: What limits equine performance? Equine Vet J 1988; 20:238.
16. Snow DH, Vogel CJ: Equine Fitness: The Care and Training of the Athletic Horse. North Pomfret, Vermont. David and Charles, Inc, 1987, pp 115, 123, 102, 92, 100, 217, 56, 198.
17. Physick-Sheard PW: Cardiovascular response to exercise and training in the horse. Vet Clin North Am Equine Pract 1985; 1:383.
18. Ganong WF: Review of Medical Physiology. Los Altos, California, Lange, 1985, p 517.
19. Wilmore JH, Costill DL: Training for Sport and Activity: The Physiological Basis of the Conditioning Process. Dubuque, Iowa, Wm C Brown Publishers, 1988, pp 158, 70, 37, 361, 167.
20. Buick FJ, Gledhill N, Froese AB, et al: Effect of induced erythrocythemia on aerobic work capacity. J Appl Physiol 1980; 48:636.
21. Evans DL, Rose RJ: Cardiovascular and respiratory responses in thoroughbred horses during treadmill exercise. J Exp Biol 1988; 134:397.
22. Snow DH, Harris RC, Stuttard E: Changes in hematology and plasma biochemistry during maximal exercise in greyhounds. Vet Rec 1988; 123:487.
23. Noakes TD: Implications of exercise testing for prediction of athletic performance: A contemporary perspective. Med Sci Sports Exerc 1988; 20:319.
24. Hammond HK, Froelicher VF: Exercise testing for cardiorespiratory fitness. Sports Med 1984; 1:234.
25. Coetzer P, Noakes TD, Sanders B, et al: Superior fatigue resistance of elite black South African distance runners. J Appl Physiol 75:1822–1827, 1993.
26. Rose RJ, Evans DL, Knight PK, et al: Muscle types, recruitment and oxygen uptake during exercise in the racing camel. *In* Proceedings of the 1st International Camel Conference. Newmarket, R and W Publications, 1992, p 219.
27. Coyle EF, Feltner ME, Kautz SA, et al: Physiological and biomechanical factors associated with elite endurance cycling performance. Med Sci Sports Exerc 1991; 23:93.
28. Foreman JH, Bayly WM, Grant BD, et al: Standardized exercise test and daily heart rate responses of thoroughbreds undergoing conventional race training and detraining. Am J Vet Res 1990; 51:914.
29. Persson SGB, Ullberg LE: Blood volume in relation to exercise tolerance in trotters. J S Afr Vet Assoc 1974; 45:293.
30. McMiken DF: An energetic basis of equine performance. Equine Vet J 1983; 15:123.
31. Harris RC, Katz A, Sahlin D, et al: Measurement of muscle pH in horse muscle and its relation to lactate content. J Physiol 1984; 357:110P.
32. Snow DH, Harris RC, Gash S: Metabolic response of equine muscle to intermittent maximal exercise. J Appl Physiol 1985; 58:1689.
33. Snow DH, Harris RC: Limitations to maximal performance in the racing thoroughbred. *In* Gillespie JR, Robinson NE (eds): Equine Exercise Physiology 2. Davis, CA, ICEEP Publications, 1987, p 447.
34. Costill DL, Barnett A, Sharp R, et al: Leg muscle pH following sprint running. Med Sci Sports Exerc 1983; 15:325.
35. Coggan AR, Coyle EF: Carbohydrate ingestion during prolonged exercise: Effects on metabolism and performance. Exerc Sport Sci Rev 1991; 19:1.
36. Armstrong RB, Ogilvie RW, Schwane JA: Eccentric exercise-induced injury to rat skeletal muscle. J Appl Physiol 1983; 54:80.
37. Jones DA, Round JM: Skeletal Muscle in Health and Disease. Manchester, England, Manchester University Press, 1990.
38. Newham DJ, Jones DA, Clarkson PM: Repeated high force eccentric exercise: Effects on muscle pain and damage. J Appl Physiol 1987; 63:1381.
39. Ebbeling CB, Clarkson PM: Exercise-induced muscle damage and adaptation. Sports Med 1989; 7:207.
40. Clarkson PM, Tremblay I: Rapid adaptation to exercise induced muscle damage. J Appl Physiol 1988; 65:1.

41. Sherman WM, Armstrong LE, Murray TM, et al: Effect of a 42.2-km footrace and subsequent rest or exercise on muscular strength and work capacity. J Appl Physiol 1984; 57:1668.
42. Snow DH, Guy PS: Percutaneous needle muscle biopsy in the horse. Equine Vet J 1976; 8:150.
43. Rose RJ: Endurance exercise in the horse: A review, part 2. Br Vet J 1986; 142:542.
44. Essén-Gustavsson B, Lindholm A: Muscle characteristics of active and inactive standardbred horses. Equine Vet J 1985; 17:434.
45. Hodgson DR, Rose RJ, Dimauro J, et al: Effects of training on muscle composition in horses. Am J Vet Res 1986; 47:12.
46. Basset DR, Giese MD, Nagle FJ, et al: Aerobic requirements of overground versus treadmill running. Med Sci Sports Exerc 1985; 17:477.
47. Bouchard C, Lesage R, Lortie G, et al: Aerobic performance in brothers, dizygotic and monozygotic twins. Med Sci Sports Exerc 1986; 18:639.
48. Bouchard C, Dionne FT, Simoneau J, et al: Genetics of aerobic and anaerobic performances. Exerc Sport Sci Rev 1992; 20:27.
49. Gaffney B, Cunningham EP: Estimation of genetic trend in racing performance of thoroughbred horses. Nature 1988; 332:722.
50. Willham RL, Wilson DE: Genetic predictions of racing performance in quarter horses. J Anim Sci 1991; 69:3891.
51. Grandjean AC: Micronutrient intake of US athletes compared to the general population and recommendations made for athletes. Am J Clin Nutr 1989; 49:1070.
52. Frape DL: Dietary requirements and athletic performance of horses. Equine Vet J 1988; 20:163.
53. Lawrence LM: Nutrition and fuel utilization in the athletic horse. Vet Clin North Am Equine Pract 1990; 6:393.
54. Levine SA, Gordon B, Derick CL: Some changes in the chemical constituents of the blood following a marathon race. JAMA 1924; 82:1778.
55. Boje O: Der blutzucker wahrend und nach korperlicher arbeit. Scand Arch Physiol 1936; 74(S10):1.
56. Christensen EH, Hansen O: Hypoglykamie, arbeitsfahigkeit und ermudung. Scand Arch Physiol 1939; 81:172.
57. Bosch AN, Dennis SC, Noakes TD: Influence of carbohydrate loading on fuel substrate turnover and oxidation during prolonged exercise. J Appl Physiol 1993; 74:1921.
58. Costill DL, Coyle E, Dalsky D, et al: Effects of elevated FFA and insulin on muscle glycogen usage during exercise. J Appl Physiol 1977; 43:695.
59. Arana MJ, Rodiek AV, Stull CL: Effects during rest and exercise of four different dietary treatments on plasma glucose, insulin, cortisol, and lactic acid and packed cell volume. J Anim Sci 1988; 66:189.
60. Leaf A, Friska KB: Eating for health and performance. Am J Clin Nutr 1989; 49:1066.
61. McMahon TA, Green PR: The influence of track compliance on running. J Biomech 1979; 12:893.
62. Pratt GW Jr: Science and the thoroughbred horse. *In* Calhoun D (ed): 1989 Yearbook of Science and the Future. Chicago, Encyclopaedia Britannica, Inc, 1989, p 178.
63. Kohnke J: Health Care and Common Problems of Horses. Sydney, Australia, Vetsearch, 1989, p 40.
64. Grant BD, Balch O, Ratzlaff M, et al: The application and use of compressible plastic horse shoes—Seattle shoes. Equine Pract 1989; 11:18.
65. Bayly WM: Training programs. Vet Clin North Am Equine Pract 1985; 1:597.
66. Costill DL: Inside Running. San Francisco, Benchmark Press, 1986, p 93.
67. Harkins JD, Kamerling SG, Bagwell CA, et al: A comparative study of interval and conventional training in thoroughbred racehorses. Equine Vet J 1990; (suppl 9):14.
68. Lindholm A, Saltin B: The physiological and biochemical response of standardbred horses to exercise of varying speed and duration. Acta Vet Scand 1974; 15:310.
69. Thorton J, Essén-Gustavsson B, Lindholm A, et al: Effects of training and detraining on oxygen uptake, cardiac output, blood gas tensions, pH and lactate concentrations during and after exercise in the horse. *In* Snow DH, Persson SGB, Rose RJ (eds): Equine Exercise Physiology. Cambridge, Granta Editions, 1983, p 470.
70. Donovan CM, Brooks GA: Endurance training affects lactate clearance, not lactate production. Am J Physiol 1983; 244:E83.
71. Svedenhag J, Seger JJ: Running on land and in water: Comparative exercise physiology. Med Sci Sports Exerc 1992; 24:1155.

3

Biomechanics, Gait, and Conformation

G. DALIN AND L. B. JEFFCOTT

Introduction

This chapter will attempt to correlate the functional anatomy of the musculoskeletal system, i.e., bones, joints, ligaments, muscles, and tendons, with athletic performance and possible physiologic modifications that result from training. The principal aim of any training program is to condition all the systems of the body to maximum athletic performance while achieving the minimum damage. Knowledge of the effects of training and the ability to maximize potential in relation to the muscular and cardiorespiratory systems is extensive. However, while the importance of training effects on bone and joints is appreciated, there is relatively little published information to date. This is regrettable when one considers that surveys of wastage by insurance companies and in the racing industry have highlighted lameness and orthopedic conditions as being the most important cause of losses.[1-3] In particular, the problems in young racehorses of "bucked shins" and biomechanically induced joint injuries (e.g., traumatic arthritis) might well be prevented if there was better information on the training effects on bone and joints.

Historical Background

Excellent in-depth reviews on the evolution of equine locomotion research have been published elsewhere,[4,5] and here only a few introductory remarks will be given. Early observations on the horse's movements are found in antique paintings (e.g., cave paintings in Lascaux, France, more than 15,000 years ago) and statues, some of which show surprising insight into the details of equine locomotion. The first systematic and, in a modern sense, scientific studies on the biomechanics of the horse were carried out during the second half of the 19th century. Marey in France developed different devices to monitor the gaits, including Marey's pneumatic recorder, an India rubber ball filled with horse hair and attached under the hoof of the horse.[6] Pressure changes in the ball were transmitted through air-filled tubes to a drum-writer held by the rider. In such a way, hoof-ground contacts could be recorded. Muybridge in the United States worked with a battery of still cameras that were triggered in sequence when the horse passed. Muybridge's works were summarized in *Animal Locomotion,* published in 1887, with almost 800 plates on the movements of a number of different species.

Since these early studies, the major developments of equine locomotion studies have been the result of new photographic and electronic techniques that have become available in the last decades. Some of the methods and questions of biomechanical and locomotion research today will be presented here. For a full account of these topics, the reader is referred to reviews cited in the text.

Biomechanics

MEASUREMENT SYSTEMS INVOLVING THE HORSE

Definitions and Variables of Measurement
For the reader who is not in everyday contact with bio-

mechanics, the following short list[7-9] of definitions has been compiled:

- *Elasticity*—the capacity of a material or object to return to its original shape after application of a stress or load. Below the yield point, an elastic material returns to its original shape when the applied stress is removed.
- *Fatigue*—weakening due to repeated deformation at loads that will not break the specimen if applied only once.
- *Kinematics*—the field of kinesiology dealing with the temporal and geometric characteristics of motion.
- *Kinesiology*—the science of motion in animals, including humans.
- *Kinetics*—the field of kinesiology, which deals with the forces that produce, arrest, or modify motion.
- *Modulus of elasticity*—uniaxial stress divided by uniaxial strain in the elastic phase of a material (Young's modulus).
- *Plasticity*—the permanent deformation of a material to applied stress without total failure or breakage.
- *Safety factor*—the ratio between a material's failure stress (or strain) and the magnitude of stress (or strain) experienced during functional activities.
- *Strain*—change in dimension of a material caused by an applied force, measured as ε = change in length divided by original length. In a material subjected to tension, strain is positive. In a material under compression, strain is negative.
- *Strain rate*—the rate of deformation (strain) to an applied load (stress) per second.
- *Strength*—resistance to breakage.
- *Stress*—force applied to a material expressed as pressure or force per unit area perpendicular (normal stress) or parallel (shear stress). The SI unit is newtons per square meter (N/m^2) or pascals (Pa).
- *Toughness*—the capacity to store energy prior to fracture.
- *Viscoelastic*—a substance in which material properties vary over time. The relationship between stress and strain is time-dependent.

Force Plates and Force Shoes
The forces produced between hoof and ground have been studied by force plates, force shoes, and pressure-sensitive mats. The more advanced equipment measures the three independent ground reaction force (GRF) components, i.e., vertical, longitudinal (forward-backward) horizontal, and transverse (mediolateral) GRF components. Less sophisticated systems measure only the vertical forces (Fig. 3–1).

Force Plates. These have been used in studies of walk, trot, canter, jumping, and lameness. For practical use and to ensure reliable and repeatable data acquisition, a force plate has to fulfill a number of criteria[10]:

- Independent measurement of force in three orthogonal planes
- Low "cross-talk" between force components

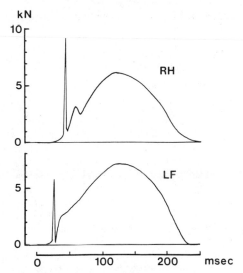

Figure 3-1. *Vertical forces (kN) trace for the stance phase of the left forelimb (LF) and right hindlimb (RH) in a Swedish warmblood trotting on asphalkt at 6.6 m/s.*

- High-frequency response
- Linear response over a sufficient range and sensitivity of force measurement
- Uniform response over the platform's surface
- Resolution of the point of application of the GRF
- Proper dimensions of the platform's surface

The GRF measurements are often "normalized" to the body mass of the horse and to the duration of the stance phase. Averaged GRF patterns can then be calculated from several recordings and comparisons made, for instance, between horses before and after treatment or between different speeds. Characteristic peak amplitudes and times of occurrence of the peaks are often used.

The major disadvantage of force plates is that data can be collected only when a hoof is placed on the plate correctly. Using a 60 × 90 cm force plate, the probability of hitting the force plate decreases from about 1 in 2 at a walk (2 m/s) to about 1 in 4 at a trot (4 m/s) and further to 1 in 6 at a canter (5 m/s).[11,12] At higher speeds, only 1 in 20 attempts result in useful data.[5] Furthermore, each successful recording contains only one hoof-ground contact.

In studies of GRF patterns in normal walking horses, Merkens and colleagues[5,13,14] in Utrecht found an almost complete symmetry between contralateral pairs of limbs with regard to amplitude and timing of GRF peaks. They also showed that during walk no more than one limb at a time contributed to either the deceleration or acceleration longitudinal horizontal force and that the total vertical force of the concurrently loaded limbs during a complete stride fluctuated between 7 and 12 N/kg of body mass.[14] Recordings made in three successive years revealed that the similarity of the GRF patterns within horses was greater than the differences between horses.[13] From analyses of walk GRF patterns of normal

and lame horses, the Utrecht group developed a method for GRF evaluation of lame horses.[15]

At a trot, the contralateral limb GRF patterns are almost completely symmetrical in unloaded horses but asymmetrical in ridden horses.[11] The mean peak vertical GRF in 13 unloaded horses trotting at 4 m/s was 11.6 and 10.2 N/kg of body mass in the fore- and hindlimbs, respectively.

GRF measurements at a canter (5 m/s) showed the highest peak vertical forces to occur in the trailing forelimb (14.8 N/kg of body mass), followed by the lead forelimb (11.6 N/kg of body mass), lead hindlimb (11.1 N/kg of body mass), and trailing hindlimb (9.4 N/kg of body mass).[12]

Force Shoes. Force shoes provide continuous recording of the forces during a number of strides and can be used on different track surfaces. Special shoes have been developed for recording vertical[16] as well as horizontal[17] forces. The force shoes used to have the disadvantage of weight and the complex wiring necessary, but now lightweight shoes and sophisticated electronics are available.[18,19]

Shoes equipped with four measuring locations were used to study variations in the vertical GRF component and its point of application. In walk and trot, the vertical load was greater in the caudal than in the cranial area of the hoof surface, and the point of application moved cranially during the stance phase.[20]

Pressure-Sensitive Mats. An alternative methods of gait analysis of horses was introduced in the 1980s known as the *Kaegi Equine gait analysis (EGA) system*.[21] This equipment uses a large series of pressure sensors in parallel lines over a 4-m measurement zone which are linked to a computer. Pressure recordings over time and distance are made, and an individual weight-bearing profile similar to the GRF profile can be generated. The only reference on the application of the EGA system involved evaluation of a series of warmblood normal (n = 50) and lame (n = 100) horses.[22] A total of 14 variables were measured for individual or pairs of limbs. At a speed of 3.5 m/s, peak vertical force was 6521 N for the forelimb and 5533 N for the hindlimb. The stance phase accounted for 37.6 percent (hindlimb) of the stride cycle. In the lame horses, there was an increased degree of weight bearing on the sound limb, a longer stance phase, and reduced single support and suspension phase. There was good repeatability of measurements, and the effects of nerve blocks and analgesics were well documented. The system appears to have considerable potential but requires more research to make it applicable to practice.

Strain Gauges

Strain gauges are used to measure in vivo bone strain but also can be used in transducers to measure muscle force as transmitted by tendons and in force plates and force shoes. They are made from materials, commonly metal foils, that change electrical resistance in proportion to the deformation of the material to which the gauge is attached. The change of resistance reflects a one-direction deformation, and combinations of three strain gauges are commercially available. In rectangular rosette strain gauges, the three elements are placed at 45 degrees to each other. Rosette strain gauges can therefore provide data on magnitude and orientation of principal strains irrespective of the gauge's orientation relative to the primary axis of strains.

In studies of bone strain, the gauges are glued onto the bone's surface. The selection of strain recording sites must be given careful thought[23]:

- The site must be surgically accessible without major soft-tissue trauma.
- Space limitations must be considered.
- Local effects on bone from muscles, tendons, and ligaments should be minimized.
- The anatomic site should be easy to identify for repeated experiments.

Midshaft bone is often used for strain recordings because this site often provides a reliable assessment of strains (and forces) transmitted along the bone diaphysis as a result of the loads applied. However, bending movements may interfere, a problem that is solved by placing three strain gauges around the midshaft perimeter.

The strain gauges are glued onto the bone recording site, and the lead wires are passed to a connector placed on the skin surface at some distance from the measuring site. During recordings, the strain gauges are connected to a Wheatstone bridge amplifier. The deformation of the strain gauge leads to resistance changes which are converted into a voltage output. These strain signals are either recorded as analog signals for later processing or are immediately converted to digital data for computer processing and analysis. Because of low signal noise, in vivo strain signals do not usually require filtering.[23]

On the basis of measurements of the bone's cross-sectional geometry and from the strain gauge recordings, the distribution of principal strains can be determined in the plane where the gauges are situated. From the principal strain data, calculations of the strains and stresses along the longitudinal and transverse axes of the bone can be made, as well as the magnitude and direction of the principal stresses.[24] Typical peak strains measured in long bones of horses are -2000 to -2500 $\mu\varepsilon$, with peak strains of -4000 $\mu\varepsilon$ on the dorsal aspect of the metacarpus of horses at a 14-m/s canter.[25]

Accelerometers

Accelerometers are used to measure accelerations and decelerations in different parts of the limbs and can give valuable information on the gait, especially if they are used in conjunction with other methods that measure the timing of the stride cycle.[26]

Noninvasive Bone Measurement

In the horse, "bone quality" involves the provision of the minimal amount of bone distributed in such a way as to maximize overall strength. An assessment of quality of bone must involve different facets of its material components and geometric structure. The basis of noninva-

sive bone measurement is to provide an assessment of total bone strength in terms of

- Stiffness or elasticity
- Mineral density
- Geometric configuration

There are essentially two types of bone that can be investigated—cortical and cancellous. The measurement of cortical bone, which is dense and compact, gives a good indication of long bone strength. Cancellous bone has a faster turnover and more rapidly reflects generalized changes in the skeletal system (e.g., osteoporosis). However, from the point of view of the athletic horse, the main changes to be identified are increasing strength of cortical bone resulting from the biomechanical effects of training rather than early detection of metabolic bone changes.

A wide range of techniques are available to quantify aspects of bone density, mass, and strength.[27] In the horse, the most frequently used are radiography, scintigraphy, single-photon absorptiometry, and ultrasound velocity.

Radiography

PLAIN RADIOGRAPHY. Plain radiography has been the traditional means of assessing skeletal maturity in the horse. This has principally involved assessment of growth plate closure, particularly that of the distal radial physis. Closure times have been correlated with unsoundness in young racehorses,[28,29] but the technique is not precise. The assessment of cortical density is imprecise because a change of greater than 30 to 40 percent in bone mineral content is required for visual evaluation by radiography. However, the situation can be improved, to some extent, by using the techniques of radiographic photodensitometry and radiogrammetry.

RADIOGRAPHIC PHOTODENSITOMETRY. Radiographic photodensitometry involves measuring the optical density of bone from a radiograph and comparing it with the optical density of a known thickness of a standard material (e.g., aluminum step wedge). This considerably improves the accuracy of the technique and should mean that changes in bone mineral content of 10 to 20 percent can be detected. A computerized system has been devised which improves clinical reproducibility to within 3.5 percent for the human forearm.[30] Bone mineral content of the equine third metacarpus has been estimated in this way by determining a radiographic bone aluminum equivalent (RBAE).[31]

RADIOGRAMMETRY. Radiogrammetry involves the measurement from a radiograph of cortical thickness, medullary cavity width, and overall bone diameter. It has been used successfully in humans[32] and in a study of equine metacarpal bones.[31] It may have clinical potential, provided that a careful and standard radiographic technique is employed.

Scintigraphy

Nuclear medicine can be used to image the skeletal system to provide information on location of bone activity as a means of identifying bone growth, new bone deposition, and bone pathology. The technique is based on the detection of a radiolabeled phosphate compound in bone and soft tissues. Intravenous injection of a technetium phosphate compound (e.g., ^{99m}Tc-MDP) is followed by its uptake into the mineral matrix of bone after passage through the vascular and extravascular fluid components. The level of uptake is related to the degree of bone turnover. This is measured 2 to 3 hours after injection with a gamma camera that is interfaced with a computer for storage and image analysis.

Scintigraphic detection of bone stress remodeling and fracture is well established in human medicine and may be used to detect pathologic changes of repetitive bone stress long before any evidence is visible radiographically.[33] Stress-induced injuries have been demonstrated by scintigraphy in the dorsal aspect of the metacarpus of racehorses.[34]

Photon Absorptiometry

SINGLE-PHOTON ABSORPTIOMETRY. The principle of the technique is to scan a bone with a narrow beam of low-energy photons from a monoenergetic radionuclide source and to measure the degree of attenuation of the beam by bone relative to its attenuation by tissue by means of a scintillation detector system. A direct relationship is established between the number of extra photons absorbed and the bone mineral content (BMC). The amount of mineral per unit area in the path of the photon beam (m_b) is calculated by the formula[35]

$$m_b = \frac{r_B \ln (I_0/I)}{\mu_B r_B \mu_S r_S} \text{ g/cm}^2$$

where r = microscopic density (g/cm^3) for bone (r_B)
and soft tissue (r_S)
μ = mass absorption coefficient (cm^2/g) for bone
mineral (μ_B) and soft tissue (μ_S)
I_0 = intensity of the beam through the uniform tissue
I = the reduced intensity through bone

For the horse, a system using americium (^{241}Am) as the source of monoenergetic (60 keV) photons has been developed.[27] The accuracy and reproducibility of the estimate of BMC by scanning is around 2 percent, which is much better than by direct radiography or radiographic densitometry. The limb containing the bone being scanned must be surrounded by a soft-tissue-equivalent material so that the surfaces facing the source and detector are flat and reasonably parallel. Both the photon source and the radiation counting device move in unison to scan the bone transversely. The transmitted intensity of the beam is reduced as it traverses the bone, and a logarithmic plot of counts per second is made.

One major disadvantage of single-photon absorptiometry is that it provides the mineral content per unit length of bone scanned (BMC, g/cm) and takes no account of differences in bone size. In other words, single-photon absorptiometry measures the mineral content in a 1.0-cm-thick slab or cross section of the bone. Thus it is really only useful in monitoring sequential changes in

an individual, where changes in the cross-sectional area of the bone can be considered negligible.

DUAL-PHOTON ABSORPTIOMETRY. Dual-photon absorptiometry is a newer technique which can quantify more accurately bone mineral content, particularly where there is variable thickness of overlying soft tissue. It is considerably more expensive than single-photon absorptiometry but provides a more sensitive indicator of general skeletal mass.[36,37] The technique uses high-purity and high-activity gadolinium (^{153}Gd), which is a dual-energy source of photons at approximately 44 and 100 keV. Scans of the human spine are made in a rectilinear fashion, and the results are expressed as grams per square centimeter. It takes 15 to 45 minutes to perform a scan of the spine, depending on the activity of the source and the precision required. The precision of measurement is considered to be 2 to 3 percent, and the radiation dose is relatively low at 10 to 20 mrem. However, this method still suffers from not taking into account the third dimension of the bone volume, and again, sites are mostly a combination of cortical and trabecular bone. Work in the horse using dual photon absorptiometry has been confined so far to excised bones.[38,39]

Ultrasound Velocity. The modulus of elasticity is the property of a material that relates to its bending strength and stiffness and ultimately to its fracture threshold. The measurement of ultrasound velocity in bone is used to assess bone quality because the velocity of sound is directly related to the modulus of elasticity (or stiffness) and density of bone provided the extensional (i.e., longitudinal) wave velocity is measured[40]:

$$E = rC^2$$

where E = modulus of elasticity
r = compact bone density or specificity gravity
C = velocity of ultrasound

Ultrasound velocity in bone is dependent on its density, water content, and probably its porosity, as well as the direction of the ultrasound path and the orientation of fibers in the bone matrix.[41]

TRANSMISSION ULTRASOUND VELOCITY. Transmission ultrasound velocity involves passing an ultrasound beam through the bone from a transmitting to a receiving transducer (Fig. 3–2). The velocity C of the ultrasound (m/s) can be derived from the distance D the two transducers are apart and the time of flight t of the sound. Corrections need to be applied to compensate for overlying soft tissues. If it is assumed that the sonic pathway is directly from one transducer to the other, the velocity determined is referred to as *apparent velocity* C_a:

$$C_a = \frac{D}{t} \text{ m/s}$$

C_a may be correct for a uniform section of cortical bone but is inaccurate for the metacarpal shaft, which is not uniform, but cylindrical with an outer cortex ($C \approx 3000$

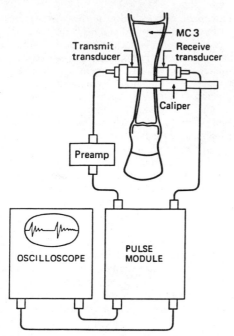

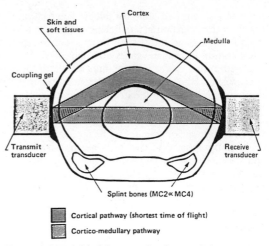

Figure 3-3. *Simplified diagram of pathways of ultrasound through the metacarpal shaft. (From McCartney and Jeffcott. Med Biol Eng Comput 1987;25:620, with permission.)*

Figure 3-2. *Schematic diagram of transmission ultrasound velocity measurement through the shaft of the third metacarpal bone of the horse. [From Jeffcott and colleagues. Equine Vet J 1988 (suppl 6):71, with permission.]*

m/s) surrounding a medullary cavity ($C \approx 1500$ m/s). In this situation, the fastest pathway for the sound will be entirely via the cortex. It is possible to estimate the pathway and correct C_a to give a transverse cortical bone ultrasound velocity C_b.[42] Not only can the cortical pathway be determined, but by measuring a later pulse which travels directly through the medulla, the ratio of the medulla to cortex also can be estimated (Fig. 3–3). From this information, the cortical cross-sectional area (CSA) of the shaft can be derived.

Combined Ultrasound Velocity and Photon Absorptiometry. The BMC measured by photon absorptiometry can be used to derive the bone mineral density (BMD) if the cortical cross-sectional area is known. The ultrasound velocity technique provides an estimate of this area, and thus

$$BMD = BMC/CSA \text{ g/cm}^3$$

The estimation of BMD provides a volumetric estimate of mineral content and allows for animals of different size to be compared and changes in growth to be assessed objectively. Using a bone model[43] for cortical bone involving the microscopic collagen density ($r_c = 1.0$ g/cm^3) and microscopic bone mineral density ($r_m = 3.2$ g/cm^3), the compact bone density (CBD) or specific gravity can be estimated:

$$CBD = r_c + (1 - r_c/r_m) BMD \text{ g/cm}^3$$

Furthermore, a modulus of elasticity E can be derived using the Helmholz equation:

$$E = CBD \times C^2 \text{ N/m}^2$$

where C = ultrasound velocity

The strength of a bone is related to its geometry and the elastic strength of the material of which it is composed. BMD and CBD are measures of the degree of the bone's mineralization and E of its elastic stiffness. In this way the mechanical properties of the whole bone can be evaluated in vivo.

Invasive Bone Measurement
Bone Biopsy. In humans it is well established that the technique of bone biopsy and subsequent histomorphometric analysis form a sound basis for assessing bone quality, quantity, and metabolism.[44] In addition, a useful estimate of mechanical strength of bone also may be gained by determining the amount of cortical and cancellous bone histomorphometrically.[45] The dynamic process involved in bone remodeling can be assessed by introducing a fluorochrome as an intravital marker. While there is great potential in horses for assessment of skeletal metabolism and the effects of exercise, this has not yet been achieved.

A simple method of biopsy using the wing of the ilium in standing or anesthetized horses has been used in studies of bone metabolism in growing horses.[46] A core is collected from the wing of the ilium some distance from the tuber coxae and consists of a central cancellous portion between two cortices. An integral part of the procedure is intravital bone labeling using fluorochromes administered with a known time interval between labels.

Muscle Biopsy. The use of muscle biopsies for estimation of muscle fiber types has been an important tool in exercise physiology since the initial work of Lindholm and Piehl.[47] This topic will be amply covered elsewhere, but there have not been any studies using muscle biopsy to estimate the specific biomechanical effects of training as opposed to general workload (i.e., treadmill speed, duration, incline, etc.).

Biochemical Methods

Alkaline phosphatase (AP) is an enzyme considered essential in mineralization, and concentrations in serum can reflect osteoblastic activity. It is a useful but somewhat insensitive marker of bone turnover unless the bone-specific isoenzyme can be assayed.

Hydroxyproline (Hp) is produced during the formation of bone collagen and is released during the process of bone resorption by osteoclasts. It is not biologically recycled and therefore cannot be used in the formation of new bone collagen. Ultimately, it is excreted in the urine and therefore is of some value as a marker of bone turnover. However, the situation is complicated by the necessity to adjust the diet of patients to overcome the dietary contribution to concentrations in urine.

Osteocalcin (or bone Gla protein) may be a more sensitive indicator of the mineralization process because it is released into the circulation during bone formation.[48] It has definite advantages over AP and Hp because it is specific for bone and can be measured easily by radioimmunoassay.

Serum calcium and phosphorus are of no use as screening tests in the diagnosis of osteopenia because the size of serum calcium and phosphorus pools bear no direct relationship to bone mineral content. However, they may be invaluable in the identification of certain conditions which may be responsible for osteopenia.

Other markers, including parathyroid hormone (PTH), urine cyclic adenosine monophosphate (AMP), vitamin D, and calcitonin, have been used,[49] but they all have limited usefulness in clinical terms.

Electromyography

The analysis of muscular activity by electromyography (EMG) is a most useful tool in locomotion research, especially if combined with other kinesiologic techniques. The muscular action potentials, indicative of active contraction, are detected by the electrodes, and the signal is transmitted via wires and cables or telemetry for amplifying and further processing. From EMG recordings, the time and magnitude of muscular action can be analyzed. The assessment of force from EMG is, however, most problematic because the force exerted by a muscle depends on a number of factors. EMG techniques recently have been reviewed by Gans.[50]

EMG has not been used extensively in horses, which is partly due to the methodologic problems involved. Skin surface electrodes are impractical for use in horses, and fine-wire electrodes are inserted into the muscles studied. The presence of electrodes does not normally cause any pain, and the electrodes are well tolerated during movement. EMG has been used in combination with high-speed cinematography in studies of limb and neck biomechanics at the walk, trot, and canter to correlate muscle activity with the mechanical actions of the muscles.[51–54]

MEASUREMENT INVOLVING THE TRACK

The effects of racetrack design on a horse's performance and health have focused on two areas: geometric design of the track and the mechanical properties of different track surfaces. The recommendations for geometric design have been based mainly on kinematic studies of racehorses and now include banking of curves and incorporation of transition curves.[55–57]

The studies of hoof-surface interaction and variations in forces between different surfaces mainly have been carried out with force-measuring shoes or by accelerometers attached to the hoof.[58] Much valuable information has also been gained by simulating hoof forces using a drop hammer on different surfaces.[59] Shock forces transmitted through the extremities are considered to play a significant role in induction of injury, and a reduction of the impact forces would be a major step forward for track designers.

BIOMECHANICAL EFFECTS OF EXERCISE AND EXERCISE-INDUCED INJURIES

Bone Structure and Function

Galileo first recognized the relationship between applied load and bone morphology. In 1683, he noted a direct correlation between body weight and bone size. In 1892, the German anatomist Julius Wolff reported that "every change in the function of a bone is followed not only by certain definite changes in its internal architecture, but in its external conformation as well, in accordance with mathematical laws." Since then, there have been some elegant studies carried out in both humans and animals to investigate the response of bone to a variety of biomechanical situations. However, it is only in the last few years that any investigations on horses have been undertaken to try to monitor the effects of training. The specific effects of exercise on bone have been shown to depend not only on the animal's age but also on the duration and intensity of training.

Bone has a dual role to support the body (skeletal homeostasis) and as a source of calcium (mineral homeostasis). It is a dynamic tissue in which changes continue to take place throughout life to maintain optimal strength and to adapt to external forces. This involves a continual and coordinated activity of forming (by osteoblasts) and removing (by osteoclasts) bone which is termed *remodeling*. The actual structure of bone is very complex, but its basic makeup is a collagen framework hardened by hydroxyapatite mineralization to give it strength. Bone is a unique tissue in that it is capable of mechanical adaptation and changes in its quantity, quality, and geometry in response to loads imposed on it.

The effects will differ between cancellous and cortical bone. The material properties of bone will be influenced by such factors as anatomic location, age, species, and pathologic and loading conditions.

The skeleton of the horse reflects the load-bearing competence of its individual components; in other words, bones are capable of adapting to the prevailing biomechanical stresses (i.e., load bearing). In racehorses, the extent of load bearing is essentially determined by the training regimen to which they are subjected. The objective of training is to increase skeletal strength while limiting the possibilities of exercise-induced injury. Although the actual mechanisms of response to loading are poorly understood, it is clear that bone readily adapts to either imposed stress or the lack of any stress by forming or losing tissue. Bone hypertrophy (i.e., modeling) occurs when stress is applied. Lack of exercise has been shown, particularly in humans, to be one of the most significant factors in stimulating bone turnover, initially seen as remodeling, but leading eventually to osteoporosis.[60] The withdrawal of any functional loading of the bone also results in rapid loss, although this can be reversed by exposure to short daily periods of suitable dynamic loading.[61]

The effects of loading and unloading of bone are well known, but the means by which the specific signals are recognized at the cellular level are not yet understood. It is now believed that there is a limiting strain range called the *minimum effective strain* (MES) that turns these mechanically controlled responses "on" and "off."[62] Published data suggest that to switch on a modeling response, approximately 1500 to 3000 $\mu\epsilon$ is required. However, a much smaller threshold strain range (~100 to 300 $\mu\epsilon$) is necessary for the mechanical control of remodeling. It also has been shown that bone requires stimulation by appropriate strain rates for optimal maintenance of strength.[63] Bones resist compression, twisting, and bending in many directions and can be trained to resist these forces. A dose-response curve has been produced[64] that shows that strains below a certain peak magnitude are associated with bone loss, while those above that level not only protect the existing bone tissue from resorption but also provide an osteogenic stimulus resulting in deposition of an amount of new bone proportional to the degree of "overstrain" engendered. Once a loading regimen has been repeated so that it is recognized by the bone, subsequent repetitions apparently do not affect the nature or magnitude of the adaptive response. This, of course, has important connotations for training of racehorses in trying to reduce exercise-induced lameness by limiting excessive amounts of fast work.

Skeletal Adaptation to Fast Exercise. The effects of exercise on cortical bone have been examined in growing (1- to 2-year-old) and adult horses at both submaximal and maximal intensities.[65,66] These studies reveal that submaximal exercise even for prolonged periods (<6 months) in young and adult horses does not dramatically alter the mass or density of cortical bone in the metacarpus. In contrast, training at high speeds results

in significant increases of ultrasound speed in both adult thoroughbred and standardbred horses. This increase in ultrasound speed is only about 1.5 percent (~50 m/s) and is thought to reflect a small increase in bone density due to a reduction in bone porosity.

Maximal exercise in young thoroughbreds (15 months old) at speeds above 12 m/s results in not only a rise in ultrasound speed but also more substantial increases in bone mass. This intense type of exercise causes a decrease in intracortical porosity which is reflected in high ultrasound speed readings. However, the increase in ultrasound speed is never greater than 1 to 2 percent and differs from the nonexercised horses only by 3 or 4 percent (<120 m/s). These small changes may have an important effect on bone strength because bone strength is proportional to the density cubed.

A more dramatic change in response to fast exercise is the alteration in distribution of compact bone that occurs in young horses. Histomorphometric examination of bone samples from these horses reveals that both modeling and remodeling of bone have been changed substantially. First, intracortical bone remodeling is significantly reduced by decreasing bone porosity. Second, the cross-sectional morphology of the metacarpal shaft is altered, resulting in greater bone formation on the dorsal periosteal and endosteal surfaces. It appears that an increase in bone formation on the dorsal periosteal surface does not occur at any appreciable rate until speeds greater than 12 m/s are achieved. It has been postulated that the signals that regulate intracortical bone density may be different from the signals that cause enlargement of the cortex. There is now increasing evidence that important changes in the density of subchondral bone also occur as a result of high-speed exercise.

The change in shape of the metacarpal bone due to high-speed exercise is important in adaptation of the bone to the rigors of fast galloping and also helps to reduce the risk of bone damage (e.g., "bucked shins").[67] The adult thoroughbred third metacarpal bone has a thick dorsal cortex compared with that of standardbreds.[68] This difference between the two breeds is not necessarily genetically related, since there is evidence that the normal growth pattern of the thoroughbred does not always involve specific enlargement of the dorsal cortex. However, it is clear that intense exercise of young thoroughbreds will dramatically enlarge the size and shape of the dorsal cortex when compared with nonexercised age-matched controls. The response of the metacarpus to the forces of compression is to enlarge the cross-sectional area. This reduces local bone stress, because stress is equal to the force (i.e., load) divided by the area over which the force acts. If the horse's metacarpus were subjected simply to axial compressive forces (i.e., no bending) during galloping, then the alteration in cross-sectional area would be uniform. This, however, is not the case, since substantially more bone is laid down on the dorsal cortex than at other sites. We can assume, therefore, that some bending forces on the metacarpus must occur during galloping in addition to compression. Bending increases the local strain on the dorsal cortex and leads to preferential enlargement of the bone in this axis. The bending is thought to occur only at the fast gallop, since it has not been possible to measure it at slower speeds. The standardbred's cannon bone does not have an enlarged dorsal cortex, which indicates that the bending forces probably do not occur at a fast trot or pace.

An understanding of the microstructure of equine bone is particularly valuable for appreciation of the biomechanical effects on the skeleton.[69] There are a number of other structural factors in bone, which have not yet been fully investigated, that may be influenced by training. For example, the alignment of collagen fibers within the bone contributes significantly to the compressive strength of the cannon bone. It is feasible that the collagen formed in trained horses is better aligned than that in untrained horses, thus contributing to the structural strength of the bone. The collagen cross-linkage of bone is also an important factor that can regulate bone mineralization and bone strength. Increases in the number of collagen cross-links also may contribute to the bone-strengthening effect of training.

It is clear, therefore, that controlled fast work over short distances will improve the biomechanical strength of the metacarpus of young horses. Further studies are required to determine the minimum amount of fast work that will result in an improvement in the strength of the metacarpus and also the duration and speed of fast exercise that provide an unacceptable risk of causing bone damage.

"Bucked Shins"—An Exercise-Induced Injury. The cause of "bucked shins" (shin soreness) was originally attributed to tearing of the periosteum and subsequent subperiosteal hematoma.[70] More recently, biomechanical injury has been proposed as a more likely cause of "bucked shins" involving a fatigue failure of the bone on the dorsal aspect of the metacarpus. Microfracturing in the outer layer of the dorsal cortex is proposed as the instigating factor leading to local inflammation and pain.[71] The major risk factors involved in "bucked shins" in order of precedence are high-speed work, immaturity, too much work too soon, and low bone strength/density. Over 90 percent of "bucked shins" cases exhibit the first signs during the fast-work stages of their preparation.[72]

Bone that is repetitively loaded will suffer fatigue, during which the bone loses strength and will ultimately fracture.[73] Bone that is under very large loads will fatigue quickly, whereas bone under smaller loads will take longer to fatigue (i.e., the greater the load or strain, the fewer cycles required to cause fatigue). On the other hand, the fatigue life of bone is positively related to its density (i.e., the denser the bone, the more cycles required to cause fatigue). However, the situation in young racehorses is more complex. We have already seen that the metacarpus of young horses responds to intense exercise by producing more bone on its dorsal surface. This bone is of low density initially, since mineralization of the newly formed bone is fairly slow. The bone therefore will have much lower fatigue life than that of fully mineralized bone. For a given load, this bone will deform more than fully mineralized bone, thus setting up

large shear forces between areas of new, low mineralized bone and older, fully mineralized bone. These larger shear forces may result in more rapid fatigue of the bone, which leads to microfracturing. This is followed by an inflammatory reaction resulting in periostitis with serum oozing underneath the periosteum. The inflammation and damage to the bone matrix stimulates the formation of periosteal new bone (generally woven bone).

Training to Maximize Bone Quality and Minimize Lameness. Although it is possible to train a horse without the horse getting "bucked shins," it is unlikely that horses can be trained without some degree of shin soreness occurring. Alteration of current training and racing practices could result in a reduction in the occurrence of "bucked shins," as well as a reduction in the occurrence of many other orthopedic injuries (e.g. carpal chips, traumatic arthritis, etc.). These, together with improvements in track structure and design, are thought to be important factors that will affect the incidence of "bucked shins" in the future.

An incremental training program that increases the length, speed, and repetition of galloping has been suggested as an alternative training program. It has been shown in other species that small numbers of high-intensity loads per day can result in enhanced bone growth. Therefore, the distance over which horses gallop need only be short (200 to 400 m). We know that the faster the speed at which this work is done, the greater is the bone's response. In order to control this response and not promote excessive risk of "bucked shins," the horses should be started at a slow gallop and the speed progressively increased after periods of 4 to 5 weeks. As galloping speed increases, so does the risk of "bucked shins," so close surveillance is required. This type of training program involves a tradeoff between maximizing the bone response and minimizing the incidence of "bucked shins." Acute "bucked shins" occurs from excessive strain in a bone that is relatively small. As a result of training, the bone enlarges, which means that for a given load (speed), there will be less strain. The strain in an adult thoroughbred at full gallop is around 3500 $\mu\varepsilon$, whereas it may be more than 5000 $\mu\varepsilon$ in a 2-year-old. If the bone strain is kept at 3000 to 3500 $\mu\varepsilon$ during a gallop, the risk of "bucked shins" should be low.

The proposed advantages of such a training program include a reduction in the incidence of "bucked shins" and, as a result, an improvement in welfare for the horse. It is envisaged that other types of exercise-induced bone and joint problems may occur less often, which could add substantial benefits. The other factor is that reductions in these orthopedic conditions may greatly enhance the horse's useful racing life and thereby reduce the substantial wastage that occurs in the racing industry.

CONCLUSIONS. In summary, galloping exercise at maximum speed results in important adaptational changes in the size and shape of the metacarpus to provide extra bone strength. The extent of these changes will vary among individual horses, and in some instances, the end result will be exercise-induced injury such as "bucked shins." Enlargement of the dorsal cortex also will result from "bucked shins" because the acute inflammation produced activates the periosteum and results in a rapid production of bone. This bone is often of a type that will gradually need to be modified to provide suitably strong (organized) bone by the process of remodeling.

Joints

Despite the important role of synovial joints in equine orthopedics, our current knowledge of their function during training and racing is sparse. The reasons are clear: To investigate moving joints is difficult and to make physiologic measurements within the joint almost impossible. The effects of exercise on articular structures have therefore mainly been studied in experimental animals and have focused on articular cartilage.

Synovial joints are complex organs which include a number of different tissues (e.g., subchondral bone, articular cartilage, ligaments, joint capsule, and synovial fluid). Their function is to provide a low-friction junction between skeletal bones. In the horse's limbs, joints withstand high-impact forces and provide stability at maximum loads during the stance phase and a fraction of a second later act as high-speed low-friction "hinges" during the swing phase. In addition to the active muscle contractions controlled by the central nervous system, joint movements are guided and limited by passive structures (e.g., articular conformation, ligaments, and muscles/tendons).

Subchondral Bone. Subchondral bone is the platform on which articular cartilage abuts to form a stable connection between them (the chondro-osseous junction). The trabeculae of the cancellous subchondral bone are oriented according to the compressive and tensile stresses acting in the joint. In the young, growing animal, the deeper layers of the articular cartilage form the articular–epiphyseal cartilage complex, which is the growth cartilage of the epiphysis. During the period of endochondral bone formation, the deeper layers of the articular cartilage receive their nutritional supply partially from epiphyseal vessels. When growth is complete, this route of supply ceases.

Articular Cartilage. Articular cartilage is hyaline cartilage, which gives a smooth articular surface for the gliding and rolling movements between opposing bones. It also provides the stiffness necessary for the compressive, tensile, and shear stresses between the two joint surfaces. The articular surface is smooth in the young animal and gradually gets rougher with age. Mechanical factors (i.e., stress, wear and tear, and aging) seem to influence surface smoothness.[74]

Morphologically, articular cartilage is divided into four zones, which reflect differences in cellular and matrix composition, metabolism, and loading. Cartilage thickness varies within and between joints but is thickest in regions of high loading. Articular cartilage consists of chondrocytes, which synthesize the components of the cartilage matrix, and the extracellular matrix, which forms more than 95 percent of the tissue volume. There is an intricate interaction between matrix and chondrocytes. Thus the composition of matrix varies between pericellular, territorial, and interterritorial matrix. There are no blood vessels or nerves in articular cartilage, and the supply of nutrients is from synovial fluid and matrix water exchange. Cartilage matrix normally has a water content of 70 to 80 percent, and this is increased closer to the articular surface. The major matrix constituents are collagen ($\sim$50 percent of dry substance), proteoglycans ($\sim$40 percent of dry substance), and noncollagenous proteins. The biochemical composition of articular cartilage in the horse is similar to that in other species.[75]

Collagen is the main matrix constituent and is responsible for the tensile properties of articular cartilage.[76] Collagen type II fibers form the bulk of articular collagen (90 to 95 percent), and some additional minor collagens assist in stabilizing the type II network. The volume of articular cartilage is constrained by the collagen network. Close to the articular surface, collagen fibers are arranged densely, parallel to the surface, while the fibers in the deepest zones have a tendency to be oriented more or less perpendicular to the articular surface.

Proteoglycans are major macromolecules of the ground substance responsible for the compressive stiffness of articular cartilage.[76,77] They consist of a protein core with glycosaminoglycan (GAG) side chains. Most proteoglycans ($\sim$85 percent) aggregate with hyaluronic acid filaments via link proteins. GAG polymer side chains are repeating disaccharide dimers (i.e., chondroitin-6-sulfate, chondroitin-4-sulfate, and keratan sulfate) containing negatively charged groups. GAG chains thus repel each other but attract water. Cartilage stiffness and compressibility are highly dependent on these characteristics of proteoglycans.

Joint Loading and Articular Cartilage. The mechanical characteristics of articular cartilage are determined ·by the content, properties, and interactions of its structural constituents.[78] The mechanical properties vary between loaded and unloaded parts of the joint. Cartilage areas subjected to high stress levels show higher proteoglycan content and are stiffer. Experimental and theoretical analyses concerning the structure and function of articular cartilage suggest that the proteoglycans are responsible for the biomechanical characteristics in compression, whereas the properties, content, and orientation of collagen are the prime determinants of the tensional properties.[79] When cartilage is subjected to compressive loads, proteoglycans are squeezed and water is expressed from the cartilage. When pressure is relieved, cartilage expands and is rehydrated from the synovial fluid and from unloaded cartilage. Physiologic loading and motion are therefore essential to maintain the normal nutrition and metabolism of articular cartilage provided by exchange with synovial fluid. Disturbances of this mechanism result in early changes of degenerative joint disease. With increasing loads, larger articular surface areas are involved (i.e., the load is spread to reduce stress). The maximum cartilage compression is about 40 percent of original rest height.

Experiments on tensile properties, compressive stiffness, and physicochemical measurements of matrix indicate that the functional integrity of articular cartilage is dependent on

- Low hydraulic permeability and high swelling tendency of the hydrophilic proteoglycan component
- Entrapment and confinement of this hydrodynamic gel within the collagen fiber network.[80]

At rest, the proteoglycans are maximally hydrated, which is approximately 20 percent of the potential because the swelling pressure of the proteoglycans is balanced by hydrostatic pressure of the collagen network. When loaded, the articular cartilage undergoes immediate elastic deformation with no decrease in cartilage volume. Cartilage "creep" then occurs when the volume of compressed cartilage decreases as water is forced from compressed to uncompressed matrix regions or out of articular cartilage. The rapid elastic deformation depends on the collagen fibers, while the creep component of the response depends on the proteoglycans.[81,82] When loading is removed, water is imbibed again by the proteoglycan activity into the cartilage.

Effects of Exercise. It is generally accepted that continued or repetitive joint loading is necessary for the well-being of articular cartilage and that cellular synthetic activity is profoundly influenced by the level of mechanical load.[83,84] There is, however, a shortage of studies on the effects of loading on the functional properties of articular cartilage. Recent studies have shown that the chondrocyte plays a central role in the response to exercise, and more studies are needed on the complex interaction between chondrocytes and matrix during load bearing. Cartilage response depends on the motion and loading pattern of the joint. Intermittent and cyclical compression stimulates cell synthesis, whereas continuous or static compression tends to inhibit synthesis.

Reduced Loading. Reduced loading (e.g., immobilization) leads to atrophy or degeneration of the cartilage. The effects depend on the method of immobilization, the species, and the age of the animal.[85] Lack of load bearing decreases proteoglycan content of articular cartilage and leads to water accumulation in the tissue,[86] with decreased stiffness and increased deformation rate. Disturbances of proteoglycan synthesis also result in qualitative changes. After remobilization, most changes are reversible.

Increased Joint Loading. Increased joint loading induces different responses depending on the rate and amplitude of the loads. *Enhanced cyclic loading,* as in moderate running exercise, increases the content of proteoglycans in the cartilage matrix[83,87] and causes a slight stiffening of the cartilage. These structural and functional adapta-

tions are considered to improve the biomechanical properties of articular cartilage. *Very strenuous exercise* injures articular cartilage by increasing fibrillation of the cartilage and reducing proteoglycan content and quality.[88] Cartilage no longer responds with improved biomechanical properties, and overload results, which can lead to degenerative joint disease.[79] *Peak overloading* has been shown to induce cartilage breakdown (i.e., accelerated catabolic processes).[89]

It has been suggested that cartilage is the first structure in the joint that responds negatively to increased levels of stress and motion.[79] Mechanical forces, however, are also likely to destroy cartilage indirectly through insults to be subchondral bone, the synovium, or the chondrocytes.[90]

Degenerative Joint Disease. Traumatically induced degenerative joint disease (DJD, osteoarthritis) appears to be the most common cause of joint problems in horses, owing to their use as athletes.[91] Horses show more lesions in areas of higher load (e.g., dorsal aspect of carpal bones, proximal phalanx, distal metacarpus). DJD involves a progressive degeneration of articular cartilage and includes cartilage changes (e.g., swelling, fibrillation, blister formation, loss of thickness, and erosions), resorption and sclerosis of subchondral bone, and synovitis. Depending on the type of joint and lesions involved, the pathogenesis shows some variations.[92] However, the initial injury is usually mechanical in nature, with an imbalance between load applied and the tissues' capacity to withstand that load. Acute or repetitive overload of joint structures may lead to DJD as a result of direct articular cartilage damage, subchondral bone changes, synovitis and capsulitis, or acute fracture, disruption of ligaments, and capsular tearing.[93] Apart from accidental injuries, overload trauma may result from such factors as fatigue, speed, poor conformation, and poor track conditions.

Soft-tissue injury, including synovitis, may be the inciting cause of DJD but also may occur secondarily to articular cartilage damage due to the release of degradation products into the synovial fluid.[94] The interaction between synovium and articular cartilage is complex, and in synovitis, inflammatory mediators such as interleukines and prostaglandins, metalloproteases, lysozyme enzymes, and free radicals have effects on the metabolism and physicochemical properties of articular cartilage. Interleukin 1 (IL-1) activity has been shown to be present in the synovial fluid from cases of equine DJD, and IL-1 activity could be relevant in the pathogenesis of DJD in horses.[95,96]

Physical and biochemical cartilage damage, on the other hand, leads to the release of breakdown products into the synovial fluid which induce synovitis. Irrespective of the site of initial damage, a vicious circle is established resulting in the development of DJD. High concentrations of GAG which reflect cartilage degradation and GAG release are found in synovial fluid from horses with DJD.[97,98] Measurements of synovial and serum concentrations of proteoglycan may enable cartilage degeneration to be detected and monitored and treatments to be refined in equine DJD.

To prevent and treat equine DJD, a deeper knowledge of the mechanisms of etiology and pathogenesis is required, including basic studies of the physical and biochemical events in normal and diseased joints as well as the importance of biomechanical factors and training regimens. Studies in these areas are essential to provide the racing industry with means to reduce one of the most important causes of losses early in the careers of racehorses.

Tendons and Ligaments

Despite the fact that overuse injuries in tendons and ligaments are common in racehorses, the biomechanics of tendons and ligaments has not received the same attention as that of bone and articular cartilage.[99] The dual role for tendons, to transmit forces and to store elastic energy, makes their mechanical behavior complicated. Tendon load can be expressed as tendon force or as tendon deformation caused by the force. Tendons have been equipped with force transducers, and displacements of their origin/insertion also have been used to assess stress and strain.[100,101] Forces and strains have been reviewed by Jansen and coworkers.[102]

So far, no in-depth studies are available on the effects of training and conditioning on the strength and quality of tendons in horses.

Locomotion and Gait

MEASUREMENT AND ANALYSIS SYSTEMS

Parameters of Measurement

Basic stride and gait descriptions consist of *linear and temporal variables*. Temporal variables (e.g., stride duration) are calculated mainly from frame numbers in high-speed cinematographic or video recordings. Some temporal variables also can be derived from force plate and measuring shoe recordings. Linear gait variables (e.g., stride length) can be measured from well-defined reference points in film and video registrations.

Joint Kinematics. Joint kinematics, i.e., angular displacement, is mainly investigated by applying reference points to the skin of horses at standardized positions in relation to the joints under study. The positions of the reference points under locomotion are determined from high-speed cinematography, video, or other optoelectronic systems. At slow gaits, electrogoniometry has been used for some joints.[103–105]

The *reference points* used in gait analysis are glued onto the skin of the horse over well-defined osteologic structures to ensure repeatability between sessions and to enable comparisons between horses to be made. Skin displacement is, however, an important source of error in skin marker–based kinematic gait analysis. In walking and trotting horses, skin displacements are negligible around the distal joints but substantial around the carpal and tarsal joints (<2 cm) and in the proximal limb reach amplitudes up to more than 17 cm (greater tro-

chanter).[106] The marked skin displacements in the proximal parts of the limbs necessitate the establishment of correction models for use in modern automatic kinematic analysis equipment.

High-Speed Cinematography and High-Speed Video Systems

Among the methods available for the measurement of kinematic variables, high-speed cinematography is the method most commonly used. The advantages and disadvantages of the method have been discussed in detail.[107] The major drawback of high-speed cinematography is the delay from recording to analysis. The superior temporal and picture resolution, i.e., the high frame frequencies (<500 Hz) and the quality of 16-mm photographic film, in combination with the quality of modern electromechanical cameras still makes this the technique of choice for research purposes. This is especially so with the availability of automatic film analysis systems capable of tracking high numbers of references from frame to frame.

TrackEye (Innovativ Vision AB, Linköping, Sweden) is an analysis system which has been applied recently to equine locomotion studies in conjunction with high-speed cinematography.[108] TrackEye covers the process from digitizing of images, automatic target tracking, and analysis. The system has reduced the time for film analysis substantially. It includes an image workstation for processing of video images and a high-resolution film-to-video scanner. Images are stored on a video disk system, and a tracking module is able to follow reference markers automatically. Analyses include calculations of marker displacements, distances, and joint angles, velocities, and accelerations. The system is now used for basic locomotion research and for studies on lameness and medication and on the correlation between conformation and performance.

High-speed video systems have not been used very much in equine locomotion research[109] but will be of great interest once the time and image resolution have been improved.

Optoelectronic Systems

A modified CODA system (Cartesian Opto-electronic Digital Anthropometer, Movement Techniques Ltd., Loughborough, U.K.) has been used in a number of kinematic studies in Utrecht. The CODA-3 scanner uses three beams of visible light. The outer two bundles are focused to vertical lines and sweep around vertical axes, and the middle one is focused horizontally and rotates around a horizontal axis. Three hundred sweeps are made every second. In the original version, prisms attached to the reference markers reflect the light back to photodiodes in the scanner units, and the position of the reference points is derived by triangulation. In a modified version, the original reflective markers have been replaced by photodiodes detecting the light sweeps and communicating to the central recording/analysis unit. Displacement data of markers/diodes are used to calculate three-dimensional marker coordinates for further analysis of joint kinematics, etc. The resolution of the system using diodes was 0.2 to 2.6 mm in a 6-m-wide recording field at a measuring distance of 13 m.[110]

In the automated SELSPOT system (Selective Electronic Co., Partille, Sweden), light-emitting diodes are used as markers, and position-sensing photodiodes act as sensors. Both optoelectronic systems described here require the attachment of diodes to the horse's body and limbs, which may interfere with the normal gait of the animal, especially at higher speeds.

Treadmills in Locomotion Research

The first high-speed treadmill for equine locomotion analysis was developed during the seventies.[111] Treadmills are now commonly used for exercise physiology research, but some of them are less suitable for gait analysis because they disturb normal locomotion too much. Even in treadmills designed for locomotion studies, differences occur between overground and treadmill stride characteristics, and these differences need to be mapped.[111–113]

NORMAL LOCOMOTION

The Stride and the Gaits

The descriptive terminology of stride and gaits is still somewhat confusing. The terminology used here is mainly based on recent suggestions for a standardized terminology.[114–116] The *stride* is the basic repeated series of movements of the individual limb. The *stride length* is the linear distance that the hoof moves during one stride cycle or the distance between two successive hoof imprints of the same foot. The *stride duration* is the time for one complete gait cycle or the time between any two identical events of a cycle. The number of strides per unit time is the *stride frequency.*

The stride consists of two phases: the *stance phase,* when the foot is in contact with the ground, and the *swing phase,* when the foot is lifted and brought forward to be placed on the ground again (Fig. 3–4). In the analysis of the stance phase, it has been arbitrarily divided into an anterior part, the *restraint stage,* and a posterior part, the *propulsion stage.*[114,117] In between these two stages is the *midstance position,* which, in the forelimb, is when the metacarpus is in the vertical position and, in the hindlimb, is when the hoof is right under the hip joint.[114]

The various stride characteristics are repeated in a strikingly stable cyclic pattern.[114,117,118] The timing of the gait components is very precisely controlled within the central nervous system. This is well illustrated by the example from a thoroughbred racehorse galloping at 18 m/s: With a stride duration of 425 ms, the stance phase lasts 95 ms, during which the vertical force between hoof and ground reaches a maximum of more than double the weight of the horse. During the stance phase, the extremity joints provide maximum stability, in sharp contrast to their fast movements during the swing phase. During the 330-ms swing phase, the hoof leaves ground contact, accelerates forward, and reaches a maximum

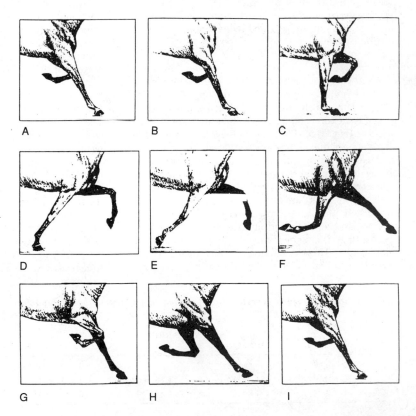

Figure 3-4. *The sequence of right forelimb movement during one stride cycle of a trotting horse. The stance phase lasts from (a) to (e) and consists of the restraint stage from (a) to (c) and the propulsion phase from (c) to (e). The swing phase lasts from (e) to (a). (a) heel contact; (b) full contact; (c) midstance position; (d) beginning of heel-off; (e) toe-off; (f) beginning of hoof acceleration; (g) midswing, and (h) end of hoof deceleration. [From Fredericson and colleagues. Acta Vet Scand 1972 (Suppl 37):1, with permission.]*

A   B   C

D   E   F

G   H   I

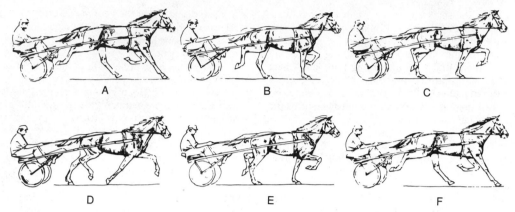

Figure 3-5. Trot. The gait characteristics of the racing trot recorded at a speed of 12 m/s. Left stride stance phase (a) to (e); advanced placement at landing, single limb support (a) to (b); bipedal support (b) to (d); advanced completion at takeoff, single limb support (d) to (e); left suspension phase (e) to (f). (From Drevemo and colleagues. Equine Vet J 1980;12:60, with permission.)

speed versus ground of more than double that of the horse's center of gravity and then decelerates to almost zero ground speed before landing 7.6 m ahead of the preceding hoof imprint.

A *gait* can be defined simply as the repetitive limb coordination pattern used in locomotion. Horses have many different gaits. Here we will deal principally with those of importance to the athletic horse, i.e., the trot, pace, canter, and gallop. *Asymmetrical gaits* are those gaits in which the limb movements of one side do not exactly repeat those of the other side (e.g., canter, gallop). *Symmetrical gaits* are those in which the limb movements of one side are repeated by the opposite side half a stride later (e.g., trot, pace).

Trot and Pace

Trot and pace are *symmetrical gaits,* i.e., the limb movements of one side are repeated by the opposite side half a stride later. In the *trot,* the diagonal limbs move together, and contralateral pairs of limbs are 50 percent out of phase (Fig. 3–5). Each pair of diagonal feet is named after the hindlimb involved (left and right diagonal). The diagonal feet are synchronously lifted, brought forward, and again placed on the ground. The horse is in ground contact twice and without ground contact twice in each gait cycle; i.e., there are two stride stance phases and two suspension phases. At slow speeds, the diagonal feet tend to land and take off at the same time. At faster speeds, there is a tendency for the forelimb to land and take off first. These differences between diagonal limbs at landing and takeoff are referred to as *advanced place-*

ment or *diagonal disassociation*. This means that for each diagonal there is an initial period of single support, a period of bipedal support or overlap, and finally, another period of single support. Another characteristic of speed is that the horses place their feet closer to the projection of the median plane on the ground, their diagonal width decreases, and they show line gait. Some data on trot are summarized in Table 3–1.

In the *pace,* the fore- and hindlimbs on the same side work synchronously, and the contralateral limbs are 50 percent out of phase. There are few studies on pace, but some data are given in Table 3–1. The tendency in standardbreds to trot or pace appears to be genetically determined; about 20 percent of the offspring sired by trotters were registered as pacers, while fewer than 1 percent of those sired by pacers were registered as trotters.[119]

Canter and Gallop

The gallop is a much more complex gait than the trot and pace, with many possible limb coordination patterns. In the horse, two main types are identified: the *canter* or the "three-beat gallop" (Fig. 3–6) and the "four-beat gallop," normally referred to as *gallop* (Fig. 3–7). Canter is seen at lower speeds and is characterized by the stance phases of the lead hindlimb and the diagonal trailing forelimb occurring simultaneously. In the gallop, the lead hindlimb normally lands and takes off in advance of the diagonal trailing forelimb.

The gait cycle of gallop can be divided into the *stride stance phase,* which begins with the landing of the

Table 3-1. *Selected Stride Characteristics of the Individual Limb in the Trot and Pace*

	No. of horses	Speed (m/s)	Stride length (m)	Stride duration (s)	Stance phase (s)	Swing phase (s)
Trot	8[160]	8.8–12.6	—	0.544–0.428	0.152–0.112	0.402–0.316
	30[114]	11.3–12.4	4.88–6.09	0.503–0.411	0.127–0.101	0.391–0.294
Pace	20[161]	14.4–15.3	6.44–7.00	0.457–0.437	0.110–0.103	—

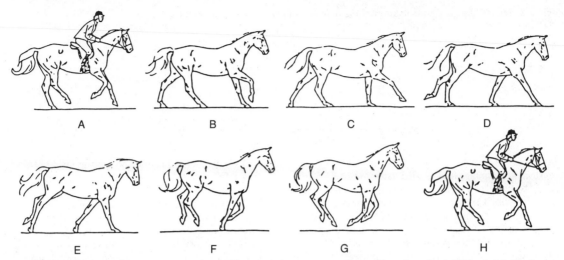

Figure 3-6. *Right lead transverse canter. The gait characteristics during one complete stride cycle at 6 m/s (360 m/min). Nonlead hindlimb landing (a); lead hindlimb and nonlead forelimb landing simultaneously (b); nonlead hindlimb takeoff (c); lead forelimb landing (d); lead hindlimb and nonlead forelimb takeoff (e); lead forelimb takeoff (f); suspension phase (g); nonlead hindlimb landing (h), and stride stance phase (a–f). [From Hellander and colleagues. Svensk Vet Tidn 1983 (suppl 3):75, and the artist, Bo Furugren, with permission.]*

trailing hindlimb and ends when the lead forelimb leaves the ground, and the *suspension phase,* when there is no limb contact with the ground. During the stride stance phase, one or more limbs are in contact with the ground. The time during which more than one limb is on the ground is the *overlap.*

Gallop can be *rotary,* i.e., when the feet are placed

on ground in a circular order (in a right lead rotary gallop the order would be RH, LH, LF, RF), or *transverse* (right lead transverse gallop: LH, RH, LF, RF). Transverse gallop is the type normally used, but rotary gallop is seen, for example, in accelerating racehorses. Some data on canter and gallop are summarized in Table 3–2.

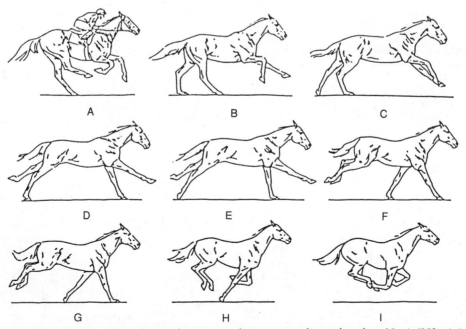

Figure 3-7. *Right lead transverse gallop. The gait characteristics during one complete stride cycle at 16 m/s (960 m/min). Nonlead hindlimb landing (a); lead hindlimb landing (b); nonlead hindlimb takeoff (c); nonlead forelimb landing (d); lead hindlimb takeoff (e); lead forelimb landing (f); nonlead forelimb takeoff (g); lead forelimb takeoff (h); suspension phase (i), and stride stance phase (a–h). [From Hellander and colleagues. Svensk Vet Tidn 1983 (suppl 3):75, and the artist, Bo Furugren, with permission.]*

Table 3-2. Selected Stride Characteristics of the Individual Limb in the Canter and Gallop

No. of horses	Speed (m/s)	Stride length (m)	Stride duration (s)	Stance phase (s)	Swing phase (s)
48[162]	5.1–19.3	2.97–8.16	0.613–0.384	0.209–0.070	0.442–0.301
34[163]	8.8–14.1	4.46–7.19	0.550–0.445	0.150–0.080	0.425–0.330
17[164]	11.1–16.4	5.3–7.0	0.50–0.38	—	—
3[165]	15.0–17.1	6.66–7.38	0.455–0.425	0.112–0.098	0.337–0.318

Effects on Gait of Growth, Training, and Lameness

Growth and Training. Gait is affected by the use of the horse. Training of certain skills means that the neuromotor functions undergo modifications, and the horse "learns" to jump, the dressage movements, or to trot or gallop in a more effective way. In the young animal, growth and training effects are hard to distinguish, but scale and training effects have been reported in trotting foals and young horses[120,121] and also for walk, trot, and canter.[122,123]

In young standardbred stallions, an intense 5-months prerace training program resulted in only minor significant changes in a few kinematic measurements.[124] Even in horses bred and trained for different use, striking similarities are found between groups. In a comparison of horses trained for dressage and for racing, most kinematic variables at the extended canter did not differ significantly.[125] The jumping horse has attracted substantial interest, and descriptions are available on show jumping[126–130] and steeplechase techniques.[131]

Lameness. Gait analysis is an old tool in the clinical evaluation of lame horses. The introduction of modern objective gait analysis systems for equine lamenesses diagnosis has, however, been delayed for economical and methodologic reasons. Numerous case reports are available, but more systematic attempts to use new techniques have been sparse.[132–136]

Conformation

SUBJECTIVE AND OBJECTIVE JUDGING OF CONFORMATION

Conformation is the body shape, form, or outline of an animal.[137,138] When selecting horses for breeding, racing, etc., conformational details have long been used as markers of such qualities as performance and soundness. Traditionally, conformation has been judged subjectively against an ideal or standard of perfection.[137] In studies where several judges evaluated the same horses, good agreement was achieved for some overall type traits, but large discrepancies were revealed for most conformational details.[139–141] Magnusson's studies[141] of the subjective method showed that the length and inclination of the skeleton parts, as well as the joint angles, were difficult to judge correctly. The agreement among judges improved when judging the type, harmony, balance, and similar overall impressions. Magnusson concluded that because of the great errors in subjective

judging, this method cannot be used in study of the relationships between conformation, performance, and soundness.[141]

In their classic work, *De l'Extérieur de Cheval,* Goubaux and Barrier[142] in 1884 suggested that photogrammetric methods be used to measure joint angles. To overcome the disadvantages of subjective judging, protocols were developed for measurements on live horses[143–145] and from photographs using reference points.[146,147]

Objective methods provide absolute figures on body measurements, such as length, width, circumference, and joint angles. Measurements should be correct, repeatable, and easy to perform. Measurements on live horses are very precise, and the following equipment is used[141]:

- *Reference points* marked with paper slips glued to the skin of the horse. When choosing reference points, a number of criteria must be fulfilled. The reference points must be easy to determine by palpation, be primarily situated on skeletal structures near the ends of bones, and points and lines between them as far as possible should coincide with the outlines and axes used in subjective judging of the conformation (for comparison).
- *Measuring tape* to measure the circumference of the carpus, cannons, and the chest and for some distances.
- *Boxlevel measuring standard* to measure height at the withers, back, and croup. With an additional crossbar, lengths of the head, body, forelimbs, etc. and depth of chest and width of breast and pelvis can be measured.
- *Calipers* used to measure width of the head, cannon bones, and cannons.
- *Goniometer* to measure joint angles and inclination of the shoulder and pelvis (water level on one arm).

The equipment used for photography and photogrammetric analyses may vary, but when using a conventional 24 × 36 mm system camera, a lens with at least 200-mm focal distance is required.[141] The median plane of the horse should be at right angles to the focal axis of the camera, which is directed horizontally toward the heart region. Standardized positioning is very important to reduce variance in measurements. For objective analyses, a standard for the position of the horse therefore must be used both when applying markers and when taking measurements. The position is described as follows by Magnusson[141]:

The horse shall stand in a natural, unaffected and relaxed manner on a horizontal level ground surface, uninfluenced by the manager. The forelimbs shall be vertical and equally loaded. . . . The hindlimb under registration [facing the camera] shall have the cannon vertical and, the contralateral limb placed somewhat more forward. Weight on the hindlimbs shall be equally distributed. [The judging of limb axes is also commended:] When judging the limb axes from in front and behind, the horse shall stand in a natural manner. This makes it necessary to study approximately 10 spontaneous standing positions before the standing conformation is recorded.

To enable comparisons to be made between horses of different size, measurements for individual horses are often expressed as percentages of height at the withers and details of the limb as percentage of the total length of the limb. In a study of standardbred trotters, adjustment for general size reduced the variation of conformation by 25 percent, on average.[141]

The early objective conformation studies focused on draft and cavalry horses, but today the interest is directed toward sport horses and the relation between conformation and different performance traits. This has resulted in a number of traditional and established ideas on horse conformation being questioned and abandoned, while others have been verified. It is also quite clear that much more research into the relation between conformation, performance, and soundness is needed.

BREED AND SEX VARIATIONS

Conformation varies between individuals, sexes, breeds, and age groups and is also affected by training and nutritional states. There is, however, little scientific information on what is to be considered normal variation of conformation in adult and growing horses. Not even thoroughbreds have been subjected to modern in-depth studies of how different conformational traits vary and their relation to performance and soundness.

Breed Differences. Results from objective studies of large groups of horses are available for standardbred trotters[141] and warmblood riding horses.[148] The results from these studies have shown that some traits that have conventionally been regarded as disadvantageous may in fact be regarded as normal. For instance, more than 80 percent of the horses in both breed groups show outwardly rotated hindlimbs. In Swedish warmblood riding horses, 60 percent had bench knee conformation and 50 percent had toe-in in the forelimbs.[148]

In comparisons between breeds, warmblood trotters were shorter, narrower, and had less depth of chest than warmblood riding horses.[149] When French trotters were compared with thoroughbreds, they had the same height at the withers, but the trotters were broader and more compact and had larger ilium, femur, and scapulum angles relative to the horizontal plane (the radius was shorter and the cannon bone thicker).[150]

Sex Differences. There are significant differences for many conformational traits. In standardbred trotters, stallions are taller, broader, and have a greater width and circumference of the cannon and carpus.[141,145,149] Furthermore, they have a flatter croup, smaller hip angle, and significantly more outwardly rotated limb axes. Mares have a greater width of the pelvis, longer body, and longer distance between the last rib and the pelvis.[141] While there was a difference between stallions and mares, the geldings most often had a mean value between the two sex groups.[141] Corresponding sex differences have been reported for Swedish warmblood riding horses.[148]

CONFORMATION AND PERFORMANCE

A great deal has been written on the relationships of conformation to performance traits, but very little on a scientific basis. Most studies of objectively measured conformational traits include comparisons between groups of good and bad performers. There is also a lack of data on how conformation is affected by intensive training.

In a study of 500 standardbred trotters, up to 5 to 9 percent of the variation in the performance traits could be explained by conformation; the better-performing horse was a light-weight, gracile type with a not too long head, tall withers, and normal size of hooves and was not tied in at the knees or hocks and had outwardly rotated limb axes and large shoulder and stifle angles.[141]

Good and poor show jumpers were compared in a study of 103 horses; the good show jumper was characterized by wider breast and pelvis, greater chest girth, longer pelvis, and smaller angle between the femur and the horizontal plane.[150] The authors, however, cautioned against distinguishing a good jumper from a poor one on the basis of conformation alone. In a comparison between show jumpers and dressage horses, it was found that show jumpers had a larger height at the withers and that height at the withers and large hock angles were correlated with competitive performance in show jumpers and dressage horses.[151]

In a study of 356 Swedish warmblood horses, Holmström and colleagues[148] objectively recorded the conformation of 33 elite dressage horses, 28 elite show jumpers, 295 riding school horses, and 195 unselected 4-year-old horses. The show jumpers and dressage horses were higher at the withers and had more sloping scapulas and larger hock angles. The show jumpers had a smaller pelvic inclination and smaller hip and fetlock angles. The dressage horses had a shorter neck and tibia, a larger elbow angle, and a larger angle between the femur and the horizontal plane.

Still, conformation is given much attention when selecting horses, and the traditional subjective judging needs to be critically evaluated and improved by the use of quantitative methods. It is clear that there is a great need for further investigations into correlations between conformation, movement, and ability to perform.

CONFORMATION AND SOUNDNESS

There are few research results available on the relation between conformational traits and soundness. The most common reason for unsoundness is injuries to skeleton, joints, and tendons of the limbs.[1-3] The correlation between conformation and orthopedic health has therefore attracted considerable interest in the judging of conformation. For reviews of the present opinions among veterinary orthopedic surgeons, the reader is referred to recent textbooks.[138]

Some authors state that every divergence from correct limb conformation causes increased stress to different parts of the limb.[152,153] Straight shoulders are considered to predispose to joint diseases because of reduced shock absorption.[154] Excessive angulation of the hock joints ("sickle hocks") is said to predispose to bone spavin[153] and to curb.[138,155]

In his study of 4-year-old standardbred trotters, Magnusson described in detail the relationships between conformational traits and symptoms of orthopedic unsoundness in 500 horses and concluded: "The trotters of middle size with long limbs, normal size of hooves, not tied in at the knees and, above all not with curby, sickle hocks and straight fetlock angles were found to have a better chance of remaining sound than horses with opposite characteristics. It seems important to prefer straight limb- and toe-axes."[141] Among the 500 trotters, 7.8 percent displayed a marked hindquarter asymmetry, and the affected horses performed significantly worse than the normal horses.[156]

In investigations of the development and epidemiology of osteochondrosis, standardbred trotters with hock joint osteochondrosis were heavier, had a higher weight gain, and had a larger circumference of the carpus and cannon compared with unaffected horses.[157,158] A relationship was found between the degree of outwardly rotated hindlimb axes and the appearance of osteochondrosis lesions in the hock and plantar osteochondral fragments in the fetlock joints.[157-159]

Conclusion

It is hoped that this chapter has given the reader an appropriate overview of skeletal function as it relates to training of horses, biomechanical stress, and the importance of gait/conformation. Although much has been achieved in recent years, this is still an area of sports medicine that requires a much greater input of research. The dramatic influence of new technology has made noninvasive, telemetric, and cinematographic measurement of skeletal function much more possible. The development of many of these techniques to become everyday tools for trainers and practicing veterinarians will soon be within our sights. We believe that the next 10 to 20 years will see some dramatic improvements in monitoring the efficiency of the locomotory system to produce sounder horses with a reduction in wastage due to orthopedic problems.

A few examples where research input will be particularly productive:

- *Bone biopsy.* This will involve development of more sophisticated means of assessing bone strength, weakness, and fatigue coupled with a better understanding of the structure of bone and its response to nutrition, training, and biomechanical loading.
- *Joints.* There will be a better appreciation of articular cartilage and its function following training with resultant establishment of methods for early diagnosis due to injury.
- *Tendons and ligaments.* This is another exciting area for research, where the need is to investigate tendon/ligament function in order to understand the injury and repair process.
- *Neuromuscular function.* The means of studying neuromuscular function and thereby adapting training programs to produce more effective skeletal function will ultimately reduce the risks to injury and lameness.
- *Locomotor/gait analysis.* There are still enormous possibilities for practical assessment of performance potential as technology for recording continues to advance.
- *Conformation.* Detailed studies of specific conformation types in relation to performance have been largely underused and underrated in most parts of the world. There are clear indications that more epidemiologic studies could have important bearing on performance, longevity, and breeding for the future.

Research involving skeletal function is traditionally difficult and expensive, but it cannot fail to be rewarding. The bottom line will be to assist in reducing the present, unacceptably high prevalence of exercise-induced lameness or reduced performance.

References

1. Vaughan LC, Mason BGE: A clinicopathological study of racing accidents in horses. London, Horse Race Betting Levy Board, 1975.
2. Jeffcott LB, Rossdale PD, Freestone J, et al: An Assessment of wastage in thoroughbred racing from conception to 4 years of age. Equine Vet J 1982; 14:185.
3. Rossdale PD, Hopes R, Offord K, et al: Epidemiological study of wastage among racehorses 1982 and 1983. Vet Rec 1985; 116:66.
4. Leach DH, Dagg AI: Evolution of equine locomotion research. Equine Vet J 1983; 15:87.
5. Merkens H: Quantitative Evaluation of Equine Locomotion Using Force Plate Data. Ph.D. thesis, Utrecht, 1987.
6. Marcey E-J: Le mouvement. Paris, Masson, 1894.
7. Vincent JFV (ed): Biomechanics—Materials: A Practical Approach. Oxford, Oxford University Press, 1992.
8. Biewener AA (ed): Biomechanics—Structures and Systems: A Practical Approach. Oxford, Oxford University Press, 1992.
9. DeCoster TA: Biomechanical principles related to the muskuloskeletal system. In Bronner F, Worrell RV (eds): A Basic Science Primer in Orthopedics. Baltimore, Williams & Wilkins, 1991, p 149.
10. Biewener AA, Full RJ: Force platform and kinematic analysis. In Biewener AA (ed): Biomechanics—Structures and Systems: A Practical Approach. Oxford, Oxford University Press, 1992, p 46.
11. Schamhardt HC, Merkens HW, van Osch GJVM: Ground reaction force analysis of horses ridden at the walk and trot. In Pers-

son SGB, Lindholm A, Jeffcott LB (eds): Equine Exercise Physiology 3. Davis, CA, ICEEP Publications, 1991, p 120.

12. Merkens HW, Schamhardt HC, van Osch GJVM, et al: Ground reaction force analysis of Dutch warmblood horses at canter and jumping. In Persson SGB, Lindholm A, Jeffcott LB (eds): Equine Exercise Physiology 3. Davis, CA, ICEEP Publications, 1991, p 128.

13. Merkens HW, Schamhardt HC, Hartman W, et al: Ground reaction force patterns of Dutch warmblood horses at normal walk. Equine Vet J 1986; 18:207.

14. Merkens HW, Schamhardt HC: Distribution of ground reaction forces of the concurrently loaded limbs of the Dutch warmblood horse at the normal walk. Equine Vet J 1988; 20:209.

15. Merkens HW, Schamhardt HC, Hartman W, et al: The use of H(orse) INDEX: A method of analysing the ground reaction force patterns of lame and normal gaited horses at the walk. Equine Vet J 1988; 20:29.

16. Frederick FH, Henderson JM: Impact force measurement using preloaded transducers. Am J Vet Res 1970; 31:2279.

17. Björck G: Studies on the draughtforce of horses. Acta Agr Scand 1958 (suppl 4).

18. Roepstorff L, Drevemo S: Concept of a force-measuring horseshoe. Acta Anat 1993; 146:114.

19. Ratzlaff MH, Wilson PD, Hyde ML, et al: Relationships between locomotor forces, hoof position and joint motion during the support phase of the stride of galloping horses. Acta Anat 1993; 146:200.

20. Barrey E: Investigation of the vertical hoof force distribution in the equine forelimb with an instrumented horseboot. Equine Vet J 1990 (suppl 9):35.

21. Auer JA, Butler KD Jr: An introduction to the Kaegi equine gait analysis system in the horse. In Proceedings of the Annual Convention of the American Association of Equine Practice, 1986, vol 31, p 209.

22. Titje S: Das EGA-System (Equine Gait Analysis)—eine Möglichkeit zur Bewegungs-analyse und Lahmheitsuntersuchung beim Pferd. Thesis, München, 1992.

23. Biewener AA: In vivo measurement of bone strain and tendon force. In Biewener AA (ed): Biomechanics—Structures and Systems: A Practical Approach. Oxford, Oxford University Press, 1992, p 123.

24. Carter DR: Anisotropic analysis of strain rosette information from cortical bone. J Biomech 1978; 11:199.

25. Davies HMS, McCarthy RN, Jeffcott LB: Surface strain on the dorsal metacarpus of thoroughbreds at different speeds and gaits. Acta Anat 1993; 146:148.

26. Benoit P, Barrey E, Regnault JC, et al: Comparison of the damping effect of different shoeing by the measurement of hoof acceleration. Acta Anat 1993; 146.109.

27. Jeffcott LB, Buckingham SHW, McCarthy RN, et al: Noninvasive measurement of bone: A review of clinical and research applications in the horse. Equine Vet J 1988 (suppl 6):71.

28. Mason TA, Bourke JM: Closure of the distal radial epiphysis and its relationship to unsoundness in two-year-old thoroughbreds. Aust Vet J 1973; 49:221.

29. Gabel AA, Spencer CP, Pipers FS: A study of correlation of closure of the distal radial physis with performance and injury in the standardbred. J Am Vet Med Assoc 1977; 170:188.

30. Price RI, Retallack RW, Gutteridge DH, et al: Quantitative in-vivo determination of bone mineral using computerized roentgenographic densitometry. Australas Phys Eng Sci Med 1983; 6:128.

31. Meakim DW, Ott EA, Asquith RL, et al: Estimation of mineral content of the equine third metacarpal by radiographic photometry. J Anim Sci 1981; 53:1019.

32. Ekman B, Ljungquist KG, Stein U: Roentgenographic-photometric method for bone mineral determination. Acta Radiol 1970; 10:305.

33. Roub LW, Gumerman LW, Hanley EN, et al: Bone stress: A radionuclideimaging perspective. Radiology 1979; 132:431.

34. Foreman JH, Hungerford LL, Twardock AR, et al: Scintigraphic appearance of dorsal metacarpaland metatarsal stress changes in racing and nonracing horses. In Persson SGB, Lindholm A, Jeffcott LB (eds): Equine Exercise Physiology 3. Davis, CA, ICEEP Publications, 1991, p 402.

35. Sorenson JA, Cameron JR: A reliable in vivo measurement of bone mineral content. J Bone Joint Surg 1967; 49A:481.

36. Kroiner B, Pros Nielsen S: Measurement of bone mineral content (BMC) of the lumbar spine: I Theory and application of a new two dimensional dual-photon attenuation method. Scand J Clin Lab Invest 1980; 40:485.

37. Riggs BL, Wahner HW, Dunn WL, et al: Differential changes in bone mineral density of the appendicular and axial skeleton with aging. J Clin Invest 1981; 67:328.

38. Lawrence LA, Ott EA: The use of noninvasive techniques to predict bone mineral content and strength in the horse. In Proceedings of the 9th Equine Nutrition Phys Society, 1985, p 110.

39. McCarthy RN, Jeffcott LB, McCartney RN: Ultrasonic transmission velocity and single photon absorptiometric measurement of metacarpal bone strength: An in vitro study in the horse. Equine Vet J 1988 (suppl 6):80.

40. Katz JL: The structure and biomechanics of bone. Soc Exp Biol Symp 1980; 34:137.

41. Lees S, Ahern JM, Leonard M: Parameters influencing the sonic velocity in compact calcified tissues of various species. J Acoust Soc Am 1983; 74:28.

42. McCartney RN, Jeffcott LB: Combined 2.25 MHz ultrasound velocity and bone mineral measurements in the equine metacarpus and their in vivo applications. Med Biol Eng Comput 1987; 25:620.

43. Greenfield MA, Craven JD, Huddleston A, et al: Measurement of the velocity of ultrasound in human cortical bone in vivo. Radiology 1981; 138:701.

44. Melsen F: Histomorphometric Analysis of Iliac Bone in Normal and Pathological Conditions. Ph.D. thesis, Denmark, Aarhus, 1978.

45. Vesterby A, Mosekilde L, Gundersen HJG, et al: Biologically meaningful determinants of the in vitro strength of lumbar vertebrae. Bone 1991; 12:219.

46. Savage CJ, Jeffcott LB, Melsen F, et al: Bone biopsy in the horse: I. Method using the wing of ilium. J Vet Med 1991; 38:776.

47. Lindholm A, Piehl K: Fiber composition, enzyme activity and concentration of metabolites and electrolytes in muscles of standardbred horses. Acta Vet Scand 1974; 15:287.

48. Melick RA, Farrugia W, Quelch KJ: Plasma osteocalcin in man. Aust NZ J Med 1985; 15:410.

49. Orwoll ES, Belsey RE: The laboratory evaluation of osteopenia. Clin Lab Med 1984; 4:763.

50. Gans C: Electromyography. In Biewener AA (ed): Biomechanics—Structures and Systems: A Practical Approach. Oxford, Oxford University Press, 1992, p 175.

51. Wentink GH: Biokinetical analysis of the movement of the pelvic limb of the horse and the role of the muscles in the walk and the trot. Anat Embryol 1978; 152:261.

52. Aoki O, Tokuriki M, Kurakawa Y, et al: Electromyographic studies on supraspinatus and infraspinatus muscles of the horse with and without rider in walk, trot and canter. Bull Equine Res Inst 1984; 21:100.

53. Tokuriki M, Aoki O, Niki Y, et al: Electromyographic activity of cubital joint muscles in horses during locomotion. Am J Vet Res 1989; 50:950.

54. Tokuriki M, Aoki O: Neck muscles activity in horses during locomotion with and without a rider. In Persson SGB, Lindholm A, Jeffcott LB (eds): Equine Exercise Physiology 3. Davis, CA, ICEEP Publications, 1991, p 146.

55. Dalin G, Drevemo S, Fredricson I, et al: Ergonomic aspects of locomotor asymmetry in standardbred horses trotting through turns. Acta Vet Scand 1973 (suppl 44):111.

56. Fredricson I, Dalin G, Drevemo S, et al: Ergonomic aspects of poor racetrack design. Equine Vet J 1975; 7:63.

57. Fredricson I, Dalin G, Drevemo S, et al: A biotechnical approach to the geometric design of racetracks. Equine Vet J 1975; 7:91.

58. Barrey E, Landjerit B, Wolter R: Shock and vibration during the hoof impact on different track surfaces. In Persson SGB, Lindholm A, Jeffcott LB (eds): Equine Exercise Physiology 3. Davis, CA, ICEEP Publications, 1991, p 97.

59. Drevemo S, Hjertén G: Evaluation of a shock absorbing woodchip layer on a harness race-track. In Persson SGB, Lindholm A, Jeffcott LB (eds): Equine Exercise Physiology 3. Davis, CA, ICEEP Publications, 1991, p 107.

60. Mazess RG, Whedon GD: Immobilisation and bone. Calcif Tissue Int 1983; 35:265.

61. Aloia JF, Cohn SH, Ostuni JA, et al: Prevention of involutional bone loss by exercise. Ann Intern Med 1978; 86:356.

62. Frost HM: Vital biomechanics: Proposed general concepts for skeletal adaptation. Calcif Tissue Int 1988; 42:145.

63. Lanyon LE: Functional strain as a determinant for bone remodelling. Calcif Tissue Int 1984; 36:556.

64. Rubin CT, Lanyon LE: Regulation of bone mass by mechanical strain magnitude. Calcif Tissue Int 1985; 37:411.

65. McCarthy RN, Jeffcott LB: Treadmill exercise intensity and its effect on cortical bone in horses of various ages. In Persson SGB, Lindholm A, Jeffcott LB (eds): Equine Exercise Physiology 3. Davis, CA, ICEEP Publications, 1991, p 419.

66. McCarthy RN, Jeffcott LB: Effects of treadmill exercise on cortical bone in the third metacarpus of young horses. Res Vet Sci 1992; 52:28.

67. Nunamaker DM: The bucked shin complex. In Proceedings of the Annual Convention of the American Association of Equine Practice, 1987, vol 32, p 457.

68. Nunamaker DM, Butterweck DM, Provost MT: Some geometric properties of the third metacarpal bone: A comparison between the thoroughbred and standardbred racehorse. J Biomech 1989; 22:129.

69. Riggs CM, Evans GP: The microstructural basis of the mechanical properties of equine bone. Equine Vet Educ 1990; 2:197.

70. Stashak TS (ed): Adam's Lameness in Horses. Philadelphia, Lea & Febiger, 1987.

71. Stover SM, Martin RB, Pool RR, et al: Contribution of microfractures to dorsal metacarpal disease (abstract). In Proceedings of the Annual Convention of the American Association of Equine Practice, 1992.

72. Buckingham SHW, Jeffcott LB: Shin soreness: A survey of thoroughbred trainers and racetrack veterinarians. Aust Equine Vet 1990; 8:148.

73. Nunamaker DM, Butterweck DM, Provost MT: Fatigue fractures in thoroughbred racehorses: Relationship with age, peak bone strain and training. J Orthop Res 1990; 8:604.

74. Jurvelin J, Helminen HJ, Lauritsalo S, et al: Influences of joint immobilization and running exercise on articular cartilage surfaces of young rabbits. Acta Anat 1985; 122:62.

75. Vachon AM, Keeley FW, McIlwraith W, et al: Biochemical analysis of normal articular cartilage in horses. Am J Vet Res 1990; 51:1905.

76. Kempson GE: Mechanical Properties of Human Cartilage. Dissertation, University of London, 1979.

77. Armstrong CG, Mow VC: Variations in the intrinsic mechanical properties of human articular cartilage with age, degeneration and water content. J Bone Joint Surg 1982; 64A:88.

78. Myers ER, Armstrong CG, Mow VC: Swelling pressure and collagen tension. In Hukins DWL (ed): Connective Tissue Matrix. London, Macmillan, 1984, p 161.

79. Jurvelin J: Biomechanical Properties of Knee Articular Cartilage under Various Loading Conditions. Thesis, University of Kuopio, 1991.

80. Poole CA: The structure and function of articular cartilage matrices. In Woessner JF Jr, Howell DS (eds): Joint Cartilage Degradation. New York, Marcel Dekker, 1993, p 1.

81. Bader DL, Kempson GE: The relationship between the mechanical properties and structure of adult human articular cartilage. Scand J Rheum 1986 (suppl 60):24.

82. Mizrahi J, Maroudas A, Lanir Y, et al: The "instantaneous" deformation of cartilage: Effects of collagen fibre orientation and osmotic stress. Biorheology 1986; 23:311.

83. Tammi M, Säämänen A-M, Jauhiainen A, et al: Proteoglycan alterations in rabbit knee articular cartilage following physical exercise and immobilization. Connect Tissue Res 1983; 11:45.

84. Behrens F, Kraft EL, Oegema TR: Biochemical changes in articular cartilage after joint immobilization by casting or external fixation. J Orthop Res 1989; 7:335.

85. Tammi M, Paukkonen K, Kiviranta I, et al: Joint-loading–induced alterations in articular cartilage. In Helminen HJ, Kiviranta I, Säämänen A-M, et al (eds): Joint Loading: Biology and Health. Bristol, England, Wright, 1987, p 64.

86. Kiviranta I, Jurvelin J, Tammi M, et al: Weight-bearing controls glycosaminoglycan concentration and articular cartilage thickness in the knee joints of young beagle dogs. Arthritis Rheum 1987; 30:801.

87. Kiviranta I, Tammi M, Jurvelin J, et al: Moderate running exercise augments glycosaminoglycans and cartilage thickness of ar-

ticular cartilage in the knee joint of young beagle dogs. J Orthop Res 1988; 6:188.

88. Vasan N: Effects of physical stress on the synthesis and degradation of cartilage matrix. Connect Tissue Res 1983; 12:49.

89. Radin EL, Ehrlich MG, Chernak R, et al: Effect of repetitive impulsive loading on the knee joints of rabbits. Clin Orthop 1978; 131:288.

90. Evans CH, Brown TD: Role of physical and mechanical agents in degrading the matrix. In Woessner JF Jr, Howell DS (eds): Joint Cartilage Degradation. New York, Marcel Dekker, 1993, p 187.

91. Burton-Wurster N, Todhunter RJ, Lust G: Animal models of osteoarthritis. In Woessner JF Jr, Howell DS (eds): Joint Cartilage Degradation. New York, Marcel Dekker, 1993, p 347.

92. McIlwraith CW, Vachon A: Review of pathogenesis and treatment of degenerative joint disease. Equine Vet J 1988; xx(suppl 6):3.

93. Richardson DW: Degenerative joint disease. In Robinson NE (ed): Current Therapy in Equine Medicine. Philadelphia, WB Saunders Co, 1992, p 136.

94. Bertone AL: Noninfectious synovitis. In Robinson NE (ed): Current Therapy in Equine Medicine. Philadelphia, WB Saunders Co, 1992, p 134.

95. Morris EA, McDonald BS, Webb AC, et al: Identification of interleukin 1 in equine osteoarthritic joint effusions. Am J Vet Res 1990; 51:59.

96. Alwan WH, Carter SD, Dixon JB, et al: Interleukin 1–like activity in synovial fluids and sera of horses with arthritis. Res Vet Sci 1991; 51:72.

97. Alwan WH, Carter SD, Bennett D, et al: Cartilage breakdown in equine osteoarthritis: Measurement of keratan sulfate by an ELISA system. Res Vet Sci 1990; 49:56.

98. Alwan WH, Carter SD, Bennett D, et al: Glycosaminoglycans in horses with osteoarthritis. Equine Vet J 1991; 23:44.

99. Genovese RL, Simpson BS: Tendon and ligament injuries. In Jones WE (ed): Equine Sports Medicine. Philadelphia, Lea & Febiger, 1989, p 241.

100. Riemersma DJ, Schamhardt HC, Hartman W, et al: Kinetics and kinematics of the equine hindlimb. Am J Vet Res 1988; 49:1344.

101. Stephens PR, Nunamaker DM, Butterweck DM: Application of a Hall-effect transducer for measurement of tendon strain in horses. Am J Vet Res 1989; 50:1089.

102. Jansen MO, van den Bogert AJ, Riemersma DJ, et al: In vivo tendon forces in the forelimb of ponies at the walk, validated by ground reaction force measurements. Acta Anat 1993; 146:162.

103. Taylor BM, Tipton CM, Adrian M, et al: Action of certain joints in the legs of the horse recorded electrogoniometrically. Am J Vet Res 1966; 27:86.

104. Adrian M, Grant B, Ratzlaff M, et al: Electrogoniometric analysis of equine metacarpophalangeal joint lameness. Am J Vet Res 1977; 38:431.

105. Ratzlaff MH, Grant BD, Adrian M: Quantitative evaluation of equine carpal lameness. J Equine Vet Sci 1982; 2:78.

106. van Weeren PR, van den Bogert AJ, Barneveld A: A quantitative analysis of skin displacement in the trotting horse. Equine Vet J 1990 (suppl 9):101.

107. Fredricson I, Drevemo S, Dalin G, et al: The application of high-speed cinematography for quantitative analysis of equine locomotion. Equine Vet J 1980; 12:54.

108. Drevemo S, Roepstorff L, Kallings P, et al: Application of TrackEye in equine locomotion research. Acta Anat 1993; 146:137.

109. Martinez-del Campo LJ, Kobluk CN, Greer N, et al: The use of high-speed videography to generate angle-time and angle-angle diagrams for the study of equine locomotion. Vet Comp Orthop Trauma 1991; 4:120.

110. van Weeren PR, Bogert AJ, van den, Barneveld A, et al: The role of the reciprocal apparatus in the hindlimb of the horse investigated by a modified CODA-3 opto-electronic kinematic analysis system. Equine Vet J 1990; 9:95.

111. Fredricson I, Drevemo S, Dalin G, et al: Treadmill for equine locomotion analysis. Equine Vet J 1983; 15:111.

112. Leach DH, Drevemo S: Velocity-dependent changes in stride frequency and length of trotters on a treadmill. In Persson SGB, Lindholm A, Jeffcott LB (eds): Equine Exercise Physiology 3. Davis, CA, ICEEP Publications, 1991, p 136.

113. Barrey E, Galloux P, Valette JP, et al: Stride characteristics of

overground versus treadmill locomotion in the saddle horse. Acta Anat 1993; 146:90.

114. Drevemo S, Dalin G, Fredricson I, et al: Equine locomotion: I. The analysis of linear and temporal stride characteristics in trotting Standardbreds. Equine Vet J 1980; 12:60.

115. Leach DH, Ormrod K, Clayton HM: Standardised terminology for the description and analysis of equine locomotion. Equine Vet J 1984; 16:522.

116. Leach D: Recommended terminology for researchers in locomotion and biomechanics of quadrupedal animals. Acta Anat 1993; 146:130.

117. Fredricson I, Drevemo S, Moen K, et al: A method of three-dimensional analysis of kinematics and coordination of equine extremity joints. Acta Vet Scand 1972; 37:1.

118. Drevemo S, Dalin G, Fredricson I, et al: Equine locomotion: 3. The reproducibility of gait in standardbred trotters. Equine Vet J 1980; 12:71.

119. Cothran EG, MacCluer JW, Weitkamp LR, et al: Genetic differentiation associated with gait in American standardbred horses. Anim Genet 1987; 18:285.

120. Leach DH, Cymbaluk N: Relationships between stride length, stride frequency, velocity, and morphometrics of foals. Am J Vet Res 1986; 47:2090.

121. Drevemo S, Fredricson I, Hjérten G, et al: Early development of gait asymmetries in trotting standardbred colts. Equine Vet J 1987; 19:189.

122. Muir GD, Leach DH, Cymbaluk N, et al: Velocity-dependent changes in intrinsic stride timing variables of quarter horse foals. In Persson SGB, Lindholm A, Jeffcott LB (eds): Equine Exercise Physiology 3. Davis, CA, ICEEP Publications, 1991, p 141.

123. Back W, van den Bogert AJ, van Weeren PR, et al: Quantification of the locomotion of Dutch warmblood foals. Acta Anat 1993; 146:141.

124. van Weeren PR, van den Bogert AJ, Back W, et al: Kinematics of the standardbred trotter at 6, 7, 8 and 9 m/s on a treadmill before and after 5 months of prerace training. Acta Anat 1993; 146:154.

125. Clayton HM: The extended canter: A comparison of some kinematic variables in horses trained for dressage and for racing. Acta Anat 1993; 146:183.

126. Fredricson I, Gernandt A, Hedlund G, et al: Horses and Jumping. New York, Arco Publishing Co, 1972.

127. Leach DH, Ormrod K, Clayton HM: Stride characteristics of horses competing in grand prix jumping. Am J Vet Res 1984; 45:888.

128. Clayton HM: Terminology for the description of equine jumping kinematics. J Equine Vet Sci 1989; 9:341.

129. Clayton HM, Barlow DA: Stride characteristics of four grand prix jumping horses. In Persson SGB, Lindholm A, Jeffcott LB (eds): Equine Exercise Physiology 3. Davis, CA, ICEEP Publications, 1991, p 151.

130. Deuel NR, Park J: Kinematic analysis of jumping sequences of Olympic show jumping horses. In Persson SGB, Lindholm A, Jeffcott LB (eds): Equine Exercise Physiology 3. Davis, CA, ICEEP Publications, 1991, p 158.

131. Leach DH, Ormrod K: The technique of jumping a steeplechase fence by event horses. Appl Anim Behav Sci 1982; 12:15.

132. Leach D: Locomotion analysis technology for evaluation of lameness in horses. Equine Vet J 1987; 19:97.

133. Merkens HW, Schamhardt HC: Evaluation of equine locomotion during different degrees of experimentally induced lameness: I. Lameness model and quantification of ground reaction force patterns of the limbs. Equine Vet J 1988 (suppl 6):99.

134. Merkens HW, Schamhardt HC: Evaluation of equine locomotion during different degrees of experimentally induced lameness: II. Distribution of ground reaction force patterns of the concurrently loaded limbs. Equine Vet J 1988; (suppl 6): 107.

135. Back W, Barneveld A, van Weeren PR, et al: Kinematic gait analysis in equine carpal lameness. Acta Anat 1993; 146:86.

136. Buchner F, Kastner J, Girtler D, et al: Quantification of hindlimb lameness in the horse. Acta Anat 1993; 146:196.

137. Ensminger NE: Horses and Horsemanship. Danville, IL, The Interstate Printers and Publishers, Inc, 1969.

138. Stashak T: The relationship between conformation and lameness.

In Stashak T (ed): Adams' Lameness in Horses, 4th ed. Philadelphia, Lea & Febiger, 1987.

139. van Vleck LD, Albrechtsen R: Differences among appraisers in the New York type appraisal program. J Dairy Sci 1965; 48:61.

140. Grundler C: Aussagewert verschiedener Hilfsmerkmale zur Beurteilung des Zucht-und Gebrauchswertes von Warmblutpferden. Dissertation, München, 1980.

141. Magnusson L-E: Studies on the conformation and related traits of standardbred trotters in Sweden. Ph.D. thesis, Skara, Sweden, 1985.

142. Goubaux A, Barrier G: De l'Extérieur de Cheval. Paris, Asselin et Cie, 1884.

143. Schmaltz R: Anatomische Notizen: V. Konstruktion and Grösse der Standwinkel an den Beinen des Pferdes. Berl Munch Tierarztl Wochenschr 1906; 14:257.

144. Schöttler F: Wachstumsmessungen an Pferden. Jb Wiss Prakt Tierzucht 1910; 5:1.

145. Rösiö B: Die Bedeutung des Exteriurs und der Konstruktion des Pferdes für seine Leistungsfähigkeit Dissertation, Berlin/Uppsala, 1927.

146. Kronacher C, Ogrizek A: Exterieur und Leistungsfähigkeit des Pferdes mit besonderer Berücksichtigung der Gliedmassenwinkelung und Schrittlängen-verhältnisse. Z Tierzucht Zuchtbiol 1932; 23:183.

147. Langlois B, Froideveaux J, Lamarche L, et al: Analyse de liaisons entre la morphologie et l'aptitude au galop, au trot et au saut d'obstacles chez le cheval. Ann Genet Sel Anim 1978; 10: 443.

148. Holmström M, Magnusson L-E, Philipsson J: Variation in conformation of Swedish warmblood horses and conformational characteristics of elite sport horses. Equine Vet J 1990; 22:186.

149. von Lengerken G, Werner K: Das Exterieur der Zucht-und Renntraber in der DDR. Wiss Z Univ Halle 1969; 18(MH5):505.

150. Langlois B, Froideveaux J, Lamarche L, et al: Analyse de liaisons entre la morphologie et l'aptitude au galop, au trot et au saut d'obstacles chez le cheval. Ann Genet Sel Anim 1978; 10: 443.

151. Müller J, Schwark HJ: Merkmalsvarians und genetische Bedingtkeit von im Turniersport erfassten Leistungsmerkmalen. Züchterische Weiterentwicklung der Sportpferderassen. In Vorträge des III International Wiss Symposium, Leipzig, 1979, p 45.

152. Churchill EA: Lameness in the standardbred. In Harrison JC (ed): Care and Training of the Trotter and Pacer. Columbus, OH, The United States Trotting Association, 1968.

153. Rooney JR: Biomechanics of equine lameness. Cornell Vet 1968; 58:49.

154. Ainslie T: Ainslie's Complete Guide to Harness Racing. New York, Trident Press, 1970.

155. Beeman M: Correlation of defects in conformation to pathology in the horse. In Proceedings of the Annual Convention of the American Association of Equine Practice, 1973, vol 19, p 177.

156. Dalin G, Magnusson L-E, Thafvelin BC: Retrospective study of hindquarter asymmetry in standardbred horses and its correlation with performance. Equine Vet J 1985; 17:292.

157. Sandgren B, Dalin G, Carlsten C, Lundeheim N: Development of osteochondrosis in the tarsocrural joint and osteochondral fragments in the fetlock joints of standardbred trotters: II. Body measurements and clinical findings. Equine Vet J 1993 (suppl 16):48.

158. Sandgren B, Dalin G, Carlsten J: Osteochondrosis in the tarsocrural joint and osteochondral fragments in the fetlock joints in standardbred trotters: I. Epidemiology, Equine Vet J 1993 (suppl 16):62.

159. Dalin G, Sandgren B, Carlsten J: Plantar osteochondral fragments in the metatarsophalangeal joints in standardbred trotters: Result of osteochondrosis or trauma? Equine Vet J 1993 (suppl 16):62.

160. Fredricson I, Drevemo S: Variations of resultant joint coordination patterns in fast-moving standardbreds. Acta Vet Scand 1972 (suppl 37):67.

161. Wilson BD, Neal RJ, Howard A, Groenendyk S: The gait of pacers: I. Kinematics of the racing stride. Equine Vet J 1988; 20:341.

162. Hellander J, Fredricson I, Hjertén G, et al: Galoppaktion I—Basala gångartsvariabler i relation till hästens hastighet. (Basic gait

variables of canter and gallop in relation to horse velocity.) Svensk Vet Tidn 1983 (suppl 3):75.

163. Deuel N, Park J: Gallop kinematics of Olympic three-day event horses. Acta Anat 1993; 146:168.

164. Leach DH, Sprigings E: Gait fatigue in the racing thoroughbred. J Equine Med Surg 1979; 3:436.

165. Pratt GW, O'Connor JT: A relationship between gait and breakdown in the horse. Am J Vet Res 1978; 39:249.

166. Fredricson I, Drevemo S, Moen K, et al: A method of three-dimensional analysis of kinematics and coordination of equine extremity joints. Acta Vet Scand 1972 (suppl 37):1.

Energetics and Performance

M. D. EATON

Appropriate production and utilization of energy are essential to the athletic horse and play a critical role in performance. Energy is required for the synthesis of the structural and functional components of any living organism and is indispensable for muscular contraction. Energy is required to pump ions and organic molecules across membranes to maintain the ionic gradients needed for generation of action potentials and electrical conductance in the nervous system. An undersupply or underproduction of energy will lead, at the very least, to suboptimal performance or, at the most, to a cessation of bodily functions necessary for survival. When the energy demand is low, it is important that "excess" energy derived from food sources can be stored within the body in a form that can be utilized readily at a later time.

Maintenance of energy balance is governed principally by an integrated network of oxidation-reduction reactions. *Oxidation* is the loss of electrons from an atom or molecule, while an acceptance of electrons is termed *reduction*. Hydrogen atoms are the principal carriers of electrons. Carbohydrates and fats are the major stores of fuel in the body and hence are the major electron donors. In aerobic reactions, oxygen is the final electron acceptor, whereas in the absence of oxygen (anaerobic reactions), glucose or glycogen can be split into two or more parts, and one of these parts can be oxidized by another. Energy flux is influenced by energy demand, substrate availability, and the presence of appropriate enzymes, coenzymes, and intermediary electron carriers.

The athletic horse has an enormous capacity to perform work, as reflected by mass-specific aerobic and anaerobic capacities that are almost twice those reported for human beings. Athletic performance requires the efficient utilization of large amounts of energy, transformed via metabolic pathways from chemical to kinetic energy (muscular contraction). All pathways are designed to produce adenosine triphosphate (ATP), which is the ultimate substrate utilized by muscle. ATP has a high-energy phosphate bond which, when cleaved, produces the energy required for muscular contraction. The continuous supply of ATP to contracting muscles is reliant on the integrative function of many body systems, including the gastrointestinal tract and the cardiovascular, respiratory, and musculoskeletal systems.

When muscles contract, there is a coupling of actin and myosin to form cross-bridges. At the head of each myosin filament is an ATP molecule that during contraction becomes hydrolyzed and releases energy. This reaction is represented as

$$ATP + H_2O \rightarrow ADP + P_i + H^+ + energy$$

where   ADP = adenosine diphosphate

The energy is utilized when the cross-bridges change their orientation compared with the axis of the myosin core, thus pulling the actin filaments along the myosin filaments. This process is repeated millions of times during muscular contraction. However, additional energy is also required during muscular relaxation. This also is supplied from ATP and is required to restore the ionic gradients necessary to initiate the contractile process. Since the ATP stores within muscle are limited, providing energy sufficient to maintain muscular activity for only a few seconds,[1] this energy source must be regenerated rapidly by either aerobic or anaerobic phosphorylation if exercise is to continue.

Energy Production

AEROBIC ENERGY SUPPLY

Oxygen Availability. Aerobic production of ATP occurs within the mitochondria via a series of single-step oxidation reactions (Fig. 4–1). In this case, oxygen is not directly involved, since the reactions are dehydrogenations. The coenzymes nicotinamide-adenine-dinucleotide (NAD) and flavin-adenine-dinucleotide (FAD) act as hydrogen carriers (i.e., they are reduced to $NADH_2$ and $FADH_2$). These coenzymes are essential for aerobic phosphorylation, but their concentrations within the muscle are low. Therefore, $NADH_2$ and $FADH_2$ must be reoxidized via the electron-transport chain in which oxygen acts as the final hydrogen acceptor to form water.

Small reserves of oxygen (O_2) are available to the exercising muscle: stored in myoglobin within the muscle (MbO_2), in hemoglobin within the circulatory system (HbO_2), or as O_2 dissolved in the bodily fluids. Since these stores provide sufficient O_2 for only a few seconds of exercise, oxidative phosphorylation is reliant on delivery of O_2 to the exercising muscles via the cardiorespiratory system. Based on this relationship, the availability of O_2 to the exercising muscle limits the rate of oxidative phosphorylation.

Aerobic Pathways: The TCA Cycle and Oxidative Phosphorylation. Pyruvate is derived from anaerobic metabolism of glucose and glycogen within the cytoplasm (see Fig. 4–1), and it is transported into the mitochondria via the activity of pyruvate dehydrogenase, which converts pyruvate to acetyl-coenzyme A (acetyl-CoA). Acetyl-CoA enters the tricarboxylic acid (TCA) cycle by combining with oxaloacetate (OAA). In the cycle there is a series of dehydrogenations and decarboxylations that consumes the acetyl group of the acetyl-CoA but allows recovery of the initial OAA. Also produced in the cycle are 2 CO_2 molecules, the transfer of 8 H atoms to form 3 $NADH_2$ and 1 $FADH_2$ molecules, and 1 ATP molecule. The $NADH_2$ and $FADH_2$ then undergo oxidative phosphorylation. Each molecule of $NADH_2$ combines with O_2 to form H_2O in a reaction linked to a pathway that combines 3 ADP and 3 P_i molecules to form 3 ATP molecules. A similar reaction with $FADH_2$ produces 2 ATP molecules. The end result of the TCA cycle and oxidative phosphorylation is that for each molecule of acetyl-CoA, 12 molecules of ATP are produced.

Fat Utilization: Beta-Oxidation. Fatty acids (FAs) are incorporated indirectly into the TCA cycle and oxidative phosphorylation and therefore must be utilized via aerobic pathways (see Fig. 4–1). FAs are transformed into

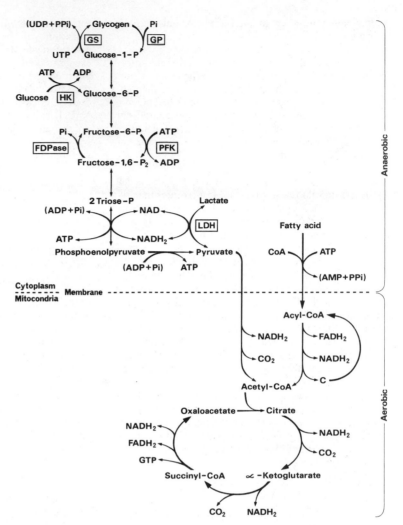

Figure 4-1. Glycolysis, fatty acid oxidation, and the tricarboxylic acid cycle in a muscle cell. Adenosine triphosphate (ATP), guanosine triphosphate (GTP), uridine triphosphate (UTP), adenosine diphosphate (ADP), adenosine monophosphate (AMP), coenzyme A (CoA), orthophosphate (P_i), pyrophosphate (PP_i), glucose-1-phosphate (G-1-P), glucose-6-phosphate (G-6-P), fructose-6-phosphate (F-6-P), fructose-1,6-diphosphate (F-1,6-P_2), nicotinamide-adenine-dinucleotide (NAD), flavin-adenine-dinucleotide (FAD), glycogen synthetase (GS), glycogen phosphorylase (GP), hexokinase (HK), phosphofructokinase (PFK), fructosediphosphatase (FDPase), lactate dehydrogenase (LDH).

acetyl-CoA esters that are dehydrogenated to liberate H atoms, which then combine with NAD and FAD to form $NADH_2$ and $FADH_2$. These are subsequently used in oxidative phosphorylation. This process involves the splitting off of C_2 fragments, thereby leaving a shorter acetyl-CoA ester that can be dehydrogenated. The C_2 fragments are then utilized in the TCA cycle as acetyl-CoA. For a typical FA, such as palmitic acid, approximately 129 molecules of ATP are produced for each molecule of FA.

ANAEROBIC ENERGY SUPPLY

ATP. Stores of ATP in the body are limited and contribute very little to the total energy supply. In human beings, the total stores of ATP are about 0.25 mol, which would supply only sufficient energy for 3 minutes at rest[2] or less than 1 second of maximal exertion.[1] As mentioned previously, although ATP provides the energy for muscular activity, ADP must be reconstituted if exercise is to continue. In addition to the aerobic mechanisms described above, a number of anaerobic pathways exist for the production of ATP.

ADP. ATP can be synthesized from ADP, and this reaction is catalyzed by myokinase:

$$2ADP \xrightarrow{\text{myokinase}} ATP + AMP$$

where   AMP = adenosine monophosphate

This reaction occurs in the working muscle but provides only small amounts of ATP.

Phosphocreatine. Phosphocreatine, or creatine phosphate (CP), is a high-energy phosphagen that acts as an immediate substrate for ATP synthesis:

$$ADP + CP \rightarrow ATP + creatine$$

The stores of CP are also limited and are capable of supplying energy for a few minutes at rest or only seconds during intense exercise.[1]

Glycogenolysis. Glycogen is metabolized to glucose-1-phosphate (G-1-P) by phosphorylase. The G-1-P is converted to glucose-6-phosphate (G-6-P), which then enters the anaerobic glycolytic pathway (described below). The glycogen reserves in the horse are substantial, for example, up to 700 mmol glycosyl units per kilogram of muscle (dry weight), and are the largest fuel source for anaerobic metabolism.[3]

Glucose. Glucose is phosphorylated to G-6-P in the cell cytosol by hexokinase in a reaction that requires the utilization of an ATP molecule. G-6-P is converted to fructose-6-phosphate (F-6-P), which is subsequently converted to fructose-1,6-diphosphate (F-1,6-P$_2$) with the utilization of another ATP molecule. F-1,6-P$_2$ is subsequently metabolized to 2 pyruvate molecules with the production of 4 ATP molecules and 2 NADH$_2$ molecules. Thus the anaerobic glycolytic pathway has a net yield of 3 molecules of ATP from 1 molecule of glycogen or 2 molecules of ATP from 1 molecule of glucose. The end stage of this anaerobic pathway is the conversion of pyruvate to lactate in a reaction catalyzed by lactate dehydrogenase that also will reoxidize the NADH$_2$. Alternatively, the pyruvate can enter the mitochondria and participate in the TCA cycle.

The anaerobic production of energy provides a rapid means of producing limited supplies of energy. The aerobic pathways are more complex and significantly slower but yield approximately 13 times more ATP per glucose unit than anaerobic pathways.

INTEGRATION OF AEROBIC AND ANAEROBIC PATHWAYS

The control of these pathways is complex and is achieved by a number of regulatory systems. The relative concentrations of substrates and end products, the availability of enzymes, and the effect of feedback mechanisms that either activate or inhibit enzyme activity are all involved.

The most important regulators are the availability of O$_2$ and the ratio of ATP/ADP. With the onset of exercise, the reserves of O$_2$ stored in hemoglobin and myoglobin, and also stores of ATP and CP are utilized. If sufficient O$_2$ is available, the aerobic pathways reoxidize most of the NADH$_2$ produced in the cytoplasm, and energy production can continue principally via aerobic pathways. If energy demand increases, there will be a persistent decline in the ATP/ADP ratio, providing a continued stimulus for the glycolytic pathway, with a corresponding increase in NADH$_2$ and pyruvate. The primary controller of this pathway is the effect of the ATP/ADP ratio on the activity of phosphofructokinase (PFK) and fructose diphosphatase (FDPase); a low ATP/ADP ratio will activate PFK and inhibit FDPase, thus stimulating glycolysis with up to a 100-fold increase in the production of pyruvate from glycogen. At low to moderate intensities of exercise, the great majority of pyruvate produced will enter the TCA cycle. Similarly, beta-oxidation will be stimulated to provide energy via aerobic means. However, there is a critical intensity of exercise at which insufficient O$_2$ is available for oxidative phosphorylation, and a proportion of the NADH$_2$ is reoxidized via pyruvate being metabolized to lactate. An exercise intensity increases, a greater proportion of the NADH$_2$ is reoxidized via pyruvate, and thus a greater proportion of the energy is supplied by anaerobic pathways. Eventually, at intensities greater than maximal oxygen uptake, any further increases in energy supply can occur only via anaerobic pathways.

Sources of Energy

The major fuels for muscular contraction and their stores within the body are outlined in Table 4–1. These estimates are the ones provided by McMiken.[4]

CARBOHYDRATES

Carbohydrate (CHO) is stored principally as glycogen in the muscles and liver, while blood glucose provides an immediate energy supply. One glucose molecule can yield up to 38 ATP molecules. One mole of glucose (180 g) can liberate 2824 kJ (674 kcal) when oxidized, of which 70 percent is used to produce 38 mol ATP, with the remainder of the energy lost as heat.[2]

During short bouts of high-intensity exercise, muscle glycogen concentrations have been shown to decrease by approximately 20 to 30 percent. In a study by Snow and Harris,[3] horses galloping 1600 m in 113 to 122 seconds (13 to 14 m/s) during training exhibited a mean decrease in glycogen concentration from resting values of 618 mmol/kg dry weight to postexercise values of 493 mmol/kg dry weight. A similar study by Hodgson and colleagues,[5] in horses competing in 800- and 1200-m trial races, found that glycogen was depleted by 167 and 158 mmol/kg dry weight, respectively. Nimmo and Snow[6] compared horses galloping over distances of 506 and 3620 m and found that the rate of glycogen utilization ranged from 149.4 to 18.8 μmol/g per minute, respectively, indicating that the rate of energy production was greatest at the faster speeds. Since the muscle glycogen concentration decreases only by approximately one-third during a single bout of high-

Table 4-1. Energy Stores

Fuel	Energy	
	kJ	kcal
ATP	38	9
Creatine phosphate	188	45
Glycogen	75,300	17,988
Fat	640,000	152,889

Note: These values were calculated by McMiken[4] and are estimations for a 500-kg horse with a muscle mass of 206 kg, adipose tissue of 25 kg, and a liver of 6.5 kg.

intensity exercise, it is unlikely that glycogen availability limits this type of performance.

During exercise of moderate intensity, where horses trotted on a treadmill at 7 m/s and the mean exercise time was 56 minutes, muscle glycogen concentration dropped from preexercise values of 530 mmol/kg to 470 mmol/kg dry weight.[7] Thus the rate of glycogen utilization was 1.1 μmol/g per minute.

Prolonged exercise results in the greatest depletion of muscle glycogen. In endurance horses competing in an 80-km ride, the muscle mean glycogen concentration fell by 56 percent.[8] Hodgson and colleagues[9] studied horses in rides ranging from 40 to 160 km and found similar values for glycogen utilization.

Several studies have examined the glycogen depletion patterns of different muscle fiber types. As exercise intensity is increased, there is a progressive recruitment of the faster-contracting, more powerful fibers. During high-intensity exercise, there is a preferential depletion of glycogen in type IIb muscle fibers,[5,10] with little depletion occurring in type I fibers. Exercise at a moderate intensity to fatigue[7] resulted in all type I and approximately half the type IIa fibers having a low glycogen content, while the type IIb fibers retained a high level of glycogen. During prolonged low-intensity exercise, in rides ranging from 40 to 160 km, as the distance of the ride increased, there was a progressive fiber type recruitment from type I and then type IIa, followed by type IIb,[9] and there may be complete depletion of the type I fibers.[8]

FAT

Lipids are stored within the muscle as well as in extramuscular depots as adipose tissue, where triglycerides undergo hydrolysis to glycerol and free fatty acids (FFAs). One mole of stearic acid (285 g), when oxidized, yields approximately 11,000 kJ, which produces 146 mol ATP; that is, 69 percent of the energy is used for ATP production, with the remaining 31 percent lost as heat.[2] Thus fat is an efficient energy source for exercising horses. High-intensity exercise relies on CHO as the main fuel source, with fat likely to be of little importance. However, during low-intensity exercise, fat has been shown to be a major energy source. A study by Essén-Gustavsson and colleagues[7] demonstrated an increase in plasma FFAs from 175 μmol/liter at rest to 600 μmol/liter after exercise for 56 minutes, indicating a mobilization of fat as a fuel source. Rose and colleagues[11] found that in a 3-day event, after the steeplechase and roads-and-track section, the FFAs increased from 156 μmol/liter before the event to 586 μmol/liter, while in an 80-km endurance ride, the FFAs increased from 47 to 1254 μmol/liter after the ride. However, Snow and colleagues[8] failed to demonstrate a decrease in the lipid content of muscle in horses competing in an 80-km endurance ride.

Further proof of fat acting as a fuel for low-intensity exercise is evident from measurement of the respiratory quotient R. The respiratory quotient is determined by measuring CO_2 and O_2 concentrations in expired respiratory gases, and $R = CO_2$ produced $/O_2$ utilized. The R value for fat oxidation is 0.71, the R value for CHO oxidation is 1.0, while a value of 0.72 to 0.99 indicates a mixture of both fat and CHO metabolism. R values greater than 1.0 indicate anaerobic metabolism producing lactate that is eventually converted to CO_2. Horses exercising for 90 minutes on a treadmill[12] had R values of 0.81 to 0.90, while at the end of a high-speed exercise test the R values range from 1.22 to 1.36.[13]

In some studies, high-fat diets have been shown to have a paradoxical effect on glycogen stores.[14–17] Horses fed a fat-supplemented diet (approximately 10 to 12 percent of the digestible energy was derived from fat) increased resting muscle glycogen concentration by 18 to 52 percent. Vegetable oils are the most readily available sources of fat that can be used as a dietary supplement. The effects of high-fat diets on performance are equivocal, with some authors reporting improved performance and others reporting no change. Meyers and colleagues[14] and Oldham and colleagues[18] demonstrated a greater capacity for exercise during an incremental treadmill exercise test, while Harkins and colleagues[17] demonstrated improved racetrack performance after fat supplementation. The improvement in performance was thought to be due to either the increased glycogen stores or the high-fat diets inducing an increase in fat utilization which promoted a "glycogen sparing" effect. However, often these improvements were small and the findings questionable. Several studies[7,19,20] did not demonstrate a significant improvement in oxygen uptake or run-to-fatigue time during an incremental exercise test on a treadmill when horses were fed a high-fat diet.

PROTEIN

Protein also can act as an energy source, although under normal conditions it probably makes a negligible contribution to energy requirements during exercise. Amino acids are deaminated, enter the urea cycle, and eventually are metabolized to enter the TCA cycle at various points.

Energy Expenditure

OXYGEN UPTAKE

Definition and Components of Oxygen Uptake. Oxygen uptake ($\dot{V}_{O_2}$) is a measurement of the body's total aerobic metabolic rate. Normally, $\dot{V}_{O_2}$ is measured in liters per minute or milliliters per kilogram of body weight per minute and therefore represents a rate of consumption and not a finite capacity. The $\dot{V}_{O_2}$ is a measure of the function of the cardiovascular and respiratory systems and involves a chain of events starting with air entering the upper airways and ending with the utilization of O_2 by the respiratory chain in the mitochondria. These events involve ventilation of the lungs, diffusion of O_2 through the alveolar wall, affinity of hemoglobin (Hb) for O_2, the perfusion of the lungs (i.e., heart rate, stroke volume, and blood pressure), peripheral circulatory factors (including muscle blood flow, capillary density, and

O_2 diffusion and extraction), and finally, O_2 utilization within the muscle, which will depend on substrate availability, myoglobin concentration, enzyme activity, the size of the muscle mass, and the muscle fiber type. The maximum rate of oxygen uptake is termed $\dot{V}_{O_2max}$.

Measurement of $\dot{V}_{O_2}$. Measurement of $\dot{V}_{O_2}$ can be performed most easily in a laboratory,[21-25] although field measurements where oxygen analyzers are mounted on a cart that travels close to an exercising horse have been performed,[26] as well as oxygen uptake measurements using telemetry.[27] Measurement of $\dot{V}_{O_2}$ involves the horse wearing a respiratory gas collection mask that ensures unrestricted breathing of fresh air but allows the collection of expired gases, which are analyzed for O_2 and CO_2 concentrations. The measurement of $\dot{V}_{O_2}$ is highly reproducible[13,24,25] (error of approximately 3 percent).

OXYGEN UPTAKE AT REST

The resting rate of $\dot{V}_{O_2}$ is approximately 3 to 5 ml/kg per minute or, for a 500-kg horse, around 1.5 to 2.5 liters/min. Measurement of resting $\dot{V}_{O_2}$ is often complicated by excitement or the anticipation of exercise, and therefore, the basal values are probably around 2 ml/kg per minute.

OXYGEN UPTAKE DURING SUBMAXIMAL EXERCISE

Speed. In humans[28,29] and horses,[21,30] there is a linear relationship between $\dot{V}_{O_2}$ and speed during submaximal intensities of exercise, where aerobic energy supply can meet all the energy demand (Fig. 4–2). Thus the net energy consumption per kilogram per meter is constant and independent of speed. When the speed is increased so that $\dot{V}_{O_2}$ approaches $\dot{V}_{O_2max}$ and anaerobic energy supply becomes of increasing importance, this linearity is lost.

In horses, the linear relationship of $\dot{V}_{O_2}$ and speed is

$$\dot{V}_{O_2} \text{ (ml/kg/min)} = 8.24 \times \text{speed (m/s)} - 4.08$$
$$(r = 0.94)$$

for horses exercising on a horizontal treadmill at speeds from 1 to 13 m/s where gait was not restricted (Eaton and colleagues, unpublished data). The negative y intercepts found in some studies[22,30] indicate that at very low speeds there is a nonlinear relation of $\dot{V}_{O_2}$ and speed. This nonlinearity may be due partly to the horse exercising at unnatural speeds (see the following discussion on economy of locomotion), errors involved in measuring low rates of $\dot{V}_{O_2}$, and effects of excitement and apprehension during low-intensity exercise. These results may vary from values that would be obtained for horses exercising on a track as a result of differences in gait selection and track surface and alterations in the normal pattern of locomotion due to the treadmill.

During thoroughbred and quarter horse racing, the intensity of exercise (i.e., speeds greater than 15 m/s) will be such that a proportion of the energy supplied will be delivered anaerobically and the horses will be

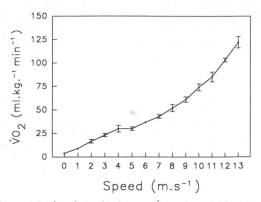

Figure 4-2. *The relationship between $\dot{V}_{O_2}$ and speed. There is a linear relationship between $\dot{V}_{O_2}$ and speed for horses exercising on an uninclined treadmill at speeds from rest to 13 m/s. At speeds of 5 to 7 m/s, there is a loss of linearity due to the horses being forced to exercise using extended gaits.*

exercising at intensities greater than those which produce $\dot{V}_{O_2max}$. In endurance rides of 40 to 100 km (speeds of 2 to 6 m/s), virtually all the energy requirements will be supplied aerobically. Endurance horses exercising at these speeds carrying a rider would have a $\dot{V}_{O_2}$ of approximately 40 to 80 ml/kg per minute (i.e., 30 to 60 percent of $\dot{V}_{O_2max}$).

Load. In virtually all types of equine athletic performance, the horse is forced to carry a load, which is either a rider or driver, and thus the energy requirements are increased. Armsby[31] demonstrated that for a horse at rest, energy expenditure increased to a degree proportional to the weight of the load. Pagan and Hintz[26] demonstrated a similar increase in horses exercising on a track at speeds of 1 to 6 m/s. They concluded that while the amount of energy expended by horses was related to speed, it also was proportional to the body weight of the riderless horse or the combined weight of the horse plus rider. Therefore, a 450-kg horse carrying a 50-kg rider would expend about the same amount of energy as a 500-kg horse without a rider. In horses exercising on a treadmill (mean speed 7.2 m/s) carrying a load equivalent to 10 percent of body weight, the $\dot{V}_{O_2}$ increased from 24.4 to 28.0 liters/min, but there was no significant difference in O_2 cost between the loaded and unloaded states (53 and 55 ml/kg per minute, respectively). The increase in $\dot{V}_{O_2}$ due to the load is achieved by an increase in the ventilation.[22] The implications of these findings have direct application to racing. If a jockey were forced to ride 1 kg overweight, the effect of this on energy demand would be negated if the horse were to lose 1 kg prior to the race (providing this weight loss could be achieved without any deleterious effects on performance and there was no effect of wind resistance or the pattern of locomotion).

Slope. The effect of slope on $\dot{V}_{O_2}$ is substantial (Fig. 4–3). These results are from thoroughbred horses exercising on a treadmill at speeds ranging from 1 to 13 m/s.

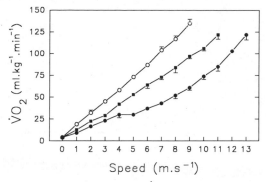

Figure 4-3. *The effect of slope on* $\dot{V}_{O_2}$. *Horses exercising on a treadmill increase* $\dot{V}_{O_2}$ *as the incline of the treadmill increases. At some speeds, exercising on a 10 percent incline will double the energy expenditure compared with exercise on the flat* (● = *0 percent incline;* ■ = *5 percent incline, and* ○ = *10 percent incline*).

At 8 m/s at 0 and 10 percent inclines, the mean heart rate (HR) was 133 and 198 beats/min, respectively. The treadmill velocity at which a plasma lactate concentration of 4 mmol/liter (V_{La4}) was reached was 11.8 and 7.0 m/s at 0 and 10 percent slopes, respectively.

In horses trotting (mean speed 5.2 m/s) on a treadmill, the $\dot{V}_{O_2}$ increased by 13.4 liters/min (76 percent) when the slope of the treadmill was increased from 0 to 6.25 percent.[22] This increase in $\dot{V}_{O_2}$ was brought about by an increase in oxygen extraction and ventilation (primarily due to an increase in tidal volume). The effect of slope will play an important role in determining energy expenditure in athletic horses, especially during endurance rides and the cross-country phase of 3-day events. At some speeds, exercising on a 10 percent gradient will more than double the energy expenditure if the speed remains constant.

In human beings, the effects of a downhill grade on energy cost are substantial, although little research has been done in this area with horses. In human beings running at 15 km/h on the flat, the energy consumption was estimated at 63 kJ/kg (15 kcal/kg), while on a −6.25 percent slope it was 46 kJ/kg (11 kcal/kg). Once the downhill slope was steeper than −10 percent, the energy utilization increased and was greater than running on the flat.[29] In athletic horses it is likely that a slight downhill slope will cause a lowering of energy demand, but at some unknown incline the energy expenditure will increase, and this effect may be exaggerated by the presence of a rider and variable gaits.

Duration. The effect of exercise duration on energy expenditure will vary with the intensity of exercise and the development of fatigue. In a study of prolonged submaximal exercise[12] where horses exercised on a 2 percent incline at 3 m/s for 90 minutes, the $\dot{V}_{O_2}$ did not alter between 5 and 75 minutes of exercise, with a slight decrease occurring after 90 minutes. The mean HR (121 beats/min) remained unchanged throughout the run.

Another experiment[32] where the initial treadmill speed was set to give a HR of 150 beats/min demonstrated significant changes in cardiorespiratory measurements during 30 minutes of exercise. There were increases in $\dot{V}_{O_2}$ by 15 percent and cardiac output by 25 percent (due to increases in HR by 14 percent and stroke volume by 11 percent). These responses were thought to be related to the fact that the horses were not completely successful in thermoregulating during the prolonged exercise, since rectal temperature continued to rise throughout the experiment. As the intensity of exercise increases, inducing more rapid disturbances in thermoregulation and the circulatory system, the duration of exercise will become more critical in energetic homeostasis.

Temperature. Changes in energy demand due to temperature are related to the effects of thermoregulation (e.g., fluid shifts, increased blood flow to the skin, sweat production) rather than to effects on economy per se. Although it is possible that blood flow to the muscles may decline when horses exercise in a hot environment, this has not been proven. Obviously, there will be an optimal temperature range for enzyme activity, muscular contraction, and O_2 diffusion, but it is unlikely that in the exercising horse this would impose any direct effects on energy utilization except in extreme environmental conditions. Aspects of thermoregulation are discussed in Chapter 9.

Track Surface. The condition of the ground underneath the horse can have a substantial effect on the energetic demand, especially in horses exercising at high intensities or for prolonged periods. A heavily mudded track surface will increase the energy expenditure because extra effort is required to lift the hooves out of the soft track. Also, there will be changes in the pattern of locomotion associated with the feet slipping each time they strike the ground. Uneven ground may have a similar effect, in that it may alter the pattern of limb movement (e.g., stride length may decrease) so that the energy cost of locomotion increases. It is difficult to quantify precisely these effects on energy expenditure, but race times for both thoroughbreds and endurance horses are significantly longer in heavy conditions.

MAXIMAL AEROBIC POWER

$\dot{V}_{O_2max}$ occurs when the oxygen uptake does not increase despite an increase in the workload (Fig. 4–4). Elite human athletes have $\dot{V}_{O_2max}$ values of 70 to 90 ml/kg per minute,[33] while thoroughbred racehorses have values reported in the range of 140 to 187 ml/kg per minute.[24,25,34,35] In humans, $\dot{V}_{O_2max}$ has been considered the "gold standard" by which prolonged exercise capacity can be judged. Harkins and colleagues[36] demonstrated a negative correlation between $\dot{V}_{O_2max}$ and the time taken for horses to run distances ranging from 1200 to 2000 m. In addition, there is anecdotal evidence of a relationship between $\dot{V}_{O_2max}$ and racing performance, although this is yet to be proven.

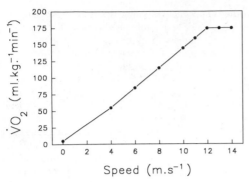

Figure 4-4. *Maximal oxygen uptake. Horses exercising on a treadmill set at a 10 percent incline demonstrate the linear relationship between speed and $\dot{V}_{O_2}$ up to the speed where maximal oxygen uptake is reached (in this case at 175 ml/kg per minute at 12 m/s). Once maximal oxygen uptake is attained, further increases in speed will not elicit any further increases in $\dot{V}_{O_2}$ and the extra energy required to run at these speeds must be provided by anaerobic pathways.*

HIGH-INTENSITY EXERCISE

Supramaximal intensities are experienced when the workload is greater than that provided for by the maximal rate of oxygen uptake. At such intensities, the energy demand exceeds the aerobic energy supply, and therefore, anaerobic energy production is required. This can occur when

- The energy demand increases at such a rapid rate that the slower aerobic pathways are not able to supply the required energy and the faster glycolytic pathways are recruited.
- The total energy demand is greater than that supplied by aerobic pathways. Quarter horses, thoroughbreds, and standardbreds exercise at supramaximal intensities each time they race.

Anaerobic capacity is proportional to the maximum amount of ATP that can be supplied by anaerobic energy systems. Anaerobic energy release is critical for a rapid and high output of muscular power. Unlike $\dot{V}_{O_2max}$, the anaerobic capacity is considered a finite capacity and not a rate. A number of tests are used to measure anaerobic capacity in humans, but many of these cannot be used in horses. One test that has been used recently to measure anaerobic capacity in horses is the maximal accumulated oxygen deficit (MAOD).

MAOD. Oxygen deficit refers to the lag in $\dot{V}_{O_2}$ that occurs at the beginning of exercise (Fig. 4–5). The *maximal accumulated oxygen deficit* (MAOD) is the total oxygen deficit that occurs during exercise at supramaximal intensities and is the difference between the oxygen demand and the actual $\dot{V}_{O_2}$ (Fig. 4–6). The O_2 demand is calculated by an extrapolation of the linear relationship of $\dot{V}_{O_2}$ and speed at submaximal intensities. Although few results are available measuring MAOD in horses, values ranging from 30 to 128 ml O_2 equivalents per kilogram

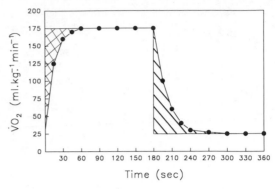

Figure 4-5. *Oxygen deficit and oxygen debt. At the start of exercise, there is a lag in oxygen uptake relative to the energy demand; this "lag" is termed the oxygen deficit. Thus, in the early stages of exercise, the energy demand is met by O_2 stores within the body and anaerobic energy supply. At the cessation of exercise, metabolism does not immediately return to resting levels; this postexercise period is characterized by excessive postexercise oxygen consumption (EPOC), also termed the oxygen debt (Cross hatch = oxygen deficit; diagonal lines = excessive postexercise oxygen consumption.)*

have been reported.[37,38] This compares with humans, where values of 42 and 90 ml O_2 equivalents per kilogram for endurance and sprint athletes, respectively, have been reported.[39,40]

MAOD is not correlated with $\dot{V}_{O_2max}$, from which it can be suggested that the capacity of anaerobic energy supply is not dependent on the rate of oxygen uptake (i.e., aerobic energy supply). Although plasma lactate concentration has been suggested to be an indicator of anaerobic energy production, many other variables affect blood lactate concentration (including the rate of lactate production and metabolism, the duration and intensity of exercise, and the movement of lactate into and out of the plasma), making such measurements of limited value when attempting to estimate anaerobic capacity.

In horses, there have been no investigations relating anaerobic capacity to performance. In humans, sprint-trained athletes had a higher MAOD than distance-trained athletes (78 and 56 ml O_2 equivalents, respectively).[41] There also was a correlation ($r = -0.76$) between MAOD and performance in a 300-m time trial but no correlation in a 600-m trial. Thus, in humans, MAOD is related to anaerobic performance, but whether such a relationship exists in horses is not known. However, in most competitive horse events other than quarter horse racing, aerobic energy delivery provides the major contribution to energy requirements.

OXYGEN UPTAKE KINETICS

In horses, the rate at which $\dot{V}_{O_2}$ can increase with the onset of exercise is remarkable, there being up to a 30- to 40-fold increase within 60 seconds. The rapid increases in ventilation, cardiac output, and hematocrit allow for the rapid increase in $\dot{V}_{O_2}$, implying that the oxi-

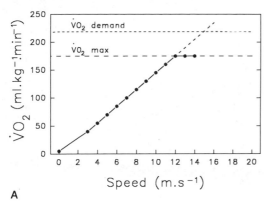

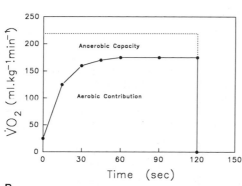

A

B

Figure 4-6. A, *Determination of O_2 deficit, calculation of O_2 demand and speed. The relationship between speed and $\dot{V}_{O_2}$ for a particular horse exercising on a treadmill at 10 percent incline is demonstrated. The $\dot{V}_{O_2max}$ is 175 ml/kg per minute, and for this horse to exercise at an intensity 125 percent of $\dot{V}_{O_2max}$, the $\dot{V}_{O_2}$ demand would therefore be 219 ml/kg per minute. Thus this horse would need to run at 15 m/s to exercise at an intensity of 125 percent of $\dot{V}_{O_2max}$. B, Determination of O_2 deficit, exercise at 125 percent of $\dot{V}_{O_2max}$. This figure demonstrates the relationship between $\dot{V}_{O_2}$ and time for a horse exercising on a treadmill at a 10 percent incline at an intensity of 125 percent of $\dot{V}_{O_2max}$, which was calculated to be at an O_2 demand of 219 ml/kg per minute at a speed of 15m/s. Initially, there is a lag in oxygen uptake, and eventually $\dot{V}_{O_2}$ reaches $\dot{V}_{O_2max}$. The exercise ceases when the horse can no longer keep pace with the treadmill. The difference in the O_2 demand and the actual oxygen uptake is termed the* maximal accumulated oxygen deficit *and is a measure of the anaerobic capacity.*

Table 4-2. Oxygen Uptake Kinetics

Intensity, $\%\dot{V}_{O_2max}$	$t_{50\%}$ $\dot{V}_{O_2max}$ (s)	$t_{75\%}$ $\dot{V}_{O_2max}$ (s)
105	9.9	24.6
115	9.2	21.1
125	11.1	20.8

*Note: The mean time (seconds) taken to reach 50 and 75 percent of $\dot{V}_{O_2max}$ ($t_{50\%}$ and $t_{75\%}$) for horses exercising at intensities of 105, 115, and 125 percent of $\dot{V}_{O_2max}$.

Rose and colleagues[37] demonstrated in horses exercising at 120 percent of $\dot{V}_{O_2max}$ that the $t_{50\%}$ $\dot{V}_{O_2max}$ was 9.8 seconds, the $t_{95\%}$ $\dot{V}_{O_2max}$ occurred by 60 seconds, and $\dot{V}_{O_2}$ had reached a steady state by 75 seconds.

ENERGY PARTITIONING

The kinetics of $\dot{V}_{O_2}$ also emphasize the fact that energy supply is not derived from one source, there being an integration of aerobic and anaerobic pathways. During low-intensity exercise, virtually all the energy requirements will be met by aerobic mechanisms, and this would be the case in endurance rides. Sports requiring sudden bursts of activity (e.g., jumping and polo) or sustained high-intensity performance (e.g., racing) will require an increased anaerobic energy component.

At the start of supramaximal exercise, the reserves of oxygen (in the lungs, hemoglobin, and myoglobin), as well as stores of ATP and phosphocreatine in muscle, will provide the immediate supply of energy for exercise lasting for a few seconds. As the exercise continues, the anaerobic processes that utilize glycogen will provide energy, and as the duration of exercise increases, the aerobic pathways will become more important. The rate of change from anaerobic to aerobic metabolism is extremely fast and becomes faster the greater the intensity of exercise, as seen by the changes in $t_{75\%}$ $\dot{V}_{O_2max}$ (see Table 4-2).

The intensity of exercise at which aerobic ATP production fails to meet energy demands and anaerobic processes commence will vary depending on a range of factors. The most important is the rate of O_2 delivery to the exercising muscle. Other factors include mitochondrial density, catecholamine levels, intracellular enzyme concentrations, prior training, nutritional status, warmup, and the rate of increase in the workload.

The proportion of energy derived from aerobic versus anaerobic sources further highlights the exercise capacity of the horse. During a run at a speed eliciting an intensity of 125 percent $\dot{V}_{O_2max}$ and lasting for nearly a minute, the majority of the energy (70 percent) was supplied aerobically.[38] This intensity can be compared with a sprint race of 1000 m (Fig. 4-7). From these data it can be suggested that horses that are considered sprinters still rely on aerobic energy delivery. Apart from the initial acceleration period, horses in longer races (e.g., 3200 m) could provide a substantial proportion of their

dative processes within the muscle are able to utilize the O_2. In a study by Eaton and colleagues,[38] $\dot{V}_{O_2}$ increased rapidly at the onset of supramaximal exercise. The mean times (seconds) taken to reach 50 and 75 percent of $\dot{V}_{O_2max}$ ($t_{50\%}$ and $t_{75\%}$) for horses exercising at intensities varying from 105 to 125 percent $\dot{V}_{O_2max}$ are shown in Table 4-2. There was a significant decrease in the time required to reach $\dot{V}_{O_2max}$ as the intensity of exercise increased. An intensity of 125 percent $\dot{V}_{O_2max}$ is calculated such that the intensity of the exercise has an O_2 demand that is 125 percent of the $\dot{V}_{O_2max}$. Because the $\dot{V}_{O_2max}$ is limited, this "extra 25 percent" must be supplied by anaerobic mechanisms.

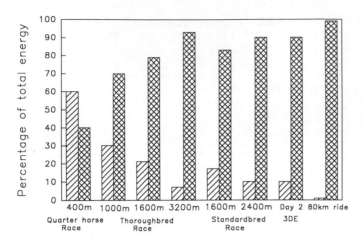

Figure 4-7. Energy partitioning. Estimates of the proportion of energy that is derived from aerobic and anaerobic pathways during competitive events (Diagonal lines = anaerobic contribution; cross hatch = aerobic contribution.)

energy requirement via aerobic pathways. Using the preceding results, it is possible to estimate that it is only in races of very short duration (i.e., 400 m lasting around 20 to 22 seconds) that anaerobic sources predominate. In humans, the anaerobic capacity assumes a more substantial role, contributing 50 percent of the energy supply in supramaximal exercise of 1 minute duration, corresponding to an intensity of 175 percent $\dot{V}_{O_2max}$.[39] The preceding discussion further highlights the importance that $\dot{V}_{O_2max}$ may have on equine athletic performance, since in most competitive events aerobic energy delivery predominates.

POSTEXERCISE METABOLISM: OXYGEN DEBT

Following exercise, metabolism does not immediately return to the resting state (see Fig. 4–5); rather, there is a period of recovery characterized by excessive postexercise oxygen consumption (EPOC). The EPOC only amounts to a small fraction of the total O_2 cost (i.e., total exercise $\dot{V}_{O_2}$ + EPOC). In humans exercising at 30 to 70 percent of $\dot{V}_{O_2max}$, the EPOC accounted for 1 to 8.9 percent of the total O_2 cost.[42] Initially, this EPOC was described as an "oxygen debt" necessary for the repayment of the O_2 deficit. However, this does not fully explain the phenomenon of EPOC. EPOC has been considered to have two phases: an initial fast phase and a slower phase. The fast phase was thought to be "alactic" and was a result of the resynthesis of high-energy phosphagens, and the slow phase was the "lactic acid" phase which was due to the oxidation of lactate. Further research has shown a dissociation of EPOC with muscle and blood lactate concentrations.

EPOC is the result of a number of functions occurring at the cessation of exercise. A component of EPOC is undoubtedly due to the rephosphorylation of creatine and ADP. However, this may only constitute 10 percent of EPOC[43] in humans and less than 1.5 percent in horses.[37] The oxidation of lactate accounts for a major part of the EPOC, while smaller fractions of lactate are involved in glycogen repletion and amino acid synthesis. The catecholamines released during exercise probably cause an elevation in postexercise mitochondrial respiratory function which contributes to EPOC. The changes in calcium ion concentrations that occur before and after exercise are also thought to contribute to the rate of postexercise mitochondrial function. The elevation of FFAs found during submaximal exercise may contribute to EPOC. Elevation of muscle temperature also may be associated with an increase in postexercise $\dot{V}_{O_2}$.

In a study by Rose and colleagues,[37] oxygen uptake was measured after a bout of exercise at 120 percent $\dot{V}_{O_2max}$. The EPOC was calculated from the area under the $\dot{V}_{O_2}$ curve and was 324.5 ml/kg (including $\dot{V}_{O_2}$ for resting metabolism). The EPOC/O_2 deficit ratio was 2.75. The fast and slow phases of the $\dot{V}_{O_2}$ recovery were completed by 1.4 and 18.3 minutes, respectively. The EPOC/O_2 deficit ratio and the duration of the O_2 recovery curve were similar to those in human studies. There was a poor relationship between alterations in muscle metabolite concentrations and recovery $\dot{V}_{O_2}$. Muscle and plasma lactate levels were still substantially elevated 20 minutes after recovery despite $\dot{V}_{O_2}$ returning to resting values.

Economy of Locomotion

The preceding discussion regarding the relationship of submaximal oxygen uptake with speed and load leads to the conclusion that the net energy cost per kilogram per meter is independent of speed and load (or body weight). This energy cost is defined as the economy of locomotion. Some authors[22,44,45] reported that the economy of locomotion in horses fell within the narrow range of 0.122 to 0.133 ml O_2/kg/m for horses walking and trotting. However, this economy changes when a greater range of speeds are used. Hörnicke and colleagues[27] found higher values for walking and trotting (0.21 ml O_2/kg/m) and for galloping (0.19 ml O_2/kg/m), whereas horses working at speeds from 5 to 13 m/s on a treadmill had an economy of locomotion ranging from 0.10 to 0.160 ml O_2/kg/m (Eaton and colleagues, unpublished data). The most likely reason for this alteration of economy with speed is the effect of gait, especially when values are derived from horses forced to work at specific speeds utilizing restricted or extended gaits on motorized treadmills.

A study by Hoyt and Taylor[21] measured $\dot{V}_{O_2}$ in ponies exercising at a variety of speeds and gaits on a treadmill. The ponies had been trained to walk, trot, and canter and to extend their gait on command. The results showed a curvilinear response of speed and $\dot{V}_{O_2}$ (Fig. 4–8).

When the ponies were forced to use extended gaits, the $\dot{V}_{O_2}$ would increase (by up to 70 percent), even though the speed remained unchanged. Thus there is a speed that is energetically optimal for each gait. This optimal value for economy was similar to the previous value of 0.122 to 0.133 ml O_2/kg/m. Hoyt and Taylor[21] then measured the speed and gait of the ponies as they moved freely over the ground at their natural paces. They found that the ponies preferred to move at speeds that were energetically optimal for each gait. This may have important implications for horses working for long periods, such as endurance horses, especially if they are forced to use extended gaits.

It is possible that the range of the energetically op-timal speeds for each gait may be altered by training. In a study by Gottlieb-Vedi and colleagues,[30] trotters exercising on a treadmill over a range of speeds (2 to 10 m/s) had a linear relationship of $\dot{V}_{O_2}$ and speed ($r = 0.95$). It is possible that the training and selection of trotters have meant that they are able to work at an extended gait without any loss in economy.

The development of unnatural gaits such as pacing also has consequences relating to energy expenditure. In an experiment where standardbred horses had been trained to pace wearing hobbles or exercise using natural gaits, while working on a treadmill between 4 to 12 m/s, there was a trend for $\dot{V}_{O_2}$ to be higher when pacing compared with trotting, although there was no statistical difference. The speed required to reach $\dot{V}_{O_2max}$ was calculated to be 13.8 and 14.6 m/s for pacing and galloping, respectively (Evans and colleagues, unpublished data). Also, there was no difference in stride frequency or stride length between gaits, since the horses attempted to achieve an optimal economy while pacing. Although these differences are small, there may be significant energy implications for horses performing at maximal intensities during races.

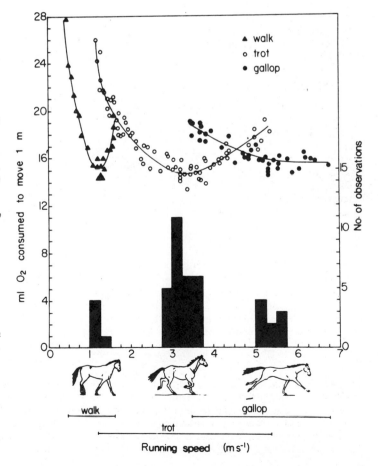

Figure 4-8. Economy of locomotion. The oxygen cost to move a unit distance (rate of O_2 consumption divided by speed while exercising on a treadmill) declined to a minimum and then increased with increasing speed in a walk and trot. It also declined to a minimum in a gallop; due to limitations in the speed of the treadmill, it was not possible to see if an increase occurred with high-speed galloping. The minimal oxygen cost to move a unit distance was almost the same in all three gaits. The histogram shows gaits where an individual horse was allowed to select its own speed while running on the ground. The horse chose three speeds that coincided with the energetically optimal speed for each gait. On a motorized treadmill, the animal must move at the speed of the treadmill, but when running on the ground, there were ranges of speeds that the horse never used for any sustained period. (From Hoyt and Taylor[21]. Reproduced with permission).

Conclusions

The efficient utilization of energy is essential to the survival and performance of the athletic horse. The regulation of energy balance is achieved by an integrated network of chemical reactions (principally by oxidation-reduction reactions). The main purpose of these reactions is to

- Provide a readily available fuel source, that is, ATP.
- Convert energy excess to the immediate demand into a form that can be stored within the body to be utilized at a later time.

The stores of readily available energy (i.e., ATP, ADP, and CP) are sufficient to last only a few seconds during high-intensity exercise. Thus ATP must be replenished continuously if exercise is to continue. If sufficient oxygen is delivered to the exercising muscle or if energy demand is low, ATP production is via aerobic pathways, while anaerobic pathways are recruited if there is an inadequate oxygen supply or if metabolic demand is high. Aerobic pathways operating via the TCA cycle and oxidative phosphorylation produce 38 molecules of ATP per molecule of glucose. Fats are also efficiently utilized by these pathways, producing large amounts of ATP. The major anaerobic pathways utilize glucose and glycogen to produce ATP, with 1 molecule of glycogen or glucose producing 3 or 2 molecules of ATP, respectively. Anaerobic pathways provide an extremely rapid means of producing limited supplies of energy, while the aerobic pathways are more complex and thus slower but far more efficient.

Oxygen uptake provides a means of accurately measuring energy expenditure. $\dot{V}_{O_2}$ increases linearly with speed, and when exercising on a 10 percent slope, the energy expenditure will be approximately twice that on the flat. The horse is unique in its capacity to utilize oxygen, as seen by the high values for $\dot{V}_{O_2max}$ and the rapid kinetics of oxygen uptake. In all but the most intense exercise, aerobic pathways contribute the majority of the energy supply. It is this phenomenal ability to utilize oxygen that allows the athletic horse to work at extremely high intensities such as those during thoroughbred and standardbred races and also for prolonged durations such as during endurance rides of 160 km.

References

1. Åstrand P, Rodahl K: Textbook of Work Physiology. New York, McGraw-Hill, 1977.
2. Bursztein S, Elwyn DH, Askanazi J, et al: Energy Metabolism, Indirect Calorimetry, and Nutrition. Baltimore, Williams & Wilkins, 1989.
3. Snow DH, Harris RC: Effects of daily exercise on muscle glycogen in the thoroughbred horse. *In* Persson SGB, Lindholm A, Jeffcott LB (eds): Equine Exercise Physiology 3. Davis, Calif, ICEEP Publications, 1991, p 299.
4. McMiken DF: An energetic basis of equine performance. Equine Vet J 1983; 15:123.
5. Hodgson DR, Rose RJ, Allen JR, et al: Glycogen-depletion patterns in horses performing maximal exercise. Res Vet Sci 1984; 36:169.
6. Nimmo MA, Snow DH: Changes in muscle glycogen, lactate and pyruvate concentrations in the thoroughbred horse following maximal exercise. *In* Snow DH, Persson SGB, Rose RJ (eds): Equine Exercise Physiology. Cambridge, Granta Editions, 1983, p. 237.
7. Essén-Gustavsson B, Blomstrand E, Karlstron K, et al: Influence of diet on substrate metabolism during exercise. *In* Persson SGB, Lindholm A, Jeffcott LB (eds): Equine Exercise Physiology 3. Davis, Calif, ICEEP Publications, 1991, p 288.
8. Snow DH, Baxter P, Rose RJ: Muscle fiber composition and glycogen depletion in horses competing in an endurance ride. Vet Rec 1981; 108:374.
9. Hodgson DR, Rose RJ, Allen JR: Muscle glycogen depletion and repletion patterns in horses performing various distances of endurance exercise. *In* Snow DH, Persson, SGB, Rose RJ: Equine Exercise Physiology. Cambridge, Granta Editions, 1983, p 229.
10. White MG, Snow DH: Quantitative histochemical study of glycogen depletion in the maximally exercised thoroughbred. Equine Vet J 1987; 19:67.
11. Rose RJ, Ilkiw JE, Arnold KS, et al: Plasma biochemistry in the horse during 3-day event competition. Equine Vet J 1980; 12:229.
12. Rose RJ, Evans DL: Metabolic and respiratory responses to prolonged submaximal exercise in the horse. *In* Saltin B (ed): Biochemistry of Exercise VI. Chicago, Human Kinetics Publishers, 1986, p 459.
13. Seeherman HJ, Morris EA: Methodology and repeatability of a standardized treadmill exercise test for clinical evaluation of fitness in horses. Equine Vet J 1990; (suppl 9):20.
14. Meyers MC, Potter GD, Greene LW, et al: Physiologic and metabolic response of exercising horses to added dietary fat. *In* Proceedings of the 10th Equine Nutrition and Physiology Symposium, 1987, p 107.
15. Webb SP, Potter GD, Evans JW: Physiologic and metabolic response of race and cutting horses to added dietary fat. *In* Proceedings of the 10th Equine Nutrition and Physiology Symposium, 1987, p 115.
16. Jones DL, Potter GD, Greene LW, et al: Muscle glycogen concentrations in exercised horses at various body conditions and fed a control or fat-supplemented diet. *In* Proceedings of the 12th Equine Nutrition and Physiology Symposium, 1991, p 109.
17. Harkins JD, Morris GS, Tulley RT, et al: Effect of added dietary fat on racing performance in thoroughbred horses. Equine Vet J (in press).
18. Oldham SL, Potter GD, Evans JW, et al: Storage and mobilization of muscle glycogen in racehorses fed a control and high-fat diet. *In* Proceedings of the 11th Equine Nutrition and Physiology Symposium, 1989, p 57.
19. Topliff DR, Potter GD, Dutson JL, et al: Diet manipulation and muscle glycogen in the equine. *In* Proceedings of the 8th Equine Nutrition and Physiology Symposium 1983, p 119.
20. Moser LR, Lawrence LM, Novakofski J, et al: The effect of supplemental fat on exercising horses. *In* Proceedings of the 12th Equine Nutrition and Physiology Symposium, 1991, p 103.
21. Hoyt DF, Taylor CF: Gait and the energetics of locomotion in horses. Nature 1981; 292:239.
22. Thornton J, Pagan J, Persson S: The oxygen cost of weight loading and inclined treadmill exercise in the horse. In Gillespie JR, Robinson NE (eds): Equine Exercise Physiology 2. Davis, Calif, ICEEP Publications, 1987, p 206.
23. Evans DL, Rose RJ: Determination and repeatability of maximum oxygen uptake and other cardiorespiratory measurements in the exercising horse. Equine Vet J 1988; 20:94.
24. Rose RJ, Hodgson DR, Bayly WM, et al: Kinetics of $\dot{V}_{O_2}$ and $\dot{V}_{CO_2}$ in the horse and comparison of five methods for determination of maximum oxygen uptake. Equine Vet J 1990; (suppl 9):39.
25. Seeherman HJ, Morris EA: Application of a standardized treadmill exercise test for clinical evaluation of fitness in 10 thoroughbred horses. Equine Vet J 1990; (suppl 9):26.
26. Pagan JD, Hintz HF: Equine energetics 2: Energy expenditure in horses during submaximal exercise. J Anim Sci 1986; 63:822.
27. Hörnicke H, Meixner R, Pollmann U: Respiration in exercising horses. *In* Snow DH, Persson SGB, Rose RJ (eds): Equine Exercise Physiology. Cambridge, Granta Editions, 1983, p 7.
28. Hill AV, Long CNH, Lupton H: Muscular exercise, lactic acid, and

the supply and utilisation of oxygen, parts 1–3. Proc R Soc Lond 1924; 96:438.

29. Margaria R, Cerretelli P, Aghemo P, et al: Energy cost of running. J Appl Physiol 1963; 18:367.

30. Gottlieb-Vedi M, Essen-Gustavsson B, Persson SGB: Draught load and speed compared by submaximal tests on a treadmill. *In* Persson SGB, Lindholm A, Jeffcott LB (eds): Equine Exercise Physiology 3. Davis, Calif, ICEEP Publications, 1991, p 92.

31. Armsby HP: The Principles of Animal Nutrition. New York, Wiley, 1903, p 502.

32. Thomas DP, Fregin GF: Cardiorespiratory drift during exercise in the horse. Equine Vet J 1990; (suppl 9):61.

33. Saltin B: The physiological and biochemical basis of aerobic and anaerobic capacities in man: Effect of training and adaptation. *In* Russo P, Gass G (eds): Proceedings of the 5th Biennial Conference at Cumberland College on Health Science and Exercise, Nutrition, and Perf, Sydney, 1985, p 41.

34. Evans DL, Rose RJ: Maximum oxygen uptake in racehorses: Changes with training state and prediction from submaximal cardiorespiratory measurements. *In* Gillespie JR, Robinson NE (eds): Equine Exercise Physiology 2. Davis, Calif, ICEEP Publications, 1987, p 52.

35. Rose RJ, Hendrickson DK, Knight PK: Clinical exercise testing in the normal thoroughbred racehorse. Aust Vet J 1990; 67:345.

36. Harkins JD, Beadle RE, Kamerling SG: The correlation of running ability and physiological variables in thoroughbred horses. Equine Vet J 1993; 25:53.

37. Rose RJ, Hodgson DR, Kelso TB, et al: Maximum O_2 uptake, ox-

ygen debt and deficit and muscle metabolites in thoroughbred horses. J Appl Physiol 1988; 64:781.

38. Eaton MD, Rose RJ, Evans DL, et al: The assessment of anaerobic capacity of thoroughbred horses using maximal accumulated oxygen deficit. Aust Equine Vet 1992; 10:86.

39. Hermansen L, Medbø J: The relative significance of aerobic and anaerobic processes during maximal exercise of short duration. Med Sports Sci 1984; 17:56.

40. Medbø JI, Mohn AC, Tabata I, et al: Anaerobic capacity determined by maximal accumulated O_2 deficit. J Appl Physiol 1988; 64:50.

41. Scott CB, Roby FB, Lohman TG, et al: The maximally accumulated oxygen deficit as an indicator of anaerobic capacity. Med Sci Sports Exerc 1991; 23:618.

42. Gore CJ, Withers RT: Effects of exercise intensity and duration on postexercise metabolism. J Appl Physiol 1990; 68:2362.

43. Gaesser GA, Brooks GA: Metabolic bases of postexercise oxygen consumption: A review. Med Sci Sports Exerc 1984; 16:29.

44. Taylor CR: What determines the cost of locomotion? A closer look at what muscles do. *In* Proceedings of the 5th Scientific Meeting of the Association of Equine Sports Medicine. Lawrence, NJ, Veterinary Learning Systems, 1985, p 15.

45. Zuntz N, Hagemann O: Untersuchungen uber den Stoffwechsel des Pferdes bei Ruhe und Arbeit. Landwirtschaftl Jb 1898; 27(suppl III).

46. Evans DL, Silverman EB, Hodgson DR, et al: Gait and respiration in standardbred horses during pacing and galloping. Res Vet Sci (submitted).

5

Hematology and Biochemistry

R. J. ROSE AND D. R. HODGSON

Since the 1960s, evaluation of the hemogram and plasma or serum biochemistry has been a cornerstone in the assessment of the athletic horse. Initially, investigations focused on the hemogram,[1-3] which was assessed manually using the hemocytometer. In more recent years, automated techniques have become available for both hematologic and plasma or serum biochemical measurements, resulting in a wider range of available measurements as well as less expense per test. This has given rise to "profiles," where a large number of measurements are done on each blood sample and the clinician hopes that various abnormalities may become apparent to explain the loss of performance or the horse's ill health. While abnormalities may be found, in many cases it is difficult to interpret the findings in the absence of a detailed physical examination.

Hematology and plasma or serum biochemistry provide access to the function of a range of body systems and are crucial tools in assessment of the athletic horse. However, it also must be remembered that with a large number of analyses, one could be outside the normal range by chance and not because of any particular pathology. It is useful, therefore, to have a degree of scepticism about minor abnormalities found on a "profile" which may have no pathologic significance. Particular care must be taken in interpretation of changes in the red cell indices (erythrocyte numbers, hematocrit, and hemoglobin) because of the labile nature of the red cell pool.

In this chapter we will examine some of the factors that can affect the interpretation of the hemogram and biochemical profile, including technical considerations, as well as the influence of exercise and training.

Blood Collection Techniques and Factors Affecting Interpretation of Results

Blood samples are usually collected from the jugular vein using evacuated collection tubes (Vacutainer, Becton-Dickinson, Cockeysville, Md.) with double-ended needles. This system allows quick and simple sample collection. For hematology, blood is collected into tubes containing ethylenediaminetetraacetic acid (EDTA) as an anticoagulant, whereas lithium or ammonium heparin are used if plasma biochemical measurements are to be performed. Tubes containing fluoride/oxalate as an anticoagulant are preferred when either plasma glucose or lactate values are to be measured. With the latter anticoagulant, hemolysis is common, and plasma samples cannot be used for other measurements. Some laboratories prefer serum to plasma samples, and plain evacuated tubes are available for serum collection.

Hematologic measurements are affected by a variety of factors, including the time of day, the relationship to feeding, the demeanor of the horse, and the relationship to exercise, whereas plasma or serum biochemical values are less subject to change as a result of diurnal variations or feeding.

ATTITUDE OF THE HORSE

The horse's demeanor and degree of excitement can have a significant effect on the resting hemogram.[1,4-6] In one study of thoroughbred horses,[7] horses were classified as either placid, timid (forceful jugular pulse and elevated heart rate), apprehensive (horse pulled back during blood collection), or excited (resisted blood collection and moved about). While only the excited horses had increases in the erythrocyte and leukocyte counts when compared with the placid group,[7] we have noted small increases in red cell indices when horses show only slight degrees of apprehension. The critical factor appears to be the time required to collect the blood sample, since Persson and colleagues[8] found that erythrocytes were mobilized from the spleen 30 to 60 seconds after the intravenous injection of epinephrine in a study using [15]Cr-labeled erythrocytes. Thus it would seem that provided blood samples are collected within 30 seconds of entering a box stall, slight temperament changes will have little influence on the hemogram. However, it is important to note that in one study of endurance horses,[9] a group of five horses that were considered apprehensive during blood collection had hematocrits that were 21 percent higher than six quiet horses in samples collected every 2 weeks throughout 12 weeks of training. Thus care must be taken when interpreting changes in erythrocytes and leukocytes, particularly when values are higher than normal. It also should be anticipated that very placid horses may have values for red cell indices that are lower than mean values for the breed.

SAMPLE HANDLING

While there have been some reports[10] that the use of evacuated blood collection tubes could damage erythrocytes, extensive experience has shown that provided needles no smaller than 21-gauge diameter are used, the evacuated tubes are quite satisfactory.

Following blood collection, blood smears for cytologic examination should be made as soon as possible and preferably within 6 hours of sample collection. If blood is stored overnight prior to analysis, there may be a small increase in the hematocrit and mean cell hemoglobin associated with enlargement of the erythrocytes.[7] This increase is usually limited to no more than 0.01 to 0.02 liter/liter (1 to 2 percent) in hematocrit values.

Exposure of the blood samples to high environmental temperatures, such as may be found if blood samples are stored in a car exposed to direct sunlight, may result in some sample hemolysis, causing serum or plasma potassium values to be falsely elevated. Even without obvious hemolysis, sample storage can cause increases in serum or plasma potassium, and therefore, elevated potassium values should first be investigated as a methodologic problem rather than a pathologic one.

SAMPLE PROCESSING AND ACCURACY

In one investigation of the repeatability of measurements of hemoglobin, hematocrit, erythrocyte counts, and leukocyte counts, the precision was found to be ±5 percent in 36 duplicate measurements. Thus, in the normal ranges for each of these measurements when sequential sampling is performed, changes would have to be greater than 0.02 liter/liter (2 percent) for hematocrit, 7.5 g/liter (0.75 g/dl) for hemoglobin, 0.5 × 10^9/liter (500/μl) for leukocyte counts, and 0.5 × 10^{12}/liter (0.5 × 10^6/μl) for erythrocyte counts before the changes could be regarded as clinically significant. In addition to the precision related to the measuring equipment, daily variation in the red cell indices in individual horses must be taken into account. Persson[11] reported up to a 30 percent variation in the resting hemoglobin values of three standardbred trotters that had daily blood samples collected for 7 days. From these findings, it is clear that some caution is required when interpreting erythrocyte indices, particularly from a single blood sample. Repeated measurements may permit greater confidence in the findings.

Plasma and serum biochemical measurements are generally performed using autoanalyzers, and the accuracy of such equipment is generally ±5 percent. Measurement of electrolytes is generally performed using ion-selective electrodes in autoanalyzers rather than flame photometry, used previously. Carlson[12] has noted that because ion-selective electrodes measure the electrolyte concentration in the water component of the plasma or serum, values are 6 to 7 percent higher than electrolytes measured by flame photometry. Flame photometry measures electrolyte concentrations in millimoles per liter of plasma or serum, where the water content is 93 to 94 percent.

EFFECT OF FEEDING

When hay is fed, there may be substantial increases in hematocrit and plasma total protein, probably associated with substantial salivary fluid production.[13] The hematocrit and total protein remain elevated for several hours. In a study where a multiple regimen (feeding every 4 hours) was used, hematocrit and total protein remained constant, whereas a single large meal resulted in substantial fluid shifts out of the extracellular space.[14] In combination with the fluid shifts after the single feed, increases were found in plasma sodium and decreases in plasma potassium for several hours after feeding. Thus blood sampling should be avoided for at least 3 hours after feeding, particularly when a large feed is given or when there is access to substantial amounts of hay.

EFFECT OF PRIOR EXERCISE AND DIURNAL VARIATION

Exercise obviously has a major impact on red cell indices, there being mobilization of erythrocytes from the spleen under the influence of catecholamines. Following exercise, there is a gradual decrease in circulating erythrocytes over a period of 1 to 2 hours to return to preexercise values. The leukocyte population may change in response to prior exercise. Allen and Powell[15] reported that in thoroughbreds after morning exercise, blood

samples collected at 4:00 P.M. had higher leukocyte numbers as well as a higher proportion of neutrophils than samples collected in the morning prior to exercise. Plasma or serum potassium values may decrease substantially below normal resting values 1 to 2 hours after exercise, and following endurance exercise, they may decrease to values below 3 mmol/liter.[16]

The Resting Hemogram and Serum or Plasma Biochemical Variables

THE RESTING HEMOGRAM

The resting hemogram is widely used by equine practitioners in an attempt to detect abnormalities that are not discernible on clinical examination. While the normal range for an individual horse may be quite narrow, normal values for a breed fall into a broad range (Table 5–1). The normal ranges for adult thoroughbred horses in training are given in Table 5–2. Most of the hematologic values for the different breeds are similar, especially the total leukocyte count. However, as groups, the red cell indices from standardbred pacers and endurance horses are lower than those for thoroughbred racehorses. This may be due to differences in plasma volumes, since plasma volume expansion may occur during training in standardbred and endurance horses because of the extensive submaximal training that is included in their work schedule.

Virtually all mature athletic horses that do not have clinical abnormalities will have hemogram values within the ranges reported in Table 5–2. While a number of factors can affect the resting hemogram, as discussed earlier in this chapter, there are some reports that resting red cell indices that are lower than "normal" may adversely affect racing performance. An Australian study[17] indicated that thoroughbred horses with red cell indices falling more than 1 standard deviation below the mean did not win races at city race courses. This observation backed up a common clinical impression that horses with red cell indices below a certain "threshold" were likely to perform suboptimally. However, it is tempting for clinicians who cannot find any other abnormalities to falsely ascribe the cause of poor performance to minor deviations from breed means. Several studies in thoroughbred racehorses have failed to demonstrate any relationship between the hematocrit prior to racing and subsequent racing performance.[5,6]

USE OF THE RESTING HEMOGRAM TO DIAGNOSE PERFORMANCE PROBLEMS

Some veterinarians advocate regular collection of blood samples every 1 to 2 weeks from horses in training. This may be helpful in the diagnosis of subclinical abnormalities, because individual normal values will fall within a much narrower range than values for the breed. Thus a hematocrit of 0.34 liter/liter may be of clinical significance in a horse that normally has values between 0.38 and 0.42 liter/liter, whereas no clinical significance could be attributed to an isolated blood sample with a

Table 5-1. Normal Hematologic Values (Mean or Mean ± SD) Reported for Adult Horses at Rest[42]

Breed and training state	RBC (× 10^{12}/liter)	HB (g/liter)	PCV (liter/liter)	WBC (× 10^9/liter)
Thoroughbreds				
Macleod and Ponder				
2- and 3-year olds	10.8	141	—	—
More than 3 years old	11.6	154	—	—
Irvine				
2-year-old, not in training	—	125	—	—
More than 3 years old, not in training	8.1	134	0.43	—
2-year-old, in training	7.4	117	0.39	—
More than 3 years old, in training	6.7	114	0.36	—
Archer and Miller				
In training	9.5 + 1.1	147 ± 9	0.41 ± 0.07	8.4 ± 2.2
Brenon				
In training	6.8	139	0.43	—
Steel and Whitlock				
In training	9.7 ± 1.3	134 ± 19	0.42 ± 0.05	10.4
Sykes				
2-year-old, in training less than 1 month	10.2	136	0.40	—
2-year-old, in training 3 to 6 months	11.0	153	0.46	—
2-year-old, in training more than 6 months	11.1	155	0.46	—
3-year-old, in training less than 1 month	10.5	145	0.43	—
3-year-old, in training 3 to 6 months	11.0	157	0.47	—
3-year-old in training more than 6 months	11.0	156	0.46	—
More than 4 years old, in training less than 1 month	10.6	148	0.44	—
More than 4 years old, in training 3 to 6 months	10.9	151	0.45	—
More than 4 years old, in training more than 6 months	10.9	152	0.45	—
Tasker				
In training	—	145 ± 11	0.40 ± 0.04	—
Stewart, Clarkson, and Steel				
In training	10.3 ± 1.5	157 ± 18	0.40 ± 0.05	—
Allen, Archer, and Archer				
2-year-old	9.9 ± 1.0	146 ± 14	0.40 ± 0.04	—
3-year-old	9.7 ± 1.1	151 ± 15	0.41 ± 0.04	—
4-year-old	9.3 ± 1.0	150 ± 17	0.41 ± 0.05	—
More than 4 years old	8.8 ± 1.1	146 ± 16	0.40 ± 0.05	—
Stewart and Steel				
In training	9.5 ± 1.3	150 ± 20	0.40 ± 0.06	—
Schalm et al.	9.6 ± 1.1	152 ± 14	0.44 ± 0.04	9.8 ± 1.4
Stewart, Riddle, and Salmon				
In training	9.1 ± 1.0	142 ± 14	0.40 ± 0.04	8.4 ± 1.2
Allen and Powell				
Before training	9.2 ± 0.8	136 ± 10	0.37 ± 0.02	9.8 ± 1.3
After 5 months of training	10.2 ± 1.2	152 ± 17	0.41 ± 0.04	9.6 ± 1.1
Revington				
Racing	9.6 ± 0.9	151 ± 10	0.42 ± 0.03	8.9 ± 1.3
Standardbreds				
Steel and Whitlock	8.7 ± 1.4	124 ± 19	0.39 ± 0.04	9.8
Tasker	—	149 ± 15	0.39 ± 0.04	—
Schalm et al.	8.3 ± 0.7	137 ± 9	0.39 ± 0.03	7.9 ± 1.0
Arabian				
Schalm et al.	8.4 ± 1.2	138 ± 21	0.39 ± 0.05	9.5 ± 2.3
Quarter horse				
Tasker	—	139 ± 22	0.38 ± 0.05	—
Schalm et al.	9.1 ± 1.4	138 ± 17	0.40 ± 0.05	9.7 ± 1.3
Equitation and polo horses				
Tasker	—	132 ± 16	0.37 ± 0.05	—
Endurance horses				
Carlson	7.3	—	0.35	7.7
Carlson et al.	—	—	0.36 ± 0.03	7.5 ± 1.2
Rose	7.9 ± 0.5	130 ± 11	0.37 ± 0.03	8.8 ± 1.9
Cold-blooded breeds				
Schalm et al.	7.5	115	0.35	8.5

Source: From Rose, R.J. and Allen, J.R. Hematologic responses to exercise and training. Vet Clin North Am Equine Pract 1985;1:465.

Table 5-2. Values for the Resting Hemogram in Normal Adult Thoroughbred Horses

Value	Range	Mean
Erythrocytes ($\times 10^{12}$/liter)	7.0–11.0	9
Hemoglobin (g/liter)	110–170	140
PCV (liter/liter)	0.32–0.46	0.40
MCV (fl)	42–47	44
MCHC (g/liter)	330–380	350
MCH (pg)	14.0–17.0	15.5
Leukocytes ($\times 10^9$/liter)	6.0–11.0	8.5
Neutrophils ($\times 10^9$/liter)	2.5–6.5	4.5
Lymphocytes ($\times 10^9$/liter)	2.0–5.5	3.5
Monocytes ($\times 10^9$/liter)	0.2–0.8	0.5
Eosinophils ($\times 10^9$/liter)	0.1–0.4	0.2
Basophils ($\times 10^9$/liter)	0–0.3	0.1

hematocrit 0.34 liter/liter. While there is some variation in the resting red cell indices, samples collected after fast exercise or epinephrine administration show little variation on repeated sampling.[11]

Carlson and colleagues[18] demonstrated that horses presented with anemia (2 standard deviations below the mean) were most likely to have intercurrent disease rather than primary anemia. Therefore, if the red cell indices are low and there is no history of blood loss, low-grade infectious or inflammatory disease should be suspected rather than a primary disorder in red cell production.

Resting hematology also can be useful in the diagnosis and prognosis of viral respiratory infections.[19] In studies in Hong Kong, horses with equine herpesvirus type 1 infections had monocyte counts higher than 0.5×10^9/liter, together with higher neutrophil and lower lymphocyte counts than normal, during the first 1 to 2 days.[19,20] Within the first 4 to 5 days, the neutrophil count decreased and the lymphocytes increased, whereas the monocytes continued to remain elevated. The other notable finding was an increase in plasma viscosity, which together with changes in monocyte numbers persisted for several months in some horses following infection with equine herpesvirus.

The neutrophil/lymphocyte (N/L) ratio also has been used as an index of disease, and some veterinarians at the racetrack regard an increase in N/L ratio as an indicator of overtraining or "training off." While such changes often appear to provide an indication of "stress," the changes in N/L ratio reflecting increased plasma cortisol,[21] care must be taken in interpreting these changes because a number of factors, such as exercise and time of collection, can affect the results.

NORMAL RESTING SERUM OR PLASMA BIOCHEMISTRY

A number of measurements are included in the usual biochemical "profile" to determine whether some of the key body systems are dysfunctioning. In this section we will discuss the most common measurements and the

significance of abnormalities for athletic performance. The normal ranges for plasma or serum biochemical indices are given in Table 5–3.

Electrolytes. Abnormal electrolyte levels in the plasma will adversely affect athletic performance, and there have been some reports that even small deviations from a narrow concentration of serum electrolytes are associated with poor racing performance.[22] However, most electrolyte disturbances are associated with clinical diseases such as diarrhea, renal disease, and electrolyte losses in sweat. More recently, Harris and Snow[23] showed that some horses with chronic rhabdomyolysis had abnormal creatinine clearance ratios for various electrolytes, although plasma concentrations were within the normal ranges. Thus measurement of clearance ratios for the different electrolytes should be considered in cases of "tying up."

Sodium concentrations are maintained within narrow limits in the plasma, and abnormalities tend to reflect relative water excess (decreased plasma sodium) or relative water deficit (increased plasma sodium) rather than net changes in sodium balance. Sodium values in plasma are affected by the total exchangeable sodium and potassium concentrations as well as the total-body water.[24] Under conditions of marginal sodium intake, horses show excellent renal sodium conservation.[25] However, a study in exercised ponies demonstrated that decreased sweat production and a greater decrease in plasma volume occurred when there was dietary sodium restriction (5 mg/kg) compared with diets where sodium was available at 25 mg/kg of body weight.[26] Therefore, it is important to ensure that adequate sodium is available in the diets of most athletic horses, and salt licks or electrolyte supplements would seem to be important.

Table 5-3. Normal Ranges for Plasma Biochemical Measurements in Mature Performance Horses

Measurement	Normal range (SI units)	Normal range (traditional units)
Sodium	134–144 mmol/liter	133–144 mEq/liter
Potassium	3.2–4.2 mmol/liter	3.2–4.2 mEq/liter
Chloride	94–104 mmol/liter	94–104 mEq/liter
Total CO_2	26–34 mmol/liter	26–34 mEq/liter
Total protein	55–75 g/liter	5.5–7.5 g/dl
Albumin	26–38 g/liter	2.6–3.8 g/dl
Globulins	20–35 g/liter	2.0–3.5 g/dl
Fibrinogen	<4 g/liter	<400 mg/dl
AST (U/liter)	150–400	150–400
CK (U/liter)	100–300	100–300
LDH (U/liter)	<250	<250
Glucose	4–8 mmol/liter	70–140 mg/dl
GGT (U/liter)	10–40	10–40
AP (U/liter)	70–210	70–210
Urea	4–8 mmol/liter	24–48 mg/dl
Creatinine	100–160 μmol/liter	1.1–1.8 mg/dl
Calcium	2.7–3.3 mmol/liter	10.8–13.2 mg/dl
Phosphate	0.75–1.25 mmol/liter	2.3–3.9 mg/dl

Potassium is a critical electrolyte because it is involved in a range of body functions, in particular neuromuscular activity. As a grass eater, the horse has evolved ingesting large amounts of potassium, about two-thirds of which is excreted in urine.[25] Therefore, when a horse is in full training on a high-grain diet, it is possible for potassium deficiencies to develop. Less than 2 percent of the total-body potassium is contained in the extracellular fluid, and therefore, serum or plasma potassium values may not reflect changes in total-body potassium. For example, in a study by Tasker,[27] food and water restriction resulted in a total-body potassium loss of 4500 mmol (16 percent of total exchangeable potassium), but serum potassium decreased to only 3.5 mmol/liter. However, in general, plasma or serum potassium values less than 3 mmol/liter indicate decreases in whole-body potassium content. Because of the difficulty in estimating potassium deficits, measurement of red cell potassium has been proposed as a method for determining intracellular potassium changes.[28,29] While there is some evidence that large decreases in intracellular potassium can be detected using this method, in general, it is too variable to be clinically useful. Hyperkalemia is an unusual disorder in athletic horses, and if values greater than 4.5 mmol/liter are found, hemolysis or incorrect sample handling should be suspected first before a pathologic disorder is diagnosed. However, in a quarter horse, the syndrome of periodic hyperkalemic paralysis, which is a familial disorder now relatively common in the United States, should be at the top of the list of differential diagnoses.

It is important to note that substantial variation can occur in plasma potassium values during the course of a day, particularly in horses that may be fed only twice daily. A study by Clarke and colleagues[14] showed that 1 hour after a large meal (4 kg), the mean serum potassium values decreased from 3.5 to 2.9 mmol/liter, returned to prefeeding values by 4 hours, but at 5 and 7 hours after feeding increased to values of 4.0 and 4.2 mmol/liter, respectively.[14] From these results, it is clear that to interpret plasma or serum potassium values correctly, it is important to collect the blood samples at the same time of the day and under the same feeding conditions.

Chloride is the major anion of the extracellular fluid (ECF) and in the sweat. Most of the chloride ingested each day, which may reach 3000 mmol on alfalfa diets,[30] is excreted in the urine. Primary alterations in athletic horses result from losses of chloride in the sweat, particularly in horses involved in prolonged exercise. Thus hypochloremia found in a resting blood sample would be due most likely to sweat electrolyte losses. Hyperchloremia is seldom found but is most common in situations that produce metabolic acidosis, because plasma concentrations of bicarbonate and chloride are inversely related. Large increases in plasma chloride (>110 mmol/liter) are most common in cases of renal tubular acidosis.[31]

Most laboratories that use autoanalyzers measure *bicarbonate* as *total carbon dioxide* (TCO_2), which, on average, is about 5 percent higher than actual bicarbonate values because the TCO_2 includes dissolved CO_2. In general, low TCO_2 values indicate metabolic acidosis and high values signify metabolic alkalosis. Acid-base disturbances are extremely rare in resting samples from athletic horses. Low TCO_2 values are occasionally found if blood samples are collected within 90 minutes of high-intensity exercise because of elevated lactate concentrations. High TCO_2 values are mostly found as a result of excessive feeding of sodium bicarbonate or because of administration of bicarbonate as a so-called milkshake to horses prior to racing.[32] Metabolic alkalosis can sometimes be found in endurance horses following extensive sweat losses in response to the depletion of extracellular chloride.

Calcium and *phosphate* are maintained within a very narrow range, and normal plasma or serum concentrations tend to be maintained, even in the face of severe dietary calcium/phosphorus imbalances. Calcium is also lost in sweat, although the extent of the losses is much less than the other major electrolytes. Changes in these electrolytes are found mostly in cases of diarrhea or renal failure.

Muscle-Derived Enzymes. The most common enzymes that are used to indicate muscle damage are aspartate amino transferase (AST) and creatine kinase (CK). In addition, lactate dehydrogenase (LDH), which is a commonly available enzyme measurement on autoanalyzers, also increases following muscle damage, although it is less specific than AST or CK. While it has been generally assumed that increases in CK and AST indicate muscle damage because elevations in these enzymes are found in horses with rhabdomyolysis, some studies have suggested that the increases may be related to the exercise load.[33,34] In some cases, remarkable rises (>30,000 IU/liter) have been reported in endurance horses without clinical evidence of muscle disorders.[34] Changes in CK are more rapid than those in AST, where the long half-life in plasma may lead to values being increased for several weeks after a single bout of muscle damage. In contrast, CK values may decrease quickly over a period of 6 to 48 hours.[35] Because of the lack of correlation between clinical muscle damage and plasma or serum muscle-derived enzyme activities, one should be careful in making a diagnosis of a muscle disorder solely on the basis of elevations in CK and AST, particularly if the elevations are relatively small. However, Valberg and colleagues[36] have shown that in horses with recurrent exertional rhabdomyolysis there were subclinical episodes of rhabdomyolysis which resulted in increases in AST and CK without clinical evidence of disease.

Liver Enzymes. The most commonly measured indicator of liver dysfunction is gamma-glutamyl transferase (GGT), although both alkaline phosphatase (AP) and sorbitol dehydrogenase (SDH) are also useful measurements when liver disease is suspected. In the acute stages of hepatocellular dysfunction, as well as in biliary tract obstruction, the liver enzymes will become elevated, AP showing the greatest elevation when there is biliary obstruction. Liver disease is uncommon in athletic horses but can be a cause weight loss and poor performance in areas where horses have access to plants with high concentrations of pyrrolizidine alkaloids. In racehorses in training, there appears to be a syndrome where routine blood sampling reveals elevations in GGT activity (in some cases to values greater than 100 IU/liter). In these horses, there is no clinical evidence of liver disease. Although many horses with elevated liver enzymes race successfully, in some cases the increase in GGT activity is associated with decreased athletic performance. The increased GGT values often decrease when the horses have a change of diet or are put out to pasture.

Protein Measurements. Measurement of total protein, albumin, globulins, and fibrinogen provide an index of hydration status, as well as indices of infection, inflammation, increased protein loss, or decreased protein production. Hyperproteinemia usually is the result of dehydration in athletic horses, but because of the large normal range (see Table 5–3), it may be difficult to detect protein increases in horses that have normal protein values in the range 55 to 60 g/liter. It is important to remember that a high plasma protein concentration also may be caused by elevations in globulins or fibrinogen. Hypoproteinemia is uncommon in athletic horses, and if it occurs, horses should be investigated by seeking possible sites of protein loss (gastrointestinal tract, kidney), which is a much more common cause of hypoproteinemia than decreased protein production. Fibrinogen is a sensitive index of inflammatory foci within the body and is a useful screening measurement in any athletic horse with poor performance to ensure that a low-grade infection is not the cause of the problem.

Measurements of Renal Function. Creatinine and urea are indices of renal function, but both measurements can be increased in response to prerenal factors, particularly dehydration and exercise. Alterations in resting levels of creatinine and urea are unusual in athletic horses, and some changes occur with training, there being modest increases in plasma or serum urea concentrations (1 to 2 mmol/liter), probably as a result of increases in dietary protein.

Hematologic Changes Associated with Exercise

THE ERYTHROCYTES

The red cell pool is under the direct influence of catecholamine concentrations, so exercise has a variable effect on red cell indices, depending on the speed and duration of the exercise bout. The splenic erythrocyte reserve is impressive, the spleen having the capacity to store up to 50 percent of the total red cells.[37] The splenic capacity for red cell storage and subsequent release during exercise is related to the type of horse, draught horses having much lower relative splenic weights than thoroughbred horses.[38] Splenic capacity also appears to alter in response to increasing age, since several studies in trotters have found that the postexercise hematocrit

and total circulating hemoglobin increase progressively from 1 to 3 years of age.[39–41]

There is a linear increase in hematocrit with increasing exercise intensity, up to exercise intensities approaching three-quarter pace (90 to 100 percent $\dot{V}_{O_2max}$).[42] In adult athletic horses, the maximal hematocrit is usually in the range 0.60 to 0.65 liter/liter, there being mean values of 0.61 liter/liter in thoroughbred racehorses. While most of this increase is related to splenic erythrocyte release, there are also substantial fluid shifts out of the plasma during exercise, and therefore, some of the increase in hematocrit is due to fluid movement.[43]

The increase in oxygen transport capacity associated with the erythrocyte release during exercise is one of the important factors in the horse's high aerobic capacity.[44] However, an upper point must be reached where the improved oxygen-carrying capacity is offset by an increase in blood viscosity, probably accounting for the dramatic effects on performance in horses with red cell hypervolemia.[39] Studies in splenectomized horses have shown a considerable reduction in exercise capacity.[37,45] Because of the reduced cardiac output, Persson and Bergsten[45] proposed that the spleen acts as a cardiovascular reserve to maintain ventricular filling at high heart rates.

Changes also occur in the erythrocytes themselves, there being small decreases in mean corpuscular volume and increases in mean corpuscular hemoglobin and mean corpuscular hemoglobin concentration. Erythrocytes are also more resistant to osmotic stress, but the cell shape and degree of deformity are unaffected.[46] It has been suggested that a large number of erythrocytes released during exercise are irregular, and these have been termed *echinocytes*.[47] However, a more recent study has found that the percentage of echinocytes is quite low and probably not of physiologic importance in altering oxygen delivery.[46]

MEASUREMENT OF TOTAL RED CELL VOLUME

In a number of studies, Persson has reported that there is a good correlation between exercise capacity of standardbred trotters and total hemoglobin or red cell volume.[11,37,40,41] Horses with values more than 2 standard deviations outside the mean had significantly lower exercise capacity, and Persson reported red cell hypervolemia as a cause of poor performance in "overtrained" horses. Measurement of total hemoglobin or total red cell volume is relatively simple and is based on the use of Evans blue, a dye that enables measurement of plasma volume using the technique of dye dilution. If the maximal hematocrit is measured after intense exercise, then the total blood volume, plasma volume, and red cell volume can be calculated. Persson[48] has reported the steps in measurement of red cell volume as follows:

1. Collect a venous blood sample (20 ml) into a tube containing EDTA within 1 to 2 minutes of near-maximal exercise so that there is complete mobilization of splenic erythrocytes. This sample is used for deter-

mination of hematocrit, as well as providing plasma for measurement of the spectrophotometric background (blank plasma).

2. A 1% (1 g/100 ml) solution of Evans blue dye is made up, and a dose of 0.25 to 0.40 mg/kg is injected intravenously via a catheter. This is equivalent to approximately 15 ml for a 450-kg horse. Because it is important to measure the exact amount of dye administered, the syringe is weighed before and after the injection.

3. Blood (20 ml) is sampled from the contralateral jugular vein 15 minutes after injection of the dye and collected into tubes containing EDTA. The blood is centrifuged, and the plasma from this sample and the blank is stored overnight in a refrigerator and then recentrifuged to reduce the plasma turbidity prior to determination of the plasma extinctions by spectrophotometry.

4. The extinctions are determined at a spectrophotometer wavelength of 620 nm. The difference between the blank and dye readings (E_x) is used for calculation of the degree of dye dilution. The plasma volume (dye dilution space) is calculated by comparison with the net extinction value (E_0) of a known dye concentration (20 μg in 25 ml of horse plasma, prepared for each new batch of dye) according to the formula

$$\text{Plasma volume (liters)} = \frac{E_0 \times EB}{E_x \times 0.8}$$

where EB is the amount of dye injected (in grams) and 0.8 is the dilution factor of the standard dye concentration.

5. The total blood volume is calculated using plasma volume and the postexercise hematocrit (PCV) according to the formula

$$\text{Total blood volume (liters)} = \frac{\text{plasma volume}}{100 - \text{PCV}} \times 100$$

The total red cell volume (CV, liters) is the difference between the total blood volume and the plasma volume. This value must be adjusted to body weight and is expressed as milliliters per kilogram.

Normal values for total red cell volume vary depending on age, with values as low as 44 ml/kg in yearlings increasing up to mean values of 63 ml/kg at 3 years of age and 74 ml/kg at 4 years of age for standardbred trotters.[48] Persson reported values of 89 ± 9 ml/kg for mature thoroughbred racehorses.

THE LEUKOCYTES

The proportions of leukocytes change depending on the intensity and duration of exercise, as well as the degree of "stress" to which the horse is subjected (Fig. 5–1). The total leukocyte count increases by 10 to 30 percent depending on the intensity and duration of exercise, but

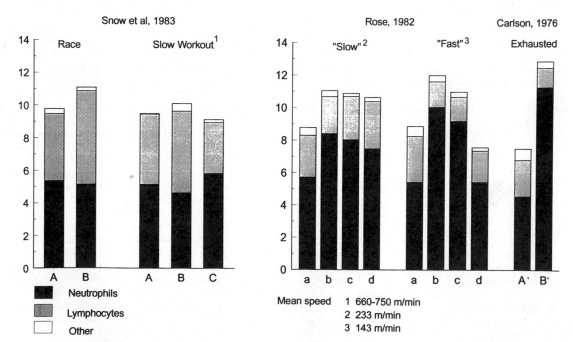

Figure 5-1. *Changes in leukocyte count after exercise. 1, Data from Snow and colleagues[51] in thoroughbreds: A = before exercise; B = immediately after exercise; C = 3 hours after exercise. 2, Data from Rose[50] in endurance horses: a = before ride; b = immediately after the ride; c = 30 minutes after ride, d = 24 hours after the ride. 3, Data from Carlson and colleagues[49] in endurance horses: A' = rest; B' = exhausted horses, after the ride.*

the extent of the increase is not as dramatic as for the erythrocyte indices.[21,49–31] Long-distance, low- to moderate-intensity exercise produces a leukocytosis that results from a neutrophilia and lymphopenia.[49,50,52] The extent of the leukocytosis is related to increases in plasma cortisol,[53] and speed is a significant factor affecting the extent of the neutrophilia and lymphopenia, with horses completing an endurance ride at a faster speed having a higher N/L ratio than slower horses. Under conditions of severe stress, such as is found in exhausted endurance horses, there is not only a greater degree of neutrophilia but also the appearance of band-form neutrophils[49] (see Fig. 5–1).

Maximal exercise results in a different leukocyte response than endurance exercise because of release of lymphocytes sequestered by the spleen. There is only a small increase in leukocytes due to an increase in lymphocyte numbers and a resultant decrease in the N/L ratio.[46,51] Lymphocytosis is transient after maximal exercise, lasting only a few hours. After this, the lymphocyte numbers decrease, resulting in an increase in the N/L ratio coincident with an increase in the plasma cortisol level.

Changes in Plasma or Serum Biochemical Values Associated with Exercise

ELECTROLYTES AND ACID-BASE STATUS

Maximal Exercise. With brief periods of high-intensity exercise, there are transient changes in plasma electrolyte concentrations, some of which may be quite marked. Following racing over distances varying from 1200 to 2400 m, similar changes occur in electrolyte and acid-base status. Sodium increases largely as a result of fluid movement out of the extracellular space. Potassium increases dramatically at high exercise loads, reaching values greater than 10 mmol/liter.[54,55] This increase in potassium has been thought to be due mainly to an accumulation of hydrogen ions in active muscle, resulting in a decrease in the reuptake by the fibers and an impairment of the Na^+,K^+-ATPase pump.[55] However, the increased plasma potassium is transient, and most studies where samples have been collected several minutes after maximal exercise have shown potassium values within the normal resting range.[56–58] Nonetheless, it has been proposed that the decreased muscle membrane potential resulting from the decreased intracellular potassium concentration, together with the increased extracellular concentration, may be a contributing factor to fatigue during high-intensity exercise.[59]

A consistent finding in most of the studies of high-intensity exercise is that despite the increase in total protein and plasma sodium, reflecting fluid movement out of the extracellular fluid, no change occurs in chloride values.[56–58] This may be due to large increases in another strong anion, lactate, with exchange of chloride across muscle cell membranes.

Bicarbonate or total carbon dioxide concentrations decrease following racing to the range 5 to 10 mmol/liter.[57,58,60] This decrease in bicarbonate is coincident with a large increase in hydrogen ion concentration, the venous blood pH decreasing to values less than 7.0.[57] However, lactate metabolism after exercise results in a rapid increase in pH and bicarbonate, with values returning to within the normal range by 90 minutes after exercise.

Prolonged Low-Intensity Exercise. Endurance exercise results in substantial sweat losses of electrolytes because horse sweat is hypertonic relative to plasma.[61,62] During the course of an endurance ride in hot conditions, it is likely that horses may lose between 5 and 10 percent of their body weight.[63] The sweat electrolyte losses result in variable changes in plasma or serum electrolyte concentrations because of the associated alterations in total-body water. Plasma or serum electrolyte changes are known to be influenced by alterations in exchangeable sodium and potassium as well as total-body water.[24] Plasma sodium has been reported to be unchanged, decreased, or increased depending on the conditions and duration of endurance ride.[64–69] In one study,[69] despite an estimated 5900-mmol loss of sodium, chiefly in sweat, plasma sodium concentrations increased from 140 to 148 mmol/liter. Moderate decreases in plasma or serum potassium have been reported following endurance exercise,[64–68,70] although small increases also have been found.[16,69,71] Despite the modest changes in plasma or serum potassium values, decreases in whole-body potassium content are likely to occur when there are substantial sweat losses, although the falls are probably only 25 to 50 percent of the decline in total exchangeable sodium. Chloride losses during endurance exercise may be substantial, because it is the principal anion lost in the sweat. During endurance exercise, most investigators have reported a decrease in plasma or serum chloride values, which in some cases may result in decreases of 10 to 15 mmol/liter.[65,72] Because of the substantial chloride losses, there may be renal retention of bicarbonate, giving rise to metabolic alkalosis.[49,73] The maximal increase in bicarbonate concentration usually is in the range 3 to 5 mmol/liter. In other cases, no change in acid-base status or a slight metabolic acidosis occurs, resulting from small increases in plasma lactate.[66] These studies led to the conclusion that administration of bicarbonate, either as a treatment or as a feed supplement, was contraindicated in endurance horses.

Speed and Endurance Phase (Day 2) of a 3-Day Event. During the speed and endurance phases of 3-day events, horses exercise over distances of around 23 to 25 km at speeds varying from 200 to 700 m/min. The electrolyte alterations found are similar to those during endurance exercise, there being variable sweat losses of fluid and electrolytes.[74] Acid-base changes reflect the different intensities of exercise during a 3-day event, there being a slight metabolic alkalosis after the second roads-and-track phases.[75] At the conclusion of the cross-country, horses had a mean base deficit of 8.5 mmol/liter due to lactic acidosis.[75]

FLUID BALANCE

Maximal Exercise. During maximal exercise, there are acute shifts of fluid out of the extracellular into the intracellular spaces, reflected by increases in total protein and albumin.[57,58] The extent of the fluid shift and fluid loss appears to be related to the duration of intense exercise, because the increase in total protein is greater for races longer than 1600 m than for those of 1200 and 1400 m.[57] In most cases, these changes in fluid movement are short-lived, there being a return to preexercise values by 30 minutes after maximal exercise.[58] The extent of fluid loss in sweat is minimal in most racehorses, there being a 5- to 10-kg body weight loss after races. However, in horses that are transported in hot conditions prior to exercise, there may be more extensive sweat losses associated with the transport. These losses may be worsened if the horses are excitable and sweat profusely due to catecholamine release.

Prolonged, Low-Intensity Exercise. During the initial part of prolonged exercise, there is an increase in plasma volume. Substantial fluid losses occur during endurance exercise, with body weight losses of 5 to 8 percent,[69,76] translating into fluid losses of 25 to 40 liters. The extent of the fluid loss depends on the ambient temperature and humidity, with the most extreme sweat losses found during hot, humid conditions. Kerr and Snow,[62] in a study of sweat loss during exercise, concluded that the average rate of body weight loss was 1.5 percent per hour during endurance exercise under warm conditions. However, it is interesting that in a range of studies of endurance exercise, the fluid losses appear to be greater during the early stages of exercise, the increase in plasma total protein and albumin being much greater from preride to midride than from midride to the end of the ride.[16,72,73] This decreased rate of fluid loss with increasing exercise duration is probably due to a decrease in the rate of sweat production which occurs with increasing exercise duration.[62]

RENAL RESPONSES TO EXERCISE

Increases in both urea and creatinine are found in response to high- and low-intensity exercise.[16,56,58,65,77] These traditional indices of renal function are also affected by prerenal factors, such as hemoconcentration. Additionally, creatinine increases during exercise as a result of increased phosphocreatine turnover, and therefore, increases in plasma or serum creatinine cannot be used as an indication of reduced glomerular filtration rate. After maximal exercise, creatinine concentrations remain elevated for 60 minutes, even though plasma total protein concentrations return to normal.[58]

Studies of renal blood flow, glomerular filtration rate, and urine flow during maximal and submaximal exercise have shown a decrease in renal blood flow and glomerular filtration rate, which was most severe during high-intensity exercise, there being a 70 percent decrease in renal blood flow.[78] The alteration in renal function is short-lived, there being a return to normal shortly after cessation of exercise.[78] However, after prolonged exercise where there has been extensive fluid loss in the sweat, the reduction in renal blood flow and glomerular filtration rate may continue because acute renal failure is a common complication of exhaustion in endurance horses. This will be reflected by persistent elevations in plasma creatinine and urea concentrations.

RESPONSE OF MUSCLE-DERIVED ENZYMES TO EXERCISE

Modest increases in muscle-derived enzymes are found in the plasma or serum in response to low- and high-intensity exercise. Following high-intensity exercise, increases are found in the activities of CK, AST, and LDH.[57,58,79] Increases in these enzymes also have been found after show jumping.[80] These increases have been suggested to reflect increases in mitochondrial membrane permeability[79] rather than muscle damage. The muscle-derived enzymes show greater elevations as a result of more prolonged, low-intensity exercise, such as endurance riding and day 2 of 3-day events.[16,74] In one study of endurance exercise, horses completing an endurance ride at an average speed of 234 m/min had mean CK values that were double those of a slow group that averaged 144 m/min. Thus both exercise duration and intensity are important in the increases in the muscle-derived enzymes that occur during exercise. In one interesting report, CK activity increased to values in excess of 30,000 IU/liter despite no evidence of clinical muscle damage.[34] In this case, the AST activity was about 6,000 IU/liter prior to exercise and did not increase further. From these results it is clear that increases in muscle-derived enzymes do not necessarily indicate clinically apparent muscle damage in exercising horses, particularly in horses after endurance exercise.

BLOOD LACTATE AND GLUCOSE CHANGES WITH EXERCISE

Lactate increases in plasma or blood because of diffusion and/or active transport from active skeletal muscle. Lactate is usually measured in plasma, and concentrations are about 40 to 50 percent higher than those in blood, although the relationship is quite variable. During all types of exercise, lactate is produced in working muscle, but high lactate concentrations do not occur until higher exercise intensities are reached. Increases in lactate occur in muscle when there is insufficient oxygen available to oxidize pyruvate in the mitochondria. To free nicotinamide-adenine-dinucleotide ($NADH_2$) of its hydrogen, pyruvate can accept the H_2 to form lactate. Lactate increases also occur when there is stimulation of glycogenolysis, with the result that an increase in pyruvate causes a rise in lactate because of a mass-action effect.[81] Thus plasma lactate increases do not necessarily signify a lack of oxygen availability.

With maximal exercise, such as thoroughbred racing, there is substantial lactate production. Over distances of 1200 to 2400 m, there is little difference in plasma lactate concentrations after racing, values ranging from 25 to 30 mmol/liter.[56,57] Values after trotting races are usually a little lower.[82] In contrast, endurance riding results in little increase in plasma lactate concentrations, values usually being less than 2 mmol/liter.[66–68,71] After the cross-country phase of a 3-day event, blood lactate values of 8 mmol/liter were found.[75] However, the lactate concentrations after the second roads-and-track phase were only 2 mmol/liter, indicating that aerobic metabolism was predominant for most of the exercise on day 2 of 3-day events.

Plasma glucose generally increases with all forms of exercise because of stimulation of hepatic glycogenolysis. However, with prolonged exercise, glucose concentrations will decrease as a result of liver glycogen depletion.[65] After short-term exercise, the degree of increase in plasma glucose concentrations is related to the intensity of exercise, with peak values in the range of 10 to 12 mmol/liter (180 to 206 mg/dl) found after racing.[57,58,83,84] The extent of the increase in plasma glucose concentration is probably related to the degree of sympathetic activity, which is related to the intensity of exercise.[85]

CHANGES IN FATTY ACIDS, TRIGLYCERIDES, AND GLYCEROL WITH EXERCISE

In human long-distance athletes, it has been estimated that at the conclusion of a marathon, nonesterified fatty acids (NEFAs) may provide as much as 90 percent of the total energy requirements.[86] Because of the delay in mobilization of NEFAs from fat depots, NEFAs are not important energy sources for short-term exercise, such as quarter horse, standardbred, and thoroughbred racing. The highest concentrations of plasma NEFAs have been reported after endurance exercise in horses,[67,68,87,88] although high concentrations also were found after the second roads-and-track phase of a 3-day event.[74] The predominant NEFAs are oleic, palmitic, linoleic, and linolenic acids.[87]

Care must be taken in interpreting NEFA concentrations in plasma because it cannot be assumed that high concentrations always reflect increased utilization of fat as an energy source. If there is mobilization of fat reserves followed by inhibition of fat utilization due to high lactate concentrations,[89] plasma concentrations may be high even though fat is not being utilized. Lypolysis results in elevated concentrations of NEFAs and glycerol,[66–68] with NEFAs being utilized by muscle and glycerol acting as a substrate for hepatic gluconeogenesis.[90] The triglycerides increase later in the exercise period than the NEFAs,[74] probably because besides being oxidized in skeletal muscle the NEFAs act as precursors for triglycerides.[63]

Hormonal Responses to Exercise

CATECHOLAMINES

Epinephrine and norepinephrine, secreted by the adrenal medulla, have important roles in increasing oxygen delivery during exercise by enhancing cardiac output, splenic erythrocyte release, and skeletal muscle blood flow. Catecholamine release is also important in the mobilization of glucose from hepatic glycogen stores. Studies in horses have shown a relationship between exercise intensity and circulating catecholamine concentrations,[85] catecholamine concentrations increasing significantly at intensities greater than half-pace. While epinephrine and norepinephrine concentrations increase in parallel, the extent of increase in epinephrine is greater than that in norepinephrine.[85] A close relationship also was found between catecholamine concentrations and plasma lactate, the relationship being exponential.[85] The half-life of catecholamines in plasma is very short, being around 30 seconds.[85] The catecholamines are intimately involved in maximal performance, several studies indicating that beta-adrenergic blocking agents decrease exercise capacity.[91,92]

GLUCOCORTICOIDS

Of the glucocorticoids, cortisol is the main one studied in examinations of changes in plasma hormone levels in response to exercise. There is substantial diurnal variation in the plasma cortisol and cortisone concentrations, values being highest in the morning and lowest in the late afternoon.[93] The half-life of cortisol in the horse is about 1 to 2 hours. A study in the United Kingdom[21] showed that the N/L ratio provided some indication of the plasma cortisol levels, higher N/L values indicating higher plasma cortisol concentrations. However, in another study, no relationship was found between absolute neutrophil and lymphocyte counts and resting plasma cortisol concentrations.[94]

Exercise results in an increase in plasma cortisol, and the extent of the increase is similar following maximal and submaximal exercise.[95,96] Exercise results in a two- to threefold increase in cortisol,[68,71,94–97] with values returning to preexercise levels by 4 hours after an acute exercise bout.[94] Cortisol values are similar after racing over distances varying from 1200 to 2400 m.[57] While the cortisol response to exercise is similar despite differing exercise conditions, one study that compared cortisol values in horses after show jumping, cross-country, trotting and galloping, and endurance riding showed that cortisol values were similar except for endurance riding, where the plasma cortisol level was about 30 percent higher than in other athletic activities.[98] In contrast, adrenocorticotropic hormone (ACTH) concentrations increase linearly with exercise load,[94] peak values being related to exercise intensity, whereas cortisol reaches peak concentrations about 30 minutes after exercise.[94]

INSULIN AND GLUCAGON

Associated with the increased rate of glycogenolysis in response to exercise, there is a decrease in plasma insulin and an increase in glucagon concentrations.[67,68,94,97,99] The lowered plasma concentrations are due to decreased insulin secretion, control being mediated via the sympathetic nervous system rather than being dependent on plasma glucose concentrations.[94] Despite a wide range of plasma glucose concentrations after different durations and intensities of exercise, there is invariably a decrease in insulin concentrations. However, in one study of endurance exercise, there was a close relationship ($r = 0.89$) between plasma insulin and plasma glucose concentrations.[97] Thus, in prolonged exercise, where plasma glucose levels can decrease substantially, there may be a more direct association between plasma glucose and insulin values. While all forms of exercise appear to depress insulin concentrations in plasma, following exercise there is a rebound hyperinsulinemia.[94]

Plasma glucagon concentrations have been measured chiefly during endurance exercise at speeds of 3 to 4 m/s,[66,67] although there is a report of values during the higher speeds of the Arab Horse Society's marathon race, where speeds may average 7 to 8 m/s.[77] In the latter study, the glucagon values were substantially higher than during endurance exercise and were 20 times those taken prior to exercise.

RENIN-ANGIOTENSIN-ALDOSTERONE

If horses are fed multiple small feeds each day, there is little change in either plasma aldosterone or renin concentrations.[14] However, a large feed results in fluid movement out of the extracellular space, and the resultant decrease in plasma volume is associated with a substantial rise in plasma renin for 0.5 to 3 hours, followed by an increase in aldosterone from 3 to 7 hours after feeding.[14] While aldosterone concentrations increase following exercise,[100,101] plasma renin level shows only a small rise.[102]

THYROID HORMONES

In reviewing the literature from a range of species, Thornton[103] concluded that single bouts of exercise, except where prolonged, may produce little change in free thyroxine or in the turnover of thyroid hormone. Optimal thyroid function is necessary for oxidation of NEFAs during prolonged exercise, but the importance of normal thyroid function during high-intensity exercise is not known. Thornton[103] concluded that the thyroxine levels necessary for optimal athletic performance may be inversely related to environmental temperature.

ATRIAL NATRIURETIC PEPTIDE

Atrial natriuretic peptide (ANP) is a hormone that is released from the walls of the atria in response to changes in atrial dimensions. The hormone causes rapid and profound vasodilation and natriuresis. Concentrations of ANP increase two- to threefold during submaximal exercise and five- to sixfold during maximal exercise.[104]

Hematologic, Biochemical, and Hormonal Changes Associated with Training

HEMATOLOGIC CHANGES WITH TRAINING

Racehorse Training. Training results in an increase in the total erythrocyte pool, Persson[11] estimating that the total hemoglobin, measured using Evans blue dye dilution,

increases by 30 percent in 2-year-old trotters during the training period prior to their first race. While some of this increase may be an age effect, it is clear that training produces an increase in the total-body capacity for oxygen carriage. The increase in total hemoglobin is not necessarily reflected in increases in resting red cell indices. In thoroughbreds, training has been reported to result in increases in the resting hematocrit, hemoglobin, and red cell count.[3,15,105] In the main, the increases in red cell indices are modest, there being a mean increase in hematocrit of between 0.04 and 0.06 liter/liter in most studies. This increase is similar to the daily variation that can be found on repeated sampling,[11] and therefore, the physiologic significance of the finding is questionable. The temperament of the horse may be one factor responsible for the increase in red cell variables because horses often become more excitable and difficult to handle as training progresses. Thus the reported increases in hematocrit, hemoglobin, and red cell count could be due to more excitement at the time of sample collection rather than reflecting an increase in total red cell mass. Clarkson[106] found that differences in the training response of the hemogram were related to the hematocrit values prior to the beginning of training. Horses with initial hematocrit values less than 0.40 liter/liter had significant increases in red cell variables following training, whereas those with hematocrit values less than 0.40 liter/liter prior to training had mean resting hematocrit increases from 0.36 to 0.43 liter/liter. Thus, while small increases in resting hemoglobin, hematocrit, and erythrocyte numbers may occur during training, such changes are too small to be used reliably as an index of increasing fitness.

The levels of 2,3-diphosphoglycerate (2,3-DPG) show small increases as a result of training.[107] The authors of this study concluded that in comparison with other effects on the oxyhemoglobin dissociation curve, such as blood pH, partial pressure of CO_2, and temperature, the increase in 2,3-DPG is of little significance for oxygen transport.

Persson and colleagues[39,108] have characterized a syndrome of red cell hypervolemia in Swedish standardbred trotters which appears to be due to overtraining. These horses are diagnosed because, after Evans blue dye administration, they have increased total red cell volume. The cause of the red cell hypervolemia is unclear, although Persson, Larsson, and Lindholm[108] have reported adrenocortical insufficiency. Horses with red cell hypervolemia have reduced exercise capacity, possibly because of increased blood viscosity with resultant decreased oxygen uptake.[109] Whether red cell hypervolemia occurs as a result of other training programs is unknown, but we have not found such cases in more than 150 racehorses (thoroughbred and standardbred) examined for poor performance using treadmill exercise testing. However, some veterinarians working at the racetrack report that horses with clinical signs of overtraining may show an increase in hematocrit and a decrease in N/L ratio in blood samples collected at rest.

There are few changes in the leukocytes during racehorse training. The total and differential leukocyte counts are similar before and after training in thoroughbreds.[15] In a study in which neutrophil and lymphocyte counts were performed before and 4 hours after a standardized exercise test, there was no change as a result of training.

Endurance Training. Endurance horses have lower resting red cell indices than thoroughbred racehorses.[42] There may be a reduction in hematocrit with training in endurance horses due to an expansion of plasma volume. McKeever and colleagues[110] reported an expansion of plasma volume by about 25 percent after as little as 1 week of training. However, a study by Rose and Hodgson[9] reported no significant changes in hematology during 12 weeks of endurance training. Neither red cell indices nor the total or differential leukocyte count changed when samples were collected every 2 weeks. Undoubtedly changes in plasma volume do occur,[110] but these must be masked by similar changes in red cell mass.

Similarly to racehorse training, the total leukocyte count is unchanged with training, and there is no alteration in the proportions of neutrophils, lymphocytes, and monocytes. It is clear that alterations in the proportions of leukocytes indicate little about the stage of fitness.

Changes in Plasma or Serum Biochemical and Hormonal Values Associated with Training

There are few changes in resting biochemical values as a result of training. While some studies have found statistically significant changes in some plasma biochemical measurements,[111,112] most of these changes are small and of little biologic significance. Certainly, there are no resting biochemical measurements that provide a clear indication of increasing fitness.[113] While there is a trend toward a decrease in the activities of some of the muscle-derived enzymes with increasing fitness,[111] the findings are variable, and results between studies are inconsistent.[9,111–113]

Resting acid-base and electrolyte status does not change with training status,[9,112,113] although postexercise plasma lactate levels decrease following training in response to a standardized submaximal exercise test.[113] Measurement of plasma or whole-blood lactate concentration following such a test is the most reliable biochemical indicator of increasing fitness, although exercise testing on a treadmill is necessary for repeatable results, with measurement of derived indices such as the speed at which lactate reaches a value of 4 mmol/liter[41] (V_{LA4}). The V_{LA4}, also called the *point of onset of blood lactate accumulation,* increases with increasing fitness and is a useful objective index of improvements in fitness. The use of lactate measurements in the assessment of fitness is discussed further in Chapter 12.

Few studies have been performed on hormonal changes as a result of training. While there is some suggestion of alterations in adrenocortical function with overtraining,[108] other studies have not found any alterations.[94] In the latter study, there were no differences in cortisol or ACTH concentrations before and after training in response to a standardized treadmill test. Furthermore, insulin concentrations were unaffected by training, and an ACTH stimulation test produced similar results before and after training. Training does produce an increase in thyroxine secretion,[114] although the significance of this finding is unclear.

Conclusions

Hematology and plasma or serum biochemical measurements are of vital importance in assessment of the athletic horse. Blood sampling is simple and relatively inexpensive while providing information about the function of a number of body systems. However, because the physiologic state of the horse can influence many of the measurements, care must be taken in interpretation. Additionally, repeatable results from resting red cell indices are difficult to achieve, although postexercise results are quite consistent. In horses with suspected anemia, sampling of blood following fast exercise would help in determining the significance of resting red cell indices.

Simple guides to the state of fitness and performance capacity cannot be achieved by the use of blood and plasma/serum measurements. However, routine monitoring of hematology and biochemistry during training may provide a mechanism for determining minor disturbances in an individual horse, where the normal range is much narrower than for the general population of horses.

References

1. Irvine CHG: The blood picture in the racehorse: I. The normal erythrocyte and hemoglobin status: a dynamic concept. J Am Vet Med Assoc 1958; 133:97.
2. Steel JD, Whitlock LE: Observations on the haematology of thoroughbred and standardbred horses in training and racing. Aust Vet J 1960; 36:136.
3. Sykes PE: Hematology as an aid in equine track practice. *In* Proceedings of the 12th Annual Convention of the American Association of Equine Practitioners, 1966, p 159.
4. Archer RK, Clabby J: The effect of excitation and exertion on the circulating blood of horses. Vet Rec 1965; 77:689.
5. Laufenstein-Duffy H: The daily variation of the resting PCV in the racing thoroughbred and the difficulty in evaluating the effectiveness of hemantinic drugs. *In* Proceedings of the Annual Convention of the American Association of Equine Practitioners, 1971, p 151.
6. Revington M: Haematology of the racing thoroughbred in Australia: I. Reference values and the effect of excitement. II. Haematological values compared to performance. Equine Vet J 1983; 15:141.
7. Stewart GA, Riddle CA, Salmon PW: Haematology of the racehorse: A recent study of thoroughbreds in Victoria. Aust Vet J 1977; 53:353.
8. Persson SGB, Ekman L, Lydin G, et al: Circulatory effects of splenectomy in the horse: I. Effect on red cell distribution and variability of haematocrit in the peripheral blood. Zentralbl Vet Med 1973; A20:441.
9. Rose RJ, Hodgson DR: Hematological and biochemical parameters in endurance horses during training. Equine Vet J 1982; 14:144.

10. Archer RK: Hematology in relation to performance and potential: A general review. J S Afr Vet Assoc 1975; 45:273.
11. Persson SGB: The circulatory significance of the splenic red cell pool. *In* Proceedings of the 1st International Symposium on Equine Hematology, 1975, p 303.
12. Carlson GP: Fluid, electrolyte and acid-base balance. *In* Kankeko JJ (ed): Clinical Biochemistry of Domestic Animals, 4th ed. New York, Academic Press, 1989, p 543.
13. Kerr MG, Snow DH: Alterations in hematocrit, plasma proteins and electrolytes in horses following the feeding of hay. Vet Rec 1982; 110:538.
14. Clark LL, Ganjam VK, Fichtenbaum B, et al: Effect of feeding on renin-angiotensin-aldersterone system of the horse. Am J Physiol 1988; 254:R524.
15. Allen BV, Powell DG: Effects of training and time of day of blood sampling on the variation of some common hematological parameters in normal thoroughbred racehorses. *In* Snow DH, Persson SGB, Rose RJ (eds): Equine Exercise Physiology. Cambridge, Granta Editions, 1983, p 328.
16. Rose RJ, Hodgson DR, Sampson D, et al: Changes in plasma biochemistry in horses competing in a 160-km endurance ride. Aust Vet J 1983; 60:101.
17. Stewart GA, Steel JD: Hematology of the fit racehorse. J S Afr Vet Assoc 1975; 45:287.
18. Carlson GP, Harold D, Ziemer EL: Anemia in the horse: Diagnosis and treatment. *In* Proceedings of the American Association of Equine Practitioners, 1983, p 279.
19. Mason DK, Watkins K, McNie J, et al: Hematological measurements as an aid to early diagnosis and prognosis of respiratory viral infections in thoroughbred horses. Vet Rec 1990; 126:359.
20. Mason D, Watkins KL, Luk CM: Hematological changes in two thoroughbred horses in training with confirmed equine herpesvirus 1 infections. Vet Rec 1989; 124:503.
21. Rossdale PD, Burguez PN, Cash RS: Changes in blood neutrophil:lymphocyte ration related to adrenocortical function in the horse. Equine Vet J 1982; 14:293.
22. Williamson HM: Normal and abnormal electrolyte levels in the racing horse and their effect on performance. J S Afr Vet Assoc 1975; 45:334.
23. Harris PA, Snow DH: Role of electrolyte imbalances in the pathophysiology of the equine rhabdomyolysis syndrome. *In* Persson SGB, Lindholm A, Jeffcott LB (eds): Equine Exercise Physiology 3. Davis, Calif, ICEEP Publications, 1991, p 435.
24. Edelman IS, Leibman J, O'Meara MP, et al: Interrelationships between serum sodium concentration, serum osmolality and total exchangeable sodium, total exchangeable potassium and total body water. J Clin Invest 1958; 37:1236.
25. Tasker JB: Fluid and electrolyte studies in the horse: III. Intake and output of water, sodium, and potassium in normal horses. Cornell Vet 1967; 57:649.
26. Lindner A, Schmidt M, Meyer H: Investigations on sodium metabolism in exercised Shetland ponies fed a diet marginal in sodium. *In* Snow DH, Persson SGB, Rose RJ (eds): Equine Exercise Physiology. Cambridge, Granta Editions, 1983, p 318.
27. Tasker JB: Fluid and electrolyte studies in the horse: IV. The effects of fasting and thirsting. Cornell Vet 1967; 57:658.
28. Muylle E, Van Den Hende C, Nuytten J, et al: Preliminary studies on the relationship of red blood cell potassium concentration and performance. *In* Snow DH, Persson SGB, Rose RJ (eds): Equine Exercise Physiology. Cambridge, Granta Editions, 1983, p 366.
29. Muylle E, van den Hende C, Nuytten J, et al: Determination of red blood cell potassium content in diarrhoea: A practical approach to therapy. Equine Vet J 1984; 16:450.
30. Groenendyk S, English PB, Abetz I: External balance of water and electrolytes in the horse. Equine Vet J 1988; 20:189.
31. Ziemer EL, Parker HR, Carlson GP, et al: Clinical features and treatment of renal tubular acidosis in two horses. J Am Vet Med Assoc 1987; 190:294.
32. Rose RJ, Lloyd DR: Sodium bicarbonate: More than just a "milkshake"? Equine Vet J 1992; 24:75.
33. Murakami M, Takagi S: Effects of continuous long distance running exercise on plasma enzyme levels in horses. Exp Rep Equine Health Lab 1974; 11:106.
34. Kerr MG, Snow DH: Plasma enzyme activities in endurance horses. *In* Snow DH, Persson SGB, Rose RJ (eds): Equine Exercise Physiology. Cambridge, Granta Editions, 1983, p 432.
35. Cardinet GH, Littrell JF, Freedland RA: Comparative investigations of serum creatine phosphokinase and glutamic-oxaloacetic transaminase activities in equine paralytic myoglobinuria. Res Vet Sci 1967; 8:219.
36. Valberg S, Jönsson L, Lindholm A, et al: Muscle histopathology and plasma asparatate aminotransferase, creatine kinase and myoglobin changes with exercise in horses with recurrent exertional rhabdomyolysis. Equine Vet J 1993; 25:11.
37. Persson SGB, Lydin G: Circulatory effects of splenectomy in the horse: III. Effect on pulse-work relationship. Zentralbl Vet Med 1973; A20:521.
38. Kline H, Foreman JH: Heart and spleen weights as a function of breed and somatotype. *In* Persson SGB, Lindholm A, Jeffcott LB (eds): Equine Exercise Physiology 3. Davis, Calif, ICEEP Publications, 1991, p 17.
39. Persson SGB: On blood volume and working capacity in horses. Acta Physiol Scand 1967; (suppl 19):1.
40. Persson SGB: Blood volume and work performance. *In* Proceedings of the 1st Internation Symposium on Equine Hematology, 1975, p 321.
41. Persson SGB: Evaluation of exercise tolerance and fitness in the performance horse. *In* Snow DH, Persson SGB, Rose RJ (eds): Equine Exercise Physiology. Cambridge, Granta Editions, 1983, p 441.
42. Rose RJ, Allen JR: Hematologic responses to exercise and training. Vet Clin North Am Equine Prac 1985; 1:461.
43. Carlson GP: Thermoregulation and fluid balance in the exercising horse. *In* Snow DH, Persson SGB, Rose RJ (eds): Equine Exercise Physiology. Cambridge, Granta Editions, 1983, p 291.
44. Evans DL, Rose RJ: Cardiovascular and respiratory responses in thoroughbred horses during treadmill exercise. J Exp Biol 1988; 134:397.
45. Persson SGB, Bergsten G: Circulatory effects of splenectomy in the horse: IV. Effect on blood flow and blood lactate at rest and during exercise. Zentralbl Vet Med 1975; A20:801.
46. Smith J, Erickson H, Debowes R, et al: Changes in circulating equine erythrocytes induced by brief, high-speed exercise. Equine Vet J 1989; 21:444.
47. Boucher JH: Evidence for pulmonary microcirculatory impediment causing hypoxemia in healthy exercising horses. Physiologist 1984; 27:28.
48. Persson SGB: Practical aspects of blood volume measurement: Procedure for determination of total red cell volume (CV) in the horse. *In* Proceedings of the International Conference on Equine Sports Medicine, 1986, p 51.
49. Carlson GP, Ocen PO, Harrold D: Clinicopathologic alterations in normal and exhausted endurance horses. Theriogenology 1976; 6:92.
50. Rose RJ: Hematological changes associated with endurance exercise. Vet Rec 1982; 110:175.
51. Snow DH, Ricketts SW, Mason DK: Hematological response to racing and training exercise in thoroughbred horses, with particular reference to the leukocyte response. Equine Vet J 1983; 15:149.
52. Snow DH: Hematological, biochemical and physiological changes in horses and ponies during the cross-country stage of driving trial competitions. Vet Rec 1990; 126:233.
53. Rose RJ: Changes in Haematology and Plasma Biochemistry of Horses in Response to Training and Endurance Exercise. Fellowship thesis, Royal College of Veterinary Surgeons, London, 1984.
54. Harris PA, Snow DH: The effects of high-intensity exercise on the plasma concentration of lactate, potassium and other electrolytes. Equine Vet J 1988; 20:109.
55. Harris PA, Snow DH: Plasma potassium and lactate concentrations in thoroughbred horses during exercise of varying intensity. Equine Vet J 1992; 23:220.
56. Keenan DM: Changes of blood metabolites in horses after racing with particular reference to uric acid. Aust Vet J 1979; 55:54.
57. Snow DH, Ricketts SW, Douglas TA: Post-race blood biochemistry in thoroughbreds. *In* Snow DH, Persson SGB, Rose RJ (eds): Equine Exercise Physiology. Cambridge, Granta Editions, 1983, p 389.

58. Judson GJ, Frauenfelder HC, Mooney GJ: Biochemical changes in thoroughbred racehorses following submaximal and maximal exercise. *In* Snow DH, Persson SGB, Rose RJ (eds): Equine Exercise Physiology. Cambridge, Granta Editions, 1983, p 408.

59. Sahlin K, Broberg S: Release of K$^+$ from muscle during prolonged dynamic exercise. Acta Physiol Scand 1989; 136:293.

60. Bayly WM, Grant BD, Breeze RG, et al: The effects of maximal exercise on acid-base balance and arterial blood gas tension in thoroughbred horses. *In* Snow DH, Persson SGB, Rose RJ (eds): Equine Exercise Physiology. Cambridge, Granta Editions, 1983, p 400.

61. Carlson GP, Ocen PO: Composition of equine sweat following exercise in high environmental temperatures and in response to intravenous epinephrine administration. J Equine Med Surg 1979; 3:27.

62. Kerr MG, Snow DH: Composition of sweat of the horse during prolonged epinephrine (Adrenalin) infusion, heat exposure, and exercise. Am J Vet Res 1983; 44:1571.

63. Rose RJ: Endurance exercise in the horse: A review, part 1. Br Vet J 1986; 142:532.

64. Carlson GP, Mansmann RA: Serum electrolyte and plasma protein alterations in horses used in endurance rides. J Am Vet Med Assoc 1974; 165:262.

65. Rose RJ, Purdue RA, Hensley W: Plasma biochemistry alterations in horses during an endurance ride. Equine Vet J 1977; 9:122.

66. Lucke JN, Hall GM: Biochemical changes in horses during a 50-mile endurance ride. Vet Rec 1978; 102:356.

67. Lucke JN, Hall GM: Further studies on the metabolic effects of long-distance riding: Golden Horseshoe Ride. Equine Vet J 1980; 12:189.

68. Lucke JN, Hall GM: Long-distance exercise in the horse: Golden Horseshoe Ride. Vet Rec 1980; 106:405.

69. Snow DH, Kerr MG, Nimmo MA, et al: Alterations in blood, sweat, urine and muscle composition during prolonged exercise in the horse. Vet Rec 1982; 110:377.

70. Deldar A, Fregin FG, Bloom JC, et al: Changes in selected biochemical constituents of blood collected from horses participating in a 50-mile endurance ride. Am J Vet Res 1982; 43:2239.

71. Grosskopf JFW, Van Rensburg JJ, Bertschinger HJ: Haematology and blood biochemistry of horses during a 210 km endurance ride. *In* Snow DH, Persson SGB, Rose RJ (eds): Equine Exercise Physiology. Cambridge, Granta Editions, 1983, p 416.

72. Rose RJ, Arnold KS, Church S, et al: Plasma and sweat electrolyte concentrations in the horse during long distance exercise. Equine Vet J 1980; 12:19.

73. Rose RJ, Ilkiw JE, Martin ICA: Blood gas, acid-base and hematological values in horses during an endurance ride. Equine Vet J 1979; 11:56.

74. Rose RJ, Ilkiw JE, Arnold KS, et al: Plasma biochemistry in the horse during 3-day event competition. Equine Vet J 1980; 12:132.

75. Rose RJ, Ilkiw JE, Sampson D, et al: Changes in blood gas, acid-base and metabolic parameters in horses during three-day event competition. Res Vet Sci 1980; 28:393.

76. White KK, Short CE, Hintz HF, et al: The value of dietary fat for working horses: II. Physical evaluation. J Equine Med Surg 1978; 2:525.

77. Lucke JN, Hall GM: A biochemical study of the Arab Horse Society's marathon race. Vet Rec 1980; 107:523.

78. Schott HC, Hodgson DR, Bayly WM, et al: Renal responses to high-intensity exercise. *In* Persson SGB, Lindholm A, Jeffcott LB (eds): Equine Exercise Physiology 3. Davis, Calif, ICEEP Publications, 1991, p 361.

79. Nimmo MA, Snow DH: Time course of ultrastructural changes in skeletal muscle after two types of exercise. J Appl Physiol 1982; 52:910.

80. Lekeux P, Art T, Linden A, et al: Heart rate, hematological and serum biochemical responses to showjumping. *In* Persson SGB, Lindholm A, Jeffcott LB (eds): Equine Exercise Physiology 3. Davis, Calif, ICEEP Publications, 1991, p 385.

81. Gollnick PD, Saltin B: Significance of skeletal muscle oxidative enzyme enhancement with endurance training. Clin Physiol 1982; 2:1.

82. Krzywanek H: Lactic acid concentration and pH values in trotters after racing. J S Afr Vet Assoc 1975; 45:355.

83. Sréter FA: The effect of systematic training on plasma electrolytes, hematocrit values and blood sugar in thoroughbred racehorses. Can J Biochem Physiol 1959; 37:273.

84. Snow DH, Mackenzie G: Some metabolic effects of maximal exercise in the horse and adaptations with training. Equine Vet J 1977; 9:134.

85. Snow DH, Harris RC, MacDonald IA, et al: Effects of high-intensity exercise on plasma catecholamines in the thoroughbred horse. Equine Vet J 1992; 24:462.

86. Costill DL: Physiology of marathon running. JAMA 1972; 221:1024.

87. Rose RJ, Sampson D: Changes in certain metabolic parameters in horses associated with food deprivation and endurance exercise. Res Vet Sci 1982; 32:198.

88. Snow DH, Fixter LM, Kerr MG, et al: Alterations in composition of venous plasma FFA pool during prolonged and sprint exercise in the horse. *In* Biochemistry of Exercise. Chicago, Human Kinetics Publishers, 1983, p 336.

89. Paul P: Effects of long lasting physical exercise and training on lipid metabolism. *In* Metabolic Adaptation to Prolonged Physical Exercise. Basel, Birkhauser-Verlag, 1975, p 156.

90. Lucke JN: Factors contributing to exhaustion in the long distance riding horse. *In* Proceedings of the Association of Veterinary Anaesthesiologists of Great Britain and Ireland, 1982, p 140.

91. Snow DH, Summers RJ, Guy PS: The actions of the beta-adrenoreceptor blocking agents propranolol and metoprolol in the maximally exercised horse. Res Vet Sci 1979; 27:22.

92. Plummer C, Knight PK, Ray SP, et al: Cardiorespiratory and metabolic effects of propranolol during maximal exercise. *In* Persson SGB, Lindholm A, Jeffcott LB (eds): Equine Exercise Physiology 3. Davis, Calif, ICEEP Publications, 1991, p 465.

93. Zolovick A, Upson DW, Eleftheriou BE: Diurnal variation in plasma glucocorticosteroid levels in the horse. J Endocrinol 1966; 25:249.

94. Church DB, Evans DL, Lewis DR, et al: The effect of exercise on plasma adrenocorticotrophin, cortisol and insulin in the horse and adaptations with training. *In* Gillespie JR, Robinson NE (eds): Equine Exercise Physiology 2. Davis, Calif, ICEEP Publications, 1987, p 506.

95. Snow DH, Mackenzie G: The metabolic effects of maximal exercise in the horse and adaptations with training. Equine Vet J 1977; 9:134.

96. Snow DH, Mackenzie G: Effect of training on some metabolic changes associated with submaximal endurance exercise in the horse. Equine Vet J 1977; 9:226.

97. Snow DH, Rose RJ: Hormonal changes associated with long distance exercise. Equine Vet J 1981; 13:195.

98. Linden A, Art T, Amory D, et al: Effect of 5 different types of exercise, transportation and ACTH administration on plasma cortisol concentration in sport horses. *In* Persson SGB, Lindholm A, Jeffcott LB (eds): Equine Exercise Physiology 3. Davis, Calif, ICEEP Publications, 1991, p 391.

99. Dybal NO, Gribble D, Madigan JE, et al: Alterations in plasma corticosteroids, insulin and selected metabolites in horses used in endurance rides. Equine Vet J 1980; 12:137.

100. Gaiani R, Mongiorgi S: La concentrazione plasmatica del l'adosterone nel cavallo trottatore a riposo e sottoposto ad allenamento. Atti Soc Ital Sci Vet 1975; 24:273.

101. Guthrie GP, Cecil SG, Darden ED, et al: Dynamics of renin and aldosterone in the thoroughbred horse. Gen Comp Endocrinol 1982; 48:296.

102. Purohit RC, Nachreiner RF, Humburg JM, et al: Effects of exercise, phenylbutazone, and furosemide on the plasma renin activity and angiotensin I in horses. Am J Vet Res 1979; 40:986.

103. Thornton JR: Hormonal responses to exercise and training. Vet Clin North Am Equine Pract 1975; 1:477.

104. McKeever KH, Hinchcliff KW, Schmall LM, et al: Atrial natriuretic peptide during exercise in horses. *In* Persson SGB, Lindholm A, Jeffcott LB (eds): Equine Exercise Physiology 3. Davis, Calif, ICEEP Publications, 1991, p 368.

105. Stewart GA, Clarkson GT, Steel JD: Hematology of the racehorse and factors affecting interpretation of the blood count. *In* Pro-

ceedings of the Annual Convention of the American Association of Equine Practitioners, 1970, p 17.

106. Clarkson GT: Haematology and Serum Iron in the Racehorse. M.V.Sc. thesis, University of Melbourne, Melbourne, Australia, 1968.

107. Stull CL, Lawrence LM: The effect of exercise and conditioning on equine red blood cell characteristics. Equine Vet Sci 1986; 6:170.

108. Persson SGB, Larsson M, Lindholm A: Effects of training on adrenocortical function and red-cell volume in trotters. Zentralbl Vet Med Assoc 1980; 27:261.

109. Persson SGB, Essen B, Lindholm A: Oxygen uptake, red-cell volume, and pulse/work relationship in different states of training in trotters. *In* Proceedings of the 5th Meeting of the Academic Society for Large Animal Veterinary Medicine, 1980, p 34.

110. McKeever KH, Schurg WA, Jarrett SH, et al: Exercise training-induced hypervolemia in the horse. Med Sci Sports Exerc 1987; 19:21.

111. Mullen PA, Hopes R, Sewell J: The biochemistry, haematology, nutrition and racing performance of two-year-old thoroughbreds throughout their training and racing season. Vet Rec 1979; 104:90.

112. Judson JG, Mooney GJ, Thornbury RS: Plasma biochemical values in thoroughbred horses in training. *In* Gillespie JR, Robinson NE (eds): Equine Exercise Physiology 2. Davis, Calif, ICEEP Publications, 1987, p 354.

113. Milne DW, Skarda RT, Gabel AA, et al: Effects of training on biochemical values in standardbred horses. Am J Vet Res 1976; 37:285.

114. Irvine CHG: Thyroxine secretion rate in the horse under various physiological states. J Endocrinol 1967; 39:313.

6

The Respiratory System: Anatomy, Physiology, and Adaptations to Exercise and Training

P. LEKEUX AND T. ART

Introduction

IMPORTANCE OF THE RESPIRATORY SYSTEM IN THE ATHLETIC HORSE

During the last decade, research in exercising horses provided growing evidence that the respiratory system may be a limiting factor for maximal performance, even in healthy animals.[1-7] Therefore, any pulmonary dysfunction, even subclinical or moderate, may significantly impair the aerobic metabolism of exercising horses. The observation that respiratory abnormalities frequently are responsible for the "poor performance" syndrome in the horse[8-10] confirms the importance of optimal pulmonary function in the athletic horse. A good understanding of the peculiarities of equine respiratory structure and function is essential for a comprehensive evaluation of the respiratory system and possible correction of its dysfunction.

FUNCTIONS OF THE RESPIRATORY SYSTEM IN THE HORSE

Gas exchange is the major function of the lung, which ensures the transport of O_2 from air into blood and of CO_2 in the reverse direction. Some parts of the respiratory system also play a role in other nonpulmonic functions, such as humidification, warming, and filtering of the inhaled air, swallowing, phonation, olfaction, blood reservoir, blood filtering, defense mechanisms against environmental aggressors, surfactant production, acid-base regulation, thermoregulation, and the synthesis, release, modification, inactivation, or removal of bioactive substances such as amines, serotonin, histamine, norepinephrine, kallikreins, eicosanoids (prostaglandins, thromboxanes, leukotrienes), neuropeptides (vasoactive intestinal polypeptide, substance P, etc.), enzymes (bradykinase, converting enzymes, etc.), cytokines (tumor necrosis factor, interleukin 2, etc.).

EXTERNAL FACTORS INFLUENCING PULMONARY FUNCTION

If the respiratory system is able to influence some nonrespiratory functions, the opposite is also true. Pulmonary function may be disturbed by factors that are not directly related to the integrity of the respiratory system, such as the quality of the inspired air, the position of the head and neck, the abdominal mass, locomotion-respiration coupling, cardiac function, the equipment used, and a range of other factors. All these factors must be taken into account when evaluating equine pulmonary function.

Structural Peculiarities of the Equine Respiratory System and Their Functional Impact

The function of an organ is highly influenced by its anatomy, and vice versa. This is particularly true with regard to the respiratory system, where external respiration induces important structural changes, mainly during exercise-induced hyperpnea. It is therefore useful to remember some structural peculiarities that do influence pulmonary function in the athletic horse. More morphologic details can be obtained from anatomic handbooks.[11]

THE AIRWAYS

The main function of the airways is to carry air from the nose to the gas-exchanging regions of the lung during inspiration and the opposite during expiration. Therefore, any change in structure that modifies the permeability of the airways to airflow also has a direct impact on pulmonary function.

Nostrils. Equine nostrils are large and mobile. Their particular structure allows expansion during inspiration, with activation of some muscles resulting in flaring of the nostrils and collapse of the nasal diverticulum. This is particularly notable and of some significance during exercise-induced hyperpnea. In addition, this can be disturbed, for example, by injury to the facial nerve which provides the motor efferents to the nostrils.

Nasal Cavities. Because of their large turbinates and important vascularization, the nasal cavities provide a large surface area for heat and water exchange, but they also provide a large source of airflow resistance. Both sympathetic and parasympathetic fibers are distributed to the nasal cavities. Their stimulation may respectively vasoconstrict and vasodilate the vascular sinuses, which can induce a decrease or increase in nasal resistance. On the other hand, factors inducing an increase of the resistance in the nasal cavities (such as injuries due to nasal intubation, a nasal septum defect due to a too narrow halter in foals, a tight nose band, etc.) will have deleterious effects during exercise. Hemorrhages resulting from upper airway endoscopy or passage of a nasogastric tube frequently are due to injuries of the nasal septum and ventral concha veins.

Pharynx. The soft palate divides the pharynx into the nasopharynx and the oropharynx. Numerous lymphoid follicles are present in the mucous membranes of the dorsal and lateral walls of the nasopharynx and the dorsal surface of the soft palate. The number and size of these follicles are particularly important in young horses and usually regress in mature horses.

The natural tendency of the soft structures of the nasopharynx to collapse during inspiration is limited by tensor muscle contraction.

The guttural pouches are paired diverticulae of the Eustachian tubes that communicate with the pharynx via slitlike openings. Their function is still unknown, and they do not seem to influence directly the passage of air through the upper airways. However, these pouches contain strategic structures such as blood vessels (internal and external carotid arteries), cranial nerves (vagus, cervical sympathetic trunk, glossopharyngeal, hypoglossal, and spinal accessory nerves), and retropharyngeal lymph nodes. Any abnormality, even subclinical, of the guttural pouches may potentially damage these highly sensitive structures and consequently induce some dysfunction. For example, a lesion of the glossopharyngeal nerve and the vagus may induce a soft palate paralysis and result in its dorsal displacement.

At a functional level, the most important structural peculiarity of the equine upper airways is the intrapharyngeal ostium, which is an opening in the soft palate formed caudodorsally by the palatopharyngeal wall, laterally by the pillars of the soft palate, and rostrally by the visible border of the soft palate. The laryngeal structures, i.e., the corniculate cartilages and the epiglottis, articulate with the ostium like a button in a buttonhole,[12] forming an airtight seal when the horse breathes (Fig. 6–1). This peculiar arrangement explains why the horse is a compulsory nasal breather. Indeed, because of this anatomic characteristic, the horse, unlike the human and canine, is not able to switch from nasal to oronasal breathing when the nasal resistance to airflow become too high, namely, during exercise-induced hyperpnea.

In horses, the displacement of the caudal border of the soft palate to a position above the epiglottis, called *dorsal displacement of the soft palate,* is not physiologic, except when it occurs during swallowing, coughing, or whinnying (see Fig. 6–1). In all other conditions, this dorsal displacement is abnormal and will induce dyspnea, especially during strenuous exercise. It induces a narrowing of the upper airways and causes a soft palate flapping, sometimes resulting in a dramatic asphyxia in racing horses.

Larynx. The structural and functional peculiarities of the equine larynx make it a potential bottleneck in the upper airways. The rostral protrusion of the laryngeal cartilages through the intrapharyngeal ostium constitutes the aditus laryngis. This pharyngeal opening is formed dorsally by the corniculate cartilages, laterally by the vocal folds, and ventrally by the epiglottis (Fig. 6–2). The aditus laryngis can vary from tight seal, i.e., full adduction of the laryngeal structures during swallowing in order to protect the lower airways from ingesta, to a maximal opening, i.e., full abduction of these structures during exercise-induced hyperpnea in order to decrease the resistance to airflow (see Fig. 6–2). This full opening is completed by a dilation of the larynx due to contraction of the intrinsic muscles, which eliminates the opening of the laryngeal ventricles.

Any impairment of this laryngeal dilatation due to structural factors (such as rostral displacement of the palatopharyngeal arch) or functional factors (such as laryngeal hemiparesis) will be responsible for inadequate ventilation during heavy exercise[13] and will generally induce abnormal respiratory noises related to the increased airflow resistance[14] (see Fig. 6–2).

Trachea. The horse's trachea is a 70- to 80-cm-long flexible tube consisting of 48 to 60 cartilaginous rings that are open dorsally (Fig. 6–3). The free ends of these plates overlap in the cervical but not in the thoracic part of the trachea.[11] Its cross section is almost circular proximally and distally (transverse diameter 5.5 cm, sagittal

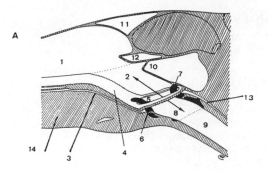

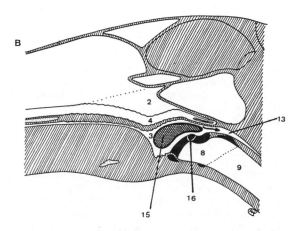

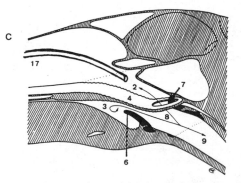

Figure 6-1. *Lateral view of the pharyngolaryngeal area during normal breathing (A), swallowing (B), and dorsal displacement of the soft palate (C). (1: nasal cavity; 2: nasopharynx; 3: oropharynx; 4: soft palate; 5: intrapharyngeal ostium ("button hole"); 6: epiglottis; 7: corniculate cartilage; 8: larynx; 9: trachea; 10: guttural pouch; 11: frontal sinus; 12: sphenopalatine sinus; 13: esophagus; 14: tongue; 15: food bolus; 16: closed larynx; 17: endoscope.) (Modified, with permission, from Cook WR: Specifications for speed in the racehorse. In The Airflow Factors. Menasha, WI, Russell Meerdink, 1989.)*

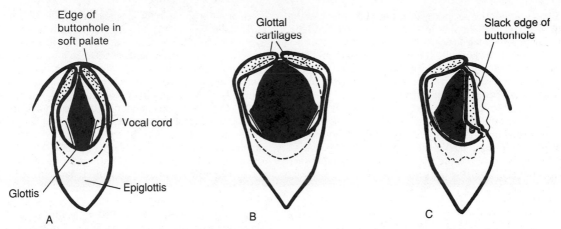

Figure 6-2. Front view of the larynx in a healthy resting (A) and exercising (B) horse and in an exercising horse with laryngeal hemiplegia (C). (Modified, with permission, from Cook WR: Specifications for speed in the racehorse. In The Airflow Factors. Menasha, WI, Russell Meerdink, 1989.)

diameter 5 cm) but is more flattened dorsoventrally (transverse diameter 7 cm, sagittal diameter 5 cm) between the two extremes. Routine endoscopic evaluations of the lower airways of horses examined for exercise intolerance show evidence that there is sometimes a sharp lateral narrowing of the intrathoracic trachea just cranial to the tracheal bifurcation.

Tracheal smooth muscles lie in the dorsal tracheal membrane. They are innervated by the autonomic nervous system.

Despite its cartilaginous structure, the extrathoracic trachea is quite compliant and is susceptible to collapse during the highly compressing transmural pressure that occurs during forced inspiration.[15] Its compliance (and therefore its collapsibility) is significantly decreased, however, by smooth-muscle contraction (due to the exercise-induced adrenal discharge) and by tracheal extension (due to exercise-induced head and neck stretching). Moreover, the resistance to collapse is also dependent on the shape of the tracheal cross section. In this regard, all horses do not seem to be equal. Indeed, the transverse

to sagittal diameter ratio[16] varies from 0.9 (i.e., circular shape) to 2 (i.e., an elliptical shape) with a mean of 1.4 (Fig. 6–4). The more ellipsoid the trachea, the more compressible it is. Therefore, horses with a transverse to sagittal diameter ratio higher than 1.5 are disadvantaged and more susceptible to exercise intolerance due to insufficient ventilation. The size and age of the horse do not influence the compliance of the trachea.[16]

Bronchi. After the bifurcation of the trachea into the right and left principal bronchi, the bronchial tree branches

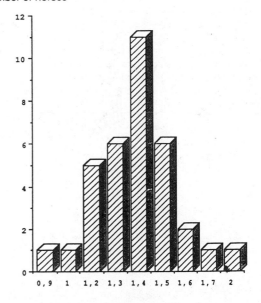

Figure 6-4. Distribution of 33 tracheas according to their transverse sagittal diameter ratio.

Figure 6-3. Cross-sectional view of the cervical trachea (1: tracheal muscle; 2: cartilage; 3: adventice; 4: mucosa; 5: connective tissue). (Modified, with permission, from Collin B: Atlas d'anatomie. Liège, Belgium, Université de Liège, 1976.)

many times to the periphery of the lung via the primary bronchi, the segmental bronchi, the bronchioles, and the terminal bronchioles (Fig. 6–5).

These intrathoracic conducting airways are also susceptible to collapse when the transmural pressure exerted on their walls is compressive. This is particularly true at the level of the small airways, which do not have cartilaginous support. However, in contrast with extrathoracic airways, where partial dynamic collapse occurs only during inspiration, the collapse of small airways occurs only during forced expiration, i.e., when the extraluminal pressure is more positive than the intraluminal pressure (Fig. 6–6).

THE LUNGS

With airway generation, the individual diameter and length of the airways decrease, but the total cross-sectional area increases. Therefore, the small airways are not a bottleneck in healthy horses and represent only a small part of the total resistance to airflow.

Respiratory bronchioles are poorly developed in the horse, and most of the gas exchange occurs at the alveolar-capillary unit, which seems to be well designed in this species. The horse's lung is highly developed and represents about 1 percent of the body weight. It contains probably more than 10^7 alveoli and probably 1000 times more capillary segments. The alveolar surface density is large and alveolar septa thin when compared with other mammals.[17]

Although the equine lung is not really divided by fissures into lobes, an apical, a diaphragmatic, and an accessory lobe in the right lung and an apical and a diaphragmatic lobe in the left lung are usually described (see Fig. 6–5). The lungs are covered by a thick pleura.

The connective-tissue septa between lobules are not complete. This allows some collateral ventilation, i.e., transfer of air between adjacent lobules via accessory pathways such as the interalveolar pores of Kohn, the canals of Lambert, and communicating respiratory bronchioles and alveolar ducts described by Martin. The advantage of this collateral ventilation is to partially compensate for reduced ventilation in areas with small airway obstructive diseases.[18] However, in horses, these accessory pathways present a high resistance to airflow and are able to provide only a maximum of 16 percent of the required volume, a very small proportion compared with the 90 percent recorded in the human lung.[19] Therefore, these pathways are probably of limited value for equine pulmonary function, except possibly for the prevention of atelectasis in horses suffering from airway obstruction.

THE BLOOD SUPPLY

The lung receives blood from two circulations (Table 6–1). The *pulmonary circulation* receives the total cardiac output from the right side of the heart. The branches of the pulmonary artery carry venous blood to the lung, accompany the bronchi, and form rich capillary plexuses on the walls of the alveoli. Here the blood is arterialized and returned to the left side of the heart by the pulmonary veins.

The equine pulmonary arteries adjacent to the bronchioles and the alveolar ducts are muscular and have a rather thick medial smooth-muscle layer (thinner than the cow and pig but thicker than the dog and sheep). This amount of smooth muscle determines the reactivity of the vessels to hypoxia and consequently explains why a horse may present a pulmonary hypertension due to an hypoxic vasoconstriction.[20]

The *bronchial circulation,* a branch of the systemic circulation, carries arterial blood for the nutrition of the airways and other lung structures. It originates from two arteries: (1) the bronchoesophageal artery, supplying the airways and interlobular septa of most of the lung, and (2) the right apical bronchial artery, supplying the airways of the right apical lobe. Bronchial arteries form a circulatory plexus in the connective tissues along the airways. Branches from this plexus penetrate the bronchial walls to form a subepithelial vascular plexus, the role of which is probably to ensure some heat dissipation. The bronchial circulation is drained by either the azygos or the pulmonary veins.

At the level of the terminal bronchioles, pulmonary and bronchial circulations anastomose. Most of these anastomoses occur at the level of the capillaries and veins rather than the arteries.[21,22]

The *lymph vessels* are numerous and arranged in two sets: a superficial one, forming a network in and under the pleura, and a deep one, accompanying the bronchi and the pulmonary vessels.

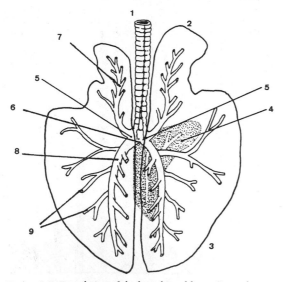

Figure 6-5. *Dorsal view of the bronchi and lungs (1: trachea; 2: right apical lobe; 3: right diaphragmatic lobe; 4: azygos lobe; 5: principal bronchi; 6: carina; 7: apical lobe bronchus; 8: diaphragmatic lobe bronchus; 9: segmental bronchi). (Modified, with permission, from Collin B: Atlas d'anatomie. Liège, Belgium, Université de Liège, 1976.)*

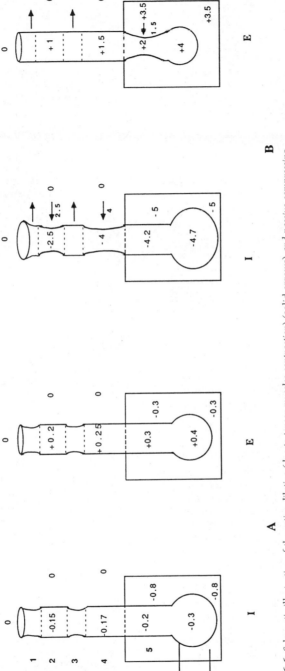

Figure 6-6. Schematic illustration of the active dilating (due to tensor muscles contraction) (solid arrows) and passive compressing (due to transmural pressure) (dashed arrows) mechanisms on the airways during resting (A) and exercising (B), inspiration (I) and expiration (E). Pressures are given in kPa. (0 = atmospheric pressure). (1: nasal cavity; 2: pharynx; 3: larynx; 4: extrathoracic trachea; 5: intrathoracic airways; 6: alveoli; 7: pleural cavity.)

Table 6-1. Comparison Between Pulmonary and Bronchial Circulations

	Pulmonary	Bronchial
Aims	• Gas exchange • Venous blood filtration • Blood reservoir	• Nutrition of airways, vessels, and visceral pleura • Thermoregulation
Structure	Right ventricle ↓ Pulmonary artery ↓ Pulmonary arterioles ↓ Pulmonary capillaries ↓ Pulmonary veins	Left ventricle ↓ Bronchial and bronchoesophageal arteries ↓ Peribronchial plexus ↓ Subepithelial plexus ↓ Pleural, vascular, and ganglia plexi ↓ Azygos veins
Blood flow (liters/min)	±99 percent of the right ventricle: 30 (280)	±2 percent of the left ventricle: 0.6 (6)
Pressure (mmHg)	Arterial: 30 (100) Capillary: 20 (80) Venous: 10 (60)	Arterial: 100 (200) Capillary: 20 (>60) Venous: 15 (60)
Capillary flow	Pulsatile	Constant
Vascular resistance (mmHg/liter/min)	0.7 (0.25)	140 (20)
Effect of hypoxia	Vasoconstriction	Vasodilation
Effect of hyperthermia	—	Vasodilation
Effect of pleural pressure changes	+++	+

Note: Data given in this table are only indicative. Exercise values are in parentheses. a: anastomoses

THE THORACIC CAVITY

Rib Cage

The thoracic cavity appears to be roughly triangular, with its caudal base formed by the diaphragm. The roof is formed by the thoracic vertebrae and the ligaments and muscles connected with them, the lateral walls are formed by the 18 ribs and the intercostal muscles, and the floor is formed by the sternum, the cartilages of the sternal ribs, and their associated muscles. A longitudinal septum, termed the *mediastinum,* extends from the roof to the floor, and the diaphragm divides the cavity into two lateral chambers, each containing a lung. The pleura provides a continuous cover over the surface of the lung (visceral pleura) and extends to provide a lining for the internal surface of the thoracic walls (parietal pleura) and to form the mediastinal cavity. Practically, all the organs in the thorax are in the mediastinal cavity, with the exception of the lungs, the caudal vena cava, and the right phrenic nerve.

Compared with the dorsoventrally flattened thorax of the primate, the horse has a rather rounded thorax. Moreover, cranially, its thorax is laterally compressed to facilitate locomotor function. The differences in size, shape, and position of the abdomen in relation to the lungs, as well as the high rigidity of the equine thorax,[23] are probably advantageous for locomotion and for stabilization of the relaxation volume of the respiratory system during postural changes.

Respiratory Muscles and Their Innervation

Inspiratory Muscles. The diaphragm is the main inspiratory muscle. It is a domed musculotendinous sheet separating the abdomen and the thorax. It consists of a cos-

tal portion, arising from the xyphoid process and the costochondral junctions of the eighth to fourteenth ribs, and a crural portion, arising from the ventral surface of the first three lumbar vertebrae and extending toward the tendinous center of the diaphragm. The apex of the dome extends to the eighth intercostal space at the level of the base of the heart. The external intercostal muscles, which join the ribs, are also active during inspiration. However, during exercise, the serratus ventralis participates in inspiration much more than do the external intercostal muscles.[24]

Other inspiratory muscles include those connecting the sternum or the ribs and the head (sternomandibularis, scalenus). When they contract, they pull the sternum or the ribs forward and participate consequently in enlargement of the thorax.[25]

Expiratory Muscles. The abdominal muscles (external and oblique abdominis, transverse and rectus abdominis, transverse thoracis) and the internal intercostal muscles are expiratory muscles. When they contract, they increase the abdominal pressure, forcing the relaxed diaphragm forward and reducing the thoracic volume.[25]

Other Respiratory Muscles. Some muscles, such as the abductor muscles which dilate the nares, the pharynx, and the larynx, are able to modify the size of the airways.

Innervation. The *phrenic nerves,* which innervate the diaphragm, come from the cervical cord and lie on both sides of the heart. In horses suffering from electrolyte imbalances (e.g., after prolonged exercise or diarrhea), the phrenic nerve may become hyperexcitable, and sometimes a diaphragmatic flutter (the thumps) may be observed (i.e., diaphragmatic contraction in phase with cardiac depolarization) This is usually transient but does respond to intravenous administration of calcium borogluconate.

The laryngeal muscles are innervated by the *recurrent nerves*. The recurrent nerve is one of the longest nerves of the body. The left laryngeal nerve originates from the brain and travels down the neck into the chest as a part of the vagus. At the level of the heart, the recurrent nerve branches off the vagus and becomes an individual nerve, which has to travel back up the neck before it finally reaches the larynx. The high incidence of left hemiplegia in the horse has been related to neural injuries due to the specific course of the left laryngeal nerve. However, this theory is challenged by the occasional occurrence of right hemiplegia.

Functional Peculiarities of the Equine Respiratory System at Rest and Adaptations During Exercise

The main respiratory processes involved in gas exchange are ventilation (i.e., how air gets to the alveoli), perfusion (i.e., how gas is removed from the lungs by the blood), ventilation/perfusion ratio (i.e., how matching of air and blood in the lung influences the gas exchange), diffusion (i.e., how gas gets across the air-blood barrier), gas transport (i.e., how gases are moved from lungs to the tissues), mechanics of breathing (i.e., how the lungs are moved), and control of breathing (i.e., how the supply of gas exchange is adjusted to the demand).

VENTILATION

Lung Volumes

Expired Minute Volume. Equine lung volumes are illustrated in Fig. 6–7. The volume of air inhaled or exhaled during a normal breath is termed the *tidal volume*.[26] Its value in the healthy resting athletic horse is about 12 ml/kg of body weight. Multiplying the tidal volume by the respiratory frequency gives the *expired minute ventilation*.

Exercise imposes a potent stress on the ventilatory pump: As speed increases, minute ventilation increases almost linearly, and the expired minute ventilation, which averages 80 liters/min at rest (Table 6–2), may reach values in the vicinity of 1800 liters/min during heavy exercise.[27] The change in minute ventilation necessary to meet the gas exchange requirements can be reached by changing tidal volume, respiratory frequency, or both.

In trotting horses, the increase in minute ventilation is achieved by a simultaneous increase in tidal volume and respiratory frequency at low exercise intensities and mainly by an increase in respiratory frequency at high exercise intensities.[28] Values as high as 133 breaths/

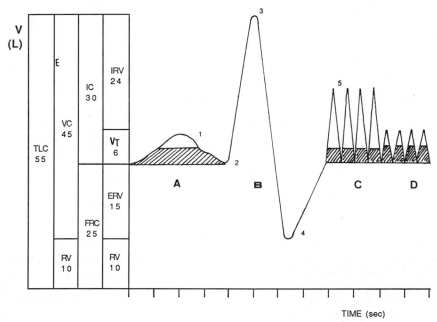

Figure 6-7. *Mean lung volumes (L) in healthy adult horses under several conditions (TLC: total lung capacity; VC: vital capacity; RV: residual volume, i.e., the volume of gas which remains in the lung after a forced expiration; IC: inspiratory capacity; FRC: functional residual capacity, i.e., the volume of air which remains in the lung after a normal expiration; IRV: inspiratory reserve volume; V_T: tidal volume; ERV: expiratory reserve volume). A, Rest breathing B, Forced breathing. C, Exercise breathing. D, Recovery breathing. (1: resting inspiratory level; 2: resting expiratory level; 3: maximal inspiratory level; 4: maximal expiratory level; 5: exercising inspiratory level.) The hatched zones represent the dead-space portion of tidal volume. This figure supposes that exercise does not change FRC, which remains to be investigated in the horse.*

Table 6-2. *Mean Respiratory Values in Healthy Thoroughbred Horses Considered Average for Their Quality, Fitness, Age (5 Years), and Size (Body Weight 470 kg) and Running on a Treadmill under Temperate Climatic Conditions (Lung and Gas Volumes are Expressed as BTPS and STPD Respectively).*

Value	Unit	Rest	Walk	Slow trot	Canter	Fast gallop	Recovery 5'
A. Ventilation*							
$\dot{V}_{O_2 max}$	%	3.3	14	18	60	100	20
V_T	liters	5.6	5.8	6.2	9.2	13.2	6.5
V_D	liters	3.4	3.4	3.5	2.6	2.6	3.5
V_A	liters	2.2	2.4	2.8	6.6	10.6	3.0
V_D/V_T	%	60	58	57	28	20	54
f	breaths/min	14	65	91	113	121	110
t_i	seconds	1.9	0.45	0.34	0.27	0.25	0.29
t_e	seconds	2.4	0.47	0.32	0.27	0.25	0.26
t_i/t_{tot}	%	44	49	52	50	50	53
$\dot{V}_E$	liters/min	78	377	564	1040	1598	715
$\dot{V}_D$	liters/min	47	219	321	291	320	386
$\dot{V}_A$	liters/min	31	158	243	749	1278	329
$\dot{V}_E/\dot{V}_{O_2}$	liters/liter	35	40	47	26	24	55
$\dot{V}_E/\dot{V}_{CO_2}$	liters/liter	43	48	51	27	23	51
mean $\dot{V}_i$	liters/s	2.9	13	19	34	53	26
mean $\dot{V}_e$	liters/s	2.3	12	20	34	53	30
$\dot{V}_{i\,max}$	liters/s	4.1	14	27	45	64	32
$\dot{V}_{e\,max}$	liters/s	4.2	18	30	52	79	39
$\ddot{V}_i$	liters/s^2	8	240	632	1124	1685	650
$\ddot{V}_e$	liters/s^2	7	225	566	1086	1595	744
B. Mechanics of breathing†							
$P_{pl\,min}$	kPa	−0.78	−1.19	−1.78	−3.19	−4.85	−1.68
$P_{pl\,max}$	kPa	−0.34	0.31	0.55	2.42	3.62	0.53
$max\Delta P_{pl}$	kPa	0.44	1.50	2.33	5.61	8.47	2.21
P_{in}	kPa	0.02	0.54	1.16	2.61	4.26	1.71
$\Delta P_{\dot{V}=0}$	kPa	0.24	−0.29	−0.90	−2.42	−3.88	−1.90
C_{dyn}	liter/kPa	23	−20	−6.8	−3.8	−3.4	−3.4
R_L	Pa/liter/s	25	26	30	48	57	27
R_{UA}	Pa/liter/s	20	21	23	38	46	21
R_{LA}	Pa/liter/s	5	5	7	10	11	6
W_{vis}	J	1.4	6.2	14	36	82	14
$\dot{W}_{vis}$	J/min	17	403	1274	4068	9922	1540
$\dot{W}_{vis}/\dot{V}_E$	J/liter	0.22	1.07	2.2	3.9	6.2	2.2
$\dot{W}_{vis}/\dot{V}_{O_2}$	J/liter	7.7	42	106	102	148	118

min have been reported in standardbred horses running on a treadmill.[29] Values for tidal volume of racing trotting horses are rare; tidal volumes of about 12 liters have been reported for horses trotting at 10 m/s, with a respiratory frequency of 87 breaths/min.[30]

In galloping horses, the respiration and the locomotion are compulsorily coupled.[31] Step and respiratory frequencies average 110 to 130 per minute with maximum values of 148 per minute.[32,33] Therefore, when the horse gallops, the increase in minute ventilation with increasing speed is due mainly to the increase in tidal volume rather than in respiratory frequency. Tidal volumes between 12 and 15 liters are reported in fast galloping horses.[2,5,33,34] An extreme value of 29.7 liters has been observed in a horse decoupling the 1 : 1 step/respiratory frequency ratio for a 2 : 1 ratio.[35]

Although frequently suggested, a relationship between stride length and tidal volume amplitude has not been demonstrated until now.[36]

Alveolar and Dead Space Ventilation. Only a part of the inspired volume reaches the area of the lung where gas exchange takes place; this is the *alveolar ventilation.* The remaining part of the minute ventilation is wasted in the regions of lung where no gas exchange occurs; this is the *physiologic dead space ventilation,* which includes the conducting airways (anatomic dead space) and the alveoli that are ventilated but not perfused (alveolar

Table 6-2. Continued

Value	Unit	Rest	Walk	Slow trot	Canter	Fast gallop	Recovery 3'
C. Gas exchange[†]							
$\dot{V}_{O_2}$	ml/kg/min	4.7	20.2	25.5	85.1	142.5	27.7
$\dot{V}_{CO_2}$	ml/kg/min	3.8	17.0	23.4	80.9	146.8	29.8
R	—	0.82	0.85	0.92	0.95	1.03	1.07
Venous P_{O_2}	mmHg	39	32	30	25	16	62
Venous P_{CO_2}	mmHg	47	49	50	64	96	43
HCO_3^-	mmol/liter	28.8	28.9	27.5	26.6	23.0	19.2
Arterial P_{O_2}	mmHg	95	101	99	83	69	115
Arterial P_{CO_2}	mmHg	45	44	43	46	50	32
$(A\text{-}a)\Delta_{O_2}$	mmHg	4	2	4	16	29	6
pH_a	—	7.39	7.40	7.40	7.39	7.26	7.36
PCV	%	38	42	44	48	58	56
Hb	g/liter	140	150	160	175	220	220
Arterial S_{O_2}	%	97	97.5	97	95	90	98.5
Arterial C_{O_2}	liter%	20	22	22	25	28	33
Venous C_{O_2}	liter%	14	11	11	7	5	21
$C(a\text{-}v)_{O_2}$	liter%	6	11	11	18	23	12
Alveolar P_{O_2}	mmHg	99	103	103	99	98	121
Alveolar P_{CO_2}	mmHg	44	43	42	45	49	31
Fme_{O_2}	%	16.2	17.0	17.7	14.9	14.3	18.4
Fme_{CO_2}	%	2.6	2.6	2.5	4.6	5.4	2.1
Fet_{O_2}	%	14.0	14.5	14.5	13.9	13.9	17.2
Fet_{CO_2}	%	6.3	6.1	6.0	6.4	7.0	4.5
D. Pulmonary hemodynamics[§]							
HR	beats/min	35	75	103	155	210	83
SV	liters	1.05	1.07	1.12	1.39	1.36	1.32
$\dot{Q}$	liters/min	37	80	115	215	285	110
PaPmax	mmHg	37	69	78	99	152	53
PaPmin	mmHg	22	30	39	47	50	26
PaPm	mmHg	28	43	52	65	82	35
Pw	mmHg	16	25	30	37	49	20
P (aP-w)	mmHg	12	18	22	28	33	15
PVR	mmHg/liter/min	0.32	0.22	0.19	0.13	0.11	0.14
$t^{\circ}a$	°C	37.5	37.9	38.1	38.7	41.3	39.7
$\dot{V}_{O_2}/HR$	ml/kg/beat	0.06	0.25	0.25	0.55	0.68	0.34
$\dot{V}_A/\dot{Q}$	liters/liter	0.84	1.98	2.11	3.48	4.48	3.00

[*]$\dot{V}_{O_2max}$ %: percent of maximal oxygen uptake; V_T: tidal volume; V_D: physiologic dead space; V_A: alveolar volume; V_D/V_T: ratio of dead space tidal volume; f: breathing frequency; t_i: inspiratory time of the breathing cycle; t_e: expiratory time; t_i/t_{tot}: ratio of inspiratory to total time for the breathing cycle; $\dot{V}_E$: minute volume; $\dot{V}_D$: dead space ventilation; $\dot{V}_A$: alveolar ventilation; $\dot{V}_E/\dot{V}_{O_2}$: ventilatory equivalent for oxygen uptake; $\dot{V}_E/\dot{V}_{CO_2}$: ventilatory equivalent for carbon dioxide output; mean $\dot{V}_i$: mean inspiratory flow or inspiratory drive; mean $\dot{V}_e$: mean expiratory flow; $\dot{V}_{i\,max}$: peak inspiratory flow; $\dot{V}_{e\,max}$: peak expiratory flow; $\ddot{V}_i$: volume acceleration at the onset of inspiration; $\ddot{V}_e$: volume acceleration at the onset of expiration.

[†]$P_{pl\,min}$: peak intrapleural pressure recorded during inspiration; $P_{pl\,max}$: peak intrapleural pressure recorded during expiration; $max\Delta P_{pl}$: maximum change in intrapleural pressure; P_{in}: inertial pressure; $\Delta P_{\dot{V}=0}$: intrapleural pressure gradient between the two points of zero flow; C_{dyn}: dynamic lung compliance; R_L: total pulmonary resistance; R_{UA}: upper airway resistance; R_{LA}: lower airway resistance; W_{vis}: viscous work of breathing; $\dot{W}_{vis}$: minute work of breathing; $\dot{W}_{vis}/\dot{V}_E$: work of breathing per ventilated liter; $\dot{W}_{vis}/\dot{V}_{O_2}$: work of breathing per liter of oxygen uptake.

[‡]$\dot{V}_{O_2}$: oxygen uptake; $\dot{V}_{CO_2}$: carbon dioxide output; R: respiratory exchange ratio; venous P_{O_2}: venous oxygen partial pressure; venous P_{CO_2}: venous carbon dioxide partial pressure; arterial P_{O_2}: arterial oxygen partial pressure; arterial P_{CO_2}: arterial carbon dioxide partial pressure; HCO_3^-: bicarbonate content; $(A\text{-}a)\Delta_{O_2}$: alveolar-arterial oxygen gradient; pH_a: arterial pH; PCV: packed cell volume; Hb: blood hemoglobin concentration; arterial S_{O_2}: percent saturation of hemoglobin with oxygen; arterial C_{O_2}: arterial oxygen content; venous C_{O_2}: venous oxygen content; $C(a\text{-}v)_{O_2}$: arteriovenous oxygen content gradient; alveolar P_{O_2}: alveolar oxygen partial pressure; alveolar P_{CO_2}: alveolar carbon dioxide partial pressure; Fme_{O_2}: mixed expired oxygen fraction; Fme_{CO_2}: mixed expired carbon dioxide fraction; Fet_{O_2}: end-tidal oxygen fraction; Fet_{CO_2}: end-tidal carbon dioxide fraction.

[§]HR: heart rate; SV: stroke volume; $\dot{Q}$: cardiac output; PaPmax: maximal pulmonary artery pressure; PaPmin: minimal pulmonary artery pressure; PaPm: mean pulmonary artery pressure; Pw: pulmonary artery wedge pressure; P (aP-w): pulmonary driving pressure; PVR: pulmonary vascular resistance; $t^{\circ}a$: arterial blood temperature; $\dot{V}_{O_2}/HR$: oxygen pulse; $\dot{V}_A/\dot{Q}$: global ventilation/perfusion ratio.

dead space). The dead space to tidal volume ratio averages 50 to 60 percent in the resting horse,[37,38] a percentage twice as large as reported in other athletic species such as humans and dogs.

For a given minute ventilation, the lower the physiologic dead space ventilation, the higher is the alveolar ventilation and the better is the gas exchange. However, the evidence that adequate gas exchange is maintained with very low tidal volume and very high respiratory frequency (600 breaths/min, i.e., high-frequency or jet ventilation) suggests that factors such as mass convection, convective dispersion, and molecular diffusion may provide an adequate gas transport between the atmospheric air and the alveoli despite a very high dead space to tidal volume ratio.[39,40]

Exercise-induced changes in alveolar ventilation and dead space to tidal volume ratio in horses depend on the type of exercise performed.[2,41–43] During mild to moderate exercise, the dead space volume does not change significantly.[43] Therefore, the increase in tidal volume will increase the alveolar ventilation and decrease the dead space to tidal volume ratio.

If the exercise is prolonged at a constant rate, the dead space ventilation will increase by a simultaneous increase in respiratory frequency and in the dead space to tidal volume ratio.[42,43] This adaptation probably reflects the thermoregulatory role of the respiratory system.

Lastly, during intense effort, there is a decrease in the same ratio from about 60 to 20 percent.[38,42] In absolute terms, the physiologic dead space is reduced from 3.5 liters at rest to 2.5 liters during heavy exercise. Because the anatomic dead space averages 2.5 liters at rest[41]

and is expected to remain unchanged during exercise, the exercise-induced difference in the dead space (1 liter) is probably attributable to the disappearance of the alveolar dead space (i.e., alveoli that are ventilated but not perfused) induced by the recruitment of previously nonfunctional pulmonary capillaries.[38]

Distribution of Ventilation

The distribution of ventilation is not uniform in the lung, even in healthy horses. This occurs for two different reasons. The main reason is that the intrapleural pressure changes are not uniform all over the thoracic cage. Because of gravitational effects, pressure is more negative in the dorsal than in the ventral part of the lung.[44] Consequently, the dorsal alveoli are more distended, less compliant, and receive less air during inspiration at any ventilatory rate.

A second reason may be the occurrence of some inequalities in the regional small airways resistance and/or alveoli compliance; inhaled air preferentially enters the areas of the lungs with low resistive airways and highly compliant alveoli. Figure 6–8 displays how the alveoli that follow highly resistive airways (B), or which have a lower compliance, will fill up much more slowly than the others (A).[45] This ventilatory asynchronism is moderate in healthy horses and does not have significant effects on gas exchange at low respiratory frequencies. However, in horses with significant asynchronism (i.e., subclinical small airways disease) and with a high respiratory frequency (i.e., during exercise), this phenomenon will significantly impair gas exchange and may result in poor performance[46] (see Fig. 6–8).

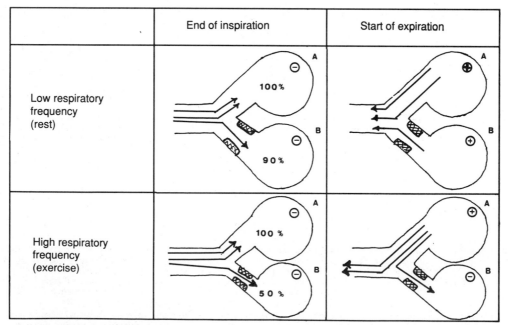

Figure 6-8. *Schematic illustration of the negative effect of ventilatory asynchronism on alveolar ventilation. The higher the respiratory frequency, the lower is the ventilation in obstructed alveoli (B), which receive less fresh air because of the high resistance of their conducting airways. At the start of expiration and because of the pressure gradient due to the dephasage, some expired air from the normal alveoli (A) may momentarily become (poor quality) inspired air for the obstructed alveoli (B).*

Factors that Tend to Reduce Ventilatory Asynchronism. The interdependence between adjacent lung regions tends to limit the nonuniform changes in regional ventilation.[19] These mechanical interactions are the result of the intricate mesh of interconnecting elastic and collagenous tissue fibers in the lung.

Collateral ventilation between adjacent lung areas is also potentially able to reduce the nonuniformity of the ventilation distribution. However, in the horse, these collateral pathways, because of their high resistance to airflow, are of limited usefulness at low respiratory frequencies and probably of no functional importance at all at high respiratory frequencies.[19]

Factors that Tend to Increase Ventilatory Asynchronism. All factors that either interfere with the properties of the lungs such as decrease in the compliance of the alveoli (interstitial edema), increase in the resistance of small airways (collapse, bronchospasm, hypersecretion, blood), or increase in respiratory frequency (during exercise) are likely to increase the ventilatory asynchronism and impair the gas exchange.

Exercise, by increasing the respiratory frequency, probably magnifies the regional differences in ventilation (see Fig. 6–8). The lobules, which have a long time constant for filling, do not fill adequately before expiration begins, and consequently, ventilation/perfusion mismatching and hypoxemia result. Moreover, because of the interdependence between adjacent lung areas, the lobules with increased airflow resistance and/or decreased compliance are stretched and compressed by the surrounding lung parts.[47] This may induce abnormal stresses on the tissues of these lobules. It has been suggested that exercise-induced pulmonary hemorrhage could sometimes be a consequence of this pulmonary overstretching.[48]

PULMONARY PERFUSION

The lungs are perfused by the pulmonary artery, which supplies the gas-exchange regions. The distribution of blood flow throughout the lung depends on the pressure difference between the pulmonary artery and the pulmonary vein and the vascular resistance and, in horses as in other species, is influenced by the gravitational forces. Blood flow to the conducting airways, interlobular septa, and pleura is supplied by the bronchial artery, and the filtrated fluid is drained by the lymphatic circulation.

The differences between pulmonary and bronchial circulations are emphasized in Table 6–1. The pulmonary vascular resistance is very low; it is estimated at only one-seventh the resistance of the systemic circulation. Consequently, the mean pressure throughout these vessels is much less than in the systemic circulation (26 versus 124 mmHg). While the vascular resistance in the systemic circulation is totally due to the precapillary vessels, the pulmonary vascular resistance is equally distributed between the pre- and postcapillary vessels. Because of the peculiar distribution and the low value of

the pulmonary vascular resistance, pressure in the pulmonary capillaries remains pulsatile.

During strenuous exercise, pulmonary blood flow increases five- to eightfold.[3,49–51] A marked simultaneous pulmonary hypertension is a feature of exertion in horses and ponies; the mean pulmonary arterial pressure rises about threefold, from 28 mmHg at rest to about 84 mmHg at a fast gallop, with maximal reported values of 100 mmHg.[4,52–57]

The pulmonary right-to-left shunt of the cardiac output is approximately 1 percent at rest. It may decrease up to 0.4 percent during heavy exercise.[4]

Factors Influencing Pulmonary Vascular Resistance
Factors capable of modifying the pulmonary vascular resistance are either extravascular or intravascular. Changes in lung volume represent the main *extravascular factor*. The pulmonary vascular resistance increases at extreme lung volume because of the compression of the lung vessels during forced expiration (small lung volume) or during forced inspiration (lung distended).[58] The increase in blood viscosity related to the exercise-induced rise in packed cell volume is another extravascular factor influencing pulmonary vascular resistance; each increase of 1 percent in the packed cell volume induces an increase of 4 percent in the pulmonary vascular resistance.[59]

Vasoactive compounds or changes in the local composition of blood are *intravascular factors* that regulate the pulmonary vascular resistance by modifying vascular smooth-muscle tone. Pulmonary vascular resistance decreases when blood flow and/or pulmonary arterial pressure increases.[59] This results from the combination of dilatation of the perfused vessels (increase in their cross-sectional area and consequently decrease in their flow resistance) and recruitment of previously unperfused vessels. Therefore, despite the substantial increase in packed cell volume, there is an approximately threefold decrease (from 0.32 to 0.11 mmHg/liter/min) in pulmonary vascular resistance with strenuous exercise (see Table 6–2).

Factors Influencing Pulmonary Perfusion Distribution
Gravitational Factors. It has been shown that there is a vertical gradient of pulmonary blood flow, with the ventral regions receiving more perfusion per unit lung volume than the dorsal regions.[60] According to the relative magnitudes of pulmonary arterial, venous, and alveolar pressures, blood flow in the lung can be divided into four zones.[58]

In *zone 1*, at the top of the lung, there is no blood flow, because the mean pulmonary arterial pressure is too low to overcome the hydrostatic pressure imposed by the column of blood connecting the pulmonary artery to the apical blood vessels. Therefore, alveolar pressure exceeds both pulmonary arterial and venous pressures, and the collapsible capillaries remain closed. However, because the mean pulmonary arterial pressure is about 15 to 18 mmHg (i.e., 20 to 25 cmH$_2$O), it may be sufficient to perfuse the vertical height of the lung above the heart (20 to 25 cm in the horse). This zone is probably small in most horses. Because this lung region is unperfused, it does not participate in gas exchange and represents the so-called alveolar dead space. During exercise, the increased pulmonary arterial pressure probably improves the recruitment of the vessels in zone 1 and therefore makes the distribution of perfusion more homogeneous. The alveolar dead space is estimated to be 0.8 to 1 liter in the resting horse or about 3.5 percent of the functional residual capacity and is very likely to disappear in the exercising horse.[38]

In *zone 2,* pulmonary arterial pressure is greater than the alveolar pressure, the latter being, in turn, greater than venous pressure. Therefore, the capillary is open for a part of its length, until the point where alveolar pressure exceeds intravascular pressure. Consequently, blood flow in zone 2 is determined by the respective values of alveolar and arterial pulmonary pressures (and is independent of venous pressure); it therefore increases down this zone of lung, according to the progressive increase of pulmonary arterial pressure as a result of the hydrostatic gradient.

In *zone 3,* both pulmonary arterial and venous pressures exceed alveolar pressure; capillaries are perfused throughout their length and are increasingly distended down this zone.

A *fourth zone* is sometimes described in which the pulmonary blood flow decreases as a result of a compressing interstitial pressure on the vessel. Although it is well established that pulmonary blood flow is distributed in a vertical direction with respect to gravity, Hakim et al.[61] have suggested that in humans there also could be a gradient from center to periphery. Because local or peripheral vascular resistance rises in proportion to distance from the lung hilum, the center of each lobe will be better perfused than its periphery. The hypothesis that the same is true in the other species remains to be investigated.

Humoral and Neural Factors. Although predominantly passive mechanical forces determine regional blood flow distribution, the smooth muscles in arteries and veins respond to vasoactive compounds. The magnitude and mechanism of these responses depend on numerous factors such as the preexisting level of pulmonary vascular tone and the integrity of the pulmonary vascular endothelium.[62]

A modest autonomic innervation, with both adrenergic and cholinergic components, is found in the muscular vessels of the pulmonary circulation. Stimulation of the sympathetic nervous system constricts the blood vessels of the lung, whereas parasympathetic stimulation causes vasodilation.

Hypoxic Vasoconstriction. The modification of ventilation in some regions of the lung or in the whole lung also influences pulmonary perfusion. In unventilated regions of the lung, alveolar hypoxia occurs, inducing a local hypoxic vasoconstriction. This constriction provides a mechanism to redistribute pulmonary blood flow from less-ventilated to well-ventilated regions and therefore improves the ventilation/perfusion ratio and the gas exchange. The magnitude of the response to hypoxia depends on the thickness of the pulmonary arterial smooth-muscle layer; the response of the horse is intermediate between such species as cattle and pigs, where the response is quite vigorous, and sheep and dogs, where the response is minimal.[18,20] The mechanism for the occurrence of this constriction is still unclear. A combination of the action of a vasoactive agent with cellular mechanisms has been evoked as a possible cause. Hypoxic vasoconstriction is generally advantageous when occurring locally but may become unfavorable when occurring throughout the whole lung, as in acute hypoxia.

The exercise-induced pulmonary hypertension does not seem to be due to hypoxic pulmonary vasoconstriction.[63]

Bronchial Circulation

The bronchial circulation receives approximately 1 to 2 percent of the cardiac output from the left side of the heart. It supplies the airways, large pulmonary blood vessels, septa, pleura, and other lung structures. However, the lung does not suffer from a partial obstruction of the bronchial circulation. The numerous anastomoses between the pulmonary and bronchial circulations may provide blood flow to the bronchial circulation.[39]

Inversely, when the pulmonary perfusion is locally impaired, the bronchial circulation may proliferate and maintain some blood flow throughout the lung, thus contributing partly to gas exchange.[64] Such proliferations also may occur during pulmonary inflammation. Because they can be extensive in the dorsocaudal regions of the lungs, which are the regions that sometimes bleed during exercise, they have been related to the occurrence of exercise-induced pulmonary hemorrhage. In addition, the role played by pulmonary and/or the bronchial hypertension in exercise-induced pulmonary hemorrhage is strongly suspected but has not been demonstrated so far.

Postpulmonary shunts may result from anastomoses between pulmonary and bronchial circulations and theoretically may be partly responsible for the fall in the arterial O_2 partial pressure observed during exercise. However, a shunt of 1 percent, which is a reasonable approximation, would reduce arterial O_2 partial pressure by 5 mmHg, while the actual decrease during exercise is much larger.[4]

Lymphatic Circulation

Fluid filtration occurs between the capillaries and the interstitial tissue. The alveolar endothelium is less permeable than the capillary endothelium. Therefore, the fluid does not leak into the alveoli unless the epithelium is damaged or unless there is a considerable accumulation of fluid in the interstitial tissue. Fluid filtered from the capillaries moves through the interstitium toward the perivascular and peribronchial tissues, where lymphatic vessels are located. During exercise, the marked increase in the pulmonary arterial pressure probably induces an increase in the rate of fluid filtration across the capillary walls of the lung. The fact that this condition is not associated with pulmonary edema suggests that, in horses as in other species,[65] there is a substantial capacity of the lymphatic system to drain the pulmonary interstitial space.[59] Moreover, the "pumping" action associated with the large and frequent pressure changes in the equine thoracic cage during exercise could contribute to the adequacy of the lymphatic drainage.

VENTILATION/PERFUSION RATIO

Gas exchange ultimately depends on optimization of the ventilation/perfusion ratio; efficient gas exchange occurs in the lung regions where the ratio is 0.8 to 1.0.

Most lung regions have a ventilation/perfusion ratio of 0.8, but regions exist that are excessively perfused (ventilation/perfusion ratio < 0.8) or ventilated (ventilation/perfusion ratio > 0.8). When ventilation is impaired (i.e., partial airway obstruction), the ventilation/perfusion ratio decreases, and in extreme cases of total airway obstruction, the ventilation/perfusion ratio is 0. This corresponds to a right-to-left shunt. If perfusion is inadequate—pulmonary vasoconstriction or hypotension—the ventilation/perfusion ratio will increase, and in extreme cases of underperfusion due to emboli or in zone 1, the ventilation/perfusion ratio becomes infinite (Fig. 6–9).

In quiet, resting horses, the ventilation/perfusion ratio is not influenced by the gravitation; i.e., it is uniform from the top to the bottom of the lung, suggesting that the gradient in lung ventilation is matched by the gradient in lung perfusion.[60] In heavily exercising horses, there is only a very slight mismatch of ventilation and perfusion. This mismatch accounts for 25 percent of the increase in the alveolar-arterial pressure difference in O_2.[4]

The physiologic characteristics of the ventilation/perfusion ratio of horses contrast with those in humans. In the latter, the ventilation/perfusion ratio is nonuniform at rest, and a true mismatching occurs during exercise.[66]

In subjects suffering from airway disease, exercise will enhance ventilation/perfusion mismatching, mainly by the impairment of ventilation. This is particularly true in horses, where the collateral ventilation has little ability to compensate for the nonpermeability of small airways.[19] Therefore, the lobules that take a longer time to fill will have an inadequate ventilation/perfusion ratio and hypoxemia, and sometimes hypercapnia will result.

PULMONARY DIFFUSION

Composition of the Respiratory Gases
The ambient O_2 partial pressure, i.e., the relative contribution of the O_2 pressure to the total pressure of the ambient gas mixture, is about 20.93 percent of the total pressure exerted by the air (760 mmHg at sea level). CO_2 partial pressure in ambient air is negligible (0.03 percent) (Fig. 6–10).

After passing through the nasal cavities and the upper airways, air is saturated with H_2O. At normal body temperature (37°C), the partial pressure of the water vapor represents about 6.1 percent of the total pressure, or

47 mmHg. Therefore, the other gases exert a total pressure of only 713 mmHg (or 760 − 47 mmHg). Therefore, the actual O_2 pressure in the trachea decreases from 159 mmHg (room air) to 149 mmHg.

The alveolar air is quite different from the inspired air because CO_2 is continuously expelled into and O_2 taken from the alveoli. Alveolar air composition is not constant owing to cyclic variations depending on the respiratory phase (alveolar partial pressure of O_2 increases during inspiration and decreases during expiration). Consequently, the following values for alveolar air composition are mean values: 13.6% O_2, 5.3% CO_2, 74.9% nitrogen, and 6.2% H_2O. However, after expiration, the remaining air in the lungs will be mixed with the air of the next inspiration, damping the variation in alveolar gas composition (see Fig. 6–10).

Alveolar Diffusion
Diffusion is the passive process whereby O_2 passes from alveoli to capillary blood and CO_2 passes in the reverse direction. As indicated by the following formula, the rate of diffusion v is influenced by the pressure gradient of the gases between alveoli and capillary ($P_A − P_{cap}$), by the physical properties of the gases (D = diffusion coefficient), by the surface area available A, and by the thickness X of the alveolar-capillary barrier:

$$v = \frac{D \times A\,(P_A - P_{cap})}{X}$$

The alveolar-arterial pressure gradient is not constant; on the one hand, it decreases progressively as the blood passes through the alveolar capillary, and on the other, it varies according to the stage of the respiratory cycle. The maximal pressure gradients that can be encountered are about 60 and 6 mmHg of O_2 and CO_2, respectively. The coefficient of diffusion of O_2 in the horse averages 0.45 liter/min/mmHg.[11] CO_2 is 25 times more diffusible than O_2.

The horse, along with other active animals, appears to have an appropriately enlarged alveolar-capillary surface area.[67] Moreover, during exercise, this area is enlarged by the recruitment of unperfused vessels induced by the increase in pulmonary arterial pressure.

At rest and moderate exercise levels, no measurable diffusion limitation is observed in the healthy horse. The alveolar-arterial O_2 tension difference averages 4 mmHg. In contrast, during heavy but not necessarily maximal exercise (from 60 percent of $\dot{V}_{O_2max}$), arterial hypoxemia and hemoglobin desaturation occur in horses.[3,68] Simultaneously, the alveolar-arterial O_2 tension difference widens and may reach values as high as 30 mmHg.[38]

Hypoxemia is primarily related to one of the following factors: (1) decrease in the partial pressure of O_2 in the inspired air, (2) right-to-left vascular shunts, (3) ventilation/perfusion mismatching, (4) diffusion impairment, or (5) alveolar hypoventilation. Right-to-left shunts and mismatching of ventilation and perfusion have been shown to be accessory factors in producing hypoxemia during exercise.[4] A mild ventilation/perfusion ratio inequality accounts for 25 percent of the wid-

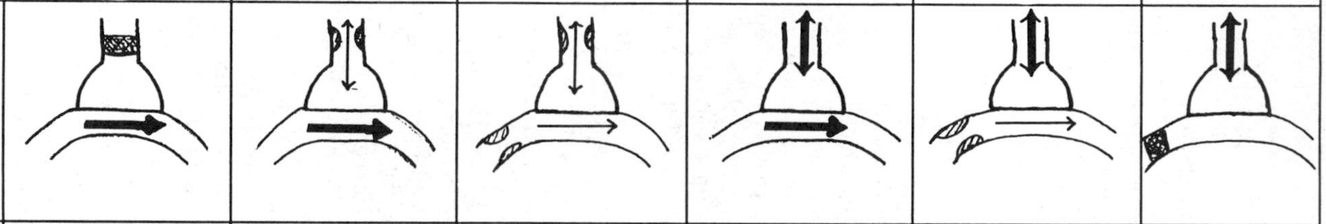

	A	B	C	D	E	F
Ventilation	O	↓	↓	N	N	N
Perfusion	N	N	↑	N	↓	O
V/Q	O	↓	↑	↑	↑	∞
Gas exchange	O	↓	↓	N	↓	O
Examples	Total airway obstruction (shunt)	Partial airway obstruction (airway dysfunction)	Partial airway and vascular obstruction (hypoxic vasoconstriction)	No obstruction (healthy animal)	Partial vascular obstruction (vascular dysfunction)	Total vascular obstruction (alveolar deadspace)

Figure 6-9. Illustration of several cases of ventilation-perfusion mismatching at the bronchoalveolar level (O: zero; N: normal).

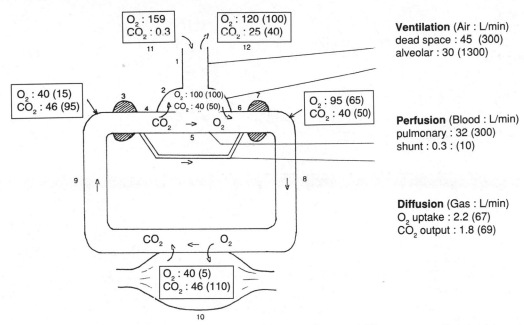

Figure 6-10. *Partial pressures of gases (mmHg) in relation to ventilation, perfusion, and diffusion processes (liters/min) in resting and exercising (data between brackets) conditions (1: airways; 2: alveoli; 3: right heart; 4: pulmonary artery; 5: pulmonary capillaries; 6: pulmonary veins; 7: left heart; 8: arteries; 9: veins; 10: locomotor muscles; 11: inspired air; 12: expired air).*

ening of the alveolar-arterial O_2 tension difference. Alveolar-capillary diffusion disequilibrium is responsible for the remaining 75 percent of this widening. Actually, during heavy exercise, different and opposite factors may influence the diffusion capacity. Capillary transit time is greatly shortened, as is the time for O_2 equilibration (Fig. 6–11). This will impair diffusion.

On the other hand, other changes actually improve diffusion. First, a mixed venous O_2 pressure as low as 16 mmHg has been reported during a fast gallop.[69] Because the alveolar O_2 pressure remains steady (Figs. 6–11 and 6–12), the pressure gradient between the capillary blood and the alveolar air is increased, improving O_2 extraction and diffusion. Second, the increased blood flow results in functional new alveoli previously unperfused at rest and therefore increases the exchanging alveolar surface. It also distends the pulmonary capillaries and thus increases the capillary blood volume. In humans, the capillary blood volume is able to expand about three times its resting value with only a four- to fivefold increase in pulmonary blood flow.[70] In horses, the blood flow increases eightfold, and it can be presumed that the capillary blood volume expands considerably more than that in humans. Lastly, the increase in the packed cell volume promotes O_2 diffusion by increasing the number of binding sites available.

The fact that the horse shows evidence of diffusion limitation during heavy exercise[4] suggests that the physiologic adjustments improving the pulmonary diffusion are overcome by the short capillary blood transit time, which averages 0.4 to 0.5 s in this species.[71] However, other athletic species have a short transit time during

exercise (0.29 s in the dog, 0.35 s in the pony, and 0.5 s in humans), but neither the dog nor the pony demonstrates diffusion limitation during exercise.[72] Therefore, it may be hypothesized that these species are able

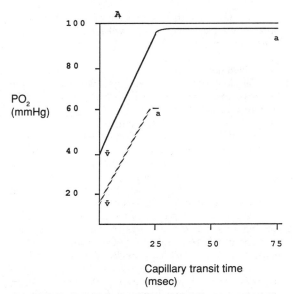

Figure 6-11. *Schematic illustration of O_2 diffusion across the alveolar-capillary membrane in resting (solid line) and exercising (dashed line) conditions. The capillary transit time (ms) is decreased about 3-fold during strenous exercise (A: alveolar air; v̄: mixed venous blood; a: arterialized blood).*

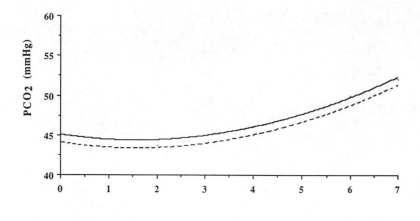

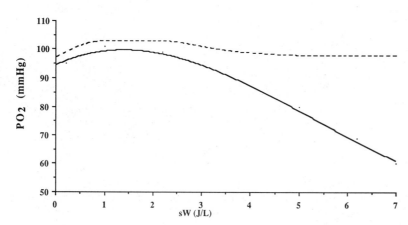

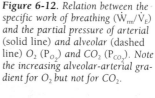

Figure 6-12. *Relation between the specific work of breathing ($\dot{W}_{rm}/\dot{V}_E$) and the partial pressure of arterial (solid line) and alveolar (dashed line) O_2 (P_{O_2}) and CO_2 (P_{CO_2}). Note the increasing alveolar-arterial gradient for O_2 but not for CO_2.*

to compensate for their short capillary transit time by other physiologic adaptations, which may be absent in the horse.

Tissue Diffusion
Arterial blood enters the tissue capillary with an arterial O_2 partial pressure of 85 to 100 mmHg and an arterial partial pressure of CO_2 of 40 to 44 mmHg. The tissue O_2 and CO_2 tensions are determined by the level of metabolic activity but generally average 40 and 46 to 48 mmHg, respectively. Therefore, O_2 and CO_2 will diffuse down their respective pressure gradients (see Fig. 6–10). Once released into the tissues, O_2 will be bound to myoglobin, an iron-containing pigment, the main function of which is the transfer of O_2 within the muscle cells.

Because the arterial O_2 partial pressure in blood returning from all tissues averages 16 mmHg during heavy exercise, it may be assumed that O_2 tension at the level of the exercising muscle is much lower. The dramatic decrease in O_2 tension in the tissues increases the driving pressure for oxygen diffusion at this level. Overall, the release of O_2 from hemoglobin at the level of the working muscles is promoted by the right shift of the oxyhemoglobin dissociation curve resulting from acidosis, hypercapnia (venous P_{CO_2} = 96 mmHg), and hyperthermia ($t°a$ = 41.3°C). Tissues with high aerobic

metabolic needs are more vascularized than others, and accordingly, the surface area for gas exchange is greater.

GAS EXCHANGE

Oxygen Uptake
Under steady conditions, oxidative metabolism supplies the body with essentially all the metabolic energy needed to maintain the supply of high-energy phosphate compounds required for homeostasis. Oxygen molecules enter the body and pass through each of the serial transport steps of the respiratory system (ventilatory convection, pulmonary diffusion, circulatory convection, and peripheral tissue diffusion) at a rate that is exactly matched to the rate at which they are consumed by oxidative phosphorylation in the mitochondria. The measurement of the rate of the whole-body aerobic metabolism at steady state, or O_2 uptake, is therefore a direct measure of the rate at which the pulmonary gas exchanger is functioning to meet the body's demand. The O_2 transport system functions as a cascade delivery system in which the difference in concentration of O_2 at the top of the cascade (ambient air) and the bottom (mitochondrial inner membrane) drives the flux of O_2 through the system and the reverse for CO_2.

When the demand for O_2 is set in the peripheral tissues, e.g., in the muscle during exercise, gas exchange rates at each of the respiratory system's transport steps must adjust proportionally in order to maintain the supply of O_2 to the muscles. With increasing exercise intensity, there is a nearly linear increase in the rate of O_2 uptake to a certain point, beyond which O_2 uptake remains constant at higher speed[27,42,53] (Fig. 6–13). At intensities above that at which the rate of O_2 uptake plateaus, termed $\dot{V}_{O_2max}$, the turnover rate of high-energy phosphate compounds continues to increase, but the source of metabolic energy that enables this increased turnover to occur is anaerobic glycolysis, with subsequent increases in the concentration of lactate in the muscle and blood. Such exercise is termed *supramaximal*. It is generally assumed that $\dot{V}_{O_2max}$ represents the athlete's capacity for the aerobic resynthesis of high-energy phosphate compounds and provides therefore a quantitative statement of an individual's capacity for aerobic energy transfer. Compared with mammals of similar size, horses achieve a higher $\dot{V}_{O_2max}$ per kilogram by building and maintaining more of the following structures in the O_2 transport chain: heart size, hemoglobin, and peripheral capillary bed. Additionally, they have a larger skeletal muscle mass that contains a higher density of mitochondria than do domestic animals of the same size.[72a] In horses $\dot{V}_{O_2max}$ is probably not reached until heart rate exceeds 200 beats/min.[42] The measurement of $\dot{V}_{O_2max}$ in horses has the disadvantage of requiring sophisticated equipment, but it is undoubtedly the more accurate index for the assessment of fitness and training adequacy in the athletic horse.[27,53]

Carbon Dioxide Output

The principal end products of aerobic catabolism are CO_2 and H_2O. At rest, these products are voided approximately as produced. Because of their chemical composition, each foodstuff requires different amounts of O_2 in relation to CO_2 produced during oxidation. A respiratory value that is potentially diagnostic of foodstuff is obtained by simultaneously measuring both CO_2 output and O_2 uptake and taking their ratio:

Moles of CO_2 produced per unit time/moles of O_2 consumed per unit time

When measured at the lungs, this ratio is called the *respiratory exchange ratio R*. An R near 1.0 indicates that the cells are catabolizing mostly carbohydrates, whereas an R near 0.7 indicates predominantly lipid catabolism. Under steady-rate exercise conditions (up to 80 percent of $\dot{V}_{O_2max}$ in trained subjects), the exchange of O_2 and CO_2 measured at the lungs reflects the actual gas exchange from nutrient metabolism in the peripheral tissue.

Strenuous exercise, above 80 percent of $\dot{V}_{O_2max}$ in trained subject, presents a situation in which R can rise significantly above 1.00. The lactic acid (LA) generated during exhaustive exercise is buffered by sodium bicarbonate in the blood to maintain the acid-base balance in the reaction

$$HLA + NaHCO_3 \rightarrow$$
$$NaLA + H_2CO_3 \rightarrow H_2O + CO_2$$

During this process, carbonic acid, a weaker acid, is formed. In the pulmonary capillaries, carbonic acid

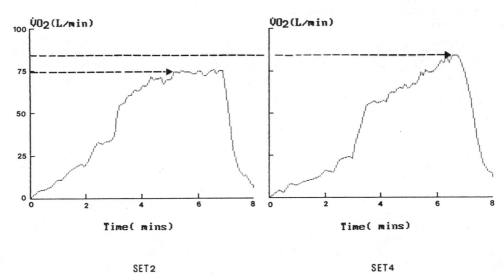

Figure 6-13. *Oxygen uptake ($\dot{V}_{O_2}$) curves obtained from the same horse (weight 512 kg, age 5 years) on a breath-by-breath basis (each point is the mean of 10 respiratory cycles) during a standardized treadmill exercise before (SET2) and after (SET4) a 6-week period of training. The test consisted in an exercise of increasing speed (1.7, 4, 8, 9, 10, 11 m/s, 1 minute for each speed) on a treadmill inclined at 6 degrees. The gallop started at the third minute of the test. $\dot{V}_{O_2max}$ was reached at 9 m/s during SET2 and was not reached during SET4.*

breaks down to its components, CO_2 and H_2O, and CO_2 exits through the lungs. This buffering process adds extra CO_2 to that quantity normally released during energy metabolism, and the R moves above 1.00.

BLOOD GAS TRANSPORT

Oxygen

The partial pressure of O_2 represents the relative pressure exerted by the gas in a mixture of gases (in air or in liquids); the saturation of O_2 represents the percentage of the total hemoglobin binding sites occupied by O_2; the O_2 content represents the total amount of O_2 in the blood, which is primarily O_2 bound to hemoglobin with lesser amounts dissolved in the plasma.

O_2 Dissolved. Once O_2 passes through the alveolar-capillary barrier, it either dissolves in the plasma or combines with hemoglobin, the latter being its main form of transport. At rest, the complete equilibration between alveolar and capillary O_2 tensions occurs before the blood leaves the capillary. Oxygen has low solubility in plasma; only 0.3 ml of O_2 will be dissolved in 100 ml of plasma when alveolar partial pressure of O_2 is 100 mmHg. However, the O_2 dissolved in the plasma determines the arterial partial pressure of O_2 and therefore plays an important role in both O_2 diffusion and O_2 blood transport.

O_2 Bound to Hemoglobin. Each molecule of hemoglobin can reversibly bind up to four molecules of O_2, forming the oxyhemoglobin complex. Beyond its primary role of O_2 transport, hemoglobin provides a sink for O_2 and therefore contributes to the maintenance of an adequate pressure gradient during alveolar-capillary diffusion. In resting horses, hemoglobin concentration is about 140 to 150 g/liter. Each gram of hemoglobin is able to hold 1.36 to 1.39 ml of O_2.

O_2 Content. The oxygen content of blood is mainly determined by the hemoglobin concentration and its sat-

uration with O_2. When hemoglobin is saturated with O_2, 100 ml of blood carries about 20 ml of O_2, compared with the 0.3 ml of O_2 dissolved per 100 ml of plasma.

The saturation of hemoglobin depends on the arterial O_2 partial pressure, which depends, in turn, on the amount of O_2 dissolved in the plasma. Above an O_2 partial pressure of approximately 70 mmHg, the oxyhemoglobin curve is flat, and any increase in partial pressure will add little O_2 to hemoglobin. The hemoglobin is nearly saturated; only a few (3 to 5 percent) of the binding sites are still available. Below an O_2 partial pressure of 60 mmHg, the oxyhemoglobin curve shows a sharply decreasing slope. This partial pressure is encountered in the tissues (mean partial pressure of O_2 about 40 mmHg). In this state, blood loses about 25 percent of its O_2 to the advantage of the tissues. When the metabolism is high, i.e., during exercise, the tissue partial pressure of O_2 is still less, and more O_2 will be released. Lastly, increases in blood temperature, [H^+], partial pressure of CO_2, and intracellular concentration of certain organic phosphates (2,3-DPG) induce a right shift of the curve, promoting a higher O_2 release at the level of the metabolizing tissues.

Figure 6–14 shows the oxyhemoglobin dissociation curve of horses, which is slightly different from the classic curve reported for human beings. The affinity of equine hemoglobin for O_2 is higher than in humans but less influenced by the temperature modifications.[73]

When the number of erythrocytes—and therefore the amount of hemoglobin—is reduced, as in anemia, the O_2 content is reduced despite normal arterial O_2 partial pressure and hemoglobin saturation. On the contrary, when the packed cell volume increases, as during exercise in horses, the O_2 content increases, even if the arterial O_2 partial pressure is reduced (see Table 6–2). The increase in the packed cell volume and the consequent increase in hemoglobin due to splenic contraction are an adaptation to exercise specific to the horse, providing almost 50 to 60 percent more binding sites for O_2 during exercise.[74] This represents a compensatory adjustment for the fall in arterial O_2 partial pressure and

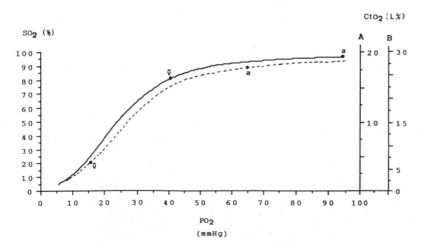

Figure 6-14. Oxyhemoglobin dissociation curve in resting (solid line) and heavily exercising (dashed line) horses. The shift of the curve to the right is due to exercise-induced hyperthermia and acidosis [P_{O_2}: partial pressure for O_2; S_{O_2}: percent saturation of hemoglobin for O_2; Ct_{O_2}: O_2 content at rest (A) (hemoglobin = 140 g/liter) and during exercise (B) (hemoglobin = 220g/liter)]. Values for arterialized (a) and mixed venous ($\bar{v}$) blood are also illustrated on the curves.

hemoglobin desaturation. However, too great an increase in packed cell volume may be disadvantageous from a hemodynamic point of view because it increases the blood viscosity.[75]

Carbon Dioxide

Carbon dioxide results from metabolic processes occurring in the tissues, and once produced, it diffuses from the cells into the capillary blood. In resting conditions, when the blood leaves the tissues, the partial pressure of CO_2 has increased from 40 mmHg in arterial blood to 46 mmHg. Approximately 5 percent of the CO_2 is dissolved in the plasma; this fraction determines the partial pressure of CO_2. The remaining CO_2 is transported in two chemical combinations. Most of the CO_2 combines reversibly with H_2O, forming carbonic acid, which then dissociates into bicarbonate and hydrogen ion:

$$H_2O + CO_2 \leftrightarrow H_2CO_3 \leftrightarrow HCO_3^- + H^+$$

Between 60 and 80 percent of the CO_2 is transported as HCO_3^-. The reaction may occur in the plasma but occurs mainly in red cells, where the presence of carbonic anhydrase accelerates the process several hundred fold. The reverse reaction occurs when the blood reaches the lungs.

The formation of carbamino compounds (15 to 20 percent of the total CO_2 blood content) by coupling of the CO_2 to the $-NH$ groups of proteins (mainly hemoglobin) is the last form of transport for CO_2. At high intensities of exercise, i.e., 100 percent of $\dot{V}_{O_2max}$, the large muscular mass produces an extraordinary amount of CO_2, and the lung seems unable to completely eliminate it. The development of a relative CO_2 retention that is observed in horses even when running without a mask is unique among mammals.[69] Human athletes develop a compensatory hyperventilation during heavy exercise to ensure high alveolar O_2 partial pressure, which in turn hastens the rate of equilibrium of alveolar gases with mixed venous blood but also provokes a decrease of the arterial partial pressure of CO_2 (about 30 mmHg).[76] Obviously, in exercising horses, there is a lack of truly compensatory hyperventilation, contributing to the development of exercise-induced hypercapnia.[69,72a]

MECHANICS OF BREATHING

Volume changes in the respiratory apparatus imply that work is being performed on the respiratory system, mainly expanding or compressing the gas in the lungs and displacing it in and out of the airways. The driving forces exerted by the respiratory muscles are opposed mainly by static forces (elastic, gravitational, and surface) and flow-resistive forces (viscous and turbulent resistance of the gases and viscous resistance of the tissues); the inertial forces, negligible at rest, are also of importance in running horses.

Therefore, at each stage of the respiratory cycle, the change in pleural pressure (ΔP_{pl}) is the sum of the elastic (P_{el}), frictional (P_{fr}), and inertial (P_{in}) pressure changes. It is determined by the change in lung volume (ΔV_T),

lung compliance (C), airflow ($\dot{V}$), respiratory resistance (R), volume acceleration ($\ddot{V}$), and inertance (I) of the respiratory system:

$$\Delta P_{pl} = P_{el} + P_{fr} + P_{in} = \Delta V_T/C + R\dot{V} + I\ddot{V}$$

The study of the relationship between the pressures exerted on the respiratory system (which are the causes) and the changes in volume and airflow that result (which are the effects) is the basis of the mechanics of breathing (Fig. 6–15).

Breathing Strategy in the Horse

The equine species differs from the other species with regard to breathing strategy.[26,77,78] Unlike humans, horses at rest breath around, rather than from, the relaxed volume of the respiratory system (i.e., the equilibrium position where the tendency of the lung to recoil inward is equal to the tendency of the chest wall to recoil passively outward).[77] Inversely to other species, the second part of exhalation is active in the horse, and consequently, the very first part of inhalation is passive. The physiologic reason for this strategy is still unknown, but it has been hypothesized that it could minimize the work of breathing. Indeed, the equine chest wall is very stiff compared with other species.[23] This implies that the work done to overcome this stiffness during inspiration (called the *elastic work*) will be proportionally higher. Breathing

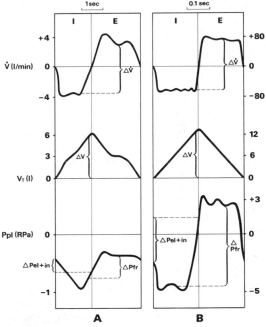

Figure 6-15. *Simultaneous recording of flow ($\dot{V}$), volume (V_T), and pleural pressure (P_{pl}) curves at rest (A) and during exercise (B). Scales are different on the two graphs [I: inspiration; E: expiration; P_{fr}: frictional forces; P_{el+in}: elastic and inertial forces; total pulmonary resistance (R_L) = $\Delta P_{fr}/\Delta\dot{V}$; dynamic lung compliance (C_{dyn}) = $\Delta V/\Delta P_{el+in}$].*

around, rather than from, the relaxed respiratory volume implies that the energy stored during the latter active part of expiration will be restored during the first passive part of inhalation. Thus the abdominal muscles, by performing positive work during expiration, share the total work of breathing with the inspiratory muscles.

A direct consequence of this specific breathing strategy is that the pattern of the respiratory airflow is bi- or polyphasic.[26,77,78] Exercise induces a sharp increase in the peak respiratory airflow and enlarges the flow-volume loops (Fig. 6–16), the shape of which tend towards an increasingly rectangular pattern. The fact that, at a fast trot, a plateau occurs during inspiration and expiration suggests a flow limitation when ventilation increases.[78]

Ventilatory muscle activity has not yet been studied directly during exercise. However, numerous indirect experiments relating measurements of pleural and transdiaphragmatic pressure changes,[79,80] respiratory airflow shape and amplitude,[78] or blood perfusion of the respiratory muscles[24,81] have helped to quantify the magnitude of the increase in ventilatory muscle activity.

Pleural Pressure
Because the visceral and parietal pleurae are maintained in close apposition, the lung and the thorax interact mechanically. The work performed by the ventilatory muscles induces changes in the pressure of the intrapleural space. During inspiration, the pleural pressure (which at rest and in quiet conditions is subatmospheric) decreases, and at the end of inspiration, when the airflow returns to 0, the pleural pressure increases slightly. During expiration, the pleural pressure increases toward its value at functional residual capacity, i.e., lung volume before inspiration (see Fig. 6–15).

There is a vertical pressure gradient throughout the thorax so that pleural pressure is more subatmospheric in the dorsal than in the ventral regions. Also, the changes in the pleural pressure during respiration are greatest in the middle and in the bottom and less in the top of the thorax. This results in preferential ventilation of the ventral regions of the lungs.[44]

The force exerted by the ventilatory muscles, especially the diaphragm, also may be estimated by measurement of the transdiaphragmatic pressure, i.e., the pressure gradient between the thorax and the gastric pressures, the latter being assimilated to the abdominal pressure.[77,79,80]

When exercise starts, the maximal pleural pressure changes increase, and in thoroughbred horses during maximal exercise, maximal pleural pressure changes as high as 8.5 kPa have been recorded.[5] In this condition, respiratory frequency is about 120 breaths/min, and therefore, such a pressure swing takes less than 250 ms.

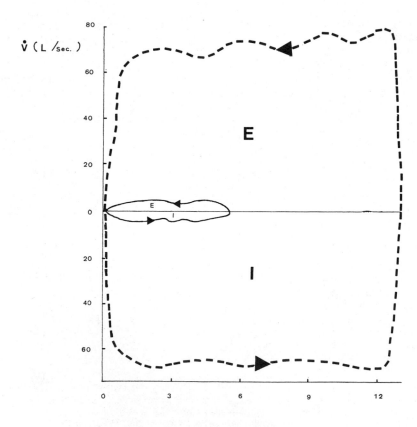

Figure 6-16. Flow ($\dot{V}$)–volume (V_T) loop in a resting (solid line) and exercising (dashed line) horse (I: inspiration; E: expiration).

Because the transformation of chemical energy into mechanical energy has a limiting rate, less tension can be maintained at high velocities of contraction than at lower speed. The force-speed characteristics of the respiratory muscles could therefore be a limiting factor to further increases in ventilation during strenuous exercise.

Pulmonary Resistance

Definition and Distribution Throughout the Respiratory System. The total pulmonary resistance quantifies the permeability of the airways to airflow. The respiratory flow must be generated mainly against the frictional resistance between the air molecules and the walls of the airways but also against the viscous drag of the tissues.

The resistance R to airflow passing through a tube is determined by the radius r and the length l of the tube, as well as by the physical properties of the gas breathed (μ), according to the following formula:

$$R = \frac{8\mu l}{r^4}$$

This points out the critical importance of the radius; if it is divided by 2, R is multiplied by 16.

During quiet breathing, 50 percent of the total pulmonary resistance results from the nasal passages, 30 percent from the remaining upper airways, and 20 percent from the intrathoracic airways[82] (Fig. 6–17). The importance of the relative contribution of the nasal cavities is not specific to horses, but this species, in contrast to others, cannot switch from nasal to oronasal breathing.

Effect of Exercise on Total Pulmonary Resistance. While not modifying significantly the relative contribution of each part of the respiratory tract to the total pulmonary resistance, exercise induces a substantial increase in this resistance.[5,82] During exercise, physiologic adjustments, such as dilatation of the external nares, full abduction of the larynx, and bronchodilation, tend to facilitate the increase in flow and decrease the resistance by enlarging the airways' cross-sectional area and therefore the airways' radius. However, despite these exercise-induced adaptations, heavy exercise induces a more than twofold increase in the total pulmonary resistance. The total pulmonary resistance is the result of two kinds of opposed factors: physiologic ones tending to decrease the resistance and physical ones (mainly frictions, turbulences, inhomogeneous distribution of the resistance along airways and alveoli, and airway cross-sectional area changes induced by compressing transmural pressures) tending to increase it. When the horse walks or trots slowly, both factors cancel each other, and the resistance remains unchanged. However, during heavy exercise, the physical factors, depending on flow amplitude and increasing total pulmonary resistance, largely override the physiologic ones, and the resistance increases. Lastly, during recovery, while the ventilatory parameters return progressively to their baseline, the physiologic factors overcome, and the resistance may be less than during quiet breathing at rest.[82]

Factors Increasing Resistance to Airflow During Exercise. FRICTION AND TURBULENCE. The importance of friction and turbulence to the increase in the total pulmonary resistance has been demonstrated by experiments where exercising horses breathed a helium-oxygen mixture. This mixture has a lesser density than air and therefore minimizes turbulence and friction. During exercise, it induced a significant increase in minute ventilation due to an increase in respiratory frequency, as well as a 50 percent decrease in the total pulmonary resistance and mechanical work of breathing.[83]

DYNAMIC PARTIAL COLLAPSE OF THE AIRWAYS. Studies of the inspiratory and expiratory components of the resistance values in trotting horses have shown that during inspiration, the extrathoracic airways account for more than 90 percent of the total pulmonary resistance, while during expiration, the intrathoracic airways are responsible for more than 50 percent of the pulmonary resistance[82] (see Fig. 6–17). This observation could be explained by the fact that during exercise, a dynamic partial collapse may occur when the pressure surrounding the airways exceeds the pressure within the lumen.[84] When a horse inhales, subatmospheric pressures in the extrathoracic airways may be as low as minus 5 kPa, while the pressure in the surrounding tissues remains atmospheric (see Fig. 6–6). During expiration, the intrathoracic pressure becomes greater than the pressure prevailing inside some of the intrathoracic airways (see Fig. 6–6). When exposed to compressive pressures, these structures tend to collapse, consequently increasing their resistance to airflow. Because of their bony support, the nasal cavities are less subject to compression than less well supported structures such as the nares, pharynx, trachea, and bronchi. If this collapse occurs

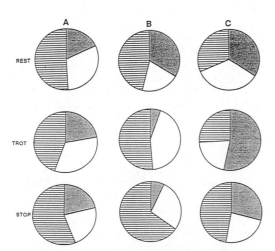

Figure 6-17. *Relative contribution of nasal* (hatched area), *laryngeal plus extrathoracic tracheal* (light area), *and intrathoracic airway* (dark area) *resistance to total pulmonary resistance under resting and exercising conditions (A: total resistance; B: inspiratory resistance; C: expiratory resistance; stop: 20 first seconds of recovery).*

normally in healthy horses, it can be expected to be dramatically worse in horses suffering from airways obstruction, a condition accompanied by substantial transmural pressures during exercise.[85]

It has been shown that both the extra- and intrathoracic parts of the trachea are sufficiently compliant to decrease their cross-sectional areas when submitted to high, but nevertheless physiologic, compressive transmural pressures.[15,16] Moreover, the shape of the cross-sectional area of the individual trachea significantly influences collapsibility; tracheae with a circular cross-sectional shape are less compressible than tracheae with a more ellipsoidal shape.[16] This is particularly important in view of the variability observed in this shape among individual horses (see Fig. 6–4), some horses being probably more susceptible than others to dynamic tracheal collapse. In other words, during intense exercise, when high levels of ventilation are reached, horses having an ellipsoidal trachea may be disadvantaged compared with those having a more circular trachea.

Lastly, the extension of the trachea decreases its collapsibility.[16] This means that hyperextension stiffens the trachea under dynamic conditions, therefore decreasing its resistance to airflow and consequently increasing the maximal airflow. This could explain the benefit of neck extension during maximal exercise; as well as providing maximal patency of the nasopharyngeal airways, the cervical extension and the consequent longitudinal extension of the trachea decrease the tracheal compliance and minimize the phenomenon of dynamic collapse.

Nonpathologic Factors Influencing Pulmonary Resistance. A major factor affecting the diameter of the tracheobronchial tree and consequently its resistance to airflow is smooth-muscle contraction or relaxation. When irritant materials such as dust are inhaled, the tracheobronchial irritant receptors are stimulated, resulting in a bronchoconstriction, the afferent of which is elicited by the parasympathetic system. A practical consequence is that any factor that will impair the mucociliary clearance also will decrease the airway permeability. For example, keeping the heads of healthy horses raised for a long time during transportation may impair the physiologic upper airway clearance and interfere with the airway permeability.[86]

A noncholinergic excitatory system, with substance P as the transmitter and activated by axon reflexes from airway receptors, also may cause bronchoconstriction. Relaxation of smooth muscle occurs following β_2-adrenergic receptor stimulation by circulating cathecolamines. The nonadrenergic, noncholinergic inhibitory nervous system is another bronchodilator system. Its efferent fibers are in the vagus, and the neurotransmitter could be nitric oxide.[87]

Dynamic Compliance

The *dynamic compliance* gives an estimate of the elastic properties of the lung. The lung has an inherent elasticity due to the elasticity of the tissue (the normal lung is an elastic structure that contains a network of elastin and collagen fibres) and the surface tension forces. The latter is lowered by the pulmonary surfactant, a complex material composed of 80 percent lipids and 20 percent proteins. The surfactant maintains alveolar stability and prevents pulmonary atelectasis.

The elastic properties of the lung are well documented by the generation of a pressure/volume relation curve constructed by plotting the different driving pressures necessary to inflate the lung up to a given level versus the lung inflation. This relationship, established during spontaneous and tidal breathing, defines the dynamic compliance (see Fig. 6–15). Although it depends on the intrinsic properties of the lung, it is also influenced by dynamic factors such as lung inflation and respiratory frequency. Dynamic compliance increases with lung inflation and may decrease with increasing respiratory frequency. The latter is especially true in lungs presenting a certain degree of subobstruction of the lower airways. Therefore, dynamic compliance measurement is sometimes used as an index of ventilatory asynchronism.

Pathologic conditions that induce lung rigidity (i.e., pulmonary edema, pulmonary hypertension, fibrosis) also induce a decrease in dynamic compliance. The dynamic lung compliance at rest is approximately equal to 23 liters/kPa. Because of technical problems associated with the determination of dynamic compliance during hyperventilation in large animals, the effect of exercise on the elastic properties of the horse's lung is not yet documented.

Pulmonary Inertance

Inertial forces are those necessary to accelerate or decelerate the air in the respiratory airways. In human beings, the inertance of the respiratory system is negligible, and so are the pressures necessary to induce accelerations and decelerations of the air in the airways (inertial pressures), even during intense exercise. In contrast, the inertial pressures are not negligible in exercising horses.[88]

Characteristics of the Equine Trachea. Tracheal length in mammals is designated by the physiologic and anatomic peculiarities of each species.[89] Horses are grass-eating animals with proportionally longer legs than other domestic grass-eating species and consequently have a longer neck. They also have a deep thorax. The anatomic consequence of this is that they also have a proportionally longer trachea than other species. Therefore, the tracheal diameter must be "chosen" in a way that its design is optimized to satisfy dominant constraints such as tracheal resistance, inertance (the longer the trachea and the smaller its section, the greater its inertance), flow limitation, dead space, and minimum work of breathing.[89] A larger diameter would be advantageous with regard to pulmonary resistance and inertance but disadvantageous for the anatomic dead space.

Physiologic Implications. During quiet breathing, respiratory frequency is about 14 breaths/min, tidal volume is about 5.5 liters, the total pressure change to which the lungs are subjected is about 0.44 kPa, and the pressure associated with volume acceleration is about 0.22 kPa.[88] During a fast gallop, respiratory frequency increases up to 121 breaths/min, tidal volume increases up to 13.2 liters, the maximal pressure change reaches values of 8.5 kPa, and total volume acceleration reaches more than 3000 liters/s.[2] The pressure required to produce these accelerations is then 4.3 kPa, or 50 percent of the total pressure change. Therefore, it appears that inertial pressures become of great importance in the exercising horse. They may even be a limiting or at least a constraining factor to any further increase in ventilation.[88]

Consequences for the Measurement of the Dynamic Compliance. The great importance of the respiratory inertial factors in the running horse also explains why the dynamic compliance becomes negative when measured during exercise[28,83] (Figs. 6–15 and 6–18). Classically, the dynamic compliance is measured at points of zero flow and is defined by the equation

$$C_{dyn} = V_T/(\Delta P_{el} - 4\Pi^2 \cdot f^2 \cdot V_T \cdot I)$$

where ΔP_{el} is the elastic pressure change. The term $4\Pi^2 \cdot f^2 \cdot V_T \cdot I$ (i.e., the inertial pressure change) is generally considered as negligible, and the equation simplified is

$$C_{dyn} = V_T/\Delta P_{el}$$

In exercising horses, $4\Pi^2 \cdot f^2 \cdot V_T \cdot I$ increases, and its absolute value may become equal to or greater than ΔP_{el}. This explains why, in these specific conditions, C_{dyn} is either overestimated, infinite, or negative.

Mechanical Work of Breathing

A classical approach to the assessment of the mechanical work of breathing is based on measurement of the area of the pressure/volume loops (see Fig. 6–18). Although it is well known that the total work of breathing is underestimated by this method, it gives a good estimation of the dynamic components of the work of breathing. It has been shown that the work per respiratory cycle, the work per liter of air ventilated, and the work per minute are increased dramatically during exercise.[90] For example, the power output (i.e., the work of breathing per minute) increases 475 times between rest and a strenuous gallop[5] (see Table 6–2).

The relationship between the mechanical work of breathing per minute and the minute volume in running

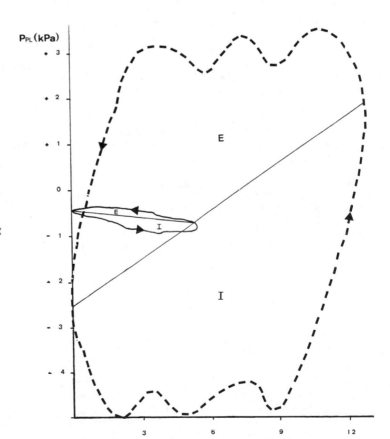

Figure 6-18. Pressure (P_{pl})–volume (V_T) loop in a resting (solid line) and exercising (dashed line) horse. The area of this loop gives an estimation of the work of breathing (I: inspiration; E: expiration; 1 kPa = 7.5 mmHg).

horses is curvilinear with an upward concavity (Fig. 6–19). The curve is of ever-increasing slope, implying that the mechanical cost of breathing for any additional units of air ventilated becomes greater with any increase in ventilation.[5,90]

The sharp increase in the work of breathing with exercise-induced hyperventilation is explained by the increase in resistive, elastic, and inertial work. The increase in the resistive work is related to the increase in the total pulmonary resistance[5,90] (see Fig. 6–19), itself due to compulsory nasal breathing,[82] to friction and turbulence,[83] and to the dynamic partial collapse of the airways.[15] The threefold increase in volume probably increases the elastic work significantly[90] owing to chest-wall stiffness. Furthermore, the length of the airways and the magnitude of flow accelerations during exercise make the inertial work nonnegligible.[88] These observations strongly suggest that the work of breathing could be a limiting or at least a constraining factor to further increases in ventilation during strenuous exercise.

Inspiratory Muscles to Total Oxygen Uptake Ratio

The ratio of the mechanical work of breathing to O_2 uptake has been calculated in galloping horses in order to evaluate the relative respiratory muscle O_2 uptake compared with total O_2 uptake. This ratio increases exponentially with the minute volume, indicating that during exercise, respiratory muscle O_2 uptake reaches a substantial percentage of the total O_2 uptake[5] (see Fig. 6–19). This suggests that in horses as in humans[91] there is a so-called critical level of ventilation above which any further increase in O_2 uptake would be entirely consumed by the respiratory muscles.

Respiration Locomotion Coupling

At the walk and trot, respiratory and step frequencies have been reported to be sometimes coupled, but this coupling is neither constant nor compulsory.[79,92] However, when the coupling exists, it seems that the "abdominal piston" acts in synergy with the respiratory pump.[79] Therefore, this strategy probably reduces the cost of breathing.

Once the horse gallops, there is a compulsory linkage between step and respiratory rates.[31,93–95] The mechanisms underlying this coupling are not yet well understood. It is probably due to a mechanical linkage, with the visceral contents acting as a piston and flexion of the back and loading of the thorax by the forelimbs contributing to the mechanical advantages of this synchronization.[31] During protraction of the forelimbs, the rib cage is pulled forward and outward, allowing inhalation. During weight bearing, the rib cage absorbs forces and is compressed, resulting in exhalation. Experimental evidence shows that in galloping horses, back flexion rather than the visceral piston mechanism assists breathing.[95]

It must be emphasized that this coupling is not absolute in healthy horses. Indeed, some galloping horses, both on the track and on the treadmill, sporadically show a "big breath" which continues for two or three strides. The reason for this remains to be investigated, but these horses seem to run better after this lung hyperinflation.

Respiratory Muscle Recruitment

In mammals, the diaphragm (separating the thorax from the abdomen) and the external intercostal muscles (joining the ribs) are the main inspiratory muscles. However, in horses, the serratus ventralis has the most important role in assisting the inspiratory effort of the diaphragm both at rest[96] and during exercise.[24] On the other hand, the transversalis is the principal muscle actively involved in expiration. Lastly, the intercostal muscles are also activated in the second part of inspiration and expiration.[96]

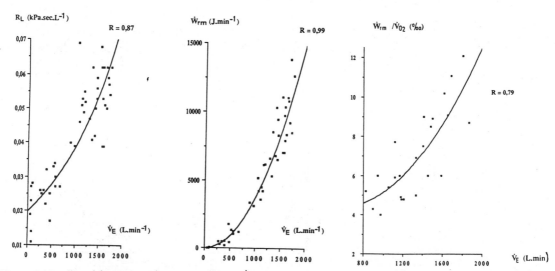

Figure 6-19. *Effect of the increase of minute ventilation ($\dot{V}_E$) on total pulmonary resistance (R_L), minute work of breathing ($\dot{W}_{rm}$), and the ratio $\dot{W}_{rm}$ to O_2 uptake ($\dot{W}_{rm}/\dot{V}_{O_2}$). This could explain why the energy cost of breathing could become excessive at high ventilatory levels.*

The study of respiratory muscle recruitment by electromyography has been performed in healthy resting horses[77,96] and in ponies during hypoxia.[97] Until now, this measurement has not been reported in exercising horses. However, during exercise, both inspiratory and expiratory muscle activity increases, and the metabolic needs of the muscles become substantial. The increase in blood flow may be related to the increase in the metabolic needs. Therefore, the activity of the ventilatory muscles in ponies has been estimated indirectly by the increase in the muscles' perfusion.[24,98,99] The ventilatory muscles comprise 5.5 percent of the total body weight and receive 10 and 15 percent of the cardiac output at rest and at maximal exercise, respectively. The increase in blood flow in these muscles is accompanied by a precipitous decrease in their vascular resistance.[24,98]

During exercise, the costal diaphragm blood flow exceeds the blood flow to all other inspiratory or expiratory muscles; it increases over 20-fold in maximally exercised ponies. Moreover, during maximal exercise, diaphragmatic blood flow reaches its upper limit,[100] and adenosine infusion, which causes a marked vasodilation in the pony's diaphragm at rest, fails to elicit any further vasodilation, indicating that vasodilator capacity is completely utilized in the pony.[101] This suggests a potential limiting factor of the ventilatory machinery during heavy exercise.

CONTROL OF BREATHING

With the exception of the changes induced by strenuous exercise, it can be assumed that the arterial blood gases and the chemical composition of the blood remain remarkably steady in healthy horses. This means that the metabolic needs are constantly matched by the alveolar ventilation. This matching is under the control of a central controller, which receives afferent information from peripheral and central receptors and which regulates, via motor neurons, the ventilatory muscles according to that information. The respiratory control center is located in the medulla, and its activity is modulated by a variety of neural inputs. Another part of the brain is also involved in controlling the respiratory rhythm, and higher conscious centers can intervene to modify the pattern of breathing.

Respiratory Control at Rest
Central Control. Breathing is controlled by neurons located in the pons and the medulla. The respiratory center in the medulla is divided into two groups of neurons. There is a dorsal group (located in the ventral portion of the nucleus tractus solitarius), which contains mainly inspiratory neurons, and a ventral group (located near the nucleus ambiguous and nucleus retroambiguous), which has both inspiratory and expiratory neurons. If the medulla is experimentally isolated from all neural inputs, the animal continues to breath rhythmically. The activity of both medullary centers is modulated by two respiratory centers in the pons: (1) the apneustic center, located in the lower pons, which stimulates the inspiratory neurons of the medulla, and (2) the pneumotaxic center, located in the upper pons, which switches off the inspiration.

Chemoreceptors and Humoral Control. Because the primary function of the lungs is the supply of O_2 and remove CO_2, it is clear that the ventilation ultimately must be controlled according to information on gas exchange. Chemoreceptors are sensors that detect changes in arterial blood gases or chemical composition. They give feedback about the results of adjustments in ventilation to the respiratory control centers. Changes in the arterial partial pressure of CO_2 and pH are detected by both peripheral and central chemoreceptors, while changes in arterial O_2 partial pressure are detected by peripheral chemoreceptors only. Therefore, at rest, sensation of the partial pressure of CO_2 and/or H^+ concentration is paramount in regulating ventilation under usual resting conditions. Small changes in arterial partial pressure of CO_2 and/or pH are more potent regulators of ventilation than changes in arterial O_2 partial pressure.

The *peripheral chemoreceptors* are located in the carotid bodies at the bifurcation of the common carotid arteries and in the aortic bodies, near the aortic arch. These chemoreceptors send afferent impulses to the control center via the vagus and the glossopharyngeal nerves. Their activity is enhanced by hypercapnia, hypoxemia, and acidosis but also by hyperthermia and decreased blood pressure. They are sensitive to the changes in arterial O_2 partial pressure but not to changes in oxyhemoglobin content. While their response to CO_2 and pH is quite linear, their response to changes in arterial O_2 partial pressure is nonlinear; they only show enhanced activity once arterial O_2 partial pressure is below 60 mmHg.

The *central chemoreceptor* tissue is located near the ventral aspect of the medulla. It lies in the intracerebral interstitial fluid and is separated from the blood by the blood-brain barrier. It apparently responds to changes in the interstitial tissue fluid pH. The latter is induced either by changes in arterial partial pressure of CO_2, giving a fast response (because CO_2 diffuses freely through the blood-brain barrier and induces a fast decrease in the interstitial fluid pH) or by a change in blood pH, giving a delayed response (because the barrier is relatively impermeable to H^+). Therefore, an acute increase in H^+ concentration is at first detected by the peripheral receptors.

Pulmonary and Airway Receptors. Three kinds of receptors with vagal afferents are located in the lungs and play a role in ventilatory control. The *pulmonary stretch receptors* are nerves ending in the tracheal and bronchial smooth muscles. Their activity is enhanced by enlargement of airway cross section, e.g., when the lung volume increases, and results in an inhibition of further inspiratory activity. The stretch receptors could be responsible for the adjustment in the pattern of breathing to minimize the energy cost of breathing. They also could prevent lung overstretching when the ventilatory demand is high, i.e., during heavy exercise.

Irritant receptors have a minor role in the control of

breathing. They are located between and below the epithelial cells of the airways (larynx, trachea, bronchi, and intrapulmonary airways). They protect the lung against various aggressions by reacting to a variety of stimulations (such as inhalation of irritant gases, dust, release of histamine) and inducing tachypnea, bronchospasm, cough, and mucus secretion.

Pulmonary C fibers ramify in the pulmonary interstitium close to the pulmonary capillaries, where they may monitor blood composition or degree of distension of the interstitium. They are probably responsible for the respiratory adjustments occurring in disease states, but this remains to be demonstrated in horses.

Muscle Spindle Stretch Receptors. As with other skeletal muscles, the ventilatory muscles have spindle stretch receptors. The density of these receptors is variable from one muscle to another; they are few in the diaphragm but numerous in the intercostals. They control the strength of the ventilatory muscle contraction.

Respiratory Control During Exercise

Gas-exchange requirements, i.e., O_2 uptake and CO_2 output, vary with the metabolic rate. Without doubt, exercise is the most potent stress to the body's oxidative machinery, i.e., to the muscle and functions concerned with external and alveolar gas exchange, gas transport, and tissue respiration. When animals exercise at increasing intensity, the O_2 uptake rises linearly to a maximum termed $\dot{V}_{O_2max}$. At this exercise intensity, all the available muscles' aerobic capacities are recruited, and with further increase in intensity, there will be no further increase in O_2 uptake. At maximal exercise, the O_2 uptake may increase more than 50 times, this increase being satisfied by an approximately 30-fold increase in the minute volume.[27,53,102]

The question of how the ventilatory rate is controlled during exercise is one of the major unresolved issues in respiratory physiology. The controversy centers around the origin of the stimulus that provides for a rapid and precise adjustment of alveolar ventilation to meet the metabolic demand. In humans, there are several theories proposing either neural stimuli or humoral stimuli or a combination of both.[103] In horses, this control seems to be different according to the exercise intensity.

Respiratory Control During Low-Intensity Exercise. During short-term moderate exercise, arterial blood gases and chemical composition do not change. This stability results because the ventilation rate increases in tandem with the metabolic rate. However, gaseous tensions are far too stable to account for the increase in ventilation on the basis of the simple negative-feedback system existing at rest. Although there is a considerable conviction that gas tensions (especially partial pressure of CO_2 and associated H^+ concentration) are involved in the control of ventilation during exercise as well, how they are involved remains enigmatic. It is likely that other drives are involved in the control of ventilation, such as mechanoreflexes originating from motion of the working

limbs and changes in cardiac output, thermoregulation, and cortical and psychological factors.[104]

The exercise-induced hyperpnea at mild and moderate exercise intensities has been thoroughly studied in ponies, showing that in this species, the hyperpnea is related to an increase in lactic acidosis[105] and to spinal afferent information.[106] Exercise-induced hyperpnea is not related to increases in arterial or venous CO_2,[107–111] a decrease in blood pH,[112] an increase in H^+ stimulation at the medullary receptors,[113] a decrease in arterial O_2 partial pressure,[114] a cardiovascular cause[109] nor an influence of limb motion.[115] However, transposition of these observations to horses is questionable because horses and ponies differ in their respiratory adjustments. While the horse become hypoxemic and sometimes hypercapnic during heavy exercise, the pony does not become hypoxemic and, on the contrary, becomes hypocapnic, with arterial partial pressures of CO_2 as low as 27 mmHg.[72]

Respiratory Control During High-Intensity Short-Term Exercise. During strenuous exercise, the horse, independent of its ability and state of fitness, demonstrates a decrease in arterial O_2 partial pressure and pH and sometimes an increase in arterial partial pressure of CO_2 (see Fig. 6–12). These chemical regulators are supposed to strongly stimulate ventilation, but the stimuli appear to be insufficient to maintain arterial blood gas homeostasis. This is not the case in other species such as humans, dogs, and ponies, which do not show hypoxemia or hypercapnia during strenuous exercise. However, it must be pointed out that in the elite, endurance human athlete at peak fitness, cardiovascular and muscular adaptations to training reach such an exceptional level that the pulmonary system may be taxed maximally or even lag behind the functional capacity of the remaining aerobic system. Such a condition may result in hypoxemia and hypercapnia during high-intensity exercise.[116]

Thus, in contrast to other species, horses do not adopt a compensatory hyperventilation, i.e., a hyperventilation that could compensate for the gas-exchange impairment due mainly to diffusion limitation and partly to ventilation/perfusion inequalities.[4,69] The reason for this hypercapnic hypoventilation in horses remains unclear, and numerous hypotheses have been put forward.

HYPOTHESES TO EXPLAIN THE LACK OF COMPENSATORY HYPERVENTILATION IN HEAVY-EXERCISING HORSES

- *Influence of the locomotion-respiration coupling on exertional ventilation.* The locomotion-respiration coupling has been suggested as a major constraint to the increase in ventilation. Although there is no doubt that respiratory frequency is totally related to step frequency in galloping horses, several experimental observations rule out the coupling as the unique reason for hypoventilation: (1) standardbred horses racing at a trot (a gait where a coupling may exist but is not compulsory) also demonstrate hypoxemia and hypercapnia,[3] (2) the magnitude of hypercapnia is poorly related to the respiratory frequency,[69] and (3) the respiratory frequency of the pony is also tightly coupled with its step frequency and, nevertheless, it adopts a compensatory hyperventilation and becomes hypocapnic during heavy exercise.[72]

- *Lesser sensitivity of the receptors.* A slight increase in ventilation in horses running at 10 m/s is observed when the CO_2 concentration in the inhaled air increases from 0 to 3 percent. However, a further increase in inhaled CO_2 up to 6 percent does not induce any further changes in ventilation when these horses are not at their maximal ventilation capacity,[34] suggesting a lesser sensitivity of the chemoreceptors. However, the underlying mechanisms of this observation remain to be elucidated.

- *Influence of force-velocity characteristics of the ventilatory muscles.* Theoretically, the compensatory hyperventilation that would be required for the homeostasis of arterial O_2 partial pressure should be ensured by either (1) a tidal volume of about 23 liters, which together with a respiratory frequency of about 120 breaths/min implies mean respiratory airflow of more than 100 liters/s, or (2) a 2 : 1 coupling between respiratory frequency and step frequency, which implies that the respiratory frequency should reach values of about 240 breaths/min.[69] In terms of respiratory muscle energetics and force-velocity characteristics, such a level of ventilation would probably be impossible to reach.

- *Negative-feedback mechanisms generated by ventilatory muscle fatigue,* (Fig. 6–20). The increase in the ventilatory level is accompanied by an exponential increase in both the work of breathing and the O_2 uptake (energy cost) of the ventilatory muscles, mainly because of the increase in lung volume, in respiratory frequency, and in the resistive, elastic, and inertial forces.[5] Consequently, the energy demand of the ventilatory muscles becomes substantial, and the energy supply may be insufficient to satisfy this demand. This could result in a negative metabolic balance at the level of the ventilatory muscles, which could lead to fatigue.[117] This phenomenon could control the pattern of breathing by a negative-feedback mechanism acting either on the respiratory centers or directly on the ventilatory muscles.[118] This negative-feedback would override all the other positive feedback, tending to further increase the ventilation.[119]

During maximal exercise, highly trained human athletes often reach the mechanical limits of the lung and respiratory muscle for producing alveolar ventilation.[120] The occurrence of muscle exhaustion has been demonstrated to occur in humans after high-intensity short-term exercise,[121] as well as during prolonged exercise.[122] This results in a progressive increase in diaphragmatic excitation-contraction decoupling.[121,123] Although it has been shown that in the horse during high-intensity short-term exercise, the occurrence of exhaustion is associated with a sudden decrease in the minute volume and the O_2 uptake,[42,124] the occurrence of muscle fatigue remains to be demonstrated in equids.

AN EXPLANATION FOR THE LACK OF COMPENSATORY HYPERVENTILATION IN HEAVY-EXERCISING HORSES. The fact that the increase in ventilation becomes limited during heavy exercise in horses may be explained by several factors. First, it has already been shown that during strenuous exercise, the horse reaches a "critical level of ventilation" above which any further increase in O_2 uptake would be entirely consumed by the respiratory muscles.[88] The advantage of not increasing ventilation further during strenuous exercise may be that extra flow-resistive and elastic work is avoided and that there is a reduction in the O_2 uptake of ventilatory muscles, consequently reducing their energy demand. In terms of performance, hypoxemia and hypercapnia could be less disadvantageous than reaching the critical level of ventilation. Second, this negative-feedback mechanism could protect the ventilatory muscles against exhaustion and irreversible damage to the contractile oxidative machinery. Third, pulmonary overstretching, i.e., high lung volume, has been shown to increase the fragility of alveolar and vessel walls.[125] By limiting the increase in lung volume, the horse could minimize the risk of tissue rupture, possibly leading to severe exercise-induced pulmonary hemorrhage.

Respiratory Control During Submaximal Prolonged Exercise. During prolonged heavy, but not maximal, exercise, the impairment of gas exchange (especially hypercapnia) seems to be progressively compensated for after several minutes of exercise.[6,69] This suggests that horses, like humans, experience a "second wind" phenomenon, i.e., the relief of hypoventilation which could be induced by diaphragmatic fatigue.[126] Several factors are put forward to explain the improvement in ventilatory muscle function after a few minutes of exercise: (1) the length of the diaphragm may be modified by recruitment of other ventilatory muscles or by changes in the functional residual capacity, resulting in an increase in its force of contraction according to its length/tension characteristics, (2) the contractile function of the diaphragm may be improved, (3) the blood flow in the working diaphragm may be redistributed, and (4) the catecholamine release may lead to increased contractility. These assumptions remain to be confirmed in the horse.

Respiration During Recovery from Exercise

After exertion, all physiologic measurements return progressively to their resting values, the speed of this return being dependent on both intensity and duration of the exercise performed, the state of fitness of the horse, and the bioclimatologic conditions.

The metabolic reasons for the excess postexercise O_2 uptake are discussed elsewhere in this book (resynthesis of phosphocreatine in the exercised muscles, catabolism or anabolism of blood lactate, persistence of high body temperature, and restoration of hormonal reserves).[102] This excess O_2 uptake is associated with an elevated minute volume that is mainly the result of an increase in respiratory frequency.[127] Obviously, 5 min-

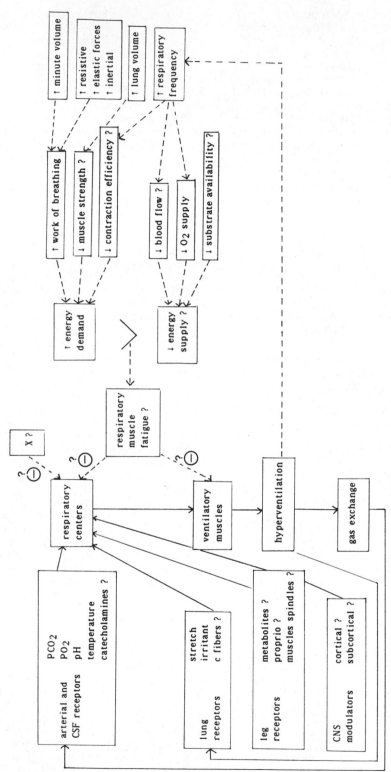

Figure 6-20. Hypotheses for the control of the ventilatory response in heavily exercising horses. The physiologic justification of such a negative-feedback mechanism (dashed line) could be to protect ventilatory muscles against exhaustion and to avoid a compensatory hyperventilation with negative metabolic balance (i.e., decreased O_2 supply to locomotor muscles due to increased O_2 supply to ventilatory muscles) (?: suspected mechanism which remains to be demonstrated in the horse).

utes after exercise, horses hyperventilate, as assessed by the high ventilatory equivalent for O_2. Despite a high dead space to tidal volume ratio, this hyperventilation results in alveolar hyperventilation and a consequent hyperoxia and hypocapnia.[3,5] In addition, the end-tidal expired gases have high O_2 (17.2 versus 14 percent at rest) and low CO_2 concentrations (4.5 versus 6.3 percent at rest).

Several explanations may be put forward to explain this posteffort hyperventilation. When the horse stops, the possible influence of the limb motion does not intervene in respiratory control, and other stimulants, such as acidosis, could become major stimulants. The resulting alveolar hyperventilation and respiratory alkalosis could be advantageous to compensate for the metabolic acidosis.

The pulmonary resistance after exercise becomes significantly lower once the ventilatory measurements return toward their resting values; this means that physiologic adjustments such as bronchodilatation or dilatation of the larynx are no longer overcome by the physical phenomena which tend to increase pulmonary resistance.[82]

The thermoregulatory role of the respiratory system also accounts for the posteffort hyperventilation that is due to an increase in the respiratory frequency rather than to an increase in tidal volume. It has been shown that ponies recovering from the same treadmill exercise test in hot and humid conditions have a significantly higher respiratory frequency than ponies recovering in dry and cold conditions.[127] This must be taken into account when horses running endurance courses are examined at the "vetgate"; when bioclimatologic conditions are hot and humid, the respiratory frequency is a poor indication of the actual ventilatory demand of the horse.[128]

Respiratory Adaptations to Training

The effects of training have received increasing attention during the last decade. The use of standardized treadmill tests has largely contributed to the improvement in knowledge in this field. However, differences in the experimental observations exist and show that physiologic adjustments to training may differ according to various factors such as the age of the athlete together with the previous stage, history, and intensity and duration of training. Indeed, during training, the multiple stages of the oxygen transport chain are stimulated and adapted, but their respective responses to training occur with different delays. The oxidative machinery of the muscles develops faster than the capillarity vascularization; hemoglobin increases only in the early stage of training; and the cardiac output increases only after several weeks of training. Adaptations to training also depend on the breed and discipline, as well as on the training programs (treadmill or field, duration and intensity). Furthermore, the kind of test used to illustrate the effects of training also influences the observations; short or prolonged exercise, standardized mild, moderate, submaximal heavy effort, or maximal exercise up to fatigue are used for this purpose. However, despite the problems associated with the study of training effects, some information is now available.

EFFECT OF TRAINING ON GAS EXCHANGE

Without doubt, training rapidly and significantly improves $\dot{V}_{O_2max}$[27,53,129,130] (see Fig. 6–13). The cardiovascular mechanisms underlying the improvement in O_2 uptake with training have already been studied, but the ventilatory mechanisms have been much less investigated. The improvement in O_2 uptake with training is related to an increase in cardiac output[1] and/or in O_2 extraction. Actually, results regarding the effects of training on arteriovenous difference in O_2 content are rather conflicting; it is reported to be unchanged during submaximal exercise,[1,3] increased during maximal exercise,[130] or decreased during maximal exercise.[53] The discrepancy between these studies is largely explained by the difference in the training programs applied, i.e., intensity and duration and the standardized exercise tests used. For example, the decrease in the arteriovenous difference in O_2 content with training during maximal exercise was simultaneous with a sharp increase in the cardiac output, which suggests that the transit time in the tissues is reduced by a significant increase in cardiac output so that adequate diffusion is less possible.[53] On the other hand, in the study reporting an increase in arteriovenous difference in O_2 content, there was no change in the cardiac output.[130]

Training does not seem to modify the exercise-induced alterations in blood gas tensions during and after heavy exercise,[3,53,131] nor the pulmonary arterial pressure and pulmonary blood flow velocity during mild standardized exercise.[132]

EFFECT OF TRAINING ON VENTILATION

Although all the systems implicated in exercise physiology (i.e., muscles, cardiovascular system, bones, and tendons) can be efficiently improved and trained, the ventilatory capacity by itself appears to be only capable of limited adaptations to training. The significant increase in the O_2 uptake induced by training is not accompanied by an equivalent increase in the minute volume. The ventilatory rate is unchanged during a maximal exercise test up to fatigue[53] or slightly lower during a standardized exercise test[27] after a period of training (Fig. 6–21). This results in a significant decrease in the ventilatory equivalent for O_2 (minute volume to O_2 uptake ratio), obvious even in the early stages of training.[27] The mechanisms underlying this training adjustment are still obscure.

In human athletes, the improvement in the ventilatory equivalent for O_2 is explained by a training-induced reduction in respiratory frequency and increase in tidal volume. Therefore, the time for gas exchange at the level of the alveoli is increased by training, and this induces a better alveolar O_2 extraction; the mean expired O_2 is about 18 percent in untrained men and 14 percent in well-trained athletes.[133,134]

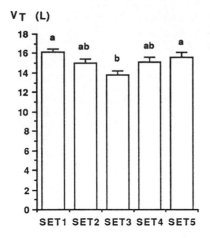

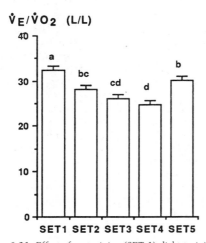

Figure 6-21. *Effect of no training (SET 1), light training (SET 2), aerobic training (SET 3), anaerobic training (SET 4), and detraining (SET 5) on ventilatory measurements [V_T: tidal volume; $\dot{V}_E/\dot{V}_{O_2}$: ventilatory equivalent for O_2; data was recorded every 3 weeks and collected at the end (11 m/s; 6-degree incline) of a standardized test on a treadmill].*

itable to the working locomotor muscles. However, these assumptions remain to be proved.

EFFECT OF DETRAINING

After a 3-week period of detraining, most of the training-modified ventilatory parameters, i.e., O_2 uptake, ventilatory equivalent for O_2, and minute ventilation during a standardized exercise, return to their pretraining level.[27,130] This indicates that while the ventilatory adaptations occur rapidly when the intensity of training is sufficient, they are nevertheless transient and highly reversible.

The Respiratory System and Its Thermoregulatory Role

Many mammals utilize the respiratory system to lose heat by evaporative cooling. To increase heat loss, they breathe (mainly expire) through the mouth instead of through the nose, and they hyperventilate by increasing the respiratory frequency and reducing tidal volume. Obviously, the horse cannot breathe through the mouth. Nevertheless, there are anatomic and physiologic characteristics that provide evidence that the respiratory system plays a role in body thermoregulation at rest, during exercise, and during recovery.

In resting ponies, changes in ambient temperature, without concomitant changes in body temperature, induce modification in respiratory frequency and tidal volume. Changes in skin and airway temperatures therefore appear capable of eliciting changes in breathing.[135]

Prolonged steady exercise induces a progressive increase in respiratory frequency with an increase in the physiologic dead space to tidal volume ratio.[42,43,136] This suggests that, in horses as in humans,[137] the respiratory system becomes increasingly involved in thermoregulation during long-term effort. Other experiments confirm the thermoregulatory role of the respiratory system in the horse during exercise. Standardbred horses exercised in extremely cold conditions ($-25°C$) reduce their respiratory frequency during the early stages of exercise and recovery.[29] Ponies performing the same test in hot and humid conditions recover with a higher respiratory frequency than in dry and cold conditions.[127]

During prolonged exercise in ponies, the bronchial circulation has been shown to increase progressively as core temperature increased with exercise duration.[138,139] Indeed, the bronchial arteries form a circulatory plexus in the connective tissues along the airways, the role of which is to ensure some heat dissipation. The same study shows a lesser modification in tracheal circulation, suggesting that the heat exchange occurs mainly at the level of the bronchi.

The Respiratory System and Its Role in Acid-Base Homeostasis

The lung can cause rapid changes in blood pH by regulating the elimination rate of CO_2. As blood flows through the tissues, CO_2 diffuses into the plasma and the

In equine athletes, the decrease in the ventilatory equivalent after training is also associated with an improvement in the alveolar O_2 extraction.[27] However, in contrast with humans, the reason for this improvement seems not to be a change in the pattern of breathing but more probably an increase in the affinity of hemoglobin for O_2. This could be explained by a training-induced shift to the left of the oxyhemoglobin curve resulting from a decrease in the extent of the exercise-induced acidosis and hyperthermia.[27]

Whatever the reason, the decrease in the ventilatory equivalent means that horses breath less air to ensure a given O_2 uptake. Theoretically, this could imply that (1) the relative energy cost of ventilation is reduced, (2) the fatigue of the respiratory muscles is delayed, and/or (3) the reduction in O_2 uptake by the muscles is prof-

erythrocytes, where carbonic acid forms and then dissociates into hydrogen and bicarbonate ions. This results in a decrease in the blood pH. In the lungs, CO_2 is expelled from the blood and the pH increases. This explains why the venous blood is more acidic than the arterial blood.

At rest, under normal conditions, the lung eliminates the CO_2 produced, so the partial pressure of CO_2 and the pH of the arterial blood remain relatively constant. In pathologic conditions, alveolar hypoventilation or hyperventilation may occur, resulting either in respiratory acidosis or alkalosis respectively.

During moderate exercise, an adequate ventilatory response is achieved, and the blood acid-base status is fairly well protected. However, during heavy exercise, the horse retains CO_2, and hypercapnia due to hypoventilation occurs, with an accompanying respiratory acidosis.[69]

Effect of Respiratory Disease on Respiratory Function During Exercise

In equine practice, respiratory diseases are as important and common as musculoskeletal diseases. While overt respiratory diseases are obvious and seldom a diagnostic challenge, most respiratory diseases are much more subtle and insidious.[10] They are liable to impair gas exchange during exercise and therefore to limit the horse's performance primarily by increasing the airway's resistance to airflow (Fig. 6–22).

NASAL DISORDERS

During inspiration, pressure within the nares is subatmospheric; these poorly supported parts therefore tend to collapse. This dynamic collapse is prevented or minimized by the alar muscles. In case of damage to the motor pathways of the facial nerve, the external nares are paralyzed, and the collapse is no longer prevented. During exercise, the nasal resistance will be increased dramatically. Because the horse is limited to nasal breathing, any partial obstruction at this level will result in exercise intolerance.

PHARYNGEAL DISORDERS

Pharyngeal Lymphoid Hyperplasia

Pharyngeal lymphoid hyperplasia appears to reflect the immature and hyperreactive condition of the submucosal lymphoid tissue present throughout the pharynx.[140] The clinical significance of this condition and its effect on the performance capability of the horse are still controversial. It appears to have little effect on upper airway function[141] and on the finishing place[140] and does not seem to impair gas exchange during exercise unless the lesions are extremely severe.[142] However, in some horses, severe pharyngitis may induce abnormal inspiratory respiratory noises during exercise. The endoscopic examination of horses suffering from this problem shows that when the nares are manually obstructed, the pharyngeal walls tend to collapse more easily than

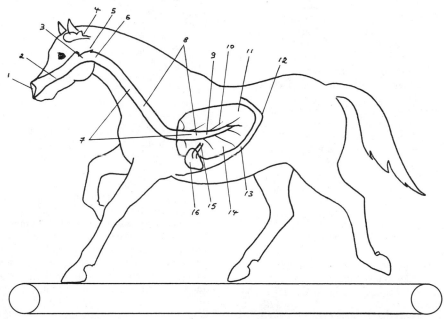

Figure 6-22. *Illustration of some subclinical respiratory problems potentially responsible for poor performance due to inadequate gas exchange [1: inadequate nostril flaring; 2: excessive nasal resistance; 3: pharyngeal dysfunction (displacement of the soft palate, epiglottic entrapment, etc.); 4: inadequate control of breathing; 5: guttural pouches infection; 6: inadequate laryngeal dilation; 7: subclinical viral infection; 8: dynamic airway collapse; 9: bronchitis; 10: ventilatory asynchronism due to exercise-induced bronchospasm or small airway disease; 11: exercise-induced pulmonary hemorrhage; 12: rib cage injury; 13: diaphragmatic fatigue; 14: ventilation-perfusion mismatching; 15: pulmonary vasoconstriction; 16: inadequate hemoglobin concentration].*

in healthy horses. The same horses reexamined after strenuous exercise show a further hypertrophy, and even hyperemia, of the lymphoid follicles. It can therefore be hypothesized that horses suffering from pharyngitis have an abnormally high pharyngeal resistance because, on the one hand, the pharyngeal lumen is reduced by the hypertrophied follicles and, on the other, a dynamic collapse of the pharyngeal walls further increases the resistance to airflow.

The stimulation of pharyngeal irritant receptors by mediators released by the lymphoid follicles also could result in reflex bronchoconstriction.[48] Lastly, follicular pharyngitis could be secondary to problems such as viremia or a poor environment, the latter being the primary cause of exercise intolerance.

Intermittent Dorsal Displacement of the Soft Palate
Normally, the soft palate lies ventral to the epiglottis during respiration. In dorsal displacement of the soft palate, the caudal free border of the soft palate is displaced to a position above the epiglottis. This causes narrowing of the nasopharyngeal airway and turbulence on inspiration and expiration.

Horses with intermittent dorsal displacement of the soft palate generally are asymptomatic at rest and during low-intensity exercise. This condition is encountered most frequently in racehorses as an intermittent event that causes temporary obstruction, abnormal respiratory noises (gurgling), mouth breathing, and sometimes asphyxia and "choking down" at high speed.

There are several etiologies for the dorsal displacement of the soft palate. It may result from or be favored by (1) anatomic problems (i.e., epiglottic hypoplasia[143] and malformation of the laryngeal cartilages), (2) functional problems secondary to nervous disorders, guttural pouch infection, pharyngitis, and chronic bronchitis, or (3) mechanical actions (i.e., retraction of the tongue, which causes both an elevation of the palate and a caudal retraction of the larynx, contraction of the sternothyrohyoideus muscles, and negative intrapharyngeal pressures during heavy exercise, causing some collapse of the unsupported structures).

Various treatments have been advocated for intermittent dorsal displacement of the soft palate, from prevention (tongue tie, figure-of-eight nose band) to surgical treatment (sternothyrohyoideus myectomy or resection of the caudal free margin of the soft palate). However, the results obviously depend on identification and treatment of the primary cause.

Rostral Displacement of the Palatopharyngeal Arch
In this condition, the caudal margin of the intrapharyngeal ostium is displaced rostrally on the corniculate processes of the arytenoid cartilages. The rostrally displaced tissue obstructs the laryngeal aperture and forms a sheet that impedes the abduction of the arytenoid cartilages.

The clinical signs resulting from rostral displacement of the palatopharyngeal arch are various. In severely affected horses, it causes dyspnea and dysphagia.

In subclinically affected horses, it produces airway obstruction and severe exercise intolerance.

GUTTURAL POUCH DISORDERS

Diseases of the guttural pouches are rare but may potentially induce secondary problems such as spontaneous epistaxis, cranial nerve damage, parotid distension, and upper airway dysfunction. The guttural pouches contain nervous structures, namely, the cervical sympathetic trunk, as well as the vagus, glossopharyngeal, hypoglossal, spinal accessory, cranial laryngeal, facial, and mandibular nerves. Therefore, uni- or bilateral infectious disorders (i.e., empyema and mycosis) can cause functional disorders such as soft palate displacement and pharyngeal or laryngeal paresis.

LARYNGEAL DYSFUNCTION

Idiopathic Laryngeal Hemiplegia
The primary lesion associated with laryngeal hemiplegia is damage to the left recurrent laryngeal nerve. This results in paralysis or paresis of the cricoarytenoidus dorsalis. With this condition, the horse cannot fully dilate the larynx on the affected side, and there is partial obstruction to airflow, inducing an increase in laryngeal resistance, mainly during inspiration[14,141,144,145] (see Fig. 6–2). Most horses with laryngeal hemiplegia are presented with a complaint of decreased exercise tolerance and abnormal inspiratory noise during exercise. In galloping horses, laryngeal hemiplegia has been shown to produce a severe hypercapnic hypoxemia,[13,145] and affected ponies have shown a dramatic decrease in athletic ability accompanied by a decoupling of respiratory and step frequencies while galloping.[146]

Laryngeal hemiplegia is not an all-or-none disease; all stages of arytenoid cartilage movement exist, from normal function to no movement. Endoscopic examination therefore shows horses with varying amounts of asynchrony or asymmetry. The following grading system is proposed to objectively describe the movements of the arytenoid cartilages.[147] Briefly, grade I represents a normal larynx, showing full and synchronous abduction and adduction; horses with grade II exhibit asynchronous movements of the arytenoid cartilages at rest, but once fully stimulated by nasal occlusion or by exercise, they recover normal and synchronous movements; horses with grade III show asynchronous movements even after respiratory stimulation; horses with grade IV show a marked asymmetry with no movements of the arytenoid cartilage at any stage of the respiratory cycle. The clinical significance, functional consequences, and laryngoplasty indications for grade II and III are sometimes difficult to assess and require functional investigations. Treadmill endoscopy in such cases may allow a rational decision regarding therapy.

Arytenoid Chondritis
Arytenoid chondritis is a chronic, progressive condition of the larynx resulting in distortion of the arytenoid cartilage(s). This abnormality is characterized by an en-

largement of the cartilage causing restriction of normal motion and decreased airway diameter and resulting in exercise intolerance and inspiratory noise during exercise.[141] In the early stage, it sometimes may be confused with laryngeal hemiplegia. Its exact pathogenesis is unknown. Arytenoid chondritis is observed mainly in thoroughbred horses between 2 and 4 years of age.

Epiglottic Entrapment
Epiglottic entrapment is the envelopment of the apex and lateral margin of the epiglottis by the ventral epiglottic mucosa and aryepiglottic folds. This condition has variable effects on exercise tolerance. Sometimes it is found incidentally in horses with no history of respiratory problems, while in other cases there is severe respiratory distress.[148,149] In these horses, endoscopy of the upper airways during exercise shows a significant reduction of pharyngeal diameter due to billowing of the entrapped tissue during expiration.

TRACHEAL DISORDERS

Tracheal diseases that cause respiratory obstruction in horses are uncommon. Tracheal obstruction, consisting of either flattening of the cartilage rings in the dorsoventral plane or cartilage rings having a scroll-like conformation, has been reported to induce respiratory distress at rest and during exercise.[150] Pathologic tracheal collapse sometimes results either from misshappen cartilagenous rings[151] or from inflammation of the tracheal membrane.[152]

LOWER AIRWAY SUBCLINICAL DISORDERS

Subclinical lower airway disorders may be due to airway hyperreactivity generated by biologic (virus, bacteria, fungal spores), chemical (ammonia, hydrogen sulfide, ozone), or physical (airborne particles) irritants. They may induce bronchospasm, mucosal edema, hypersecretion, and decreased airway clearance.[153]

Horses suffering from lower airway disorders generally have an increased airway resistance and a decreased dynamic lung compliance. The exacerbated regional differences in small airways resistance and lung compliance result in an uneven distribution of ventilation. The resulting ventilation/perfusion ratio inequalities may, in turn, induce hypoxemia. The increase in total pulmonary resistance and the poor gas exchange decrease the exercise tolerance of affected horses.

On the other hand, it has been shown that the revaccination of thoroughbred horses with an oily adjuvant inactivated vaccine against influenza and rhinopneumonia does not impair their cardiorespiratory and metabolic adjustments to strenuous exercise and to training.[124]

OTHERS

Ventilation and/or gas exchange in exercising horses also may be impaired by numerous other factors such as anemia, respiratory muscle fatigue, subclinical myopathies,

central nervous disorders, cardiovascular disorders, thoracic costal injuries, inappropriate harness, inspired air pollution, and other secondary disorders.

Exercise-Induced Pulmonary Dysfunction

EXERCISE-INDUCED BRONCHOCONSTRICTION

It has been shown that in human subjects, exercise may induce a bronchoconstriction.[154,155] This response to exercise depends both on the inspired air quality and on the bronchoreactivity of the subject, but the exact sequence of events underlying its pathogenesis is still unclear. While it has been suggested that the same phenomenon may occur in horses, this remains to be demonstrated.

EXERCISE-INDUCED DYNAMIC PARTIAL COLLAPSE OF THE AIRWAYS

The importance of the dynamic partial collapse has been shown to depend on the extent of the compressive transmural pressures and on the shape of the cross-sectional area of the airways.[15,16]

EXERCISE-INDUCED PULMONARY HEMORRHAGE

Definition, Prevalence, and Epidemiology
Exercise-induced pulmonary hemorrhage is not a clinical entity or syndrome. It is rather a clinical sign that may be the result of heavy exercise and/or pathologic changes and is defined as the presence of blood in the tracheobronchial tree following strenuous exercise. Endoscopic surveys of the lower airways in racing horses have demonstrated that a large number of horses suffer exercise-induced pulmonary hemorrhage, with a relatively low percentage showing epistaxis. All variety of competitive events elicit the occurrence of exercise-induced pulmonary hemorrhage, especially above speeds of 14 m/s. Reported incidences are approximately 30 percent in standardbred horses, 60 percent in quarter horses,[156] and up to 75 percent in thoroughbred horses.[157] Repeated endoscopic examination of horses after exercise reveals an even higher incidence of exercise-induced pulmonary hemorrhage than indicated by a single examination; 95 percent of the examined horses bled on at least one occasion.[140] It generally occurs soon after training begins and tends to have an increasing incidence with increasing age.[157] There is no apparent sex difference in exercise-induced pulmonary hemorrhage susceptibility and little geographic variation in the incidence within and between countries.

Clinical Signs
Most of the clinical signs are nonspecific. They include blood in the tracheobronchial airways and, much less frequently, epistaxis either during or after exercise when the horse is released in its stall and allowed to lower its head. Other signs are more variable and include abnormal respiratory sounds, swallowing while running,

and labored breathing. Concerning its effect on performance, it seems to incapacitate some horses and to have no apparent influence on others. There is no association between race-finishing position and exercise-induced pulmonary hemorrhage.[157–159] However, racing times are adversely influenced in the races in which horses suffering pulmonary hemorrhage were recognized.[160]

Diagnosis

Several complementary tests are available to assess the diagnosis. Blood may be detected in the trachea by endoscopic evaluation of the lower airways performed 60 to 90 minutes after the race. This blood is still visible 4 to 6 hours later. If exercise-induced pulmonary hemorrhage is strongly suspected and blood is not present in the trachea 60 minutes after exercise, a repeated endoscopic examination is recommended 1 hour later.

Cytologic examination of bronchoalveolar lavage reveals the presence of numerous hemosiderophages, neutrophils, and sometimes eosinophils. Radiographic evaluation is of limited usefulness, and interpretation is difficult. In horses suffering exercise-induced pulmonary hemorrhage, there is a vaguely discernible increase in interstitial density in the dorsocaudal lobe of the lung.[161,162] Ventilation/perfusion ratio scans show variable reduction of ventilation and a loss of perfusion in the dorsocaudal fields with collateral supply from the bronchial circulation.[163]

Necropsy Findings

Because exercise-induced pulmonary hemorrhage is rarely fatal, necropsy investigations generally have been performed on confirmed "bleeders," and the lesions observed are considered as end-stage ones. Postmortem examination shows evidence that the caudodorsal diaphragmatic lung lobes are the primary sites of hemorrhage; blue-brown–colored areas are generally distributed dorsally and laterally within the dorsal half of the caudal lobe. There is an increase in bronchial arterial vessels, i.e., neovascularization. The damaged regions receive their vascular supply almost exclusively from the bronchial arterial circulation.[164,165] The microscopic examination of these regions reveals mainly bronchiolitis and an increase in fibrous connective tissue.

Pathogenesis

While the epidemiology and end-stage pathology are firmly established, there is still little understanding of the factors that predispose horses to exercise-induced pulmonary hemorrhage, the nature of the initial lesion, and the progression of the condition to the end-stage pathology. Exercise-induced pulmonary hemorrhage is so frequently encountered irrespective of the breed, the sports discipline, the age or sex of the horse, the regions of the world, and the methods of management that it is highly improbable that it has an unique etiology. Most likely, it is the result of the coexistence of multiple factors, some favoring or predisposing to the condition and others triggering the episode of exercise-induced pulmonary hemorrhage.

Affected Vessels. Micropathologic examination of end-stage exercise-induced pulmonary hemorrhage lesions shows destruction of alveolar tissue, extensive proliferation of bronchial blood vessels, and greatly increased numbers of anastomoses between bronchial and pulmonary circulations. The extent of the anastomotic flow depends on the relative pressure in the bronchial and pulmonary vasculature and on the alveolar pressure.[166] The increase in the pressure gradient between the bronchial and pulmonary arteries could perhaps favor bronchial blood flow into the pulmonary circulation. The pulmonary capillaries could consequently be submitted to the high systemic pressure and be ruptured. However, whether the bronchial neovascularization, which is a response to inflammation and considered as integral part of pulmonary repair, occurs before or after the very first episode of exercise-induced pulmonary hemorrhage remains to be elucidated. Therefore, until now, the exact source of bleeding remains unknown. Pulmonary or bronchial vessels at the capillary or arterial level may potentially be the source of the blood.

Coagulation. Although there is evidence of coagulation alteration in any exercising horse, platelet adhesiveness may decrease more in exercise-induced pulmonary hemorrhage–positive horses than in normal horses following exercise.[167] It is questionable, however, whether this modification is sufficient to elicit spontaneous bleeding and why it occurs only at the level of the lungs.

Sites of Bleeding. Most of the affected areas appear to be distributed in the dorsocaudal bronchopulmonary segments. There are some anatomic and functional characteristics of these regions which could explain their predisposition to bleed during exercise. First, this segment is subtended by the terminal divisions of the principal bronchus. Because of its axial alignment with the principal bronchus, it is likely that this segment would be a site for deposition of inhaled particles. Second, because of the more negative intrapleural pressure at this level,[44] the alveoli of these regions are fully dilated and consequently weakened. Third, relatively smaller alveoli and thicker septa result in a regional difference in elastic properties and consequently in a greater respiratory asynchronism. Moreover, the regional decrease in the distribution of the pores of Kohn and therefore in the collateral ventilation enhances the inhomogeneity of the distribution of ventilation. Lastly, the dorsocaudal region of the lung is the least well perfused by the pulmonary circulation in the resting horse; this could favor the bronchial blood flow to enter into the pulmonary circulation via the anastomoses.

Obstructive Disorders. Chronic obstructive pulmonary disease has been suggested to be the underlying lesion in exercise-induced pulmonary hemorrhage. Using the presence of mucus or mucopurulent material in the trachea to diagnose chronic obstructive pulmonary disease, several studies failed to point out any association between exercise-induced pulmonary hemorrhage and chronic obstructive diseases.[9,140,168] Moreover, exercise-induced pulmonary hemorrhage is universally encountered, while, conversely, chronic obstructive pulmonary disease is absent in some regions of the globe.

However, the bronchiolitis found in exercise-induced pulmonary hemorrhage–positive horses could be induced by respiratory disorders other than chronic obstructive pulmonary disease. Few pathogens are known to affect horses with the wide variety of epidemiologic conditions under which exercise-induced pulmonary hemorrhage is known to occur. A ubiquitous virus with high morbidity and low mortality and affecting most of the young horses, such as the EHV1, has been suggested to be this pathogen.[169]

Small airways disease is a general feature in confirmed bleeders, as proven by thorough imaging and postmortem studies.[164,165] The inflammatory processes found in the lungs of exercise-induced pulmonary hemorrhage–positive horses suggest that local inflammatory lesions causing small airways disease are likely predisposing causes of exercise-induced pulmonary hemorrhage and may precede the hemorrhagic lesions. However, exercise-induced pulmonary hemorrhage also could occur the very first time in healthy horses and lead to secondary inflammatory lesions and small airways disease. Indeed, the instillation of autologous blood into the lungs of healthy horses has been shown to induce both physiologic and morphologic modifications, the latter being similar to those observed in horses suffering exercise-induced pulmonary hemorrhage.[170,171] Therefore, at present, the question remains open as to whether the lesions encountered in the lungs of "bleeders" are the primary cause or, on the contrary, the secondary consequence of exercise-induced pulmonary hemorrhage. It also has been suggested that exercise-induced pulmonary hemorrhage could be secondary to upper airway obstruction associated with laryngeal hemiplegia.[12]

Mechanical Stress. The occurrence of exercise-induced pulmonary hemorrhage following strenuous exercise and not after prolonged exercise of lower intensity[159] suggests that the syndrome is the result of extreme mechanical forces applied to lung tissues and vessels. During heavy exercise, alveolar pressure is likely to become highly negative,[5] while pressure in the vessels (pulmonary or bronchial) increases greatly. Consequently, transmural pressure, i.e., the pressure gradient between airways and blood vessels, is expected to reach high values. Moreover, because of the poor collateral ventilation, the transmural pressure in asynchronous regions is suspected to become sufficiently high to cause capillary rupture.

Pulmonary vascular hypertension has been rejected as a possible cause of exercise-induced pulmonary hemorrhage.[48] We assert that pulmonary edema would occur before capillary pressure could increase enough to rupture a vessel. However, both alveolar and pulmonary capillary blood pressures are subjected to frequent and cyclic variations due to respiration and cardiac contrac-

tion, respectively. Consequently, transmural pressure (between pulmonary circulation and alveoli or between bronchial circulation and alveoli) is expected to present important, irregular, and sudden variations which could cause capillary rupture rather than a continuous high value causing pulmonary edema.

In "bleeders," increased interstitial fibrosis is evident in interlobular and alveolar septa, as well as around airways and vessels. This would probably contribute to a loss of elasticity of the lung tissue in the affected regions. Because of interconnections, this loss of compliance would induce an increasing shear stress at the interface. Whether or not this fall in compliance is primary or secondary to exercise-induced pulmonary hemorrhage, once compliance decreases, it will probably favor the occurrence of new episodes of hemorrhage.

Vessel and Tissue Fragility. Several factors are likely to decrease the stress resistance of the pulmonary tissues. On the one hand, it has been shown that lung injury and hemorrhage may result from inflammatory processes, mainly due to a local release of toxic products (heparin, oxygen metabolites) by phagocytic cells like neutrophils or macrophages.[172] On the other hand, it has been shown in rabbits that a high lung volume increases stress failure of pulmonary capillaries and may cause disruption of the capillary endothelium, alveolar epithelium, and sometimes all layers of the wall.[125] If the same is true in the horse, the alveoli of the dorsocaudal regions of the lung, which are more distended because of gravitational effects, also should be more fragile.

Therefore, the presence of chronic pulmonary inflammatory processes, the increase in lung volume during high exercise intensity, or both factors together may be partly responsible for increased blood vessel fragility and therefore for the occurrence of "bleeding." This fragility of the pulmonary tissue associated with pulmonary overstretching could be another justification for the limitation in the increase in tidal volume during heavy exercise in horses.

Treatment

Many therapeutic regimens have been advocated to prevent exercise-induced pulmonary hemorrhage. Most of them have no demonstrated efficiency. Without understanding the cause of exercise-induced pulmonary hemorrhage, it will be difficult to rationalize the use of most medications. Among the proposed substances, diuretics, β_2-agonists, hormones, coagulants, hematinics, and heated saturated water vapor are the most frequently used.

Furosemide (0.3 to 0.6 mg/kg IV), if permitted, is given 3 to 4 hours prior to racing. Its effect on horses known to experience exercise-induced pulmonary hemorrhage is an area where there is a considerable disagreement. There are discrepancies, first, between the trainer's and rider's opinions and the results of the research undertaken in this field and, second, between the conclusions of the scientific studies themselves. Furosemide does not improve performance in normal standardbred horses[173] but does improve racing time in both healthy and exercise-induced pulmonary hemorrhage–positive thoroughbreds.[174] It has questionable efficacy for prevention of hemorrhage in known exercise-induced pulmonary hemorrhage–positive horses. At least 50 percent of furosemide-treated horses continue to experience pulmonary hemorrhage.[158,174–176] Nevertheless, it seems to decrease the amount of bleeding.[177]

The possible effectiveness of furosemide was first based on the assumption that exercise-induced pulmonary hemorrhage is preceded by pulmonary edema. However, there is no evidence that exercising horses suffer pulmonary edema. Standardized studies performed on horses running on a treadmill show that furosemide (1 mg/kg) induces mild transient changes in hemodynamics and cardiovascular function both at rest and during exercise[178,179] and attenuates significantly the exercise-induced rise in pulmonary arterial pressure, pulmonary arterial wedge pressure, and presumably, pulmonary capillary pressure (which is expected to be halfway between pulmonary arterial and pulmonary arterial wedge pressures) in horses running at 13 m/s.[179] These results may explain why furosemide seems to limit or reduce the extent of exercise-induced pulmonary hemorrhage.

Other treatments, therapeutic regimens, and management methods have been advocated to prevent pulmonary hemorrhage, but their efficacy has not been demonstrated and their effect on bleeding and/or performance remains controversial. The treatments include the improvement of stabling environment by reducing airborne irritants, the practice of "drawing" the horses before the race, parasympatholytic or β_2-mimetic bronchodilator administration,[176] conjugated estrogen administration, coagulants, aspirin, supplementation with hesperedin-citrus bioflavinoids,[175] and water vapor–saturated air therapy.[180]

Because mechanical factors seem to play a major role in the occurrence of pulmonary hemorrhage, all treatments which decrease intra-airway pressure changes (e.g., bronchodilators), intravascular pressure changes (e.g., diuretics), or lung tissue overstretching should decrease the incidence and/or the degree of "bleeding."

Pulmonary Function Tests in the Athletic Horse

Pulmonary function testing has several applications in the athletic horse: applied research on respiratory physiology, evaluation of pulmonary efficiency, and evaluation of the effects of the training. However, the most concrete interests of these tests are the diagnosis of subclinical respiratory problems responsible for poor performance as well as the evaluation of the degree of functional recovery after a medical or surgical treatment. At the moment, heavy equipment located in an air-conditioned laboratory equipped with a high-speed treadmill is necessary in order to provide accurate and useful information about pulmonary function in the context of sports medicine. However, in the future it could be possible to fasten a small "black box" on the horse performing work in field conditions in order to record, store, and analyze several useful functional measurements.

Errors may be important when some technical and methodologic requirements are not met. Therefore, the results of a functional test must be analyzed carefully. Physiologic variability is often important for functional measurements, and comparison between tests may only be done if they are performed in standardized conditions. This chapter does not approach the clinical examination that remains essential in each case. However, these issues are addressed in chapters 12 and 13.

GAS EXCHANGE

Blood Gases

An overall evaluation of pulmonary gas exchange can be provided by the measurement of *arterial blood gas tensions*, i.e., arterial P_{O_2} and arterial P_{CO_2}. Hypoxemia (arterial P_{O_2} lower than 80 to 84 mmHg at sea level) may be the result of limitations at the level of ventilation, perfusion, diffusion, or ventilation/perfusion matching. Hypercapnia (arterial P_{CO_2} higher than 46 to 50 mmHg) is considered to indicate alveolar hypoventilation. The interpretation of these data is complicated in the exercising horse because heavy exercise induces hypoxemia and hypercapnia. However, most healthy horses show normal blood gas values at moderate exercise (up to 50 percent of their $\dot{V}_{O_2max}$), which seems not to be the case in horses with respiratory dysfunctions.[13,181] Arterial blood must be sampled anaerobically in heparinized syringes from the carotid or facial artery and stored in ice if the measurements cannot be performed immediately. Sampling in glass syringes is recommended when the measurements cannot be done within 1 hour. The presence of air in the syringe will induce an overestimation and underestimation of O_2 and CO_2 tensions, respectively. Blood gas values also may be underestimated if they are not corrected for body temperature. This is of critical importance in heavily exercising horses, which can reach body temperatures higher than 41°C, while the data are measured at 37°C in the blood gas analyzer. Most computerized blood gas analyzers calculate the corrected values by using appropriate equations.[182]

An increase in the *alveolar arterial O_2 gradient* [(A–a)D_{O_2} higher than 10 mmHg] is also an indicator of impaired O_2 exchange due to diffusion impairment, ventilation/perfusion mismatching, or right to left vascular shunt.

Alveolar partial pressure of O_2 can be evaluated by measuring the end tidal fraction of O_2 in the expired gas with a mass spectrometer or by using this equation:

$$\text{Alveolar } P_{O_2} = [(P_B - P_{H_2O}) \times Fi_{O_2}] - \text{alveolar } P_{CO_2}$$

or its simplified version:

$$\text{Alveolar } P_{O_2} = 150 - \text{arterial } P_{CO_2}$$

P_B is the ambient barometric pressure (around 760 mmHg at sea level), and P_{H_2O} is the water vapor pressure, which varies with the temperature (e.g., 47.1 and 58.3 mmHg at 37 and 41°C, respectively).

Measurements of *hemoglobin blood concentration* (Hb) and venous blood gas tensions (venous P_{O_2} and venous P_{CO_2}) are useful in order to calculate the *arterial O_2 content* (arterial C_{O_2}) and the arteriovenous gradient in the O_2 content [$(a-\bar{v})C_{O_2}$]. In contrast with arterial O_2 partial pressure, these measurements are directly correlated with the intensity of the exercise in healthy horses. Arterial O_2 content can be calculated from the following equation:

Arterial C_{O_2} (vol%)

$$= \frac{1.39 \times Hb \times \text{arterial } S_{O_2}}{100} + 0.003 \times \text{arterial } P_{O_2}$$

The *arterial hemoglobin O_2 saturation* (arterial S_{O_2}) can be evaluated by a continuous and noninvasive monitoring using pulse oximetry.[183] However, from our experience, this technique provides accurate data only in sedated horses. Hemoglobin O_2 saturation data are often provided by automatic blood gas analyzers.

Lastly, some equipment for collecting blood samples by *radiotelemetry* from horses running in the field also has been described.[184]

O_2 Uptake, CO_2 Output, and Respiratory Exchange Ratio

These measurements are of critical importance in sports medicine and must be recorded during heavy exercise in order to reach maximal values. Three different techniques have been described for measuring $\dot{V}_{O_2max}$ in horses. The *bag-collection technique* requires the use of an airtight face mask connected to a nonrebreathing valve which allows the collection and analysis of expired gases in a large balloon.[129,185] The main disadvantages of this technique are the discomfort induced by the high resistance and dead space of the equipment, the heavy weight of the mask and valves, and the impossibility of measuring transient changes in the data. The *open-flow technique* requires the use of a loose-fitting face mask connected to flexible tubing, an airflow indicator, a high-velocity centrifugal blower, and a gas-sampling device.[102,186,187] This technique allows accurate measurements of O_2 uptake and CO_2 output with minimal discomfort for the horse. The *breath-by-breath technique* requires the use of airflow sensors placed on a tight face mask, the entry of which is connected via a narrow catheter to a mass spectrometer which allows on-line measurements of the gas concentrations[5,188] (Fig. 6–23). This technique provides a continuous and simultaneous recording of all transient changes (see Fig. 6–13) not only in gas exchange data (O_2 uptake, CO_2 output, and the respiratory exchange ratio) but also in ventilatory data (inspiratory and expiratory flows, volumes, times, etc.) (see Table 6–2).

VENTILATORY DATA

Airflow is usually measured with a pneumotachograph connected to a tight but comfortable face mask which has low dead space and as limited effects as possible on pulmonary function.[189] Volume is calculated by integration of the flow signal. This integration is preferably performed by a computer program in order to avoid the drift problems due to the electronic integrators.

Several systems have been proposed in the horse. *Fleisch and Lilly pneumotachographs* are reference techniques,[190,191] but because of their limited flow ranges, they are more suitable for measuring resting than exercising flows, which can reach 100 liters/s in horses. *Ultrasonic phase-shift flowmeters* are particularly well adapted for flow measurements, both in resting and heavily exercising horses, because of their low weight, low dead space, low resistance, high range of linearity, and low sensitivity to contamination by condensation and nasal discharge.[5,192]

Calibration of these pneumotachographs involves both flow and volume. Flow can be calibrated with a rotameter adapted to the appropriate flow range. However, from our experience, the use of an air velocity transducer (TSI Incorporated, St. Paul, Minn.) connected to a high flow modulable generator is particularly appropriate for an accurate calibration of very high flow ranges. Volume is controlled with calibrated syringes. For accuracy, it is always preferable to calibrate the equipment within the ranges of flow and volume that are expected to be measured during the test.

Most computer software associated with the flowmeters allows direct calculation of the ventilatory data given in Table 6–2. *Flow-volume loops* can be obtained by using an *xy* recorder or appropriate software in resting[77] and exercising horses.[78] Analysis of these loops may provide interesting information on uncommon patterns of breathing.[193]

Lung volume changes also can be evaluated without any face mask by using other technologies. *Inductance plethysmography* requires the use of respibands applied to the rib cage and abdomen, frequency oscillators, and a calibrator-demodulator unit (Respitrace, Ambulatory Monitoring, Ardsley, NY). The sum of the rib cage and abdominal displacement gives a signal proportional to the tidal volume.[77]

Impedance plethysmography requires the use of current and voltage electrodes applied to the thorax, a phase-sensitive detector, and a voltage-controlled oscillator. This system provides impedance changes across the thorax, which are proportional to the volume changes.[194]

These two last techniques are noninvasive and easy to use but not easy to calibrate. Several problems need to be solved before they can be accurately used in exercising horses. The *functional residual capacity* (FRC) can be measured by the closed-circuit helium dilution method or the open-circuit nitrogen washout method.[195,196] The *physiologic dead space to tidal volume ratio* (V_D/V_T) can be estimated by using the simplified equation

$$V_D/V_T = \frac{(\text{arterial } P_{CO_2} - \text{mixed-air } P_{CO_2})}{P_{CO_2}}$$

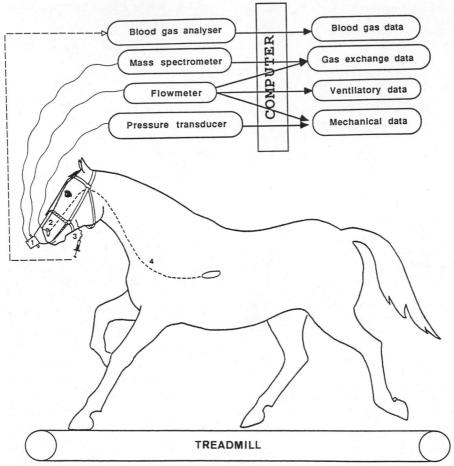

Figure 6-23. *Schematic diagram of the breath-by-breath pulmonary function testing in a horse exercising on the treadmill (1: ultrasonic sensor; 2: face mask; 3: arterial puncture; 4: esophageal balloon-catheter system; measured and calculated measurements are listed in Table 6–2).*

where mixed-air P_{CO_2} is the partial pressure of CO_2 in mixed expiratory air.

The *adequacy of the distribution of ventilation* can be evaluated by lung scans during the inhalation of radioactive gases[60] or by examining the rate of washout of nitrogen from the lungs as the horse breathes pure O_2.[197] The first method allows localization of the poorly ventilated areas of the lung but requires expensive equipment such as a gamma camera. The second method quantifies the ventilatory asynchronism which may be present in subclinical lower airway problems but requires a constant tidal volume during the measurement.

INTRAPLEURAL PRESSURE MEASUREMENTS

Intrapleural pressure can be measured by direct puncture of the pleural cavity, but this is not recommended. The most appropriate technique is to measure the pressure changes in the medial thoracic part of the esophagus, which provides accurate measurements both in resting[44] and exercising horses.[189] From our experience, the best results are obtained when a condom containing 0.5 ml of air is tightly fixed on the distal part of a semirigid polyethylene catheter (internal diameter 4 mm, external diameter 6 mm). Before the introduction of the balloon-catheter system into the esophagus via the nose, the proximal part of the catheter must be tightly connected to a pressure transducer in order to avoid an excess of air in the balloon. Indeed, a too distended balloon induces abnormally positive and damped pressure recordings. The balloon-catheter-transducer system must be calibrated by means of a water manometer.

Some interesting information about the respiratory system can be given by the measurement of intrapleural pressures changes (Ventigraph, Boehringer, Germany).[198] However, in the absence of simultaneous flow and volume recordings, it is more hazardous to conclude that an increase in pleural pressure change is due to a pathologic increase in the pulmonary resistance, a physiologic increase in the airflow, or both.

MECHANICS OF BREATHING

The simultaneous recording of flow, volume, and pleural pressure change allows the measurement of several indices of the mechanics of breathing in unsedated resting or exercising horses. When the resistance of the flowmeter is high, the mask pressure is no longer equal to atmospheric pressure and must be recorded in order to calculate the transpulmonary pressure, i.e., the gradient between intrapleural and mask pressures.

The *dynamic lung compliance* is the volume change per unit of intrapleural pressure change measured at the two points of zero flow (see Fig. 6–15). A decrease in resting dynamic lung compliance can be due to a rigidity of the lung parenchyma or, much more frequently, to a ventilatory asynchronism resulting from small airways partial obstruction. During exercise, dynamic lung compliance is overestimated and even may become negative. This is due to the fact that the inertial factors are usually neglected in its calculation. This may not be tolerated in the exercising horse because of the high air acceleration and therefore high inertial pressure changes.

The *total pulmonary resistance* is the pleural pressure change per unit of flow change recorded at isovolume, e.g., at 50 percent of inspiratory and expiratory volumes (see Fig. 6–15). An increase in total pulmonary resistance can be due to excessive intra-airway material, contraction of airway smooth muscle, inflammation of the mucosa, dynamic collapse due to a compressive transmural pressure, or dysfunction at the level of the upper airways. Because of the partitioning of the airway resistance to airflow, total pulmonary resistance is more sensitive to changes in large than in small airways.[82] In contrast with dynamic lung compliance, total pulmonary resistance can be measured accurately in exercising horses because it is measured at two points (isovolume 50 percent) where accelerations and consequently inertial pressure changes are negligible.[88]

The *work of breathing* can be estimated from the measurement of the area of the transpulmonary pressure-volume loop[90] (see Fig. 6–18). An increase in the work of breathing can be due to both an increase in total pulmonary resistance or a decrease in dynamic lung compliance.

In order to obtain accurate information, the phase compatibility between the flow and pressure signals must be tested up to 10 and preferably 20 Hz. Any dephasage must be corrected either by adapting the length of the tubings of the measuring equipment or by using appropriate software. The measurements of the data must be performed on at least 10 breathing cycles. The most appropriate method is therefore a computerized system (e.g., ACEC, Charleroi, Belgium, and Buxco Electronics, Sharon, CT) which provides continuous calculation of required data. Another inexpensive method is to adapt a highly powerful data storing and processing software such as Superscope (GW Instruments, Somerville, MA).

Some techniques allow the evaluation of the resistance to airflow without recording the intrapleural pressure. The *flow-interruptor method* is based on the fact that alveolar pressure can be evaluated at the level of the nose during repeated short-term flow interruptions. Associated with a flow measurement, this allows an evaluation of the resistance of the respiratory system.[199,200] The *forced-oscillation method* has been adapted for the equine species.[88,201,202] This method requires a loud speaker as a pressure-wave generator, a flow and pressure meter, and a fast Fourrier analyzer to measure the resistance and the reactance (i.e., the sum of compliance and inertance) of the respiratory system at several frequencies from 2 to 30 Hz. The *monofrequency forced-oscillation method* is a simplified technique which allows an evaluation of the resistance of the respiratory system by using small portable equipment connected to a face mask and easy to use in field conditions.[203] Until now, none of these three techniques has been adapted for measurements in exercising horses.

PULMONARY HEMODYNAMICS

Pulmonary vascular resistance is directly proportional to the pulmonary driving pressure (i.e., the difference between the pulmonary artery pressure and the pulmonary artery wedge pressure) and inversely proportional to the pulmonary blood flow. Pulmonary artery pressures can be measured by means of a balloon-tipped flow-directed catheter (Swan-Ganz) connected to a pressure transducer leveled at the scapulohumeral joint or a catheter-tip micromanometer (Millar, Houston, Texas) introduced into the pulmonary artery via the jugular vein and the right side of the heart.

A vasoconstriction at the level of the pulmonary arterioles will induce pulmonary artery hypertension and an increase in pulmonary vascular resistance. This may happen during alveolar hypoxia or be secondary to the action of vasoconstrictive agents.[204,205] The interpretation of these measurements is complicated in the exercising horse. Indeed, exercise induces an increase in pulmonary artery and capillary pressures[179] and a decrease in pulmonary vascular resistance due the large increase in blood flow and to the recruitment and enlargement of pulmonary vessels. Furthermore, pressure measurements in these vessels are highly influenced by the high pleural pressure changes occurring during exercise.[206]

VENTILATION/PERFUSION MATCHING

Measurement of the ventilation to perfusion matching can help to diagnose subclinical pulmonary dysfunctions in the horse. Two techniques can be used in the horse, but both require sophisticated and expensive equipment. The *radioactive isotope gas method* analyzes the topographic distribution of the ventilation/perfusion ratio by measuring the lung radioactivity by nuclear scintigraphy during steady-state inhalation and intravenous infusion of the radioactive gas krypton-81m or technetium-99m.[60,163] The *multiple inert gas elimination method* allows the determination of pulmonary dead space and shunt as well as a continuous description of the ventilation/perfusion ratio both at rest[207] and during exercise.[4] This technique measures, with a gas chromatograph, the steady-state concentration of six infused inert gases in pulmonary arterial and carotid arterial blood and in mixed expiratory gas.

DIFFUSION CAPACITY

The pulmonary diffusing capacity for O_2 can be evaluated by measuring the diffusing capacity of carbon monoxide with the single breath or the steady-state method.[208] This requires measurement of the inspired and expired concentration of carbon monoxide by an infrared analyzer after inhalation of a 0.1% CO mixture.

MUCOCILIARY CLEARANCE RATE

The tracheal mucociliary clearance rate may be impaired by subclinical viral infections or by excessive ammonium concentration in inspired air. This clearance rate can be determined in the horse from scintigraphs recorded after an intratracheal injection of technetium-99m sulfide colloid.[209]

UPPER AIRWAY FUNCTION

Upper respiratory tract dysfunctions frequently are responsible for poor performance by increasing the resistance to airflow. It is therefore crucial to make an early and precise diagnosis to ascertain if such dysfunctions are responsible for the poor performance by impairing the pulmonary gas exchange and to assess the functional efficiency of the treatment. Answers to these questions may be provided in part by upper airway videoscopic examination and upper airway resistance measurement at rest and during strenuous exercise.[14,210]

Some other techniques, such as laryngeal palpation,[12] laryngeal muscle electromyography,[211] and electrolaryngography,[212] allow detection of some laryngeal abnormalities, even when they are subclinical. However, they cannot definitely indicate if these abnormalities are responsible for gas-exchange limitation and poor performance in the horse being evaluated.

Upper airway endoscopy can be carried out by using a flexible fiberendoscope or videoendoscope. The latter technique provides a better visualization on a large monitor and allows the storage of the recording on videotapes. Endoscopic examination in the resting and postexercising horse is usually performed in an unsedated horse using a twitch for restraint and a 180-cm-long, 12-mm-diameter endoscope. This allows the detection of visible abnormalities from the nasal passages to the tracheobronchial tree, which could decrease the upper airway airflow. These include intraluminal abnormalities such as excessive secretions or blood, intramural abnormalities such as severe lymphoid hyperplasia, or narrowing of the airway and extramural abnormalities such as a compressing retropharyngeal ganglia.

Pharyngeal and laryngeal functions are not always easy to interpret in the resting horse. A momentary dorsal displacement of the soft palate which disappears by flushing this area may be due to a gag reflex induced by the introduction of the endoscope itself. Laryngeal asynchronism may be suspected by endoscopy via the right but not the left nasal passage. Some specific manipulations may be required. The thoracolaryngeal reflex, i.e., the "slap test," consists of unilateral laryngeal adduction generated by a contralateral thoracic hand slap. This reflex is supposed to be partly or totally inhibited by recurrent laryngeal neuropathy or abnormalities of the cervical spinal cord. Laryngeal abduction also can be accentuated by nasal occlusion, the rebreathing bag technique, or the injection of a ventilatory stimulant such as doxapram (40 mg/kg) or lobeline (0.2 mg/kg).[213,214] On the other hand, sedation is thought to alter coordination, synchrony, and response of pharyngeal and laryngeal movements.

Endoscopy in the exercising horse is performed on a high-speed treadmill with a 100-cm-long, 9-mm-diameter endoscope introduced in the nasopharynx and fastened to the bridle with adhesive tape or Velcro. This allows determination of the adequacy of physiologic adjustments to exercise. Incomplete laryngeal abduction and the occurrence of exercise-induced upper airway obstruction, such as dorsal displacement of the soft palate or pharyngeal mucosa collapse, can be detected.

Upper airway resistance can be evaluated by the simultaneous recording of flow and lateral tracheal pressure changes with a side-hole catheter connected to a pressure transducer.[14,82] Inspiratory and expiratory impedances are calculated as the ratio of peak tracheal pressure and flow during inspiration and expiration, respectively. A simplified technique based on the recording of intratracheal pressure also may provide useful information,[85,144] but the lack of simultaneous flow measurements makes the conclusions more hazardous. These techniques allow evaluation of the dysfunction generated by an upper airway abnormality and the efficiency of its treatment at a functional level.

Electromyographic examination of some laryngeal muscles may help to detect abnormal electrical activity associated with denervation injuries.[211] Electromyograms performed with transcutaneous needles inserted into the left dorsal cricoarytenoid muscle show abnormalities such as fibrillation potentials, positive sharp waves, bizarre high-frequency discharges, or reduced insertional activity in horses suspected of having a laryngeal neuropathy.

Electrolaryngography allows the measurement of the latency of the thoracolaryngeal reflex on the right and left sides.[212] The reflex is elicitated by a hand slap on the thorax, close to the spine. The hand carries a switch to trigger a storage oscilloscope. The motor endpoint of the reflex is recorded using surface and subdermal electrodes placed lateral to the larynx. Latency periods, calculated by a computer, greater than 45 and 90 ms are considered by Cook[212] to be pathognomonic for a laryngeal hemiparesis and hemiplegia, respectively. It must be emphasized that abnormalities recorded by these last two tests in resting horses are not always correlated with clinical signs or with exercise-induced functional abnormalities.

The *airway occlusion* test may be useful to test the possibility of oral breathing, which can be the result of a dorsal displacement of the soft palate. However, from our experience, this must always be confirmed by an endoscopic examination. Indeed, in some horses, this forced oral breathing can be due to a lack of airtightness of the palatolaryngeal junction without dorsal displacement of the soft palate.

RESPIRATORY SOUND ANALYSIS

Respiratory sound intensity can be recorded using a calibrated radiostethoscope placed over the trachea and connected to sound transducer, transmission, and recording systems.[215,216] Peak expiratory sound intensity was shown to be linearly correlated with the stride frequency and the peak expiratory flow and was considered by Attenburrow to be a useful and easy measurement for the detection and recognition of certain abnormalities in the upper airways. The *real-time stethacoustic analyzer* provides interesting information about wheezing in human patients,[217] but it is not applicable to horses in its present form.

FATIGUE OF THE VENTILATORY MUSCLES

Diaphragmatic fatigue may induce specific changes in the spectral analysis of the electromyographic signals (i.e., a shift of the power spectrum toward low frequencies)[218] and in the shape of the transdiaphragmatic pressure curves.[219] This has been demonstrated in the human but not in the horse.

Transdiaphragmatic pressure can be evaluated in the resting[77] or exercising horse[79,80] by subtraction of gastric pressure from esophageal pressure, both being measured with a balloon-catheter-transducer system. The *electromyographic signals* from the diaphragm can be measured in the horse by using paired silver electrodes built into a hollow catheter and placed in the lower esophagus close to the stomach.[77]

CONTROL OF BREATHING

In order to test the ability of the respiratory centers to induce hyperventilation in response to hypercapnia and hypoxemia, the rebreathing method can be used.[220] However, abnormalities in the control of breathing are uncommon, except in the neonatal foal, and this test does not differentiate between central and peripheral problems.

MISCELLANEOUS

Some diagnostic procedures do not really test pulmonary function, but they may provide some interesting information in horses with poor performance syndrome without clinical disease. Radiographic examination of the airways may reveal abnormalities with functional impact such as a shortening of the epiglottis,[148] a hypoplasia of the soft palate,[221] or a narrowing of the airways.[222] Information about subclinical lower airways problems and pulmonary allergic problems also can be provided by tracheobronchial aspiration,[223] bronchoal-veolar lavage,[224] serum precipitating antibody dosage,[225] and intradermal or bronchial provocation tests.[226-230]

Conclusions

The high muscle mass of horses and the formidable metabolic requirements which result from their activities during heavy exercise involve a very high CO_2 production and O_2 uptake relative to the ventilatory capabilities of this animal. Some researches indicate that the respiratory system may be the ultimate limiting factor in the racehorse. Indeed, despite the fact that numerous physiologic adjustments are brought into play, such as an enlargement of the surface of the exchanging area, an increase in cardiac output, an increase in packed cell volume, and an increase in pulmonary ventilation, arterial blood gas homeostasis is impaired in heavy-exercising horses. Although sometimes observed in elite human endurance athletes, the exercise-induced hypoxemia and hypercapnia encountered in healthy horses during strenuous exercise may be considered as unique among mammals, at least those already studied.

Some anatomic and physiologic peculiarities in horses may be put forward to explain this specific adjustment to exercise. The impairment of gases diffusion, the compulsory coupling between locomotion and respiration, the high nasal resistance associated to the compulsory nasal breathing, the dramatic increase of the mechanical work of breathing and of the respiratory muscles oxygen uptake, the force-velocity characteristics and limitation of the respiratory muscles, and the fatigue of the respiratory muscles are probably major factors partly responsible for this phenomenon. Actually, ventilation during exercise in horse seems to be a compromise between these anatomic and physiologic "constraints" and the enormous metabolic needs. It probably aims at optimizing rather than at maximizing the gas exchange at the cost of blood gas homeostasis but at the profit of the energy cost of breathing.

If the mechanisms underlying the occurrence of arterial blood gas modifications begin to be progressively elucidated, the final question of knowing whether or not the gas-exchange impairment finally has a real influence on the performance capacity of our horses remains open. The limiting role of the respiratory system is probably more important in horses racing at high speed over middle distance than in horses racing over either very short or very long distances.

Undoubtedly, if heavy exercise induces changes in arterial blood gas tensions in healthy horses, *a fortiori,* it must dramatically worsen the gas exchange in horses suffering from subclinical respiratory disease. In this case, the resulting important gas-exchange modifications might strongly diminish the effort capability of the horse.

The value of pulmonary function tests is obvious. They help to make an accurate evaluation of respiratory function and consequently are essential in the critical examination of horses suffering from poor performance syndrome. The tests used most commonly for this purpose are arterial blood gases analysis, measurement of mechanics of breathing indices, and endoscopy of the airways at rest and/or during exercise. Although these tests generally require sophisticated equipment that is only available in specialized units, they are essential to diagnose subclinical respiratory disorders and to allow rational decision making regarding therapy.

Appendix 6A

Table 6A-1. SI Conversion Table for Common Values

Data	SI units	Traditional units
Pressure	1 kPa	7.5 mmHg
	1 kPa	10.2 cmH$_2$O
	1 kPa	10 mbar
Work	1 J	0.239 cal
	1 J	10.2 cmH$_2$O × liter
Power	1 W	0.0143 kcal/min
Gas exchange	1 mmol/min	22.4 ml/min
Gas content	1 mmol/liter	2.24 ml/dl
Hemoglobin	1 mmol/liter	16.1 g/liter

Acknowledgments

We wish to thank Prof. E. Muylle for advice and C. Gresse and M. Leblond for technical assistance.

References

1. Bayly WM, Gabel AA, Barr SA: Cardiovascular effects of submaximal aerobic training on a treadmill in standardbred horses, using a standardized exercise test. Am J Vet Res 1983; 44:544–553.
2. Bayly WM, Schulz DA, Hodgson DR, et al: Ventilatory response to exercise in horses with exercise-induced hypoxemia. *In* Gillespie JR, Robinson NE (eds): Equine Exercise Physiology 2. Davis, Calif, ICEEP Publications, 1987, pp 172–182.
3. Thornton JR, Essén-Gustavsson B, Lindholm A: Effects of training and detraining on oxygen uptake, cardiac output, blood gas tensions, pH and lactate concentrations during and after exercise in the horse. *In* Snow DH, Persson SGB, Rose RJ (eds): Equine Exercise Physiology. Cambridge, Granta Editions, 1983, pp 470–486.
4. Wagner PD, Gillespie JR, Landgren GL, et al: Mechanism of exercise-induced hypoxemia in horses. J Appl Physiol 1989; 66:1227–1233.
5. Art T, Anderson L, Woakes AJ, et al: Mechanics of breathing during strenuous exercise in thoroughbred horses. Respir Physiol 1990; 82:279–294.
6. Hodgson DR, Rose RJ, Kelso TB, el al: Respiratory and metabolic responses in the horse during moderate and heavy exercise. Pflugers Arch 1990; 417:73–78.
7. Erickson BK, Pieschl RL, Erickson HH: Alleviation of exercise-induced hypoxemia utilizing inspired 79% helium 20.95% oxygen. *In* Persson SGB, Lindholm A, Jeffcott LB (eds): Equine Exercise Physiology 3. Davis, Calif, ICEEP Publications, 1991, pp 54–58.
8. Arthur RC: Respiratory problems on the racehorse. Vet Clin North Am Equine Pract 1990; 6:179–196.
9. McNamara B, Bauer S, Iafe J: Endoscopic evaluation of exercise-induced pulmonary hemorrhage and chronic obstructive pulmonary disease in association with poor performance in racing standardbreds. J Am Vet Med Assoc 1990; 196:443–445.
10. Morris EA, Seeherman HJ: Clinical evaluation of poor performance in the racehorse: The results of 275 evaluations. Equine Vet J 1991; 23:169–174.
11. Hare WCD: Equine respiratory system. *In* Getty E, et al (eds): The Anatomy of Domestic Animals. Philadelphia, WB Saunders Co, 1975.
12. Cook WR: Specifications for speed in the racehorse. *In* The Airflow Factors. Menasha, WI, Russell Meerdink, 1989.
13. Bayly WM, Grant BD, Modransky PD: Arterial blood gas tensions during exercise in a horse with laryngeal hemiplegia, before and after corrective surgery. Res Vet Sci 1984; 36:256–258.
14. Derksen FJ, Scott EA, Stick JA, et al: Effect of laryngeal hemiplegia and laryngoplasty on upper airway flow mechanics in exercising horses. Am J Vet Res 1986; 47:16–20.
15. Art T, Lekeux P: Mechanical properties of the isolated equine trachea. Res Vet Sci 1991; 51:55–60.
16. Art T, Lekeux P: The effect of shape, age, and extension on the compliance of equine tracheal segment. Vet Res Commun 1991; 15:135–146.
17. Gehr P, Erni H: Morphometric estimation of pulmonary diffusion capacity in two horse lungs. Respir Physiol 1980; 41:199–210.
18. Robinson NE: Some functional consequences of species differences in lung anatomy. Adv Vet Sci Comp Med 1982; 26:1–33.
19. Robinson NE, Sorenson PR: Collateral flow resistance and time constant in dog and horse lungs. J Appl Physiol 1978; 44:63–68.
20. Bisgard GE, Orr JA, Will JA: Hypoxic pulmonary hypertension in the pony. Am J Vet Res 1975; 36:49–52.
21. McLaughlin RF Jr: Bronchial artery distribution in various mammals and in humans. Am Rev Respir Dis 1983; 128:S57–S58.
22. Magno MG, Fishman AP: Origin, distribution and blood flow of bronchial circulation in anesthetized sheep. J Appl Physiol 1982; 53:272–279.
23. Leith DE, Gillespie JR: Respiratory mechanics of normal horses and one with chronic obstructive lung disease. Fed Proc 1971; 30:551.
24. Manohar M: Respiratory muscle perfusion during strenuous exercise. *In* Persson SGB, Lindholm A, Jeffcott LB (eds): Equine Exercise Physiology 3. Davis, Calif, ICEEP Publications, 1991, pp 1–8.
25. De Troyer A, Loring SH: Action of the respiratory muscles. *In* Fishman AP, Fisher AB (eds): Handbook of Physiology, sec 3: The Respiratory System, vol 3, part 2: Mechanics of Breathing. Bethesda, Md, American Physiological Society, 1986, pp 443–461.
26. Gallivan GJ, McDonell WN, Forrest JB: Comparative pulmonary mechanics in the horse and the cow. Res Vet Sci 1989; 46:322–330.
27. Art T, Lekeux P: Training-induced modifications in cardiorespiratory and ventilatory measurements in Thoroughbred horses. Equine Vet J 1993; 25:532–536.
28. Art T, Lekeux P: Pulmonary mechanics during treadmill exercise in race ponies. Vet Res Commun 1988; 12:245–258.
29. Dahl LG, Gillespie JR, Kallings P, et al: Effects of a cold environment on exercise tolerance in the horse. *In* Gillespie JR, Robinson NE (eds): Equine Exercise Physiology 2. Davis, Calif, ICEEP Publications, 1987, pp 235–242.
30. Gottlieb-Vedi M, Essen-Gustavsson B, Persson SGB: Draught load and speed compared by submaximal tests on a treadmill. *In* Persson SGB, Lindholm A, Jeffcott LB (eds): Equine Exercise Physiology 3. Davis, Calif, ICEEP Publications, 1991, pp 92–96.
31. Bramble DM, Carrier DR: Running and breathing in mammals. Science 1983; 219:251–256.
32. Hörnicke H, Meixner R, Pollmann U: Respiration in exercising horses. *In* Snow DH, Persson SGB, Rose RJ (eds): Equine Exercise Physiology. Cambridge, Granta Editions, 1983, pp 7–16.
33. Hörnicke H, Weber M, Schweiker W: Pulmonary ventilation in thoroughbred horses at maximum performance. *In* Gillespie JR, Robinson NE (eds): Equine Exercise Physiology 2. Davis, Calif, ICEEP Publications, 1987, pp 216–224.
34. Landgren GL, Gillespie JR, Leith DE: No ventilatory response to CO$_2$ in thoroughbreds galloping at 14 m.s^{-1}. *In* Persson SGB, Lindholm A, Jeffcott LB (eds): Equine Exercise Physiology 3. Davis, Calif, ICEEP Publications, 1991, pp 59–65.
35. Gillespie JR, Landgren GL, Leith DE: 1 : 2 ratio of breathing to stride frequencies in a galloping horse breathing 6% CO$_2$. *In* Persson SGB, Lindholm A, Jeffcott LB (eds): Equine Exercise

Physiology 3. Davis, Calif, ICEEP Publications, 1991, pp 66–70.

36. Anderson LS, Butler PJ, Snow DH, et al: The effect of gait on ventilation in the exercising thoroughbred racehorse. J Physiol 1990; 420:68P.

37. Gallivan GJ, McDonell WN, Forrest JB: Comparative ventilation and gas exchange in the horse and the cow. Res Vet Sci 1989; 46:331–336.

38. Lekeux P, Art T, Desmecht D: Effect of exercise on equine alveolar ventilation. In Proceedings of the 11th Comparative Respiratory Society Meeting, Urbana, Ill, September 1992, p S12.

39. Froese AB, Bryan AC: High frequency ventilation. Am Rev Respir Dis 1981; 123:249–250.

40. Chang HK: Mechanisms of gas transport during ventilation by high frequency oscillation. J Appl Physiol 1984; 56:553–559.

41. Pollman U, Hörnicke H: The respiratory dead space of the horse during exercise measured telemetrically. In Sansen W (ed): Biotelemetry VI. Louvain, Belgium, Université de Lourain 1984, pp 129–132.

42. Rose RJ, Evans DL: Cardiovascular and respiratory function in the athletic horse. In Gillespie JR, Robinson NE (eds): Equine Exercise Physiology 2. Davis, Calif, ICEEP Publications, 1987, pp 1–24.

43. Pelletier N, Blais D, Vrins A, et al: Effect of submaximal exercise and training on dead space ventilation in the horse. In Gillespie JR, Robinson NE (eds): Equine Exercise Physiology 2. Davis, Calif, ICEEP Publications, 1987, pp 225–234.

44. Derksen FJ, Robinson NE: Esophageal and intrapleural pressures in the healthy conscious pony. Am J Vet Res 1980; 41:1756–1761.

45. Otis AB, Mc Kerrow CR, Bartlett RA, et al: Mechanical factors in distribution of pulmonary ventilation. J Appl Physiol 1956; 8:427–432.

46. Derksen FJ, Slocombe RF, Gray PR, et al: Exercise-induced pulmonary hemorrhage in horses with experimentally induced allergic lung disease. Am J Vet Res 1992; 53:15–21.

47. Mead J, Takishima T, Leith D: Stress distribution in lungs: A model of pulmonary elasticity. J Appl Physiol 1970; 28:596–608.

48. Robinson NE: Functional abnormalities caused by upper airway obstruction and heaves: their relationship to the etiology of epistaxis. Vet Clin North Am Large Anim Pract 1979; 1:17–34.

49. Thomas DP, Fregin GF: Cardiorespiratory and metabolic responses to treadmill exercise in the horse. J Appl Physiol 1981; 50:864–868.

50. Thomas DP, Fregin GF, Gerber NH, et al: Effects of training on cardiorespiratory function in the horse. Am J Physiol 1983; 245:R160–R165.

51. Parks CM, Manohar M: Distribution of blood flow during moderate and strenuous exerixse in ponies. (*Equus cabalus*). Am J Vet Res 1983; 44:1861–1866.

52. Goetz TE, Manohar M: Pressures in the right side of the heart and esophagus (pleura) in ponies during exercise before and after furosemide administration. Am J Vet Res 1986; 47:270–276.

53. Evans DL, Rose RJ: Cardiovascular and respiratory responses to submaximal exercise training in the thoroughbred horse. Pflugers Arch 1988; 411:316–321.

54. Evans DL, Rose RJ: Dynamics of cardiorespiratory function in standardbred horses during different intensities of constant-load exercise. J Comp Physiol [B] 1988; 157:791–799.

55. Evans DL, Rose RJ: Cardiovascular and respiratory responses in thoroughbred horses during treadmill exercise. J Exp Biol 1988; 134:397–408.

56. Erickson BK, Erickson HH, Coffman JR: Pulmonary artery, aortic and esophageal pressure changes during high intensity treadmill exercise in the horse: A possible relation to exercise-induced pulmonary hemorrhage. Equine Vet J 1990; (suppl 9):47–52.

57. Erickson BK, Erickson HH, Coffman JR: Pulmonary artery and aortic pressure changes during high intensity treadmill exercise in the horse: effect of furosemide and phentolamine. Equine Vet J 1992; 24:215–219.

58. Fishman AP: Pulmonary circulation. In Fishman AP (ed): Handbook of Physiology, sec 3: The Respiratory System, vol 1: Circulation and Nonrespiratory Functions. Bethesda, Md, American Physiological Society, 1985, pp 93–166.

59. Taylor AE, Rehder K, Hyatt RE, et al: Clinical Respiratory Physiology. Philadelphia, WB Saunders Co, 1989.

60. Amis TC, Pascoe JR, Hornof W: Topographic distribution of pulmonary ventilation and perfusion in the horse. Am J Vet Res 1984; 45:1597–1601.

61. Hakim TS, Lisbona R, Dean GW: Gravity-independent inequality in pulmonary blood flow in human. J Appl Physiol 1987; 63:1114–1121.

62. Bray MA, Anderson WH: Mediators of pulmonary inflammation. In Lenfant C (ed): Lung Biology in Health and Disease, vol 54. New York, Marcel Dekker, 1991.

63. Pelletier N, Leith DE: Hypoxia does not contribute to high pulmonary artery pressure in exercising horses. In Persson SGB, Lindholm A, Jeffcott LB (eds): Equine Exercise Physiology 3. Davis, Calif, ICEEP Publications, 1991, pp 30–36.

64. Lilker ED, Nagy EJ: Gas exchange in the pulmonary collateral circulation of dogs. Am Rev Respir Dis 1975; 112:615–620.

65. Coates GO, Bradovich HO, Jerreries AL, et al: Effects of exercise on lung lymph flow in sheep and goats during normoxia and hypoxia. J Clin Invest 1984; 74:133–141.

66. Gale GE, Torre-Bueno JR, Moon RE, et al: Ventilation-perfusion inequality in normal humans during exercise at sea level and simulated altitude. J Appl Physiol 1985; 58:978–988.

67. Weibel ER: Oxygen demand and the size of respiratory structures in mammals. In Wood SC, Lenfant C (eds): Evaluation of Respiratory Processes, New York, Marcel Dekker, 1979, pp 289–346.

68. Bayly WM, Grant BD, Breeze RG: The effects of maximal exercise on acid-base balance and arterial blood gas tension in thoroughbred horses. In Snow DH, Persson SGB, Rose RJ (eds): Equine Exercise Physiology. Cambridge, Granta Editions, 1983, pp 400–407.

69. Bayly WM, Hodgson DR, Schulz DA, et al: Exercise-induced hypercapnia in the horse. J Appl Physiol 1989; 67:1958–1966.

70. Dempsey JA: Is the lung built for exercise? Med Sci Sports Exerc 1986; 18:143–155.

71. Constantinopol M, Jones JH, Weibel ER, et al: Oxygen transport during exercise in the large mammals: II. Oxygen uptake by the pulmonary gas exchanger. J Appl Physiol 1989; 67:871–878.

72. Parks CM, Manohar M: Blood-gas tensions and acid-base status in ponies during treadmill exercise. Am J Vet Res 1984; 45:15–19.

72a. Jones JH, Longworth KE, Lindholm A, et al: Oxygen transport during exercise in large mammals: I. Adaptative variation in oxygen demand. J Appl Physiol 1989; 67:862–870.

73. Clerbaux T, Serteyn D, Willems E, et al: Détermination de la courbe de dissociation standard de l'oxyhémoglobine du cheval et influence, sur cette courbe, de la température, du pH et du diphosphoglycérate. Can J Vet Res 1986; 50:188–192.

74. Persson SGB: On blood volume and working capacity in horses. Acta Vet Scand Suppl 1967; 19:1.

75. Boucher JH, Ferguson EW, Wilhelmsem CL, et al: Erythrocyte alterations during endurance exercise in horses. J Appl Physiol 1981; 51:131–134.

76. Wasserman K, Whipp BJ: Exercise physiology in health and disease. Am Rev Respir Dis 1975; 122:219–249.

77. Koterba AM, Kosch PC, Beech J, et al: Breathing strategy of the adult horse (*Equus caballus*) at rest. J Appl Physiol 1988; 64:337–346.

78. Art T, Lekeux P: Respiratory airflow patterns in ponies at rest and during exercise. Can J Vet Res 1988; 52:299–303.

79. Art T, Desmecht D, Amory H, et al: Synchronization of locomotion and respiration in trotting ponies. J Vet Med [A] 1990; 37:95–103.

80. Slocombe R, Brock K, Covelli G, et al: Effect of treadmill exercise on intrapleural, transdiaphragmatic and intraabdominal pressures in standardbred horses. In Persson SGB, Lindholm A, Jeffcott LB (eds): Equine Exercise Physiology 3. Davis, Calif, ICEEP Publications, 1991, pp 83–91.

81. Manohar M, Duren SE, Sikkes B, et al: Respiratory muscle perfusion in ponies during prolonged submaximal exercise in thermoneutral environment. Am J Vet Res 1992; 53:558–562.

82. Art T, Serteyn D, Lekeux P: Effect of exercise on the partitioning

of equine respiratory resistance. Equine Vet J 1988; 20:268–273.

83. Art T, Desmecht D, Amory H, et al: Heliox-induced changes in the breathing mechanics of ponies during exercise. In Persson SGB, Lindholm A, Jeffcott LB (eds): Equine Exercise Physiology 3. Davis, Calif, ICEEP Publications, 1991, pp 47–53.

84. Gillespie JR: The role of the respiratory system during exertion. J S Afr Vet Assoc 1974; 45:305–309.

85. Funkquist B, Holm K, Karlsson A, et al: Studies on the intratracheal pressure in the exercising horse. J Vet Med [A] 1988; 35:424–411.

86. Racklyeft DJ, Love DN: Influence of head posture on the respiratory tract of healthy horses. Aust Vet J 1990; 67:402–405.

87. Kannan MS, Johnson DE: Nitric oxide mediates the neural nonadrenergic, noncholinergic relaxation of pig tracheal smooth muscle. Am J Physiol (Lung Cell Mol Physiol) 1992; 2:L511–L514.

88. Art T, Lekeux P, Gustin P, et al: Inertance of the respiratory system in ponies. J Appl Physiol 1989; 67:534–540.

89. Leith DE: Mammalian tracheal dimensions: Scaling and physiology. J Appl Physiol 1982; 55:196–200.

90. Art T, Lekeux P: Work of breathing in exercising ponies. Res Vet Sci 1989; 46:49–53.

91. Bye PTP, Farkas GA, Roussos CH: Respiratory factors limiting exercise. Annu Rev Physiol 1983; 45:439–451.

92. Karlsen G, Brejtsen N: Synchronisation of rhythm of respiration and movement: A basis for the development of a fast trotter (in Russian). Konevodstvo I Konnyj Sport 1965; 33:22–24.

93. Attenburrow DP: Time relationship between the respiratory cycle and limb cycle in the horse. Equine Vet J 1982; 14:69–72.

94. Attenburrow DP: Respiration and locomotion. In Snow DH, Persson SGB, Rose RJ (eds): Equine Exercise Physiology. Cambridge, Granta Editions, 1983, pp 17–22.

95. Young IS, Warren RD, Altringham JD: Some properties of the mammalian locomotory and respiratory systems in relation to body mass. J Exp Biol 1992; 164:283–294.

96. Hall LW, Aziz HA, Groenendyk J, et al: Electromyography of some respiratory muscles in the horse. Res Vet Sci 1991;50:328–333.

97. Brice AG, Forster HV, Pan LG, et al: Respiratory muscle electromyogram responses to acute hypoxia in awake ponies. J Appl Physiol 1990; 68:1024–1032.

98. Manohar M: Inspiratory and expiratory muscle perfusion in maximally exercised ponies. J Appl Physiol 1990; 68:544–548.

99. Manohar M: Diaphragmatic perfusion heterogeneity during exercise with inspiratory resistive breathing. J Appl Physiol 1990; 68:2177–2181.

100. Manohar M: Blood flow in respiratory muscles during maximal exertion in ponies with laryngeal hemiplegia. J Appl Physiol 1987; 62:229–237.

101. Manohar M: Vasodilator reserve in respiratory muscles during maximal exertion in ponies. J Appl Physiol 1986; 60:1571–1577.

102. Rose RJ, Hodgson DR, Kelso TB, et al: Maximum O_2 uptake, O_2 debt and deficit, and muscle metabolites in thoroughbred horses. J Appl Physiol 1988; 64:781–788.

103. Forster HV, Pan LG: Exercise hyperpnea: Its characteristics and control. In Crystal RG, West JB (eds): The Lung: Scientific Foundations, vol 2 New York, Raven Press, 1991, pp 1553–1564.

104. Wasserman K, Whipp BJ, Casaburi R: Respiratory control during exercise. In Fishman AP (ed): Handbook of Physiology, sec 3: The Respiratory System, vol 2, part 2: Control of Breathing. Bethesda, Md, American Physiological Society, 1986, pp 595–619.

105. Erickson BK, Forster HV, Pan LG, et al: Ventilatory compensation for lactacidosis in ponies: Role of carotid chemoreceptors and lung afferents. J Appl Physiol 1991; 70:2619–2626.

106. Pan LG, Forster HV, Wurster RD, et al: Effect of partial spinal cord ablation on exercise hyperpnea in ponies. J Appl Physiol 1990; 69:1821–1827.

107. Klein JP, Forster HV, Bisgard GE, et al: Ventilatory response to inspired CO_2 in normal and carotid body-denervated ponies. J Appl Physiol Respir Environ Exer Physiol 1982; 52:1614–1622.

108. Pan LG, Forster HV, Bisgard GE, et al: Hyperventilation in ponies at the onset of and during steady-state exercise. J Appl Physiol Respir Environ Exerc Physiol 1983; 54:1394–1402.

109. Pan LG, Forster HV, Bisgard GE, et al: Cardiodynamic variables and ventilation during treadmill exercise in ponies. J Appl Physiol Respir Environ Exerc Physiol 1984; 57:753–759.

110. Forster HV, Pan LG, Bisgard GE, et al: Effect of reducing anatomic dead space on arterial P_{CO_2} during CO_2 inhalation. J Appl Physiol 1986; 61:728–733.

111. Powers SK, Beadle RE, Thompson D, et al: Ventilatory and blood gas dynamics at onset and offset of exercise in the pony. J Appl Physiol 1987; 62:141–148.

112. Pan LG, Forster HV, Bisgard GE, et al: Independence of exercise hyperpnea and acidosis during high-intensity exercise in ponies. J Appl Physiol 1986; 60:1016–1024.

113. Bisgard GE, Forster HV, Byrnes B, et al: Cerebrospinal fluid acid-base balance during muscular exercise. J Appl Physiol Respir Environ Exerc Physiol 1978; 45:94–101.

114. Forster HV, Pan LG, Bisgard GE, et al: Hyperpnea of exercise at various P_{IO_2} in normal and carotid body-denervated ponies. J Appl Physiol Respir Environ Exerc Physiol 1983; 54:1387–1393.

115. Forster HV, Pan LG, Bisgard GE, et al: Independence of exercise hypocapnia and limb movement frequency in ponies. J Appl Physiol Respir Environ Exerc Physiol 1984; 57:1885–1893.

116. Dempsey JA, Hanson PG, Henderson KS: Exercise-induced arterial hypoxaemia in healthy human subjects at sealevel. J Physiol Lond 1984; 355:161–175.

117. Leblanc P, Summers E, Inman MD, et al: Inspiratory muscles during exercise: A problem of supply and demand. J Appl Physiol 1988; 64:2482–2489.

118. Mador MJ, Acevedo FA: Effect of respiratory muscle fatigue on subsequent exercise performance. J Appl Physiol 1991; 70:2059–2065.

119. Dempsey JA: Problems with the hyperventilatory response to exercise and hypoxia. In Gonzalez NC, Fedde MR (eds): Oxygen Transfer from Atmosphere to Tissues. New York, Plenum Press, 1988, pp 277–291.

120. Johnson BD, Saupe KW, Dempsey JA: Mechanical constraints on exercise hyperpnea in endurance athletes. J Appl Physiol 1992; 73:874–886.

121. Bye PTP, Esau SA, Walley KR, et al: Ventilatory muscles during exercise in air and oxygen in normal men. J Appl Physiol Respir Environ Exerc Physiol 1984; 56:464–471.

122. Loke J, Mahler DA, Virgulto JA: Respiratory muscle fatigue after marathon running. J Appl Physiol 1982; 52:821–824.

123. Roussos C, Macklem PT: Inspiratory muscle fatigue. In Fishman AP, Fisher AB (eds): Handbook of Physiology, sec 3: The Respiratory System, vol 3, part 2: Mechanics of Breathing. Bethesda, Md, American Physiological Society, 198,6 pp 511–527.

124. Art T, Lekeux P: Effect of a booster vaccination against Influenza and Equine Herpes virus on cardiorespiratory adjustments to strenuous exercise and training in Thoroughbred horses. J Vet Med 1993; 40:481–491.

125. Fu X, Costello ML, Tsukimoto K, et al: High lung volume increases stress failure in pulmonary capillaries. J Appl Physiol 1992; 73:123–133.

126. Scharf SM, Bark H, Heimer D, et al: "Second wind" during inspiratory loading. Med Sci Sports Exerc 1984; 16:87–91.

127. Art T, Lekeux P: Effect of environmental temperature and relative humidity on breathing pattern and heart rate in ponies during and after standardised exercise. Vet Rec 1988; 123:295–299.

128. Rose RJ: An evaluation of heart rate and respiratory rate recovery for assessment of fitness during endurance rides. In Snow DH, Persson SGB, Rose RJ (eds): Equine Exercise Physiology. Cambridge, Granta Editions, 1983, pp 505–509.

129. Evans DL, Rose RJ: Maximum oxygen uptake in racehorses: Changes with training state and prediction from submaximal cardiorespiratory measurements. In Gillespie JR, Robinson NE (eds): Equine Exercise Physiology 2. Davis, Calif, ICEEP Publications, 1987, pp 52–67.

130. Knight PK, Sinha AK, Rose RJ: Effects of training intensity on maximum oxygen uptake. In Persson SGB, Lindholm A, Jeffcott LB (eds): Equine Exercise Physiology 3. Davis, Calif, ICEEP Publications, 1991, pp 77–82.

131. Butler PJ, Woakes AJ, Anderson LS, et al: The effect of cessation

of training on cardiorespiratory variables during exercise. *In* Persson SGB, Lindholm A, Jeffcott LB, (eds): Equine Exercise Physiology 3. Davis, Calif, ICEEP Publications, 1991, pp 71–76.

132. Erickson HH, Sexton WL, Erickson BK, et al: Cardiopulmonary response to exercise and detraining in the quarter horse. *In* Gillespie JR, Robinson NE (eds): Equine Exercise Physiology 2. Davis, Calif, ICEEP Publications, 1987, pp 41–51.

133. Fringer MN, Stull GA: Changes in cardiorespiratory parameters during periods of training and detraining in young adult females. Med Sci Sports 1974; 6:20–25.

134. Jirka Z, Adamus M: Changes of ventilations equivalents in young people in the course of 3 years training. J Sports Med 1965; 5:1–6.

135. Kaminski RP, Forster HV, Bisgard GE, et al: Effect of altered ambient temperature on breathing in ponies. J Appl Physiol 1985; 58:1585–1591.

136. Thiel M, Tolkmitt G, Hörnicke H: Body temperature changes in horses during riding: Time course and effects on heart rate and respiratory frequency. *In* Gillespie JR, Robinson NE (eds): Equine Exercise Physiology 2. Davis, Calif, ICEEP Publications, 1987, pp 183–193.

137. Powers SK, Howley ET, Cox R: Ventilation and metabolic reactions to heat stress during prolonged exercise. J Sports Med 1982; 22:32–36.

138. Manohar M: Tracheobronchial perfusion during exercise in ponies. J Appl Physiol 1990; 68:2182–2185.

139. Manohar M, Duren SE, Sikkes B, et al: Bronchial circulation during prolonged exercise in ponies. Am J Vet Res 1992; 53:925–929.

140. Burrell MH: Endoscopic and virological observations on respiratory disease in a group of young thoroughbred horses in training. Equine Vet J 1985; 17:99–103.

141. Williams JW, Meagher DM, Pascoe JR, et al: Upper airway function during maximal exercise in horses with obstructive upper airway lesions: Effect of surgical treatment. Vet Surg 1990; 19:142–147.

142. Bayly WM, Grant BD, Breeze RG: Arterial blood gas tensions and acid base balance during exercise in horses with pharyngeal lymphoid hyperplasia. Equine Vet J 1984; 16:435–438.

143. Haynes PF: Persistent dorsal displacement of the soft palate associated with epiglottic shortening in two horses. J Am Vet Med Assoc 1981; 179:677–681.

144. Williams JW, Pascoe JR, Meagher DM, et al: Effects of left recurrent laryngeal neurectomy, prosthetic laryngoplasty, and subtotal arytenoidectomy on upper airway pressure during maximal exertion. Vet Surg 1990; 19:136–141.

145. Belknap JK, Derksen FJ, Nickels FA, et al: Failure of subtotal arytenoidectomy to improve upper airway flow mechanics in exercising standardbreds with induced laryngeal hemiplegia. Am J Vet Res 1990; 51:1481–1487.

146. Manohar M: Right heart pressures and blood-gas tensions in ponies during exercise and laryngeal hemiplegia. Am J Physiol 1986; 251:H121–H126.

147. Hackett RP, Ducharme NG, Fubini SL, et al: Evaluation of the reliability of endoscopic examination in assessment of arytenoid cartilage movement in horses: I. Subjective and objective laryngeal evaluation. Vet Surg 1991; 20:174–179.

148. Linford RL, O'Brien TR, Wheat JD, et al: Radiographic assessment of epiglottic length and pharyngeal and laryngeal diameters in the thoroughbred. Am J Vet Res 1983; 44:1660–1666.

149. Honnas CM, Schumacher J, Dean PW: Epiglottic entrapment: The techniques for diagnosis and surgical treatment. Vet Med 1990; 613–619.

150. Mair TS, Lane JG: Tracheal obstructions in two horses and a donkey. Vet Rec 1990; 126:303–304.

151. Carrig C, Groenendyk S, Seawright A: Dorsoventral flattening of the trachea in a horse and its attempted surgical correction: a case report. J Am Vet Radiol Soc 1973; 14:32–36.

152. Hardy J: Upper respiratory obstruction in foals, weanlings and yearlings. Vet Clin North Am Equine Pract 1991; 7:105–122.

153. Willoughby R, Ecker G, McKee S, et al: The effects of equine rhinovirus, influenza virus and herpesvirus infection on tracheal clearance rate in horses. Can J Vet Res 1992; 56:115–121.

154. McFadden ER Jr, Ingram RH: Exercise-induced airway obstruction. Annu Rev Physiol 1983; 45:453–463.

155. Crimi E, Balbo A, Milanese M, et al: Airway inflammation and occurrence of delayed bronchoconstriction in exercise-induced asthma. Am Rev Respir Dis 1992; 146:507–512.

156. Hillidge CJ, Lane TJ, Johnson EL: Preliminary investigations of EIPH in racing Quarter Horse. J Equine Vet Sci 1984; 4:21–23.

157. Raphel CF, Soma LR: Exercise-induced pulmonary hemorrhage in thoroughbreds after racing and breezing. Am J Vet Res 1982; 43:1123–1127.

158. Pascoe JR, Ferraro GL, Cannon JH, et al: Exercise-induced pulmonary hemorrhage in racing thoroughbreds: A preliminary study. Am J Vet Res 1981; 42:703–707.

159. Sweeney CR, Soma LR: Exercise induced pulmonary haemorrhage in horses. *In* Snow DH, Persson SGB, Rose RJ (eds): Equine Exercise Physiology. Cambridge, Granta Editions, 1983, pp 51–56.

160. Soma LR, Laster L, Oppenlander F, et al: Effects of furosemide on the racing times of horses with exercise-induced pulmonary hemorrhage. Am J Vet Res 1985; 46:763–768.

161. O'Callaghan MW, Goulden BE: Radiographic changes in the lungs of horses with exercise-induced epistaxis. N Z Vet J 1982; 30:117–118.

162. O'Callaghan MW, Pascoe JR, Tyler WS, et al: Exercise-induced pulmonary haemorrhage in the horse: results of a detailed clinical, post mortem and imaging study: VI. Radiological/pathological correlations. Equine Vet J 1987; 19:419–422.

163. O'Callaghan MW, Hornof WJ, Fisher PE, et al: Exercise-induced pulmonary haemorrhage in the horses: results of a detailed clinical, post mortem and imaging study: VII. Ventilation/perfusion scintigraphy in horses with EIPH. Equine Vet J 1987; 19:423–427.

164. O'Callaghan MW, Pascoe JR, Tyler WS, et al: Exercise-induced pulmonary haemorrhage in the horse: Results of a detailed clinical, post mortem and imaging study: II. Gross lung pathology. Equine Vet J 1987; 19:389–393.

165. O'Callaghan MW, Pascoe JR, Tyler WS, et al: Exercise-induced pulmonary haemorrhage in the horse: results of a detailed clinical, post mortem and imaging study: III. Subgross findings in lungs subjected to latex perfusions of the bronchial and pulmonary arteries. Equine Vet J 1987; 19:394–404.

166. Modell HE, Beck K, Butler J: Functional aspects of canine bronchial-pulmonary vascular communications. J Appl Physiol 1981; 50:1045–1051.

167. Bayly WM, Meyers KM, Keck MT, et al: Effects of furosemide on exercise-induced alterations in haemostasis in thoroughbred horses exhibiting post-exercise epstaxis. *In* Snow DH, Persson SGB, Rose RJ (eds): Equine Exercise Physiology. Cambridge, Granta Editions, 1983, pp 64–70.

168. Speirs VC, van Veenendaal JC, Harrison IW, et al: Pulmonary haemorrhage in standardbred horses after racing. Aust Vet J 1982; 59:38–40.

169. O'Callaghan MW, Hornof WJ, Fisher PE, et al: Exercise-induced pulmonary haemorrhage in the horses: Results of a detailed clinical, post mortem and imaging study: VIII. Conclusions and implications. Equine Vet J 1987; 19:429–434.

170. Aguilera-Tejero E, Pascoe JR, Tyler WS, et al: Pulmonary function after instillation of autologous blood in the lungs of horses. *In* Proceedings of the 10th Comparative Respiratory Society Meeting, Urbana, Illinois, 1991, p S-6.

171. Tyler WS, Pascoe JR, Aguilera-Tejero E, et al: Morphological effects of autologous blood in airspaces of equine lungs. *In* Proceedings of the 10th Comparative Respiratory Society Meeting, Urbana, Illinois, 1991, S-7.

172. Ward PA, Mulligan MS: Lung injury by toxic oxygen metabolites. *In* Proceedings of the 10th Comparative Respiratory Society Meeting, East Lansing, Mich, 1991, pp P1–P5.

173. Tobin T, Roberts BC, Swerczek TW, et al: The pharmacology of furosemide in the horse: III. Dose and time relationships, effects of repeated dosing and performance effects. J Equine Med Surg 1978; 2:216.

174. Sweeney CR, Soma LR, Maxson AD, et al: Effects of furosemide on the racing times of thoroughbreds. Am J Vet Res 1990; 51:772–778.

175. Sweeney CR, Soma LR: Exercise-induced pulmonary hemorrhage

in thoroughbred horses: Response to furosemide or hesperidin-citrus bioflavinoids. J Am Vet Med Assoc 1984; 185:195–197.

176. Sweeney CR, Soma LR, Bucan CA: Exercise-induced pulmonary hemorrhage in exercising thoroughbreds: Preliminary results with pre-exercise medication. Cornell Vet 1984; 74:263–268.

177. Pascoe JR, McCabe AE, Franti CE, et al: Efficacy of furosemide in the treatment of exercise-induced pulmonary hemorrhage in thoroughbred racehorses. Am J Vet Res 1985; 46:2000–2003.

178. Olsen SC, Coyne CP, Lowe BS, et al: Influence of furosemide on hemodynamic responses during exercise in horses. Am J Vet Res 1992; 53:742–747.

179. Manohar M: Furosemide attenuates the exercise-induced rise in pulmonary artery wedge pressure in horses. Physiologist 1992; 35:231.

180. Sweeney CR, Hall J, Fisher JR, et al. Efficacy of water-vapor saturated air in the treatment of exercise-induced pulmonary hemorrhage in thoroughbred racehorses. Am J Vet Res 1988; 49:1705–1707.

181. Littlejohn A, Bowles F: Studies on the physiopathology of chronic obstructive pulmonary disease in the horse: 5. Blood gas and acid-base values during exercise. Ondertespoort J Vet Res 1981; 48:239–249.

182. Kelman GR, Nunn JF: Nomograms for correction of blood P_{O_2}, P_{CO_2}, pH, and base excess for time and temperature. J Appl Physiol 1966; 21:1484–1490.

183. Powers SK, Dodd S, Freeman J, et al: Accuracy of pulse oximetry to estimate HbO_2 fraction of total Hb during exercise. J Appl Physiol 1989; 67:300–304.

184. De Waal A, Littlejohn A, Potgieter GM, et al: An apparatus for collecting blood samples by radiotelemetry from horses during exercise. Vet Res Commun 1986; 10:65–72.

185. Persson SGB, Essén B, Lindholm A: Oxygen uptake, red-cell volume and pulse work relationship in different states of training in horses. In Proceedings of the 5th Meeting of the Academic Society for Large Animal Veterinary Medicine, Glasgow, UK, University of Glasgow, 1980.

186. Bayly WM, Schulz DA, Hodgson DR, et al: Ventilatory responses of the horse to exercise: effect of gas collection systems. J Appl Physiol 1987; 63:1210–1217.

187. Seeherman HJ, Morris EA: Methodology and repeatability of a standardised treadmill exercise test for clinical evaluation of fitness in horses. Equine Vet J 1990; (suppl 9):20–25.

188. Beaver WL, Wasserman K, Whipp BJ: On-line computer analysis and breath-by-breath graphical display of exercise function. J Appl Physiol 1973; 34:128–132.

189. Art T, Lekeux P: A critical assessment of pulmonary function testing in exercising ponies. Vet Res Commun 1988; 12:25–39.

190. Spörri H, Leeman W: Zur Untersuchung der Lungenmechanik bei Grosstieren (research on lung mechanics in large animals). Schw Arch Teir 1964; 106:699–714.

191. Gillespie JR, Tyler WS, Eberly VE: Pulmonary ventilation and resistance in emphysematous and control horses. J Appl Physiol 1966; 21:416–422.

192. Woakes AJ, Butler PJ, Snow DH: The measurement of respiratory airflow in exercising horses. In Gillespie JR, Robinson NE (eds): Equine Exercise Physiology 2. Davis, Calif, ICEEP Publication, 1987, pp 194–205.

193. Amis TC, Kurpershoek C: Tidal breathing flow-volume loop analysis for clinical assessment of airway obstruction in conscious dogs. Am J Vet Res 1986; 47:1002–1006.

194. Attenburrow DP, Flack FC, Portergill MJ: Impedance plethysmography. Equine Vet J 1990; 22:114–117.

195. Willoughby RA, McDonell WN: Pulmonary function testing in horses. Vet Clin North Am Large Anim Pract 1979; 1:171–196.

196. Gallivan GJ, Viel L, McDonell WN: An evaluation of the multiple-breath nitrogen washout as a pulmonary function test in horses. Can J Vet Res 1990; 54:99–105.

197. Muylle E, Van Den Hende C, Oyaert W: Nitrogen clearance in horses as a respiratory function test. J Vet Med [A] 1972; 19:310–317.

198. Deegen E, Klein H-K: Interpleural pressure measurement and bronchial spasmolysis tests in the horse performed with a transportable oesophageal pressure measuring instrument. Pferdeheilkunde 3 1987; 4:213–221.

199. Mead J, Whittenberger JL: Evaluation of airway interruption as

a method for measuring airflow resistance. J Appl Physiol 1954; 6:408–416.

200. Grobet L: Mesure de la résistance pulmonaire chez des animaux domestiques par la technique de l'interrupteur du débit aérien. M.S. thesis, Université de Liège, Liège, Belgium, 1989.

201. Gustin P, Dhem AR, Lekeux P: Measurement of total respiratory impedance in calves by the forced oscillation technique. J Appl Physiol 1988; 64:1786–1791.

202. Young SS, Hall LW: A rapid, non-invasive method for measuring total respiratory impedance in the horse. Equine Vet J 1989; 21:99–105.

203. Leninivin A, Close R, Art T, et al: Pulmonary function testing in horses by the monofrequency forced oscillation method: A preliminary study. In Proceedings of the 10th Comparative Respiratory Society Meeting, East Lansing, Mich, 1991, p P-9.

204. Dixon PM: Pulmonary artery pressures in normal horses and in horses affected with chronic obstructive pulmonary disease. Equine Vet J 1978; 10:195–198.

205. Muylle E, Nuytten J, Deprez P, et al: Pulmonary driving pressure as a pulmonary function test in horses. J Equine Vet Sci 1982; 4:57–59.

206. Amory H, Art T, Desmecht D, et al: Respiratory-induced variability of pulmonary arterial pressure measurements in cattle. Vet Res Commun 1990; 14:227–233.

207. Hedenstierna G, Nyman G, Kvart C, et al: Ventilation-perfusion relationships in the standing horse: an inert gas elimination study. Equine Vet J 1987; 19:514–519.

208. Gillespie JR, Tyler WS: Chronic alveolar emphysema in the horse. Adv Vet Sci Comp Med 1969; 13:59–65.

209. Willoughby RA, Ecker GL, McKee SL, et al: Use of scintigraphy for the determination of mucociliary clearance rates in normal, sedated, diseased and exercised horses. Can J Vet Res 1991; 55:315–320.

210. Morris EA, Seeherman HJ: Evaluation of upper respiratory tract function during strenuous exercise in racehorses. J Am Vet Med Assoc 1990; 196:431–438.

211. Moore MP, Andrews F, Reed SM, et al: Electromyographic evaluation of horses with laryngeal hemiplegia. Equine Vet Sci 1988; 8:424–427.

212. Cook WR: An electro-diagnostic test for the objective grading of recurrent laryngeal neuropathy in the horse. In Proceedings of the 37th Annual Convention of the American Association of the Equine Practitioners, New Orleans, AAEP, 1991, pp 275–296.

213. Archer RM, Lindsay WA, Duncan ID: A comparison of techniques to enhance the evaluation of equine laryngeal function. Equine Vet J 1991; 23:104–107.

214. Art T, Desmecht D, Amory H, et al: Lobeline-induced hyperpnea in equids: Comparison with rebreathing bag and exercise. J Vet Med [A] 1991; 38:148–152.

215. Attenburrow DP, Flack FC, Hörnicke H, et al: Respiratory air flow and sound intensity. In Snow DH, Persson SGB, Rose RJ (eds): Equine Exercise Physiology. Cambridge, Granta Editions, 1983, pp 23–26.

216. Attenburrow DP, Flack FC, Portergill MJ: The relationship between peak expiratory sound intensity and peak expiratory flow rate in the thoroughbred horse during exercise. Equine Vet J 1990; (suppl 9):43–46.

217. Lens E, Postiaux G, Chapelle P: Nocturnal asthma monotoring by automated spectral analysis of respiratory sounds (abstract). Clin Respir Physiol 1987; 23:S423.

218. Cohen A, Zagelbaum G: Clinical manifestations of inspiratory muscle fatigue. Am J Med 1982; 73:308–316.

219. Esau SA, Bellemare F, Grassino A, et al: Changes in relaxation rate with diaphragmatic fatigue in humans. J Appl Physiol 1983; 54:1353–1360.

220. Muir WW, Moore CA, Hamlin RL: Ventilatory alterations in normal horses in response to changes in inspired oxygen and carbon dioxide. Am J Vet Res 1975; 36:155–159.

221. Bertone JJ, Traub-Dargatz JL, Trotter GW. Bilateral hypoplasia of the soft palate and aryepiglottic entrapment in a horse. J Am Vet Med Assoc 1986; 188:727–729.

222. O'Callaghan MW, Sanderson GN: Clinical bronchography in the horse: Development of a method using barium sulphate powder. Equine Vet J 1982; 14:282–289.

223. Beech J: Technique of tracheobronchial aspiration in the horse. Equine Vet J 1981; 13:136–137.

224. Viel L: Structural-functional correlations of the lung in horses with small airway disease. Ph.D. thesis, University of Guelph, Guelph, Canada, 1983.

225. Lawson GHK, McPherson EA, Murphy JR, et al: The prevalence of precipitating antibodies in the sera of horses with COPD. Equine Vet J 1979; 11:172–176.

226. McPherson EA, Lawson GH, Murphy JR, et al: COPD in horses: Aetological studies. Responses to intradermal and inhalation antigen challenge. Equine Vet J 1979; 11:159–166.

227. Derksen FJ, Robinson NE, Armstrong PJ, et al: Airway reactivity in ponies with recurrent airway obstruction (heaves). J Appl Physiol 1985; 58:598–604.

228. Klein H-J, Deegen E: Histamine inhalation provocation test: Method to identify nonspecific airway reactivity in equids. Am J Vet Res 1986; 47:1796–1800.

229. Doucet MY, Vrins AA, Ford-Hutchinson AW: Histamine inhalation challenge in normal horses and in horses with small airway disease. Can J Vet Res 1991; 55:285–293.

230. Evans AG, Paradis MR, O'Callaghan M: Intradermal testing of horses with chronic obstructive pulmonary disease and recurrent urticaria. Am J Vet Res 1992; 53:203–208.

231. Collin B: Atlas d'anatomie. Liège, Belgium, Université de Liège, 1976.

The Cardiovascular System: Anatomy, Physiology, and Adaptations to Exercise and Training

D. L. EVANS

The cardiovascular system is a transport system consisting of a muscular pump, the heart, and a system of blood vessels that contain blood. Its principal function is transport of water, oxygen, carbon dioxide, fuels for energy production, electrolytes, hormones, and metabolic products. The cardiovascular system of the horse is uniquely designed for exceptional transport of oxygen from the lungs to the body tissues.

Horses have a high maximal oxygen consumption relative to body weight compared with most other mammals. The superior oxygen transport of the horse is due to its specialized spleen, which is able to add an extra volume of red blood cells to the circulation when it contracts after stimulus of fear or exercise. This infusion of erythrocytes increases the oxygen-transport capacity of the arterial blood and enables horses to greatly increase maximal oxygen consumption during exercise. The stroke volume of blood pumped with each cardiac contraction is over 1 liter in trained horses, and maximal rates of blood flow during exercise are about 300 liters/min. The structure and function of the equine cardiovascular system are therefore fundamental to the superior athletic performance of the horse.

Anatomy and Basic Physiology

The heart's role is to pump sufficient blood to maintain blood pressure and oxygen flow to tissues. The anatomy of the equine heart is similar to that found in other mammals (Fig. 7–1). The layout of the heart and circulatory system is illustrated in Figure 7–2. The thick-walled left ventricle pumps a stroke volume of blood into the aorta with each contraction. This establishes a wave of accelerated blood flow through the systemic arteries. Blood flow in arteries is continuous, because relaxation of the elastic arterial walls compresses the blood in the vessel, forcing it away from the heart toward the tissues.

The pressure of the blood in the arteries depends on the rate of blood flow, or cardiac output, and the amount of resistance to the flow. The main regulator of resistance is the degree of constriction or dilation of the arterioles. These vessels also regulate the rate of blood flow through the downstream capillaries, where oxygen diffuses from the hemoglobin in red blood cells to the mitochondria in tissue cells for the support of aerobic metabolism. Blood returns to the right atrium and ventricle along small and large veins. Venous blood flow depends greatly on muscular contractions, which compress the thin-walled veins. Changes in air pressures within the abdomen and thorax during breathing also assist venous return. Blood is then pumped to the lungs by the right ventricle via the pulmonary arteries. This enables removal of carbon dioxide and reoxygenation of blood for transport to working muscles.

The heart mass in thoroughbred horses is about 4 to 5 kg, or 1 percent of body weight. Trained horses have slightly higher relative heart masses (1.1 percent) than untrained horses (0.94 percent), suggesting that training causes hypertrophy of cardiac muscle.[1] There was no difference in heart mass between horses in training for 2 months and those in training for 19 months, suggesting that hypertrophy may be a rapid cardiac response to

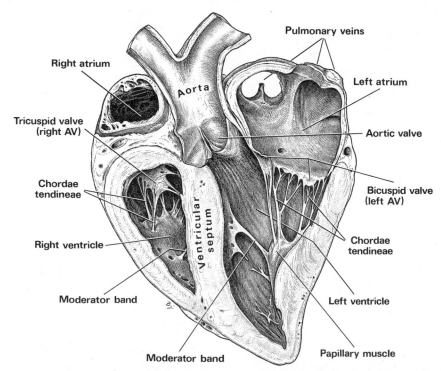

Figure 7-1. *Cross section of the equine heart showing the cardiac chambers and valves and direction of blood flow.*

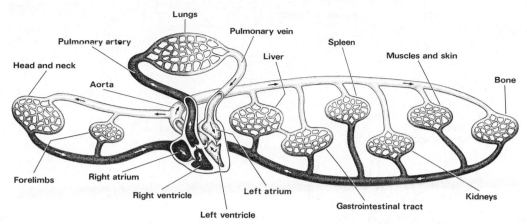

Figure 7-2. The cardiovascular system illustrating the blood flow to and from the main body systems.

training. Heart mass to body weight ratio is also a function of breed. Racing horses have a relative heart mass of 0.86, compared with 0.76 in Arabian horses and 0.62 in draft horses.[2]

The electrocardiogram (ECG) has been used to estimate the heart mass. The heart score, or mean QRS duration (ms) in the three bipolar limb leads of the ECG, has been found in one study to be highly correlated ($r = 0.9$) with postmortem heart weight.[3] An increase in heart score with age and training has been reported, but no effect of training alone on heart score was recorded in a previous study.[4]

Echocardiography has been used to assess the degree of cardiac dilation and hypertrophy due to training in endurance horses.[5] Mean calculated left ventricular mass in 53 trained endurance horses was 2.8 kg, compared with only 2.0 kg in a separate group of untrained horses.

The Cardiac Cycle

The *cardiac cycle* is the sequence of events occurring in the heart during every contraction (systole) and relaxation (diastole). The sequence and timing of blood pressures and valvular events in the equine heart and major arteries at rest are illustrated in Figure 7–3. The cyclic nature of cardiac activity depends on normal conduction of electrical impulses from the sinoatrial node, or pacemaker, through the atrial and ventricular myocardium. The conduction of impulses in the equine heart is illustrated in Figure 7–4. The diffuse distribution of the Purkinje fibers through the left ventricular wall enables

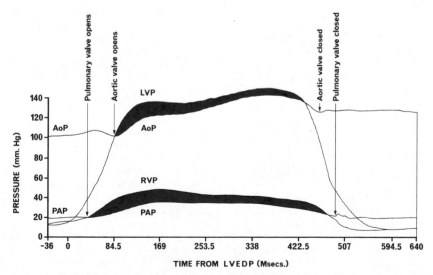

Figure 7-3. Aortic pressure (AoP), left ventricular pressure (LVP), pulmonary artery pressure (PAP), and right ventricular pressure (RVP) recorded simultaneously with intravascular transducers[6] (LVEDP, left ventricular end-diastolic pressure). Ejection begins earlier on the right side and lasts longer than on the left. The shaded areas represent the pressure gradients from the ventricles to the arterial systems.

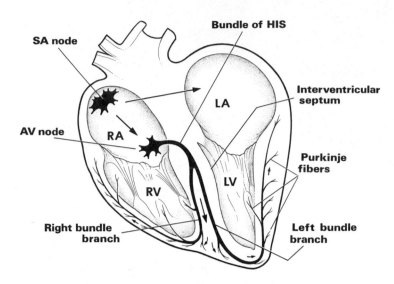

Figure 7-4. The conduction pathway of the equine heart.

rapid depolarization and development of muscular tension. However, right ventricular contraction slightly precedes left ventricular contraction. This is so because pulmonary artery pressure is lower than aortic pressure.[6]

Abnormal blood flow through the heart can cause murmurs and poor performance. *Murmurs,* or abnormal heart sounds, can be detected using a stethoscope or phonocardiograph. The significance of murmurs for athletic performance can be difficult to ascertain if there are no other signs of cardiovascular disease in the horse. Early or late systolic murmurs may be benign, but pansystolic and pandiastolic murmurs are usually significant.[7] Assessment of the cardiovascular response to exercise and measurement of maximal aerobic capacity during treadmill exercise may assist the diagnosis in doubtful cases (see Chap. 12).

Cardiovascular Adaptations to Exercise

HEART RATE

Heart Rate in the Resting Horse. The heart rate in the resting horse depends mainly on the degree of relaxation of the individual. In relaxed horses, resting heart rate is usually in the range 25 to 40 beats/min. However, sudden excitement, fear, or anticipation of exercise can elevate the heart rate rapidly to over 100 beats/min. Rapid heart rate changes in the range 20 to 110 beats/min in resting horses can be explained entirely by alterations in parasympathetic nerve activity.[8]

It has been suggested that the resting heart rate is lower in fit horses than in unfit horses.[9] However, the resting heart rate of the horse generally does not decrease after training, as in human athletes.[10-13] Use of heart rate measurements to monitor fitness is therefore restricted to measurements during or after exercise.

Measurement of Heart Rate During Exercise. Heart rate measurements during exercise in athletic horses have been used to describe the intensity of work, to measure

fitness, and to study the effects of training and detraining. There are several suitable commercial heart rate meters designed for use in exercising horses.[14-16] Heart rate during exercise also can be monitored electrocardiographically. The ECG can be obtained by wiring the horse directly to the recorder, recording the ECG on magnetic tape for examination at a later time, or by radiotelemetry.[17-20]

Commercial heart rate meters usually employ two or three electrodes incorporated into a belt or placed beneath the saddle.[14,21] Such heart rate meters enable exercise testing to be performed under racetrack conditions, facilitating assessment of the response to exercise and prescription of specific exercise loads during exercise. Records are not always perfect from such meters. The usual problem is faulty contact of the surface electrodes with the skin. However, under good conditions, the repeatability of heart rate measurements during treadmill exercise is very high.[22,23]

Heart Rate at the Start of Exercise. At the onset of exercise, the heart rate quickly increases and reaches a steady state in 2 to 3 minutes. This increase is associated with increased sympathetic nerve activity and/or catecholamine release.[8] Steady-state heart rate remains constant during submaximal work loads.[24] An overshoot of heart rate to levels above the submaximal steady-state heart rate may occur at the commencement of exercise.[25,26] Mean time taken to reach maximal heart rates after onset of exercise in thoroughbreds was 22 seconds.[27] In standardbreds trotting at speeds of 12.0 to 12.5 m/s, heart rates were not maximal until at least 700 m had been run.[28]

The kinetics of heart rate at the commencement of exercise without prior warmup is also dependent on the intensity of the exercise. In six standardbred horses, the typical overshoot was found at the start of exercise at 50 percent of $\dot{V}_{O_2max}$, but at 100 percent $\dot{V}_{O_2max}$, heart rate gradually increased during a 5-minute period of exercise[29] (Fig. 7-5). These data emphasize the impor-

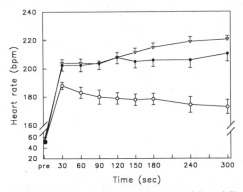

Figure 7-5. *Heart rate at the commencement of three different intensities of exercise without prior warmup in standardbred racehorses*[29] *(○, 50 %; ●, 75 %; and ▽, 100 % $\dot{V}_{O_2max}$).*

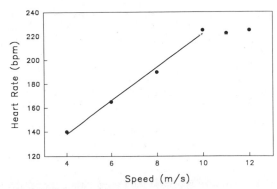

Figure 7-6. *Heart rates during a stepwise incremental tread-mill exercise test in a race-fit thoroughbred racehorse. The horse exercised for 3 minutes at 4 m/s, 2 minutes at 6 m/s, and 1 minute at 10, 11, and 12 m/s. Heart rates were recorded by te-lemetry electrocardiography during the last 15 seconds of each speed. The horse was unable to keep pace with the treadmill when the speed was increased to 13 m/s indicating fatigue and completion of the exercise test.*

tance of a suitable warmup prior to competition in horses, since oxygen consumption also increases more rapidly at the commencement of exercise if there has been prior warmup.[30]

Heart Rate During Submaximal Exercise. A linear relation-ship between heart rate and submaximal work effort has been observed in horses trotting, galloping, and swim-ming.[25,26,28,31-35] Many factors influence the position of the regression line of heart rate on work speed. These include gait,[36] length of the exercise track,[31] and tread-mill slope,[37] and the position is also influenced by the presence of a breathing mask.[38] The heart rate at a spe-cific working velocity can vary markedly between indi-vidual horses, but if standardized treadmill exercise tests are used, the heart rate versus work relationship is very precise and reproducible for individual horses at heart rates between 120 and 210 beats/min.[22,31]

This relationship is usually defined by the use of treadmill tests that involve increasing the speed or, less commonly, treadmill angle and measuring the heart rate at the completion of 1 to 2 minutes of exercise at each speed. After a suitable warmup, e.g., 3 minutes of trot-ting, the heart rate is stable after 1 minute of further exercise at higher speeds. Figure 7–6 illustrates the heart rates recorded during the last 15 seconds at each speed in a fit thoroughbred racehorse during a treadmill ex-ercise test.

The heart rate–work load relationship is also af-fected by disease states, because horses with chronic ob-structive pulmonary disease (COPD) have heart rates during submaximal exercise that are significantly higher than those found in normal horses.[36,39] Heart rate during standardized submaximal exercise is also higher in horses with cardiac disease, such as atrial fibrillation.

The time to fatigue during treadmill exercise is de-pendent on the intensity of exercise. At heart rates of 170 to 180 beats/min, seven partially trained thoroughbreds were able to exercise for an average of 24 minutes, whereas at a heart rate of 208 beats/min, equivalent to 100 percent $\dot{V}_{O_2max}$, the horses fatigued in 4 minutes.[40]

Heart rates during swimming vary greatly between horses and are usually in the range 130 to 180 beats/min.[34,41] The mean highest heart rate recorded in nine horses during show jumping was 191 ± 3 beats/min.[42]

During prolonged strenuous submaximal exercise at a constant work rate, a gradual increase in heart rate, or *cardiovascular drift,* can occur. For example, during 30 minutes of exercise, mean heart rate increased from 154 to 173 beats/min. This drift was accompanied by in-creases in minute ventilation and cardiac output, while stroke volume was unchanged.[43] In another study, horses exercising at 55 to 60 percent of individual maximal heart rate (HR_{max}) for 60 minutes had minimal changes in heart rate.[44] Heart rate during prolonged exercise in horses probably depends on the intensity of exercise, en-vironmental conditions, and possibly fitness.

Maximal Heart Rate. A loss of linearity of the heart rate on velocity regression line is typical at high work speeds (see Fig. 7–6). *Maximal heart rate* (HR_{max}) is defined as the highest heart rate measured in an incremental-speed treadmill test which results in a plateau of heart rate. If a plateau is not demonstrated, the highest heart rate re-corded in an incremental-speed treadmill exercise test is referred to as the *peak heart rate.* Alternatively, maximal heart rate can be measured in horses after 1 minute of maximal exercise after a suitable warmup.

HR_{max} can vary considerably between horses. Max-imal heart rates recorded during racing in 19 thorough-breds averaged 223 beats/min, with a range of 204 to 241 beats/min.[27] High individual variability in heart rates while racing also have been recorded in stan-dardbreds, ranging from 210 to 238 beats/min, with a mean of 221 beats/min.[45]

In humans, maximal heart rate declines with age.[46] There is no predictable relationship between age and maximal heart rate in horses. Mean peak heart rate in eight yearling thoroughbreds was approximately 240 beats/min, compared with 220 to 230 beats/min in 2- to 4-year-old horses.[47] Likewise, yearling, 2-year-old, and adult thoroughbreds had similar means (229 to 231 beats/min) and ranges (215 to 254 beats/min) of peak heart rates during an incremental treadmill exercise test.[48]

The individual HR_{max} is a highly repeatable measurement in individual horses,[22] but it is not an important measure of fitness, since it is not affected by training, despite increases in maximal oxygen consumption $(\dot{V}_{O_2max})$.[48,49]

The treadmill speed at which maximal heart rate is achieved $(V-HR_{max})$ during a stepwise test is significantly correlated with $\dot{V}_{O_2max}$ and is therefore a suitable measurement of fitness in treadmill tests that do not measure oxygen consumption.[50] In addition, the relative heart rate (as a percentage of maximal heart rate) is highly correlated with relative oxygen consumption in horses during treadmill exercise[50] (Fig. 7–7).

Submaximal Exercise Heart Rates and Fitness Measurements. Heart rate measurements during submaximal treadmill exercise have been expressed relative to treadmill speed in some studies for measurement of fitness. For example, the treadmill velocities that result in heart rates of 140 (V_{140}) or 200 beats/min (V_{200}) have been used. The V_{200} is calculated by measuring the heart rate at the end of three to four treadmill or racetrack runs, each of which results in heart rates between 120 and 210 beats/min.[38,51]

$V-HR_{max}$ also may be a useful measure of fitness. This value is obtained by substituting HR_{max} in the regression equation describing the linear heart rate on velocity relationship during submaximal exercise. Figure 7–8 shows the method of calculating V_{200} and $V-HR_{max}$.

Trained standardbred racehorses can be exercise tested on a racetrack to calculate V_{200}.[21] In this study,[21] the exercise test consisted of four steps, pacing over 1000 m. Actual test speeds were calculated for each step, but the four speeds were in the ranges 450 to 550, 600 to 700, 700 to 800, and more than 800 m/min. Rest periods between each of these steps also enabled collection of venous blood for lactate determination and calculation of HR4, another suggested index of fitness. This measurement refers to the heart rate at which blood lactate is 4 mmol/liter. It is generally higher in fitter horses.

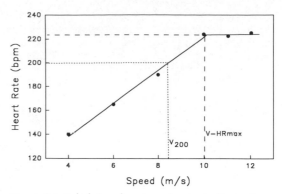

Figure 7-8. Calculation of maximum heart rate, V_{200}, and $V-HR_{max}$ from the results of a stepwise incremental-speed exercise test.

In the preceding study, V_{200} ranged from 590 to 720 m/min, and HR4 ranged from 190 to 225 beats/min (at 615 to 705 m/min, or mile rates of 2 minutes and 16 seconds to 2 minutes and 36 seconds).

A similar racetrack exercise test was used to investigate the relationship between several measures of fitness and maximal trotting velocity in Swedish trotters. Both V_{200} and the heart rate after 4000 m trotting at 10 m/s (HR10) were significantly correlated with maximal trotting velocity over 1000 m. Respective correlations were 0.6 and -0.74.[51]

A decrease in indices such as V_{140} or V_{200} indicates that the heart rate is abnormally elevated during submaximal exercise such as trotting and slow cantering. This finding in a horse in training could suggest loss of cardiovascular fitness, cardiac or pulmonary disease, lameness, or overtraining. Overtrained horses had an altered relationship between heart rate and treadmill velocity in one study, resulting in a low V_{150} (treadmill velocity at heart rate 150 beats/min).[25] A sudden decrease in V_{140} also has been reported in quarter horses during training. There was no evidence of disease or lameness in some of these horses, and it was thought that this response indicated overtraining.[52]

Measurements such as V_{200} are most useful for comparing an individual or group of horses with itself over time. Caution should be exercised if V_{200} is used to compare different horses, since the maximal heart rate can vary greatly between individuals. At a heart rate of 200 beats/min, horses with maximal heart rates of 215 and 245 beats/min are exercising at 93 and 82 percent of their respective maximal heart rates. The relative work rates are therefore quite dissimilar. In addition, there is no evidence that V_{200} is superior to measurement of one heart rate at a set treadmill speed. For example, the heart rate response to treadmill exercise at 8 m/s on a treadmill after a standardized warmup would probably give the same information as V_{200}, obviating the need for multiple exercise steps and interpolation of a regression line to the heart rate of 200 beats/min.

A racetrack fitness test based on telemetric heart rate measurements for racing standardbred horses has

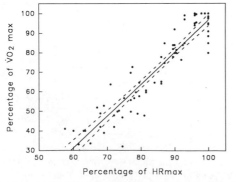

Figure 7-7. Relationship between percentage of maximal heart rate and maximum oxygen consumption in fit and unfit horses.[50]

been described.[53] This test is easier to conduct, and the results have correlated with racetrack performance. It does not require measurement of heart rate during three to four runs and subsequent calculation of velocity at a set heart rate. The horses were jogged 3 miles, then exercised for 1 mile in 170 s as a warmup, and then after 60 minutes of rest were exercised over 1 mile in 150 ± 1 s. The mean heart rate in 22 horses so tested was 202 beats/min after one-quarter of a mile and 212 beats/min at the end of the test run. The heart rate during the last quarter mile was highly correlated with fastest winning time ($r = 0.9$, $p < 0.01$).

A racetrack exercise test to measure V_{170} in ridden horses also has been described.[54] Horses were exercised over 800 m at constant speeds of 220, 270, 360, 450, and 540 m/min, and heart rates were recorded telemetrically. V_{170} differed significantly between breeds and was highly reproducible, but there was no relationship between this measurement and a subjectively derived assessment of the performance of 339 Czech warmbloods in cross-country races.

Heart Rate Recovery after Exercise. Heart rate recovery is usually very rapid in the first minute after exercise stops.[17,19,25,53] It then decreases more gradually toward normal resting values. It is therefore not possible to determine the heart rate during prior exercise by evaluating heart rate after exercise in horses.

Recovery heart rates after a standardized exercise test on a track were only moderately correlated with fastest winning time in standardbred horses ($r = 0.34$ to 0.51), with the highest correlation found at 5 minutes after exercise.[53] The author of this study also points out that the test should be carried out as part of the normal training routine and in familiar surroundings and that recovery heart rates are notoriously susceptible to rapid increases due to excitement.

Recovery heart rates are used to assess fitness of horses competing in endurance rides. Endurance riders should therefore ensure that horses to be used in competition are accustomed to the approach of strangers and cardiac auscultation. Poorly performing endurance horses have higher postexercise heart rates than the better performers.[55] Horses with heart rates less than 60 beats/min 30 minutes after exercise were found to show less evidence of dehydration and myopathy.[56] Horses with heart rates greater than 65 to 70 beats/min at the 30-minute recovery time at the midpoint of an endurance ride often develop severe dehydration and exhaustion if they are allowed to continue.[57]

It has been suggested that recovery heart rates are a suitable index of recovery between heats when using interval training. For example, it has been proposed that a recovery heart rate of 120 beats/min indicates that a horse is sufficiently recovered to undertake further heats. However, there is no evidence to support this contention, and it cannot be assumed that a horse is ready for further exercise on the basis of recovery heart rates. However, abnormally delayed recovery heart rates in the individual horse compared with normal should alert trainers to the possibility of illness or lameness.

Heart Rate and Training. In many studies, heart rates during submaximal exercise are lower after training. Heart rates during submaximal exercise may therefore provide a means of monitoring the adaptation of the cardiovascular system to chronic exercise. Thoroughbreds exercise tested at submaximal work loads on a treadmill had lower exercise heart rates after a conventional training program.[58] Exercise bradycardia, evident as a mean increase in V_{200} of 0.57 m/s, occurred after 5 weeks of treadmill training.[59]

However, not all studies conclude that significant changes occur in heart rate during submaximal exercise. Heart rates during submaximal exercise were not significantly different in standardbreds after either racetrack[12] or treadmill training.[60] In two treadmill training studies that demonstrated significant increases in maximal oxygen consumption, no significant changes were found in heart rate during submaximal exercise.[49,61] Decreasing heart rate during submaximal exercise is therefore an unreliable index of fitness in horses. The decrease in heart rate with training is often only 10 to 20 beats/min at any submaximal speed[10] (Fig. 7–9).

The use of heart rates during submaximal exercise to monitor increasing fitness also may be complicated by higher heart rates in horses at the start of training due to inadequate acclimation to the testing procedures,[10] which often include venipuncture, vascular catheteriza-

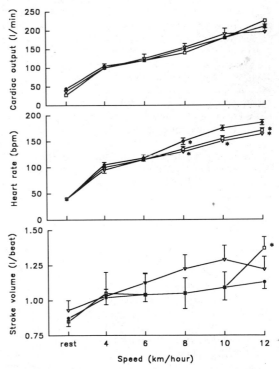

Figure 7-9. *Effect of 5 and 10 weeks of training on cardiac output (Q), heart rate (HR), and stroke volume (SV) at rest and during treadmill exercise (means ± SE). Significant differences from pretraining (*P < 0.05; **p < 0.01)[10] (●, untrained; △, partially trained; □, trained).*

tion, and wearing a mask for simultaneous measurements of respiratory function.

Maximal heart rate is not altered by training. Heart rates in thoroughbred horses during an 800-m gallop at a speed of about 800 m/min were not different after training.[58] In addition, maximal heart rates measured during treadmill exercise tests were not changed by treadmill training.[49]

Postexercise heart rates have shown no significant changes due to training in several studies.[12,13,60] However, heart rates taken within 1 to 5 minutes of completion of fast work by thoroughbreds have been lower after training in two studies.[58,62] Analysis of fitness using postexercise heart rates may be limited because of the rapid cardiac deceleration after cessation of exercise and the influence of psychogenic factors on heart rates less than 120 beats/min.[38]

The Oxygen Pulse. The *oxygen pulse* is defined as the ratio of oxygen consumption to heart rate and expresses the volume of oxygen ejected from the ventricles with each cardiac contraction. In humans, the oxygen pulse during exercise reflects the maximal aerobic capacity.[63] It is likely that this relationship also generally holds true in horses, because maximal heart rate varies only by about ±5 percent in the population. The maximal aerobic capacity in untrained and trained horses can range from 90 to 180 ml/kg/min, a difference of 100 percent. Oxygen pulse during maximal exercise could therefore be expected to range from 0.4 to 0.8 ml/kg/beat, or 180 to 400 ml/beat, in horses. Obviously, this large range must be due to individual differences in maximal stroke volume and arteriovenous oxygen content difference. Oxygen pulse increases as heart rate increases during exercise,[64] and it is therefore not possible to predict maximal aerobic capacity from oxygen pulse measurements during exercise at low heart rates. However, the close linear relationship between oxygen consumption and heart rate in horses during exercise could enable an estimation of maximal aerobic capacity, since the slope of the line would reflect the individual's oxygen pulse. Alternatively, extrapolation of this regression to an assumed maximal heart rate of 225 beats/min might be a good predictor of $\dot{V}_{O_2max}$.

STROKE VOLUME AND CARDIAC OUTPUT

Cardiac output is the product of heart rate and stroke volume. Stroke volume is the volume of blood ejected from each cardiac ventricle with each contraction. Cardiac output is therefore the volume of blood ejected from left or right ventricle each minute, expressed as liters per minute or milliliters per kilogram per minute. Increasing the cardiac output is the principal means of increasing oxygen uptake during exercise.

Oxygen uptake is the product of cardiac output and the amount of oxygen extracted from blood in the exercising muscles. It has been estimated that increases in cardiac output contribute about two-thirds of the increase in oxygen uptake that occurs during submaximal

exercise.[59] These relationships are expressed by the Fick equation:

$$\text{Oxygen uptake (liters/min)} = \text{cardiac output (liters/min)} \times C(a-v)_{O_2} \text{ (liters/liter)}$$

where $C(a-v)_{O_2}$ is the difference in oxygen concentration between arterial and mixed venous blood.[64]

Cardiac output at rest and during exercise has been measured in horses using dye dilution,[65,66] thermodilution,[10–12,68,69] an electromagnetic flow probe,[63] and direct Fick technique.[49,59,70,71] During submaximal exercise, cardiac output increases linearly with increases in work load,[10,11,64,72] principally due to tachycardia (see Fig. 7–9).

Stroke volume in the resting horse is approximately 800 to 900 ml, or about 2 to 2.5 ml/kg.[10,11,34,35,59,66,67] Stroke volumes of 2.4 ml/kg (1250 ml)[72] and 3.8 ± 0.4 ml/kg (approximately 1700 ml)[71] have been reported in fit thoroughbreds during treadmill exercise at $\dot{V}_{O_2max}$. Stroke volume increases by about 20 to 50 percent in the transition from rest to submaximal exercise[35,59,64,69] (see Fig. 7–9). It does not change as intensity of exercise increases from approximately 40 percent $\dot{V}_{O_2max}$ to 100 percent $\dot{V}_{O_2max}$.[72] This is true despite the limited time available for ventricular filling at high heart rates during exercise. Increased venous return during exercise and the increased blood volume must increase ventricular filling pressure sufficiently to prevent compromise of stroke volume.

During tethered swimming at low work loads, stroke volume decreased from 2.06 ml/kg at rest to about 1.5 ml/kg. This response may be related to decreased venous return secondary to the alterations in breathing pattern during swimming.[34] Values reported for cardiac output in fit thoroughbreds during treadmill exercise at $\dot{V}_{O_2max}$ are 789 ± 102 ml/kg/min (355 liters/min)[71] and 534 ± 54 ml/kg/min (277 liters/min).[72]

There have been few studies of the effect of training on cardiac output and stroke volume in horses. Several studies have found that training does not affect cardiac output or stroke volume measured at rest or after exercise.[10–12,59] A cross-sectional echocardiographic study of unconditioned and trained endurance horses found that the calculated stroke volume was not significantly different.[5] However, the results of this study may have been influenced by the significant differences in heart rate in the two groups, since myocardial force of contraction is partly dependent on heart rate.[65]

Stroke volume increased after training by approximately 10 percent during treadmill exercise at 12 km/h on an 11.5 percent grade in one study.[10] This response was after 10 weeks of trotting training at heart rates of 150 beats/min. However, the cardiac output during exercise was not changed, reflecting a decrease in heart rate after training during the submaximal exercise test (see Fig. 7–9). Other treadmill studies have not demonstrated significant changes in stroke volume during submaximal exercise subsequent to treadmill training.[11,59]

There have been few studies that have examined the effect of training on stroke volume and cardiac output during maximal exercise. In one study, a 23 percent increase in maximal oxygen consumption was accompanied by a significant increase in stroke volume during maximal exercise.[49] In another study that used an open-flow system for measuring oxygen consumption, stroke volume during exercise at 100 percent $\dot{V}_{O_2max}$ did not change significantly with training but decreased significantly by 11 percent from 1426 ± 50 ml to 1271 ± 68 ml after 6 weeks of detraining.[61] Studies of the effects of training on stroke volume and cardiac output during maximal exercise may be complicated by the variability of the initial state of training, as in humans.[73] Other factors that could influence the cardiovascular response to training include the training frequency, intensity, and duration.

BLOOD PRESSURE AND VASCULAR RESISTANCE

Blood pressure is the product of cardiac output and total peripheral resistance (TPR). TPR is primarily dependent on the diameter of the arterioles but is also influenced by blood viscosity. Regulation of blood pressure at the start of and during exercise is not fully understood but probably involves reflexes that originate in the brain ("central command") and the working muscle.[75] In the muscle, receptors respond to mechanical and chemical disturbances. Chemical disturbances include factors such as the decrease in arterial P_{O_2} and the increased local concentrations of metabolites such as CO_2, H^+, and lactate, which modulate "central command" signals that originate in the central nervous system. Arterial baroreceptor reflexes are also postulated to have a role in blood pressure regulation during exercise, possibly involving responses to "error" signals which necessitate establishment of a higher blood pressure.[76]

Systemic Circulation. Mean systemic arterial blood pressure found in resting horses is in the range 113 to 138 mmHg.[34,35,66,74,77] Light treadmill exercise has no significant effect on mean pressures in the carotid artery.[66] During more strenuous treadmill exercise, however, significant increases in mean systemic arterial pressure have been reported[10,11,64,74,78,79] (Fig. 7–10). At light exercise loads, falls in arterial diastolic pressure also have been reported.[11,35] A fall in mean arterial pressure also has been recorded in some horses as they commence galloping exercise, and it then increases within 2 minutes. At a speed of 548 m/min and mean heart rate of 184 beats/min, galloping thoroughbreds recorded the following systemic arterial pressures (resting values in parentheses): systolic 205 (115) mmHg, diastolic 116 (83) mmHg, mean 160 (97) mmHg, and pulse pressure 89 (32) mmHg.[77]

During forced swimming with heart rates of approximately 200 beats/min, systolic carotid artery pressures routinely reached 300 mmHg, and mean arterial blood pressure doubled from 113 ± 2 mmHg at rest. Carotid artery pressure was linearly related to work ef-

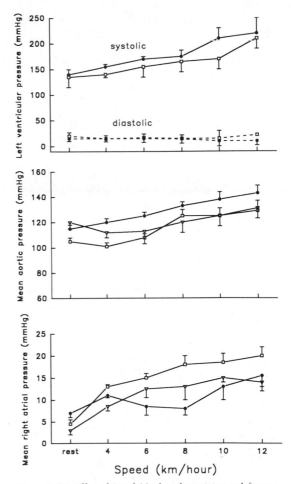

Figure 7-10. *Effect of 5 and 10 of weeks training on left ventricular (LVP), aortic (AoP), and mean right atrial (RAP) pressures at rest and during treadmill exercise (means ± SE). Significant differences from pretraining *p < 0.05; **p < 0.01. Adapted from Thomas DP, Fregin GF, Gerber NH, et al.: Effects of training on cardiorespiratory function in the horse. Am J Physiol 245:R160, 1983. With permission (●, untrained; △, partially trained; □, trained).*

fort.[34] Linear relationships between mean arterial and pulse pressures with speed on a racetrack also have been reported.[77] However, tethered swimming results in higher blood pressures than in the galloping horse. The large increases in both systemic and pulmonic blood pressures during swimming are partly attributable to the increased hydrostatic pressure on the submerged chest.[34]

Significant elevations in systolic left ventricular and mean right atrial pressures have been recorded during exercise.[10,35] The maximal rate of rise in left ventricular pressure has been used to assess left ventricular function at rest[80] and during treadmill exercise.[10,35,70] During exercise, myocardial contractility (expressed as peak time derivative of left ventricular pressure, LV dP/dt) increased with each increase in treadmill speed. In untrained adult ponies, treadmill exercise increased left ventricular end-diastolic pressure and right ventricular systolic and end-diastolic pressures.[74]

The ratio of mean arterial pressure to heart rate was used to assess total peripheral resistance during exercise in three horses.[77] Assuming constant stroke volume during the exercise test, large and significant falls in total peripheral resistance were recorded. Measurement of mean pulmonary and carotid artery pressures and cardiac output during treadmill exercise at 4 m/s also demonstrated large decreases in both pulmonary and peripheral vascular resistances. These results were presumed to be due to expansion of the vascular bed in the lungs and working skeletal muscles.[66] Similar results were reported in ponies and standardbreds in treadmill studies.[11,74] In view of the large increases in cardiac output during exercise in horses, a fall in peripheral vascular resistance is an important means of maintaining mean blood pressures within narrow limits.

Pulmonary Circulation. In 14 resting normal horses, pressures (mean $\pm$ SD) recorded in the pulmonary artery were systolic 42.23 $\pm$ 5.22 mmHg, diastolic 18.32 $\pm$ 4.13 mmHg, and mean 26.40 $\pm$ 3.83 mmHg.[81] During submaximal treadmill exercise, an increase of about 30 percent in mean pulmonary artery pressure occurred with increased treadmill speed until a plateau was reached at about 100 percent increase over control values.[78] During more intense treadmill exercise at 10 m/s on a 3 percent slope, mean pulmonary artery pressure increased from 28 mmHg at rest to 80 mmHg while heart rate was 202 beats/min.[82] The changes in pulmonary artery pressure during exercise were closely correlated with heart rate. Mean pulmonary artery pressure increased from 24 $\pm$ 1 mmHg at rest to 40 to 100 mmHg during tethered swimming.[34] The relatively high pulmonary artery pressures in exercising horses are probably not attributable to hypoxic pulmonary vasoconstriction.[83]

In resting horses, blood flow is well matched to alveolar ventilation, and strenuous exercise generally has little effect on this homogeneity.[84] Inequalities between blood flow and pulmonary alveolar ventilation were recorded during exercise at 10 m/s in two horses, but there was no relationship between this mismatching and the presence of blood in the trachea after exercise. Intrapulmonary shunting of blood was negligible both at rest and during exercise in the same study. It was concluded that neither shunting nor ventilation/perfusion mismatch explained the hypoxemia of intense exercise in horses.

The pulmonary and systemic arterial blood pressures and vascular resistances are all lower in splenectomized than in normal ponies during exercise.[85] This is despite similar cardiac outputs in the two conditions. It was concluded that increases in blood viscosity due to hemoconcentration in normal ponies may contribute substantially to the pulmonary and systemic hypertension of exercise.

Furosemide is used in some racehorses prior to racing as a prophylaxis for exercise-induced pulmonary hemorrhage (EIPH). The rationale may be that a reduction in pulmonary artery blood pressure will reduce the blood pressure in the pulmonary capillaries and therefore reduce the likelihood of hemorrhage. Furosemide does decrease blood volume and ameliorate the increase in systemic arterial blood pressure during exercise,[82,86,87] but one study indicates that the therapy neither significantly reduces pulmonary artery blood pressure during intense treadmill exercise nor prevents EIPH.[82] The possible relationships between pulmonary and bronchial arterial pressures during exercise and EIPH were discussed in Chapter 6.

Blood Pressure and Training. Values for resting arterial blood pressures measured indirectly in race-conditioned thoroughbreds have been reported.[88] Mean, systolic, and diastolic aortic blood pressures were lower during exercise after treadmill training[10] (see Fig. 7–10). Treadmill training also has resulted in higher mean right atrial pressure and a tendency to lower systolic left ventricular pressure during exercise.[10] Training also caused lower LV dP/dt_{max} at rest and during exercise. Racetrack training resulted in a decrease in mean arterial blood pressure during an exercise test.[77]

In humans, training is usually associated with a fall in peripheral vascular resistance.[73] A reduction in total peripheral resistance in the arterial circulation after training also has been reported in horses in two treadmill studies.[10,11]

BLOOD VOLUME

The total blood volume consists of the combined volume of the plasma and the cells in the blood. In resting horses, blood volume is about 9 percent of body weight. Approximately 20 percent of the blood volume is found in the pulmonary circulation and 80 percent in the systemic circulation.[6] Of the blood in the systemic circulation, 60 percent is in the veins and venules, and only 15 percent is in the arteries.

Blood volume can vary greatly during excitement and exercise. The contraction of the spleen in such circumstances adds red blood cells to the circulation, and this addition of erythrocytes can increase hematocrit from values of 35 to 45 percent at rest to 50 to 70 percent after exercise. The extent of the increase in total blood volume during exercise is dependent on work intensity, age, sex, and training state of the horse.[25] The weight of the spleen varies by over 200 percent in various breeds, and this variation may explain the differences in total blood volume between breeds of horse.[2]

Measurement of total blood volume in the horse therefore necessitates measurement of the plasma volume and the postexercise hematocrit.[25] Mean total blood volume in 10 untrained thoroughbred horses was 53.3 liters, of which only 40 percent was plasma.[61]

Plasma Volume. Plasma volume is measured in horses by injecting a known mass of a dye or other marker and subsequently measuring its concentration in the plasma after a suitable time for mixing. Evans blue dye (T1824) is frequently used. The plasma volume in the resting horse ranges from 16 to 31 liters, or 38 to 64 ml/kg of body weight.[61,89-91]

Effect of Exercise on Plasma Volume. Exercise usually results in a decrease in plasma volume. This change has been attributed to water movement from the intravascular to extravascular compartment.[89] A 13 percent decrease in plasma volume was measured within 10 minutes of completion of a 1000-m maximal gallop in six fit thoroughbred horses.[91] The decrease in plasma volume is accompanied by an increase in the total plasma protein (TPP) concentration. Total plasma protein returns to prerace values 1 hour after racing.[92] However, changes in TPP after exercise are not an accurate assessment of exercise-induced changes in plasma volume, since protein is added to the circulation during and/or after exercise. Changes in plasma osmolality may be a better indicator of changes in plasma volume after brief exercise.[91]

Maximal exercise over 600 m did not alter plasma volume or extracellular fluid volume significantly in six trained standardbreds.[89] Detection of any changes in plasma volume after maximal exercise may depend on duration of exercise and the experimental techniques used. In addition, decreases in plasma volume after exercise are quite variable, ranging from 3 to 27 percent.[91]

Effect of Training on Plasma Volume. Plasma volume in the resting horse increases after training.[90] The cardiovascular responses to an expanded plasma volume include increased right atrial pressure and stroke volume.[87] An increase in plasma volume after training may augment ventricular filling and so contribute to the increased stroke volume found with training. An expanded plasma volume is also likely to be an important mechanism for increased thermoregulatory capacity during exercise, enabling increased blood flow to the skin.

A 4.7-liter, or 29.1 percent, increase in plasma volume has been found after only 14 days of slow-speed (1.6 m/s) treadmill training.[90] Ninety percent of this increase occurred in the first week of training. This rapid increase in plasma volume coupled with constant hemoglobin concentration in blood may explain the 10 percent increase in maximal oxygen consumption that occurs over the same period at the commencement of training.[61] However, maximal oxygen consumption decreased rapidly when training was stopped, but the increased plasma volume was maintained for 6 weeks.[61]

The mechanism for the rapid increase in plasma volume with training has not been resolved, although renal water reabsorption and urea conservation have been suggested.[90] This study found that there was no change in daily water intake to explain the increase in plasma volume. Likewise, renal reabsorption of water was not associated with increased reabsorption of sodium, since the rate of sodium clearance was not altered by training and there was no change in resting aldosterone concentration in plasma.

Plasma Volume and Diet. Plasma volume can change during the day, depending on the feeding regimen adopted.[93,94] When horses were fed small portions at 4-hour intervals, there were only small changes in total plasma protein concentration and hematocrit, whereas these variables increased greatly after a single large meal. This suggests that plasma volume decreases by 10 to 15 percent for at least 1 hour after a large meal. Horses therefore should not be fed a large meal 1 to 2 hours before competition.

Plasma Volume and Athletic Performance. Plasma volume is often decreased in endurance horses during competition due to sodium and water losses in sweat.[95] Many studies in human athletes illustrate the importance of maintenance of plasma volume and body water for performance of endurance exercise.[96,97] Thermoregulation might be more efficient in horses during endurance exercise if there was forced rehydration of horses at rest stops rather than depending on horses to replace losses by voluntary drinking. The use of a solution containing 111 g glucose, 1.56 g Na, 3.22 g Cl, 1.02 g K, 170 mg phosphate, 220 mg Mg, 5 mg Mn, 108 mg Fe, 2.5 mg iodine, and "other trace elements" per liter resulted in lower heart rates and blood lactate concentration during exercise in one study.[98]

Augmenting blood volume by dextran infusion increases cardiac output during exercise at 100 percent $\dot{V}_{O_2max}$ but does not influence the measured value of $\dot{V}_{O_2}$ during exercise. This response was attributed to higher right atrial pressures after infusion.[87] An increase in cardiac output was accompanied by a decrease in the arteriovenous oxygen content difference. However, plasma volume expansion may enhance performance of endurance exercise in horses, since skin blood flow may be dependent on blood volume.

Total Red Cell Volume. The *total red cell volume* refers to the volume of red blood cells in the circulation after exercise or after an injection of epinephrine. Training results in an increase of the total red cell volume in horses. The potential for increasing oxygen-transport capacity by splenic emptying during exercise is therefore augmented by training.[99] Total red cell volume relative to body weight is also related to racing performance in Swedish trotters.[51] A correlation of 0.68 ($p < 0.001$) was found between this measurement and maximal trotting speed over 1000 m in 35 horses. This correlation was as high as found for other measurements of fitness, such as the blood lactate and heart rate response to submaximal exercise for 4000 m at 10 m/s in the same group of horses.

In a study of Swedish trotting horses, overtraining consequent to intensive training was related to adrenocortical exhaustion. Reduced plasma cortisol levels and increased total red cell volume to body weight ratio were thought to indicate overtraining.[100]

Unfortunately, the total red cell volume is not a simple measurement. It is unlikely to become a routine method of appraising the athletic horse until its relevance to performance and relationship to whole-body maximal oxygen consumption have been confirmed in other studies.

DISTRIBUTION OF CARDIAC OUTPUT

During exercise, there is redirection of blood flow to the working muscles without compromising blood flow to the central nervous system. Vasodilation in skeletal muscles and skin and vasoconstriction in the splanchnic region and nonworking muscles are characteristic responses.[86]

The effect of treadmill exercise on blood flow distribution during moderate and strenuous exercise in untrained ponies has been investigated. Blood flow to the exercising muscles increased by 31- to 38-fold during moderate exercise and by 70- to 76-fold during intense exercise. Blood flow to the cerebellum and diaphragm also increased. Large increases in blood flow to both the right and left ventricles and decreased renal blood flow also were recorded.[74] Renal vasoconstriction occurs during maximal exercise in ponies, and blood flow to the kidney is only about 20 percent of that measured in the resting horse.[101] However, no changes in renal blood flow, creatinine clearances, or filtration fraction were found during prolonged exercise at heart rates of only 55 to 60 percent of individual HR_{max}.[44] There is a reduction in blood flow to gastrointestinal organs and the spleen, but flow to the adrenal glands is more than doubled during exercise.[86] The respiratory muscles in resting ponies receive about 10 percent of the cardiac output, and this increases to about 15 percent during strenuous exercise.[101]

The distribution of tracer microspheres has been used to study the blood flow in the walls of the right and left cardiac ventricles at rest and after exercise. Total ventricular myocardial blood flow commands approximately 3 percent of the cardiac output in resting ponies, and this increases to 4 percent during maximum exercise[102] (Fig. 7–11). Left ventricular myocardial blood flow increases homogeneously and by approximately fivefold above resting values during maximal exercise, resulting in a 470 percent increase in cardiac output. This study also demonstrated that myocardium of ponies possesses considerable vasodilator reserve, since injection of adenosine, a myocardial vasodilator, resulted in greatly augmented coronary blood flow.[103]

An interaction between blood flow during submaximal exercise and feeding has been described in ponies trotting at 28 km/h on a treadmill inclined at 7 percent.[104] Eight ponies fasted for 24 hours before exercise had lower heart rates, stroke volume, cardiac output, and arterial blood pressure than ponies given a pelleted grain concentrate and *ad lib* alfalfa hay over the same period. Blood flow to the locomotor muscles, respiratory muscles, and longissimus dorsi was higher in fed ponies during exercise. These results may have implications for dietary strategies before prolonged exercise.

Long-term training has a significant effect on the vascularity of skeletal muscle. A 6-month training program of young standardbred trotters resulted in increased capillary supply to skeletal muscle fibers.[105] In contrast, no increase in muscle capillarity was observed in a shorter training program in thoroughbreds.[106]

Electrocardiogram

RESTING HORSE

The ECG has been used in athletic horses to investigate poor performance and racing ability. Poor performance is associated with atrial fibrillation, complete heart block, and premature atrial and ventricular contractions.[107,108]

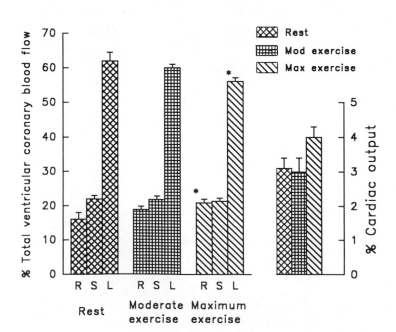

Figure 7-11. *Changes in blood flow (ml/mn per 100 g) to the ventricular myocardium, kidneys, and muscular portion of the diaphragm brought about by graded treadmill exercise in ponies. The percentage of cardiac output received by the ventricles is shown on the right-hand side of the figure (*significantly different from rest)[74] (R = right ventricle, S = septum, L = left ventricle).*

In a survey of 150 resting horses, nearly one-third had rhythm irregularities.[109] The occurrence of these dysrhythmias has resulted in some differences of opinion concerning their significance for poor racing performance. It is now generally accepted that many of the rhythm irregularities found in resting horses disappear during exercise. These dysrhythmias of physiologic origin include sinus arrhythmia, partial atrioventricular block, and sinoatrial block.[109] The occurrence of dropped beats due to partial (second-degree) atrioventricular block is attributed to a response to gradually increasing peak aortic blood pressure[6] (Fig. 7–12).

A study in thoroughbreds found a moderate but significant correlation between heart score, a correlate of cardiac mass, and race earnings per start ($r = 0.44$).[3] A large study of relationships between heart score and echocardiographic assessment of the heart in thoroughbred yearlings and prospective racing performance as 2- and 3-year-olds concluded that such measurements were not predictive of racing performance.[110] In addition, the heart scores and echocardiographic measurements in 12 yearlings with the highest performance scores as 3-year-old horses were not significantly different from those in 12 yearlings with the lowest race ratings. In another study, the heart score of a group of racehorses assessed for poor performance was similar to that measured in a different group presented for lameness or heart score evaluation.[111] It is likely that horses with comparatively small cardiac mass to body weight ratios will have limited oxygen transport and relatively

poor race performance, but routine heart score assessments do not offer a suitably accurate means of predicting race performance. The measurement is also now less popular with horse trainers and owners than in past decades.

T-wave abnormalities in the resting ECG have been described in horses during training and have been associated with poor racing performance.[111] These abnormalities have been termed *heart strain*. ECG T-wave abnormalities may return to normal after detraining, but the abnormalities recur with resumption of hard training. These abnormalities may not be significant for athletic performance because they occur as a normal response to training in some horses, and no association was found between T-wave abnormalities and Timeform rating of thoroughbreds in England.[112]

ECG DURING EXERCISE

Telemetry electrocardiography during exercise tests facilitates investigation of cardiac dysrhythmias found in resting horses. The exercise ECG shows minimal effect of the QRS complex, but PR and QT intervals shorten and P waves become superimposed on the T waves that precede them.[33] T waves also can change form during exercise.[20]

Exercise tends to exaggerate ventricular ectopic beats, facilitating the diagnosis in horses that show a normal rhythm at rest.[107,109] During exercise, second-degree atrioventricular block is usually abolished, and in

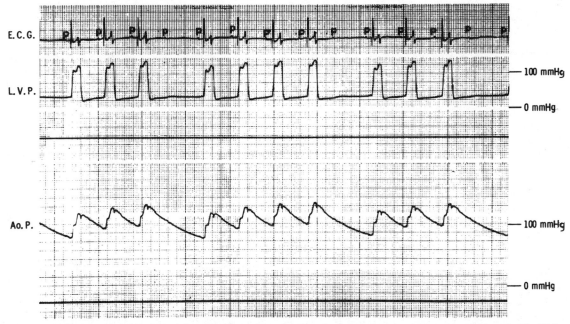

Figure 7-12. *Electrocardiogram (ECG), left ventricular pressure (LVP), and aortic pressure (AoP). Paper speed 10 mm/s. The ECG shows second-degree partial AV block, shown on the right-hand side of the figure.[74] The beats preceding the block show progressively rising peak aortic pressure. There is also a corresponding increase in peak left ventricular pressure. The missed beat effectively doubles the period of ventricular diastole, allowing the aortic pressure to continue to fall in diastole, thus reducing the postblock pressure. This is probably a baroreceptor response.[6]*

such cases, the abnormality probably does not impair performance.[33,107]

Atrial fibrillation persists during exercise,[18,107] and affected horses have higher heart rates during submaximal exercise than normal horses.[32] It is the most common cardiovascular cause of poor athletic performance.

ECG AFTER EXERCISE

The ECG after exercise also may be used to evaluate cardiac function. However, transient rhythm disturbances can occur in normal horses after exercise.[107,113] For example, brief periods of sinus dysrhythmia and partial atrioventricular block may occur after exercise. These dysrhythmias may be physiologic in origin, possibly related to vagal activity during cardiac deceleration.[7,107]

Atrial fibrillation also can occur after a race. Ten of 13 such horses had suddenly slowed during the race, and 11 of the 13 cases reverted to sinus rhythm within 24 hours, with no further evidence of poor race performance.[113] The other 3 horses had won their races, suggesting that the relationship between a diagnosis of atrial fibrillation after a race and poor performance is unclear.

Examination of the ECG after light exercise may facilitate diagnosis of atrial and ventricular ectopic beats,[107,109,113] since these dysrhythmias may be absent or infrequent at rest. However, it has been noted that there is often no histopathologic evidence of heart disease in these cases, and cardiac disease should not be diagnosed in such horses unless other signs of cardiovascular disease are detected.[107] In addition, a finding of atrial or ventricular premature beats soon after exercise does not necessarily imply that the dysrhythmia is present during fast exercise.[113]

Conclusion

The cardiovascular system of the horse has remarkable reserves of red cell volume and heart rate during exercise. These reserves are the basis of a comparatively superior oxygen-transport capacity during maximal exercise. The assessment of the cardiovascular system of equine athletes during standardized exercise tests is now routine at many centers. Such tests enable assessment of the likely influence of cardiac abnormalities, such as murmurs and dysrhythmias, on future athletic performance. Many of the normal responses to exercise and training in horses have been described, but there are still many unresolved issues. These include an understanding of possible roles of normal and abnormal cardiovascular physiology in the pathophysiology of EIPH, the physiologic mechanisms of responses to training and overtraining, and the relevance of assessments of heart rate during exercise to performance in athletic competition.

References

1. Kubo K, Senta T, Osamu S: Relationship between training and heart in the Thoroughbred racehorse. Exp Rep Equine Health Lab 1974; 11:87.

2. Kline H, Foreman JH: Heart and spleen weights as a function of breed and somatotype. *In* Persson SGB, Lindholm A, Jeffcott LB (eds): Equine Exercise Physiology 3. Davis, Calif, ICEEP Publications, 1991, p 17.

3. Steel JD: Studies on the Electrocardiogram of the Racehorse. Sydney, Australasian Medical Publishing Co, 1963.

4. Steel JD, Stewart GA, Toyne AH: Application of the heart score to the electrocardiography of Olympic athletes. Med J Aust 1970; 728.

5. Paull KS, Wingfield WE, Bertone JJ, et al: Echocardiographic changes with endurance training. *In* Gillespie JR, Robinson NE (eds): Equine Exercise Physiology 2. Davis, Calif, ICEEP Publications, 1987, p 34.

6. Holmes JR: A superb transport system: The circulation. Equine Vet J 1982; 14:267.

7. Holmes J: Prognosis of equine cardiac conditions. Equine Vet J 1977; 9:181.

8. Hamlin RL, Klepinger WL, Gilpin KW, et al: Autonomic control of heart rate in the horse. Am J Physiol 1972; 222:976.

9. Littlejohn A: Exercise-related cardiovascular problems. *In* Robinson NE (ed): Current Therapy in Equine Medicine 2. Philadelphia, WB Saunders Co, 1987, p 176.

10. Thomas DP, Fregin GF, Gerber NH, et al: Effects of training on cardiorespiratory function in the horse. Am J Physiol 1983; 245:R160.

11. Bayly WM, Gabel AA, Barr SA: Cardiovascular effects of submaximal aerobic training on a treadmill in standardbred horses, using a standardized exercise test. Am J Vet Res 1983; 44:544.

12. Milne DW, Gabel AA, Muir WW, et al: Effects of training on heart rate, cardiac output, and lactic acid in standardbred horses, using a standardized exercise test. J Equine Med Surg 1977; 1:131.

13. Skarda RT, Muir WW, Milne DW, et al: Effects of training on resting and postexercise ECG in standardbred horses, using a standardized exercise test. Am J Vet Res 1976; 37:1485.

14. Foreman JH, Rabin D: Determination of accuracy of a digitally displaying equine heart rate meter. J Equine Vet Sci 1984; 4:161.

15. Evans DL, Rose RJ: A method of investigation of the accuracy of four digitally displaying heart rate meters suitable for use in the exercising horse. Equine Vet J 1986; 18:129.

16. Physic-Sheard PW, Harman JC, Snow DH, et al: Evaluation of factors influencing the performance of four equine heart rate meters. *In* Gillespie JR, Robinson NE (eds): Equine Exercise Physiology 2. Davis, Calif, ICEEP Publications, 1987, p 102.

17. Banister EW, Purvis AD: Exercise electrocardiography in the horse by radiotelemetry. J Am Vet Med Assoc 1968; 152:1004.

18. Deegen E, Buntenkotter S: Behavior of the heart rate of horses with auricular fibrillation during exercise and after treatment. Equine Vet J 1976; 8:26.

19. Hall MC, Steel JD, Stewart GA: Cardiac monitoring during exercise texts in the horse: 2. Heart rate responses to exercise. Aust Vet J 1976; 52:1.

20. Steel JD, Hall MC, Stewart GA: Cardiac monitoring during exercise tests in the horse: 3. Changes in the electrocardiogram during and after exercise. Aust Vet J 1976; 52:6.

21. Wilson RG, Isler RB, Thornton JR: Heart rate, lactic acid production and speed during a standardised exercise test in standardbred horses. *In* Snow DH, Persson SGB, Rose RJ (eds): Equine Exercise Physiology. Cambridge, Granta Editions, 1983, p 487.

22. Evans DL, Rose RJ: Determination and repeatability of maximal oxygen consumption and other cardiorespiratory measurements in the exercising horse. Equine Vet J 1988; 20:94.

23. Seeherman HJ, Morris EA: Methodology and repeatability of a standardized exercise test for clinical evaluation of fitness in horses. Equine Vet J 1990; (suppl 9):20.

24. Engelhardt Wv: Cardiovascular effects of exercise and training in horses. Adv Vet Sci Comp Med 1977; 21:173.

25. Persson SGB: On blood volume and working capacity in horses. Acta Vet Scand 1967; (suppl 19):1.

26. Persson SGB, Lydin G: Circulatory effects of splenectomy in the horse: III. Effect on pulse-work relationship. Zentralbl Vet Med [A] 1973; 20:521.

27. Krzywanek H, Wittke G, Bayer A, et al: The heart rates of thoroughbred horses during a race. Equine Vet J 1970; 2:115.

28. Lindholm A, Saltin B: The physiological and biochemical re-

sponse of standardbred horses to exercise of varying speed and duration. Acta Vet Scand 1974; 15:310.

29. Evans DL, Rose RJ: Dynamics of cardiorespiratory function in standardbred horses during constant load exercise. J Comp Physiol [B] 1988; 157:791.

30. Rose RJ, Evans DL: Cardiovascular and respiratory function in the athletic horse. *In* Gillespie JR, Robinson NE (eds): Equine Exercise Physiology 2. Davis, Calif, ICEEP Publications, 1987, p 1.

31. Ehrlein HJ, Hornicke H, Engelhardt Wv, et al: Die Herzschlag-frequenz wahrend standardisierter Belastung als MaB fur die Leistungsfahigkeit von Pferden. Zentralbl Vet Med [A] 1973; 20:188.

32. Maier-Bock H, Ehrlein H-J: Heart rate during a defined exercise test in horses with heart and lung disease. Equine Vet J 1978; 10:235.

33. Senta T, Smetzer DL, Smith CR: Effects of exercise on certain electrocardiographic parameters and cardiac arrhythmias in the horse: A radiotelemetric study. Cornell Vet 1970; 60:552.

34. Thomas DP, Fregin GF, Gerber NH, et al: Cardiorespiratory adjustments to tethered swimming in the horse. Pflugers Arch 1980; 385:65.

35. Thomas DP, Fregin GF: Cardiorespiratory and metabolic responses to treadmill exercise in the horse. J Appl Physiol 1981; 50:864.

36. Littlejohn A, Kruger JM, Bowles F: Exercise studies in horses: 2. The cardiac response to exercise in normal horses and in horses with chronic obstructive pulmonary disease. Equine Vet J 1977; 9:75.

37. Sexton WL, Erickson HH: Effects of treadmill elevation on heart rate, blood lactate concentration and packed cell volume during graded treadmill exercise in ponies. Equine Vet J 1990; (suppl 9):57.

38. Persson SGB: Evaluation of exercise tolerance and fitness in the performance horse. *In* Snow DH, Persson SGB, Rose RJ (eds): Equine Exercise Physiology. Cambridge, Granta Editions, 1983, p 441.

39. Littlejohn A, Bowles F, Aschenborn G: Cardiorespiratory adaptations to exercise in riding horses with chronic lung disease. *In* Snow DH, Persson SGB, Rose RJ (eds): Equine Exercise Physiology. Cambridge, Granta Editions, 1983, p 33.

40. Hodgson DR, Rose RJ, Kelso TB, et al: Respiratory and metabolic responses in the horse during moderate and heavy exercise. Pflugers Arch 1990; 417:73.

41. Murakami M, Imahara T, Inui T, et al: Swimming exercises in horses. Exp Rep Equine Health Lab 1976; 13:27.

42. Art T, Amory H, Desmecht D, et al: The effect of show jumping on heart rate, blood lactate and other plasma biochemical values. Equine Vet J 1990; (suppl 9):78.

43. Thomas DP, Fregin GF: Cardiorespiratory drift during exercise in the horse. Equine Vet J 1990; (suppl 9):1.

44. Hinchcliffe KW, McKeever KH, Schmall LM, et al: Renal and systemic hemodynamic responses to sustained submaximal exertion in horses. Am J Physiol 1990; 258:R1177.

45. Asheim A, Knudsen O, Lindholm A, et al: Heart rates and blood lactate concentrations of standardbred horses during training and racing. J Am Vet Med Assoc 1970; 157:304.

46. Åstrand P-O, Rodahl K: Textbook of Work Physiology. New York, McGraw-Hill, 1977.

47. Rose RJ, Hendrickson DK, Knight PK: Clinical exercise testing in the normal thoroughbred racehorse. Aust Vet J 1990; 67:345.

48. Seeherman HJ, Morris EA: Comparison of yearling, two-year-old and adult thoroughbreds using a standardized exercise test. Equine Vet J 1991; 23:175.

49. Evans DL, Rose RJ: Cardiovascular and respiratory responses to submaximal exercise training in the thoroughbred horse. Pflugers Arch 1988; 411:316.

50. Evans DL, Rose RJ: Maximal oxygen consumption in racehorses: Changes with training state and prediction from submaximal indices of cardiorespiratory function. *In* Gillespie JR, Robinson NE (eds): Equine Exercise Physiology 2. Davis, Calif, ICEEP Publications, 1987, p 52.

51. Persson SGB, Ullberg LE: Blood volume in relation to exercise tolerance in trotters. J S Afr Vet Assoc 1974; 45:293.

52. Erickson BK, Erickson HH, Sexton WL, et al: Performance evaluation and detection of injury during exercise training in the

quarter horse using a heart rate computer. *In* Gillespie JR, Robinson NE (eds): Equine Exercise Physiology 2. Davis, Calif, ICEEP Publications, 1987, p 92.

53. Marsland WP: Heart rate response to submaximal exercise in the standardbred horse. J Appl Physiol 1968; 24:98.

54. Cikrytova E, Kostelecka B, Kovar J, et al: Standardized exercise test on a track to evaluate exercise capacity in different breeds of horses. *In* Persson SGB, Lindholm A, Jeffcott LB (eds): Equine Exercise Physiology 3. Davis, Calif, ICEEP Publications, 1991, p 37.

55. Cardinet GH, Fowler ME, Tyler WS: Heart rates and respiratory rates for evaluating performance in horses during endurance trail ride competition. J Am Vet Med Assoc 1963; 143:1303.

56. Rose RJ, Purdue RA, Hensley W: Plasma biochemistry alterations in horses during an endurance ride. Equine Vet J 1977; 9:122.

57. Rose RJ: An evaluation of heart rate and respiratory rate recovery for assessment of fitness during endurance rides. *In* Persson SGB, Lindholm A, Jeffcott LB (eds): Equine Exercise Physiology. Cambridge, Granta Editions, 1983, p 505.

58. Foreman JH, Bayly WM, Grant BD, et al: Standardized exercise test and daily heart rate responses of thoroughbreds undergoing conventional race training and detraining. Am J Vet Res 1990; 51:914.

59. Thornton J, Essen-Gustavsson B, Lindholm A, et al: Effects of training and detraining on oxygen uptake, cardiac output, blood gas tensions, pH and lactate concentrations during and after exercise in the horse. *In* Snow DH, Persson SGB, Rose RJ (eds): Equine Exercise Physiology. Cambridge, Granta Editions, 1983, p. 470.

60. Rose RJ, Allen JR, Hodgson DR, et al: Responses to submaximal treadmill exercise and training in the horse: Changes in haematology, arterial blood gas and acid-base measurements, plasma biochemical values and heart rate. Vet Rec 1983; 113:612.

61. Knight PK, Sinha AK, Rose RJ: Effects of training intensity on maximum oxygen uptake. *In* Persson SGB, Lindholm A, Jeffcott LB (eds): Equine Exercise Physiology 3. Davis, Calif, ICEEP Publications, 1991, p 77.

62. Stewart GA: Drugs, performance and responses to exercise in the racehorse. 1. Physiological observations on the cardiac and respiratory responses. Aust Vet J 1972; 48:537.

63. Wasserman K, Van Kessel AL, Burton GG: Interaction of physiological mechanisms during exercise. J Appl Physiol 1967; 22:71.

64. Waugh SL, Fregin GF, Thomas DP, et al: Electromagnetic measurement of cardiac output during exercise in the horse. Am J Vet Res 1980; 41:812.

65. Detweiller DK: Mechanical activity of the heart. *In* Svenson M (ed): Dukes' Physiology of Domestic Animals. Ithica, NY, Cornell University Press, 1984, p 131.

66. Bergsten G: Blood pressure, cardiac output and blood-gas tension in the horse at rest and during exercise. Acta Vet Scand 1974; (suppl 48):1.

67. Persson SGB, Bergsten G: Circulatory effects of splenectomy in the horse: IV. Effect on blood flow and blood lactate at rest and during exercise. Zentralbl Vet Med [A] 1975; 22:801.

68. Kubo K, Senta T, Osamu S: Changes in cardiac output with experimentally induced atrial fibrillation in the horse. Exp Rep Equine Health Lab 1975; 12:101.

69. Weber J-M, Dobson GP, Parkhouse WS, et al: Cardiac output and oxygen consumption in exercising thoroughbred horses. Am J Physiol 1987; 253:R890.

70. Manohar M, Parks C: Transmural coronary vasodilator reserve in ponies at rest and during maximal exercise. *In* Snow DH, Persson SGB, Rose RJ (eds): Equine Exercise Physiology. Cambridge, Granta Editions, 1983, p 91.

71. Butler PJ, Woakes AJ, Anderson LS, et al: The effect of cessation of training on cardiorespiratory variables during exercise. *In* Persson SGB, Lindholm A, Jeffcott LB (eds): Equine Exercise Physiology 3. Davis, Calif, ICEEP Publications, 1991, p 71.

72. Evans DL, Rose RJ: Cardiovascular and respiratory responses to exercise in thoroughbred horses. J Exp Biol 1988; 134:397.

73. Blomquist CG, Saltin B: Cardiovascular adaptations to physical training. Annu Rev Physiol 1983; 45:169.

74. Parks CM, Manohar M: Distribution of blood flow during mod-

erate and strenuous exercise in ponies (*Equus caballus*). Am J Vet Res 1983; 44:1861.

75. Mitchell JH, Kaufman MP, Iwamoto GA: The pressor reflex: Its cardiovascular effects, afferent mechanisms, and central pathways. Annu Rev Physiol 1983; 45:229.

76. Rowell LB, O'Leary DS: Reflex control of the circulation during exercise: Chemoreflexes and mechanoreflexes. J Appl Physiol 1990; 69:407.

77. Hornicke H, Engelhardt Wv, Ehrlein H-J: Effect of exercise on systemic blood pressure and heart rate in horses. Pflugers Arch 1977; 372:95.

78. Rose RJ, Allen JR, Brock KA: Effects of clenbuterol hydrochloride on certain respiratory and cardiovascular parameters in horses performing treadmill exercise. Res Vet Sci 1983; 35:301.

79. Rose RJ, Evans DL: Cardiovascular effects of clenbuterol in fit thoroughbred horses during a maximal exercise test. *In* Gillespie JR, Robinson NE (eds): Equine Exercise Physiology 2. Davis, Calif, ICEEP Publications, 1987, p 117.

80. Miller PJ, Holmes JR: Computer processing of transaortic value blood pressures in the horse using the first derivative of the left ventricular trace. Equine Vet J 1984; 16:210.

81. Milne DW, Muir WW, Skarda RT: Pulmonary arterial wedge pressures: Blood gas tensions and pH in the resting horse. Am J Vet Res 1975; 36:1431.

82. Erickson BK, Erickson HH, Coffman JR: Pulmonary artery and aortic pressure changes during high intensity treadmill exercise in the horse: Effect of furosemide and phentolamine. Equine Vet J 1992; 24:215.

83. Pelletier N, Leith DE: Hypoxia does not contribute to high pulmonary artery pressure in exercising horses. *In* Persson SGB, Lindholm A, Jeffcott LB (eds): Equine Exercise Physiology 3. Davis, Calif, ICEEP Publications, 1991, p 30.

84. Wagner PD, Gillespie JR, Landgren GL, et al: Mechanism of exercise-induced hypoxia in horses. J Appl Physiol 1989; 66:1227.

85. Davis JL, Manohar M: Effect of splenectomy on exercise-induced pulmonary and systemic hypertension in ponies. Am J Vet Res 1988; 49:1169.

86. Manohar M: Furosemide and systemic circulation during severe exercise. *In* Gillespie JR, Robinson NE (eds): Equine Exercise Physiology 2. Davis, Calif, ICEEP Publications, 1987, p 132.

87. Hopper MK, Pieschl RL Jr, Pelletier NG, et al: Cardiopulmonary effects of acute blood volume alteration prior to exercise. *In* Persson SGB, Lindholm A, Jeffcott LB (eds): Equine Exercise Physiology 3. Davis, Calif, ICEEP Publications, 1991, p 9.

88. Johnson JH, Garner HE, Hutcheson DP: Ultrasonic measurement of arterial blood pressure in conditioned Thoroughbreds. Equine Vet J 1976; 8:55.

89. Kohn CW, Muir WW, Sams R: Plasma volume and extracellular fluid volume in horses at rest and following exercise. Am J Vet Res 1978; 39:871.

90. McKeever KH, Schurg WA, Jarrett SH, et al: Exercise-training induced hypervolemia in the horse. Med Sci Sports Exerc 1987; 19:21.

91. Masri M, Freestone JF, Wolfsheimer KJ, et al: Alterations in plasma volume, plasma constituents, renin activity and aldosterone induced by maximal exercise in the horse. Equine Vet J 1990; (suppl 9):72.

92. Keenan DM: Changes of blood metabolites in horses after racing, with particular reference to uric acid. Aust Vet J 1979; 55:54.

93. Kerr MG, Snow DH: Alteration in haematocrit, plasma proteins and electrolytes in horses following the feeding of hay. Vet Rec 1982; 110:538.

94. Clarke LL, Ganjam VK, Fichtenbaum B, et al: Effect of feeding

on renin-angiotensin-aldosterone system of the horse. Am J Physiol 1988; 254:R524.

95. Carlson GP: Fluid and electrolyte alterations in endurance-trained horses. *In* Proceedings of the 1st International Symposium on Equine Haematology, 1975, p 473.

96. Nadel ER: Prolonged exercise at high and low ambient temperatures. Can J Sports Sci 1987; 12(suppl 1):140S.

97. Convertino VA: Fluid shifts and hydration state: effects of long-term exercise. Can J Sports Sci 1987; 12(suppl 1):136S.

98. Lindner A, von Wittke P, Bendig M, et al: The acceptance of an energy-rich electrolyte drink by horses in training, and its effect on heart rate and metabolism. Pferdeheilkunde 1991; 7:23.

99. Lykkeboe G, Schougaard H, Johansen K: Training and exercise change in respiratory properties of blood in race horses. Respir Physiol 1977; 29:315.

100. Persson SGB, Larsson M, Lindholm A: Effects of training on adrenocortical function and red-cell volume in trotters. Zentralbl Vet Med [A] 1980; 27:261.

101. Manohar M: Respiratory muscle perfusion during strenuous exercise. *In* Persson SGB, Lindholm A, Jeffcott LB (eds): Equine Exercise Physiology 3. Davis, Calif, ICEEP Publications, 1991, p 1.

102. Parks CM, Manohar M: Transmural distribution of myocardial blood flow during graded treadmill exercise in ponies. *In* Snow DH, Persson SGB, Rose RJ (eds): Equine Exercise Physiology. Cambridge, Granta Editions, 1983, p 105.

103. Manohar M, Parks C: Transmural coronary vasodilator reserve in ponies at rest and during maximal exercise. *In* Snow DH, Persson SGB, Rose RJ (eds): Equine Exercise Physiology. Cambridge, Granta Editions, 1983, p 91.

104. Duren SE, Manohar M, Sikkes B, et al: Influence of feeding and exercise on the distribution of intestinal and muscle blood flow in ponies. Europaische Knoferenz uber die Ernahrung des Pferdes. Pferdeheilkunde. Hippiatrika, 1992, p 24.

105. Henckel P: Training and growth induced changes in the middle gluteal muscle of young standardbred trotters. Equine Vet J 1983; 15:134.

106. Nimmo MA, Snow DH, Munro CD: Effects of nandrolone phenylpropionate in the horse: 3. Skeletal muscle composition in the exercising horse. Equine Vet J 1982; 14:229.

107. Holmes JR: An investigation of cardiac rhythm using an on-line radiotelemetry/computer link. J S Afr Vet Assoc 1974; 45:251.

108. Hillwig RW: Cardiac arrhythmias in the horse. J Am Vet Med Assoc 1977; 170:153.

109. Holmes JR, Alps BJ: The effect of exercise on rhythm irregularities in the horse. Vet Rec 1966; 78:672.

110. Leadon D, McAllister H, Mullins E, et al: Electrocardiographic and echocardiographic measurements and their relationships in thoroughbred yearlings to subsequent performance. *In* Persson SGB, Lindholm A, Jeffcott LB (eds): Equine Exercise Physiology 3. Davis, Calif, ICEEP Publications, 1991, p 22.

111. Stewart JH, Rose RJ, Davis PE, et al: A comparison of electrocardiographic findings on racehorses presented either for routine examination or poor racing performance. *In* Persson SGB, Lindholm A, Jeffcott LB (eds): Equine Exercise Physiology. Cambridge, Granta Editions, 1983, p 135.

112. Evans DL: T waves in the equine electrocardiogram: effects of training and implications for race performance. *In* Persson SGB, Lindholm A, Jeffcott LB (eds): Equine Exercise Physiology 3. Davis, Calif, ICEEP Publications, 1991, p 475.

113. Holmes JR: Cardiac arrhythmias on the racecourse. *In* Gillespie JR, Robinson NE (eds): Equine Exercise Physiology 2. Davis, Calif, ICEEP Publications, 1987, p 781.

Muscle Anatomy, Physiology, and Adaptations to Exercise and Training

D. H. SNOW AND S. J. VALBERG

As illustrated throughout this book, the horse has evolved into the supreme athlete, being capable of both high speeds and endurance. Fine neuromuscular coordination, strength, and stamina allow a thoroughbred to attain speeds in excess of 18 m/s (65 km/h), which can be maintained for about 1 minute with a stride length of up to almost 7.5 m. This is possible because the muscular system of the horse has evolved to produce powerful, efficient movement at high speeds. In most mammalian species, muscle mass makes up about 40 to 45 percent of body weight. Muscle mass in the thoroughbred, however, can comprise up to 55 percent of body weight. In other breeds, muscle mass is approximately 45 percent of body weight.[1] In addition to increased muscle bulk, elite performance is achieved by adaptations of muscle at many different levels: the gross arrangement of muscle groups, the architecture of muscle fibers and connective tissue within muscles, and the highly specialized ultrastructure of the muscle fibers themselves. Our understanding of muscle anatomy in the horse can be traced back through centuries of study of the organization and attachment of muscles and their tendons. The details of the cellular organization of muscle fibers in the horse, however, have only been characterized during the last few decades. On an ultrastructural level, much of our current understanding of the horse still relies on parallels drawn from other animal species.

This chapter is divided into three parts: (1) a general consideration of muscle structure and function, (2) muscle composition in the horse and its response to exercise and adaptations with growth, training programs, and nutrition, and (3) exertional myopathies.

Muscle Structure and Function

MUSCLE ANATOMY

Locomotor muscles in the horse are strategically located proximally on the skeleton, creating a pendulum-like effect that decreases the energy necessary to swing the limb. The arrangement of spindle-shaped muscle cells (muscle fibers) within the muscle also maximizes efficiency and power output during locomotion. In many limb muscles, muscle fibers join one or more tendinous insertions at an angle to the direction of force in a "pennate" shape. This maximizes the cross-sectional area and power output of the muscle in relation to the limited space available on the upper limb. Other muscles, *strap muscles,* maximize their range of movement by a parallel organization of muscle fibers along the direction of force. Several perpendicular tendinous insertions are usually present within this type of muscle, since most muscle fibers are only about 5 to 10 cm in length, with a cross-sectional area of 2000 to 6000 μm^2.[2,3] For efficiency, muscle fibers are grouped within the muscle so that the slower-contracting fibers commonly used for postural support are frequently located medially and the faster-contracting fibers used for higher speeds are located more superficially.

Muscles are surrounded by a loose layer of connective tissue, the *epimysium,* that lies below the external fascia and extends internally around groups of muscle fibers (fascicles) as the *perimysium.* A delicate layer of reticular fibers, the *endomysium,* envelops each individual muscle fiber. Arteries course within the perimysium and supply an average of one to three capillaries per fiber within the endomysium.[3] Nerve fibers containing both sensory and motor neurons are also present in the perimysium. Motor neurons innervate muscle fibers at a specialized site on the muscle cell membrane called the *motor end plate.* In limb muscles, one motor neuron probably innervates between 1000 and 2000 muscle fibers scattered throughout numerous fascicles.

EMBRYOLOGY

The components of limb muscle are derived from paired embryonic somites (muscle fibers) and somatopleure (connective-tissue elements). Somatic mesoderm migrates and splits sequentially to form the arrangement of individual muscles. During this process, the progressive development of myoblasts, myotubes, and finally mature muscle fibers occurs.[4] Motor neurons establish primitive neuromuscular junctions with myotubes and are essential for the continued development of muscle fibers. Elongation of the muscle fibers occurs gradually and eventually results in continuity with independently established tendons.

MUSCLE ULTRASTRUCTURE

Muscle fibers possess a number of structural adaptations which confer the ability to generate force through contraction. These include a precise alignment of contractile proteins, a cell membrane capable of propagating an electrical potential, and internal membrane structures and energy-generating pathways that can regulate the amount of calcium and adenosine triphosphate (ATP) available for excitation-contraction coupling.

Contractile Proteins

A highly repeating arrangement of filaments of noncovalently associated proteins connected in series extends the length of each muscle fiber in the form of myofibrils (Fig. 8–1). The number of myofibrils in a muscle fiber varies with its contractile type and cross-sectional area. Each myofibril is 1 to 3 μm in diameter and has a polygonal shape. The organization of numerous myofibrils in register within a cell gives skeletal muscle fibers a striated appearance under the light microscope.

Sarcomere. The repeating unit of myofilaments within the myofibril is referred to as a *sarcomere,* the fundamental unit of contraction (see Fig. 8–1). Filaments of α-actinin (molecular weight 206,000) traverse the sarcomere at each end to form the Z line. The width of the Z line varies from 50 nm in slow-contracting muscle fibers to 65 nm in fast-contracting muscle fibers. Thin myofilaments extend axially from either side of the Z line

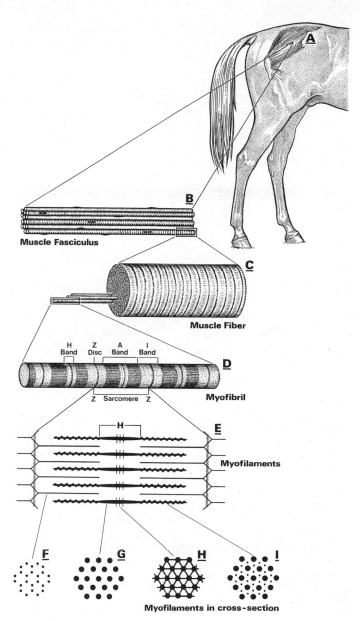

Figure 8-1. Skeletal muscle. The organization of skeletal muscle contractile proteins from the gross to the molecular level. (Adapted from Bloom W, Fawcett DW: A Textbook of Histology. Philadelphia, WB Saunders Co, 1986, p 282, with permission.)

and form a hexagonal array around overlapping thick myofilaments. Muscle contractions occur when, within each sarcomere, thin myofilaments slide over the thick myofilaments, bringing consecutive Z lines closer together. This complex arrangement of overlapping filaments permits several distinctive areas to be identified with electron microscopy. The I band contains the Z line centrally and extends to include the adjoining area of nonoverlapping thin myofilaments. Centrally, in the sarcomere, the A band is defined by the full extent of the thick myofilaments. Within the A band, the H band is defined by the central area where thick myofilaments do not overlap with thin myofilaments. In the middle of the

H band, a dark line is formed by three to five M-line filaments traversing the sarcomere (see Fig. 8–1).

Thick Myofilaments. The thick myofilaments are bipolar spindle-shaped structures 1.6 μm in length and 15 nm in diameter. *Myosin* is the primary protein in the thick myofilament with a molecular weight of 480,000. A molecule of myosin consists of a tail, formed by two identical heavy chains arranged in alpha helices, and two globular heads, each formed by a complex of one heavy chain and two different light chains (Fig. 8–2A). Two types of myosin light-chain isoforms are found in skeletal muscle, the DTNB (LC2) [5′,5′-dithiobis(2-nitro-

A

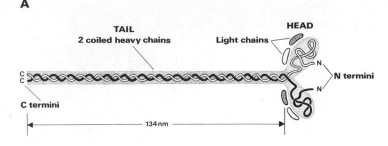

Figure 8-2. A, Myosin. A model of the myosin molecule showing the arrangement of two heavy chains and two light chains on each globular head. B, Thin filament. A model of the thin filament showing the interrelationships among actin, troponin, and tropomyosin. (Adapted from Bloom W, Fawcett DW: A Textbook of Histology. Philadelphia, WB Saunders Co, 1986, p 287, with permission.)

B

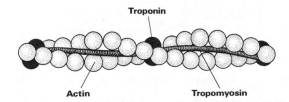

benzoate)] and the alkali light chains (LC1 and LC3). There are several different myosin heavy-chain isoforms. Although all muscle fibers are capable of synthesizing all skeletal muscle isoforms of myofibrillar proteins, fast- and slow-contracting fibers each exhibit a characteristic array of myofibrillar isoforms.[5,6]

The tails of approximately 300 myosin molecules aggregate together to form the backbone of one thick myofilament. The globular heads extend outward in a three-dimensional helical array from this backbone, leaving a central bare area without any globular heads. The globular heads contain both actin and ATP-binding sites as well as adenosine triphosphatase (ATPase) activity and are a central component of the contractile process. Histochemical stains of myosin ATPase activity differentiate three principal contractile fiber types, slow-twitch type I fibers, fast-switch type IIA fibers, and fast-twitch type IIB fibers.

Small amounts of proteins in addition to myosin can be found in the thick filaments. The C protein (molecular weight 140,000), H protein, and X protein are located in the middle one-third of each half of the A band. Their exact function is not known, but they could serve to stabilize the organization of myosin molecules. Both M protein and creatine kinase, located at the M line, may serve as structural support for the thick filaments as well as a source of ATP from creatine phosphate.

Thin Myofilaments. Thin myofilaments are 1 μm long and 8 nm in diameter, consisting primarily of *actin*. Actin is a globular protein with a molecular weight of 41,800.

Two F-actin strands twisted in a double helix form the backbone of the thin myofilament. Actin is the only myofibrillar protein identified to date that has identical isoforms in fast- and slow-contracting fibers.[5] The interaction between myosin globular heads and actin is regulated by tropomyosin and troponin (Fig. 8–2B). *Tropomyosin* is a two-stranded alpha helix with a molecular weight of about 70,000 that lies in the helical grooves formed by actin strands. *Troponin* is a complex of three noncovalently linked subunits, with a molecular weight of 76,000, that attaches at regular intervals to tropomyosin along the thin filament. Each subunit has a distinct physiologic function. The inhibitory subunit (TN-I), when bound to actin, acts together with tropomyosin to inhibit actin-myosin interaction. TN-C is the calcium-binding subunit of troponin that, in the presence of calcium, can remove the inhibitory effects of TN-I on actin-myosin binding. The precise regulatory role of the subunit TN-T, the tropomyosin-binding component, is unclear.

Sarcolemma and Sarcoplasmic Reticulum
Sarcolemma. Underneath the reticular fibers of the endomysium is a thin *basement membrane* composed of collagen type IV, laminin, fibronectin, and proteoglycan. Continuous with the basement membrane internally is a glycocalyx which coats the external surface of the underlying plasma membrane or sarcolemma. Alpha motor neurons transmit neural impulses to muscle fibers at a highly specialized area of the sarcolemma, the motor end plate. The sarcolemma at the motor end plate is highly folded and contains numerous acetylcholine receptors.

The sarcolemma serves both to maintain the intracellular milieu and to transmit neural excitatory impulses to the contractile proteins. It consists of a lipid bilayer and numerous intrinsic and extrinsic proteins. These proteins form transmembrane transport systems, kinases, adenylate cyclases, ion channels, and sodium/potassium and calcium/magnesium ATPase pumps. The sodium, potassium, and chloride ion channels together with the sodium/potassium pump provide the sarcolemma with the ability to generate an electrochemical gradient and to depolarize following neural excitation. A defective sodium channel results in abnormal muscle depolarization, as seen in horses with hyperkalemic periodic paralysis.[7]

At regular intervals along the length of the sarcolemma, tubular invaginations, *t-tubules*, traverse perpendicularly across the myofibrils at the junction of the A and I bands (Fig. 8–3). The t-tubule membranes have a lower protein content but similar lipid content as the sarcolemma and contain numerous calcium channels. The t-tubules serve to transmit electrical impulses to the interior of the muscle fiber, where, through association with the intracellular membranous system, myofibrillar contraction can be initiated.

Sarcoplasmic Reticulum. The intracellular membranous system of skeletal muscle, or sarcoplasmic reticulum (SR), is physically separate from the sarcolemma and surrounds each myofibril in a highly repeating pattern. The SR membranes contain a high concentration of calcium ATPase, the protein calsequestrin, and the calcium release channel. They function to pump calcium into the SR from the sarcoplasm, release it into the sarcoplasm to initiate contraction, and sequester it during relaxation. The efficiency of this system is demonstrated by the extremely low cytoplasmic calcium concentration in muscle during relaxation. Over the A and I bands, the SR runs parallel to the myofibrils. At the AI junction, the SR tubules change their membrane composition and converge to form *terminal cisternae* (see Fig. 8–3). The terminal cisternae run perpendicular to the myofibril on either side of the t-tubule. The t-tubule along with the two neighboring terminal cisternae form a functional as-

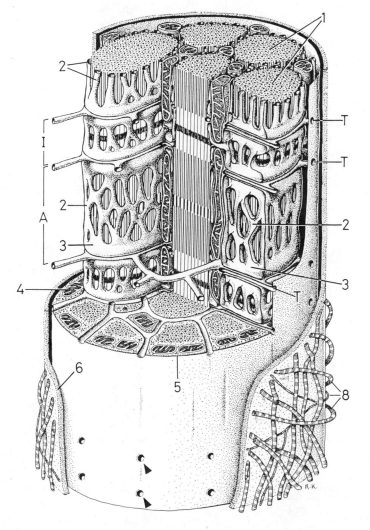

Figure 8-3. *A three-dimensional view of the internal structure of a muscle fiber. Every myofibril (1) is surrounded by a parallel arrangement of the sarcoplasmic reticulum (2) which converges to form terminal cisternae (3). Between each terminal cisterna at the AI junction is an invagination of sarcolemma called the t-tubule (T). Mitochondria (4) are present between myofibrils. The sarcolemma (5) is surrounded by a basement membrane (6), and a network of reticular and collagen fibrils (7) surrounds each muscle fiber. (Adapted from Krstic RV: General Histology of the Mammal. New York, Springer-Verlag, 1984, p 265, with permission.)*

sociation called a *triad*. The gap between the terminal cisternae and t-tubule is bridged by a tetragonal arrangement of foot processes called *junctional feet*. These feet act structurally to maintain the architecture of the triad during contraction and possibly to mediate the coupling of sarcolemmal excitation with release of calcium by the terminal cisternae into the sarcoplasm. The calcium release channel appears to be located on the terminal cisternae apposed to the foot processes.[8]

Excitation and Contraction Coupling. Neural excitation at the motor end plate results in the propagation of an electrical impulse along the sarcolemma and t-tubular system. Electrical depolarization of the t-tubule triggers the release of calcium from the terminal cisternae into the sarcoplasm precisely where thick and thin myofilaments overlap. Calcium then binds to the TN-C subunit of troponin, resulting in a conformational change moving tropomyosin deeper into the groove of the actin helix and exposing the myosin binding site on the actin filament. The globular head of myosin forms a cross-bridge with actin, activating myosin ATPase and releasing ATP. The actin filaments are displaced toward the center of the A band, and further binding of the primed myosin globular heads to actin occurs. Several cycles of cross-bridge formation and cross-bridge breaking are repeated per contraction, which shorten each half of the sarcomere in a rachet-like fashion. Relaxation occurs when calcium ions are pumped into and sequestered in the sarcoplasmic reticulum. Low calcium concentrations in the sarcoplasm and regeneration of ATP allow the troponin-tropomyosin complexes to cover the binding sites on the actin filaments during relaxation.

Cytoskeleton

Muscle cells have a well-developed cytoskeleton which plays a central role in maintaining cell shape during contractions and in sarcoplasmic flow. Intermediate filaments of dystrophin, spectrin, actin, vinculin, and ankyrin provide support for the sarcolemmal membrane. Their importance is emphasized by the severe muscular dystrophy that occurs in the absence of dystrophin.[9] These intermediate filaments appear contiguous with other intermediate filaments such as desmin and vimentin that bind myofibrils in register at the Z line[10] (Fig. 8–4). Large elastic filaments such as titin have been identified which link thick and thin myofilaments and may account for the elastic-like quality of muscle fibers.[11] To date, the distribution of only one cytoskeletal protein, tubulin, has been studied in the horse.[12]

Other Organelles

Skeletal muscle fibers contain hundreds to thousands of nuclei which are located directly underneath the sarcolemma. The number of myonuclei per fiber is established at birth. Small *satellite cells,* which are situated between the basement membrane and the sarcolemma, have nuclei that are easily confused with myonuclei. These satellite cells become very important in muscle repair. A varying complement of smooth and rough endoplasmic reticulum, golgi apparati, and lysosomes is usually found near myonuclei. Numerous proteins, including myoglobin and the enzymes involved in glycolysis, are distributed in the sarcoplasm. Glycogen granules and to a varying extent lipid droplets are also distributed throughout the sarcoplasm between the myofilaments and under the sarcolemma. Enzymes involved in oxidative metabolism are located within the mitochondrial membranes. Mitochondria in horse muscle are concentrated in subsarcolemmal locations, particularly in association with capillaries. A lesser distribution of mitochondria is found between myofibrils. The volume density of mitochondria varies in different horse muscles from 2 to 24 percent.[13] Equine mitochondria are generally cylindrical in

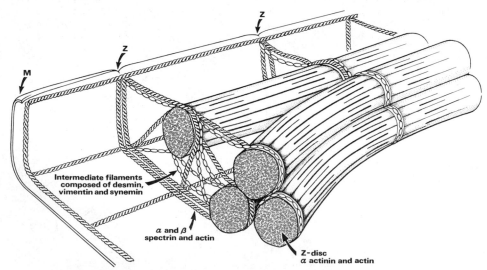

Figure 8-4. *A model of the cytoskeleton linking the myofibrils to the sarcolemma. (Adapted from Lazarides E, Capetanaki YG: In Emerson C, Fischman DA, Nadal-Ginard B, Siddiqui MAQ (eds): Molecular Biology of Muscle Development. New York, Alan R Liss 1985, p 756.)*

shape but may produce transverse extensions at the level of the I band.[14]

Equine Muscle Composition: Response to Exercise and Adaptations with Training

MUSCLE COMPOSITION

Skeletal muscle metabolism and contractility have been studied both in vivo and in vitro using a range of biochemical, histochemical, and physiologic techniques. Muscle samples for analysis have come from specimens ranging from gross dissection to small biopsies obtained from the live animal. Details on properties of individual fibers can be obtained by dissecting out single fibers[15,16] or quantitative histochemistry.[17] The former is more difficult in the horse than in human muscle. Today our knowledge is being increased by the use of noninvasive techniques such as nuclear magnetic resonance imaging (NMRI). It is the technique of muscle biopsy which, since the excellent pioneering work of Lindholm,[18] has enabled our understanding of equine muscle to expand tremendously over the last 20 years. Throughout this section, unless stated otherwise, the muscle involved is the middle gluteal, the most frequently examined muscle of the horse.

Percutaneous Muscle Biopsy

Specimens satisfactory for histochemical, biochemical, and ultrastructural studies can be obtained by muscle biopsy. These biopsies can be obtained either by the more invasive open surgical technique or percutaneously by a special biopsy needle[19,20] (Fig. 8–5). The latter method is generally used because of its ease, safety, and relatively atraumatic nature, allowing longitudinal and cross-sectional studies to be readily carried out. In addition, repeated sampling can be carried out during and following exercise bouts without any adverse effect on performance. A needle also has been designed that allows simultaneous sampling at two depths within a muscle.[21,22] Following removal of the core of muscle, the tissue is replaced by regeneration of myofibers rather than by fibrous tissue. If contractile properties are to be investigated, samples should be obtained by open excision biopsy.[23]

The following percutaneous biopsy technique[24] has been described:

> Prior to biopsying, an area of skin of approximately 2.5 cm² is closely shaved, washed and cleaned with surgical spirits or equivalent. One ml of local anesthetic is then injected subcutaneously along the line of the proposed incision and into the fascia overlaying the muscle, but not into the muscle itself. An incision about 1 cm long is made through the skin and, where necessary, the fascia. The needle together with the cutting cylinder is then inserted into the muscle. Once within the muscle, the cutting cylinder is partially withdrawn, so that the window is opened up. The window is positioned so that it is upward or sideward, and pressed firmly against the muscle to catch a small piece of muscle within the needle. Finally, the cutting cylinder is pushed down to detach the trapped muscle. This can be repeated several times so that between 50 and 200 mg of muscle is obtained. The needle is carefully withdrawn and the excised muscle is removed with the stylet. Good technique allows a cylindrical-shaped piece to be obtained. The incision is allowed to heal without suturing. This procedure can be carried out without tranquillizers and minimal restraint.

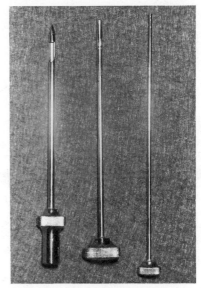

Figure 8-5. Muscle biopsy needle for collecting muscle biopsies percutaneously.

The preparation of specimens for histochemical, biochemical, and ultrastructural studies from a sample can be readily carried out.[24] Both authors have carried out thousands of biopsies with negligible untoward effects. Very occasionally, a hematoma may result if a larger blood vessel is accidentally cut during biopsying or if the horse is suffering from a disorder of hemostasis.

Fiber Types

As mentioned earlier in this chapter, the muscle fibers that make up a muscle are not identical in type. That muscles vary in color from red to white has likely been known since the beginning of such observations. However, the full significance of these differences was not apparent until Ranvier[25] observed in 1974 that color and histologic features of the whole muscle correlated with their speed of contraction. The red coloration is due to the ferroprotein myoglobin. Numerous studies have now been carried out examining the relationships among biochemical, structural, and physiologic properties of muscle, leading to a thorough but still incomplete understanding of their function. Diversity in muscle composition allows a graded response to varying demands ranging from posture maintenance to rapid movement.

Histochemical methods developed in the 1960s and 1970s have shown that most mammalian muscles consist of a mosaic of muscle fiber types with varying metabolic and contractile properties. The properties of a particular fiber are determined by its innervation, all fibers from the same alpha motor neuron having similar although not identical properties.[6] With these histochemical reactions, a plethora of classification systems dependent on the number of characteristics examined and the subdivisions used within each characteristic have been developed. Currently in the horse the two most commonly used nomenclatures for classification are those dependent on examination of only the contractile properties of the fibers and one in which this is combined with oxidative capacity.

Myosin-ATPase Differentiation. On the basis of myosin-ATPase activity at pH 9.4, two distinct fiber types exist. Those with low activity have been named *type I fibers,* and those with high activity are called *type II fibers* (Fig. 8–6A). Physiologically, these have been shown to be relatively slow and fast contracting, respectively, and therefore are also referred to as *slow-* and *fast-twitch fibers.* In addition, the type I fibers have a slower relaxation time and are more fatigue resistant than the type II fibers. The histochemical ATPase reaction seems to be correlated with the myosin heavy rather than light chain, the former having the active site.

The type II fibers can be further divided into the subtypes IIA, IIB, and IIC according to the lability of myosin ATPase following preincubation at either acidic or alkaline pH[26,27] (Fig. 8–6B). Unfortunately, due to unknown technical problems, reliable differentiation following preincubation often can be difficult in the horse,[28,29] since optimal conditions can vary both within and between laboratories.

Transformations between type I and various type II fibers can occur under appropriate stimuli. A continuum exists between the type IIA and IIB fibers[17] (Fig. 8–7A). Type IIC fibers can be found in muscles of very young animals but are rare in mature animals. If found later, they are considered to be transitional.

The variations between the myosin-ATPase activity of type I and II fibers and even within type II subtypes are due to differences in the myosin molecule, producing isomyosins as described earlier. Using specific antisera for type I and type II myosin, equine type I fibers reacted with type I antisera, while both IIA and IIB fibers reacted with fast myosin antisera and type IIC with both.[30] To overcome the problems associated with subdivision of type II fibers using conventional myosin-ATPase histochemistry, an indirect immunocytochemical method has been tried.[29] Unfortunately, with the antibodies used, differentiation of type II subtypes was not possible. Similarly, analysis in single fibers of myosin heavy chains and myosin light chains by gel electrophoresis does not always differentiate between the two subtypes of equine type II fibers.[23] This provides further support for a continuum of type II fibers.

Speed of Contraction. Recently, contractile characteristics of the different fiber types have been studied in the horse.[23] Using skinned single muscle fibers from the equine soleus, a heterogeneous muscle in this species, the $\dot{V}_{max}$ of shortening was determined. In contrast to small animals, where a three- to fivefold difference in $\dot{V}_{max}$ between fiber types is seen, the horse has a 10-fold difference, the type IIB fibers shortening more rapidly than would be expected from normal scaling. $\dot{V}_{max}$ was found primarily to be associated with fiber type rather than diameter or force generation. This higher $\dot{V}_{max}$ for

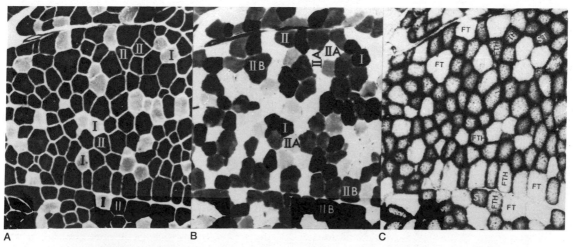

Figure 8-6. *Histochemical stains illustrating (A) type I and II fibers with myosin ATPase activity at pH 9.4, (B) type I, IIA, and IIB fibers with myosin ATPase activity at pH 9.4 following acid preincubation, and (C) succinic dehydrogenase activity showing low and high oxidative fibers (ST = slow twitch, high oxidative; FT = fast twitch, low oxidative; FTH = fast twitch, high oxidative).*

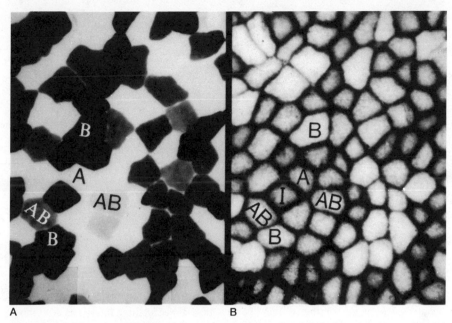

Figure 8-7. *Biopsy specimen from the middle gluteal illustrating continuum of activity for (A) myosin ATPase activity and (B) succinic dehydrogenase activity (I = type I; A = type IIA; B = type IIB; AB = type IIAB, a fiber considered to be intermediate between types IIA and IIB).*

type IIB fibers indicates that there is a sacrifice of efficiency for increased mechanical power, since this is higher in fibers with a high $\dot{V}_{max}$ than in those with a lower $\dot{V}_{max}$.

Metabolic Differentiation. In addition to fiber typing based solely on myosin-ATPase activity, divisions have been made in the horse solely on metabolic properties[31] or, more commonly, in combination with myosin-ATPase activity at pH 9.4. Usually, only oxidative capacity is determined as a metabolic marker, since it is accepted that type I fibers have relatively low and all type II fibers have high glycolytic activity.[32] For the assessment of oxidative capacity, fibers are incubated for determination of either succinic dehydrogenase or NADH-diaphorase activity and classed as either having high or low activity (see Fig. 8–6C). In combination with myosin-ATPase activity at pH 9.4, this allows fibers to be classified into three categories: slow-twitch high oxidative (ST), fast-twitch high oxidative (FTH), and fast-twitch low oxidative (FT) fibers (see Fig. 8–6C). These divisions correspond to the SO, FOG, and FG classification used by some workers.

A fairly clear distinction usually can be made between high and low oxidative fibers (see Fig. 8–6C) in the untrained horse, but as training progresses, differentiation becomes more difficult because there is a continuum of activity similar to that seen for myosin-ATPase activity of type II fibers (see Fig. 8–7B). Because type IIB fibers commonly have either low or high oxidative capacity in the trained state, some workers using a type I, IIA, and IIB classification subdivide the IIB fibers into

low and high oxidative categories. The oxidative differences shown histochemically also have been supported by biochemical studies on pools of single fibers.[16] However, histochemical reactions for oxidative capacity only provide a relative indication between fibers. Biochemical studies have shown that citrate synthase activity in type I and IIA fibers of different horses could vary as much as twofold, while histochemical staining showed a high content in all type I and IIA fibers.[33] Because of the ability of type IIB fibers to have varying oxidative status, it is important to realize that the subdivision of type II fibers using the two classification methods is not identical.[24,34] The properties of type I and type II fibers are outlined in Table 8–1.

As well as using the preceding enzyme reactions to classify fiber types, other enzyme activities have been investigated.[35,36] Van den Hoven and colleagues[36] studied numerous soluble cytoplasmic enzymes using the complex semipermeable membrane technique.

Other Features. Histochemical stains also have been used to show other differences between fiber types. Using the periodic acid–Schiff (PAS) reaction, glycogen content has been found to be lower in type I than in type II fibers,[19,37] while with stains for lipid, content has been found to be highest in the most highly oxidative fibers.[38,39] Capillarization of fibers has been studied using the PAS reaction following glycogen removal with α-amylase.[24] Capillary number can then be expressed either in terms of per fiber or per unit area of fiber type. High oxidative fibers have a greater capillarization than low oxidative fibers.[2,3,40] Not surprisingly, a relationship ex-

Table 8-1. Characteristics of Muscle Fiber Types in the Horse

	Type I	Type IIA	Type IIB
Speed of contraction	Slow	Fast	Very fast
Maximal tension developed	Low	High	High
Myosin ATPase activity at pH 9.4	Low	High	High
Myosin ATPase activity at pH 9.4 (after acid preincubation)	High	Low	Intermediate
Oxidative capacity	High	High to intermediate	Intermediate to low
Lipid content	High	Intermediate	Low
Glycolytic capacity	Low	High	High
Glycogen content	Intermediate	High	High
Muscle fibers per motor unit	Low	High	High
Fatiguability	Low	Intermediate	Intermediate to high

ists between the capillary supply and the functional and dimensional capacities of the cardiocirculatory system as well as structural and biochemical properties of the muscle.[3]

Fiber Areas. Fiber areas also can be determined from histochemical preparations. As described previously[24] and recently examined in detail,[41–43] care has to be taken in selecting sections for this determination, since uneven muscle fiber contraction may occur within samples collected by needle biopsy. A more accurate indication of fiber size can be obtained by measurement of the minimum diameter, since this is not affected by any oblique orientation of the section. Today, measurement of fiber areas can be carried out rapidly using digitized planimetry and specialized software packages. From muscle biopsy investigations it has generally been found that fiber areas vary according to type, with the type I fibers being the smallest and the type IIB low oxidative the largest,[24,44] although this can vary between muscles and even within a muscle.[42] Fiber area measurements also depend on the histochemical preparation used, since sections reacted for myosin-ATPase activity result in areas 10 to 20 percent less than those reacted for succinic dehydrogenase.[45]

Ultrastructural Differentiation. Differences also can be seen between fiber types at the ultrastructural level.[20] High oxidative fibers have many more subsarcolemmal and intermyofibrillar mitochondria than low oxidative fibers. Although histochemically type I fibers generally appear more highly aerobic than type IIA fibers, an examination of the semitendinosus revealed that the type IIA fibers had slightly higher mean volume density of mitochondria than type I fibers.[46] It also has been shown that horse muscle has a high mitochondrial content, helping explain its exceptionally high $\dot{V}_{O_2max}$.[47] Type I fibers have an abundant supply of lipid droplets, while fewer are seen in the type II high oxidative fibers, with low oxidative fibers not surprisingly having negligible amounts. Glycogen is found as "particles" consisting of glycogen, water, and enzymes associated with its synthesis and degradation and is seen as either discrete granules or rosette formations throughout the sarcoplasm.[20]

With respect to the contractile properties, type II fibers, which have a greater requirement for rapid Ca^{2+} turnover, have a more prominent sarcoplasmic reticulum. Z- and M-band width also can vary between types. In some species, fiber typing has been carried out on the basis of these ultrastructural differences.

Fiber Type Populations within Muscles

Varying functional requirements result in muscle fiber type composition differing between muscles. This has been illustrated in the horse in a study where six limb muscles were compared.[48] Similar findings have been seen in examinations of the same or other limb muscles.[19,35,44] The ease of sampling and its importance in locomotion[19,50,51] have resulted in the middle gluteal being most frequently biopsied.

Although a mosaic of fiber types is found within most muscles, this pattern can vary even within the same muscle due to different activity profiles. This variation within one muscle has been referred to as *compartmentalization*. In electromyographic studies in a number of species, this compartmentalization is related to recruitment patterns during the different phases of locomotion. In most muscles, the highest proportion of fast-twitch fibers is found superficially, with an increasing proportion of slow-twitch fibers in the deeper parts. Because of important considerations on how representative and reproducible fiber composition is from a biopsy sample, detailed analysis of a number of limb muscles has been carried out.

In the horse, the middle gluteal has been studied most extensively with respect to fiber variation[42,43,44,52–56] (Table 8–2). All have shown the nonuniformity of this muscle, which is divided into dorsal and ventral parts by a tendon that runs from the crest of the ilium to the greater trochanter.[57,58] The two compartments have separate points of origin and insertion. The ventral compartment is innervated by the cranial gluteal nerve and the dorsal by the caudal gluteal nerve. The dorsal region is visually considerably darker than the ventral. These differences suggest functional differences during locomotion.[57,58] Within each compartment there is generally an increasing proportion of type I fibers with increasing depth, and almost complete diappearance of type IIB fi-

Table 8-2. Mean ± SD Percentage of Each Fiber Type at Different Depths Within the Middle Gluteal Muscle (3 Horses, 10 Sample Sites per Horse at Each Depth)

Sampling Depth	Type I	Type IIA	Type IIB
2 cm	21.6 ± 8	36.5 ± 5	42.0 ± 9
4 cm	35.5 ± 9	35.0 ± 4	29.5 ± 8
6 cm	49.5 ± 10	34 ± 7	16.35 ± 9
8 cm	61.5 ± 12	34 ± 10	4.5 ± 6
F values			
F depth	88.18*	0.96	12.14*
F site	3.67†	1.11	4.43‡

Note: Variance ratios of a two-way ANOVA testing variation in fiber types attributable to different sampling depths (F depth) and different sample site (F site): $*p < 0.001$; $†p < 0.01$; $‡p < 0.05$.
Source: Adapted from Lopez-Rivero JL, Serrano AL, Diz AM, et al: Variability of muscle fiber composition and fiber sizes in the horse gluteus medius: An enzyme-histochemical and morphometric study. J Anat (in press), with permission.

bers occurs as the proportion of high oxidative fibers increases. Whether there is a similar change at a similar depth but progressing from cranial to caudal is presently equivocal due to differences in findings.[49,53,56] In addition to an increasing proportion of type I and oxidative fibers, a change in fiber size occurs.[59] In superficial sites type I fibers have the smallest area, with type IIB the largest, while in deeper sites the predominant type I fibers are the largest. Biochemical variation also occurs through the muscle.[60] Not surprisingly, the deeper within the muscle one goes, the higher are the citrate synthase (CS) and 3-hydroxy acyl-CoA-dehydrogenase (HAD) activities and the lower are the phosphorylase and lactate dehydrogenase (LDH) activities. This diversity within the middle gluteal muscle suggests that the deeper portions have a more postural function, while the more superficial portions are recruited with increasing work loads. This nonhomogeneity also has been described in a number of other muscles.[32,49,54]

Nonuniformity of fiber types within a muscle is an important consideration when trying to compare fiber composition in longitudinal and cross-sectional studies. If a constant site has to be sampled, allowance has to be made for the overall size of the muscle. For example, when comparing results in a foal with those in an adult, sampling depth at the same site should be approximately 2.5 cm in the foal and approximately 5 cm in the adult. In addition, frequent sampling from the same animal also requires confidence that a similar site can be sampled. When biopsying the middle gluteal muscle in the adult horse, most workers have adopted a site 10 to 15 cm caudodorsal from the tuber coxae and at an angle of 45 degrees at a depth of 5 to 10 cm in the adult. It has been found that samples taken at a uniform depth and within about a 5-cm radius of this point give reproducible results.[61,62] However, recently it has been found that even taking samples at a constant depth but 4 cm dorsal, caudal, ventral, and cranial from an initial site results in some variation.[56] Although this difference may require caution when fiber typing is done in an attempt to eval-

uate performance potential, a relatively small difference does allow repeated sampling in short time frames, e.g., in recovery studies following bouts of exercise. It also has been found that at a similar site no difference exists between samples taken from the right or left middle gluteal of normal muscle.

Muscle Fiber Recruitment

For smooth, coordinated locomotion, muscles are recruited in an orderly manner, with both extensors and flexors being involved during each stride cycle. Within a particular muscle, only certain portions may operate, having different and often complex functions due to functional compartmentalization. Even within a recruited muscle not all fibers are stimulated, since it is not generally necessary for muscle to generate maximum tension. Fibers are selectively recruited in a specific pattern that varies according to the gait, speed, and duration of exercise. This occurs through the differential stimulation of alpha motor neurons in line with the size principle.[63] The smallest-diameter motor neurons, which have the lowest threshold, innervate the type I fibers, while the largest innervate the type IIB fibers. For the maintenance of posture and for exercise at low speeds, it is only generally necessary to recruit type I fibers, which are fatigue-resistant. As the speed of movement increases, the development of more tension to generate the required torque is necessary, and type IIA fibers are recruited. The very forceful contractions required for rapid acceleration and maintenance of high speeds or for jumping result in the additional recruitment of first the type IIB high oxidative and then the low oxidative fibers.

One of the techniques used to study fiber recruitment patterns has involved the examination of glycogen depletion patterns using either semiquantitative or quantitative analysis. This has been used in the horse in a number of investigations involving varying intensities and durations of exercise.[38,39,50,64–68] All have confirmed the general recruitment pattern outlined above.

RESPONSE TO EXERCISE

The energetic basis of muscle contraction and hence performance has been described in detail in Chapter 4, and therefore, the following will consider mainly changes thought to be associated with the production of fatigue. In general, the relative importance of aerobic and anaerobic processes in producing ATP depends on the intensity of the exercise and hence the muscle fibers recruited and the influence of training in modifying their metabolic profiles.

The ability to maintain performance at a required level is limited by the onset of fatigue. One of the major causes of this is believed to be the impairment of muscle fiber function. This does not occur suddenly in all fibers leading to complete cessation of activity, but rather in a selective manner causing a reduction in performance. Impairment of muscle function could occur for a variety of reasons, including

1. Depletion of substrate for energy production

2. Interference in energy (ATP) production due to alterations in the internal milieu of the fiber
3. Changes in neuromuscular irritability due to changes in electrolyte gradients
4. Interference with the contractile process due to alterations in Ca^{2+} uptake or release by the sarcoplasmic reticulum
5. Decreased blood flow and/or excessive increase in muscle temperature

In many cases it is likely that a combination of these factors operate. To date, our understanding of the likely contributing factors to muscle fatigue in the horse has come from the collection of biopsy samples following different intensities and durations of exercise.

Fatigue with High Intensities of Exercise
The effects of high-intensity exercise on muscle and blood changes have been studied by exercising horses on a treadmill,[69–77] running on a track,[16,51,66,78–81] or doing draught work.[68,82–84] Overall, the metabolic changes seen with the highest-intensity exercise are greater than reported in humans and other species and are a further indication of the horse as an elite athlete. These changes can be associated with the disproportionally high $\dot{V}_{O_2max}$ and muscle enzyme activities of this species.[85]

Lactate Accumulation. It is now accepted that with almost all intensities of exercise a degree of anaerobic metabolism and production of lactate occurs. At the lower intensities, very little or no change is seen in blood lactate concentration, since removal keeps pace with production.[86] However, as intensity of exercise increases and progressively more type II fibers and then especially type IIB low oxidative fibers are recruited, energy production becomes increasingly dependent on anaerobic metabolism and consequent formation of lactate. With repeated bouts of exercise, muscle lactate concentrations in excess of 200 mmol/kg of dry weight have been recorded,[79] with the associated proton accumulation leading to a marked decline in muscle pH. Single bouts of exercise lead to lower muscle lactate concentrations, which are related to both intensity and, at higher work loads, duration of exercise.[51,72,78,80,81,87] Lactate concentrations in excess of 200 mmol/kg of dry weight have been reported after a race.[88] The greater anaerobic demands of galloping compared with trotting races, because of faster speeds, has been well illustrated.[88] Mean muscle lactate concentrations of 82 and 148 mmol/kg of dry weight were found after standardbred and thoroughbred races, respectively. A high correlation exists between lactate accumulation and the percentage of type IIB fibers in the muscle.[69,88]

With increasing intensity of exercise there is at first only a gradual increase in blood or plasma lactate concentration, but a point is reached where a sharp rise in circulatory levels occurs. This point is referred to as the *anaerobic threshold* or, more correctly, the *onset of blood lactate accumulation* (OBLA) and generally occurs between a blood lactate concentration of 2 and 4 mmol/liter. For comparative purposes, OBLA generally has

been given an arbitrary setpoint of 4 mmol/liter by many workers in both equine and human exercise physiology. OBLA occurs at an intensity of exercise below $\dot{V}_{O_2max}$, the point depending on the fitness of the horse.

At lower intensities of exercise, peak concentrations of blood or plasma lactate are seen immediately on the cessation of exercise.[75,89,90] However, a point is reached where lactate efflux mechanisms are probably saturated, and rapid accumulation of intracellular lactate and its consequent effects on pH commence. When this situation occurs, peak blood and plasma lactate concentrations are not seen until between 5 and 10 minutes after exercise (Fig. 8–8). It has been suggested that in horses, saturation of lactate removal occurs at concentrations of 10 and 15 mmol for whole blood and plasma, respectively.[75] In thoroughbred racing, blood lactate concentrations on the order of 25 mmol/liter are seen over distances of 1000 to 2400 m.[91] In some horses, concentrations may exceed 30 mmol/liter. Similar concentrations have been recorded after harness racing[92] and national hunt racing.[93] This order of blood lactate concentration results in venous blood pH declining to about 7.0.[91] With repeated bouts of high-intensity exercise, blood lactate concentration can exceed 40 mmol/liter.[79] Following cessation of high-intensity exercise, lactate disappearance normally occurs at a linear rate,[75] which can be hastened by submaximal exercise.[94] Training also may increase the rate of removal of lactate.[95]

Acidosis in muscle can lead to impairment of glycolysis and the respiratory capacity of mitochondria, and both may be associated with a decline in muscle [ATP]. Evidence for a disturbance in mitochondrial function comes from both biochemical[77] and ultrastructural studies[96–98] (Fig. 8–9) on equine muscle samples collected immediately after high-intensity exercise and during the recovery period. Following exercise, a vari-

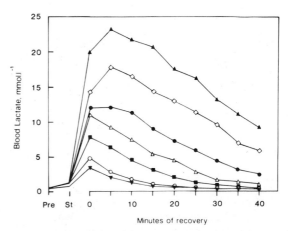

Figure 8-8. *Time course of the mean changes in blood lactate concentration following 2 min treadmill exercise [▼, 6 m/s; ○, 7 m/s; ■, 8 m/s; △, 9 m/s; ●, 10 m/s; ◇, 11 m/s; ▲, 12 m/s; n = 6 (except 12 m/s, n = 5)]. (From Harris RC, Marlin DJ, Snow DH, et al: Muscle ATP loss and lactate accumulation at different work intensities in the exercising thoroughbred horse. Eur J Appl Physiol 1991; 62:235.)*

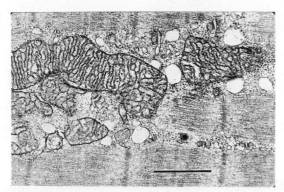

Figure 8-9. *Muscle fiber ultrastructure after maximal exercise. Note the dilated mitochondria and sarcoplamic reticulum (× 27,000). (Courtesy of L. J. McCutcheon.)*

able swelling of mitochondria with rounding and increased prominence of individual cristae occurs. Restoration to normal ultrastructural appearance occurs about 1 hour after completion of exercise and at the same time as muscle pH and temperature return to normal.[98] In addition to mitochondrial changes, swelling of the sarcoplasmic reticulum has been observed in the preceding studies. This may be associated with impaired SR function, as recently indicated by up to a 50 percent reduction in Ca^{2+} uptake by equine muscle following maximally fatiguing exercise.[99] The mechanisms that could lead to SR dysfunction could not be identified, but it was postulated that both decreased pH and muscle temperatures in excess of 43°C could be important.

Nucleotide Depletion. In addition to finding the expected high muscle and blood lactate concentrations after maximal exercise, a decline in muscle [ATP] also has been shown in many investigations. Overall, most reports have supported the initial observation by Snow and colleagues that a decline in muscle [ATP] occurs after a certain intensity of exercise. This decline also has been seen

after both trotting and galloping races.[16,50,88,81] A marked decline in phosphocreatine (PCr) to approximately 30 percent of baseline values also has been measured in a number of the previously described studies. The exact decline in PCr is difficult to determine, since rapid recovery occurs after the cessation of exercise. It has been suggested that the decline in muscle [ATP] is associated with accumulation of muscle lactate and a decline in muscle pH[79] (Fig. 8–10). The decline in muscle [ATP] was less after 800 m compared with 2000 m of maximal exercise.[80] In an actual racing situation, a decline in [ATP] was seen in all horses. This decline was very variable (range 14 to 50 percent) and not related to finishing position, although there was an indication that greater losses occurred over the longer distances.[81] From studies using different intensities of exercise and duration, it would appear that the decline in muscle [ATP] occurs after muscle lactate exceeds 40 to 80 mmol/kg of dry muscle and muscle pH falls below 6.8.[72,87] With repeated bouts of exercise, an almost 50 percent decrease in muscle [ATP] can occur.[79] However, based on single muscle fiber studies, it is likely that the decline in some type IIB fibers is considerably greater.[100] A study on pooled single fibers dissected from biopsy samples collected after racing found greatest ATP depletion in type IIB fibers with little change in type I fibers.[16] In type IIB fibers, mean ATP content in some horses was only 50 percent of resting values.

This decline in muscle [ATP] is paralleled by an increase in muscle inosine monophosphate (IMP) content as the ATP is degraded by a series of enzymatic reactions from ADP to AMP and then IMP. This decline in muscle [ATP] probably occurs more readily in equine muscle than in that of other species due to the high AMP deaminase activity in equine muscle.[101] AMP deaminase activation can occur for a number of reasons, including lowered pH. With exercise associated with anaerobic metabolism, a buildup of protons leads to a change in muscle pH from a resting level of 7.11 to as low as 6.25 estimated after repeated bouts of maximal exercise.[102] However, it has been suggested that since ATP reduction

Figure 8-10. *Comparison of the changes in muscle adenosine triphosphate (ATP) content at the end of 2 minutes of treadmill exercise with the increase in muscle lactate content. The linear regression line shown was computed using the data obtained at 9, 10, 11, and 12 m/s, at which speeds significant loss of ATP from muscle has been established [▲, end of warmup exercise; ■, 6, 7, and 8 m/s; ●, 9, 10, 11, and 12 m/s; y = 2.813 (SE 2.121) − 0.079 (SE 0.012)·x; r = 0.82; p < 0.001]. (From Harris RC, Marlin DJ, Snow DH, et al: Muscle ATP loss and lactate accumulation at different work intensities in the exercising thoroughbred horse. Eur J Appl Physiol 1991; 62:235.)*

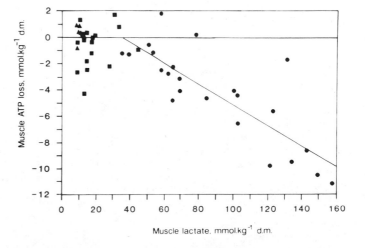

and IMP formation commence at a pH above the optimal of 6.5 for equine AMP deaminase,[103] this might not be the main explanation for AMP deaminase activation. Rather, it is thought that a sudden increase in [AMP] triggers this set of events.[87]

It has been suggested that adenine nucleotide degradation provides a mechanism for the displacement of the myokinase reaction and maintenance of a high ATP/ADP ratio. This may be essential for maintaining the contraction process and delaying the onset of fatigue.[87] However, this process cannot be completely successful, since undoubtedly the first fatigued fibers are those with the lowest ATP content. Performance studies using repeated bouts of exercise have indicated a relationship between running time and muscle ATP content[77,79] and maintenance of speed with normal ATP content. Whether the decline in [ATP] is a major contributory factor in fatigue is still uncertain, but it does seem probable that the very low levels in some fibers would impair the optimal functioning of many of the ATP-dependent processes, such as contraction, reuptake of Ca^{2+} by SR, and the Na^+, K^+ pump.

Recovery of normal muscle ATP content does not occur rapidly after the cessation of high-intensity exercise, taking over 1 hour depending on the extent of the initial depletion.[79,80] Restoration is dependent on the purine nucleotide cycle and reamination of IMP. Resynthesis of ATP follows a similar pattern to that of removal of lactate from muscle and blood, and therefore, it is uncertain which of these factors may be of importance in influencing performance if exercise is undertaken before a return to baseline values.

The deamination of adenine nucleotides also leads to the production of ammonia, which is released into the circulation. High concentrations of plasma ammonia following intense exercise have been reported by a number of investigators.[71,72,104] The threshold for a rise in the plasma ammonia level occurs at a higher intensity than that for lactate and at the point when ATP decline commences. A high correlation between plasma ammonia concentration and muscle ATP loss has been reported,[72] indicating that the former can be a useful practical indicator of ATP loss (Table 8–3). Other degradation products of purine nucleotides found in plasma, hypoxanthine and uric acid, are not considered as reliable indicators, and peak values occur later after exercise.[72,79,80,105]

Potassium. Although intramuscular potassium concentrations have not been measured after high-intensity exercise, alterations in plasma potassium indicate that as in humans, losses occur from recruited muscle fibers.[106] With increasing intensity of exercise, there is a progressive increase in plasma potassium concentration, and for short-duration activity, this is highly correlated with lactate production. This is a reflection of the greater and more frequent recruitment of muscle fibers. During maximal efforts leading to plasma lactate concentrations in excess of 30 mmol/liter, plasma potassium concentrations above 10 mmol/liter occur.[89] With duration of exercise greater than 2 minutes, a plateau for plasma potassium concentration is reached. This is thought to reflect an equilibrium between release from active muscle and reuptake by inactive fibers which are under beta$_2$-adrenergic receptor control. However, at the very highest work loads (lasting less than a few minutes), there is a continual rise until the onset of fatigue, since reuptake cannot match release[107] (Fig. 8–11). This efflux from muscle is solely due to electrical activity of the exercising muscle and is thought to be independent of acidosis or glycogen breakdown.[108] Immediately on the cessation of exercise there is a rapid decline in plasma potassium as almost immediate reuptake into now inactive muscle occurs. In humans, both the rise in plasma potassium concentration during exercise and the decline during recovery have exponential time courses with a halftime of 25 s.[108] The large changes in intramuscular potassium concentration will result in altered sarcoplasmic membrane potential and could be a contributory factor to fatigue in maximal exercise.[107,109,110]

In addition to the preceding major changes which may contribute to fatigue, there are a number of other metabolic changes occurring within muscle which may result in reduced performance capacity.

Glycogen. Although a decline in muscle glycogen concentration occurs rapidly with maximal exercise, this is not thought to be a contributory factor in fatigue. Not surprisingly, the extent of glycogen utilization is related to the amount of lactate produced.[76] Single bouts of exercise at maximal intensity only cause a reduction in whole-muscle glycogen on the order of 30 percent,[51,66,68,78,80] while with repeated bouts, reductions of up to 50 percent may occur.[79] From studies using both single bouts of exercise of varying duration[51,66,78,80] and repeated bouts of high-intensity exercise,[79] the highest proportion of glycogen is utilized during the initial stages or first bout of exercise. This is probably due to the higher anaerobiosis earlier in exercise, before there is complete circulatory adjustment and before enhanced utilization of blood-borne glucose as a substrate. In the early stages of maximal exercise, glycogen utilization rates may reach 160 mmol glucosyl units per kilogram of dry muscle per minute.[80] Marked liver glycogenolysis leading to high blood glucose concentration occurs with maximal exercise due to a dramatic increase in sympathetic activity.[111] Immediately following maximal galloping, the blood glucose level can exceed 10 mmol/liter.[91] Verification of high blood glucose utilization awaits measurement of arteriovenous difference over a bed of active muscle.

Histochemical studies of glycogen depletion have shown that after both racing and repeated bouts of exercise leading to ATP depletion, glycogen was still present in even the fibers with highest anaerobic capacity (IIB).[50,64,66,67] If exercise intensity is high enough to recruit all fibers, glycogen utilization and hence depletion will occur most rapidly in the type IIB low oxidative fibers as they use this substrate to produce ATP with an associated formation of lactate.

Table 8-3. Muscle and Blood Metabolites Before and After 2 Minutes of Exercise at Varying Intensities on a Treadmill at 5° Incline (Thoroughbreds, Mean ± SD, n = 6)

	Preexercise	Speed, m/s						
		6	7	8	9	10	11	12
Muscle ATP (mmol/kg dm)	22.8 ± 1.3	22.4 ± 1.8	22.2 ± 1.7	21.8 ± 1.7	21.6 ± 2.0	20.4 ± 2.1	18.0 ± 2.9	13.8 ± 1.9
Muscle lactate (mmol/kg dm)	9.7 ± 1.3	19.1 ± 7.5	23.9 ± 11.1	43.7 ± 13.9	57.3 ± 13.1	76.5 ± 31.0	97.0 ± 28.7	132.9 ± 19.5
Muscle pyruvate (mmol/kg dm)	0.4 ± 0.1	0.5 ± 0.2	0.3 ± 0.2	0.5 ± 0.2	0.6 ± 0.3	0.8 ± 0.4	0.7 ± 0.4	1.0 ± 0.5
Blood lactate (mmol/liter)	0.5 ± 0.2	3.5 ± 1.4	4.9 ± 2.1	7.9 ± 2.9	11.1 ± 2.2	13.6 ± 3.8	17.8 ± 6.2	23.8 ± 3.3
Plasma ammonia (μmol/liter)	75 ± 24	110 ± 40	114 ± 14	145 ± 35	178 ± 72	315 ± 92	536 ± 215	792 ± 397

Source: Adapted from Harris RC, Martin DJ, Snow DH, et al: Muscle ATP loss and lactate accumulation at different work intensities in the exercising thoroughbred horse. Eur J Appl Physiol 1991; 62:235, with permission.

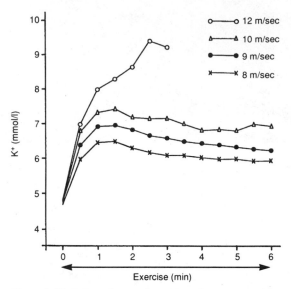

Figure 8-11. Estimated mean plasma potassium concentrations in horses in response to exercise. (From Harris P, Snow DH: Plasma potassium and lactate concentrations in thoroughbred horses during exercise of varying intensity. Equine Vet J 1992; 23:220, with permission.)

Free Fatty Acids and Carnitine. During maximal effort, intramuscular glycogen or blood-borne glucose degradation is likely to be responsible for over 90 percent of ATP synthesis. Whether the uptake of free fatty acids (FFAs) has a small role as a substrate for oxidative metabolism is uncertain. However, from the examination of plasma FFA profiles before and immediately after strenuous exercise, it has been suggested that they may contribute as an energy source.[112]

Associated with the mitochondrial uptake of FFAs is the substance carnitine, a low-molecular-weight, water-soluble quaternary amine. In resting muscle, total carnitine consists of approximately 88 percent free carnitine, 7 percent acetylcarnitine, and 5 percent acylcarnitine.[113] In addition to carnitine facilitating FFA uptake during submaximal exercise, a decrease in free carnitine with an almost equal increase in acetylcarnitine seen with high-intensity exercise has led to the suggestion that carnitine also regulates the acetyl-CoA/CoA ratio in sprint exercise.[114,115] It does this by buffering excess production of acetyl units, which could have several advantages for cells functioning at intensities above the onset of blood lactate accumulation.

Amino Acids. Anaerobic metabolism also results in an increase in muscle pyruvate content[72,81,102] and an increased formation of alanine from pyruvate.[72,74,116] In addition to alanine, changes in other amino acids have been determined.[74,116] Leucine and isoleucine increase slightly, while glutamate decreases by approximately 50 percent. The increase in the branched-chain amino acids leucine and isoleucine may be due to increased influx into muscle as a result of marked increase in plasma concentrations.[116] The decline in glutamate is a reflection of the increase in alanine resulting from the transamination of pyruvate. Some protein breakdown during both high-intensity and submaximal exercise is supported by increased concentration of phenylalanine.

Muscle Temperature. Associated with increasing intensity of exercise and increasing metabolic activity is a progressive rise in muscle temperature.[51] Temperatures in excess of 43°C have been recorded.[99] Although moderate increases in temperatures are considered favorable for metabolic activity, the very high levels seen at highest intensities of exercise may be a contributory factor to fatigue, e.g., altering Ca^{2+} uptake by SR.

Prolonged Low-Intensity (Submaximal) Exercise
During this type of activity, energy production is essentially the result of aerobic metabolism, with free fatty acids (FFAs) and glycogen being the dominant fuels. Although the body contains abundant lipid supplies to maintain energy supplies for days during low-grade or maintenance activities, when work loads such as in endurance rides are required, fatigue sets in before complete utilization of lipid depots has occurred. This is so because glycogen depletion has occurred within the liver and active muscle,[50,37] and oxidation of FFAs cannot supply sufficient ATP turnover in the absence of pyruvate. During prolonged activity, glycogen depletion patterns have shown a progressive recruitment of muscle fiber types[36,37,50,65] (Fig. 8–12). Because of the relative low intensity of exercise, initial activity only requires recruitment of type I and some type IIA fibers, but as they become depleted of glycogen, recruitment of new fibers occurs until fatigue sets in, after all fibers (including type IIB) become glycogen depleted. At the point of fatigue, both biochemical and histochemical studies have shown negligible muscle glycogen.[37] At this stage, only very low intensity exercise can be maintained, since energy is dependent on utilization of FFAs by oxidative fibers.

Following glycogen depletion, repletion occurs in the reverse order to depletion, i.e., initially in type IIB, then in type IIA, and finally in type I fibers.[37,65] Complete repletion may take up to 72 hours.

With increased durations of low-intensity exercise, FFAs assume increased importance as a substrate for muscular work. Uptake of circulating FFAs is aided by an appreciable increase in circulating concentrations.[37,117] In line with this, it would be expected that intramuscular triglyceride depots would be used. This has been shown biochemically,[39,118] although the extent is quite variable between animals.

MUSCLE ADAPTATION: EFFECTS OF AGE AND TRAINING

It is likely that muscle is the most adaptable of all tissues, being able to show a wide range of both immediate (exercise) and long-term (age, training, nutrition) responses. With the appropriate artificial (e.g., electrical) or natural stimuli, changes can occur in the metabolic and contractile properties and size of muscle fibers. This has led to the terms *plasticity* and *malleability* being used

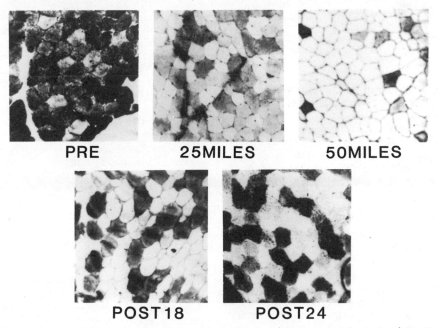

Figure 8-12. *Muscle glycogen depletion and repletion patterns in response to endurance exercise (post 18 and post 24 = 18 and 24 hours after exercise, respectively). (From Snow DH, Baxter P, Rose RJ: Muscle fiber composition and glycogen depletion in horses competing in an endurance ride. Vet Rec 1981; 108:374, with permission.)*

to describe the adaptability of skeletal muscle. The time course of many of the changes that occur within muscle of many species has been described.[119] One of the best but less appreciated examples of the plasticity of muscle is its ability to respond as an excellent energy reserve during malnutrition by providing amino acids as precursors for hepatic gluconeogenesis. This leads to atrophy of fibers, which can be reversed on restoration of normal nutrition.

Changes in Early Life (Growth)

Muscle tissue of foals at birth is more mature than that of humans and many other animal species. Differentiation of slow- and fast-contracting muscle fibers is well established at 158 days of gestation.[120,121] Growth occurs mainly via a marked increase in the length and cross-sectional area of existing muscle fibers after birth. Fibers lengthen through the insertion of new sarcomeres to existing myofibrils near tendinous attachments. Growth hormone, insulin, and thyroid hormone have an essential role in stimulating this development. Intermittent active stretching of sarcomeres, such as occurs during isometric contractions, and testosterone both prompt an increase in fiber diameter. Increased fiber diameters are mainly due to the enlargement and subsequent splitting of myofibrils at the Z line.[122]

Differences in composition between muscles is already apparent in the prenatal phase. Individual differences between animals within one muscle appear to develop during early growth, since the proportion of type II fibers can increase differently.[120] Exactly when, how, and why this occurs requires investigation. It is likely

mainly to be genetically controlled, since activity of different breeds in early life is similar.

Rapid growth during the first 3 months of life also affects the metabolic pathways in skeletal muscle. During this phase, oxidative capacity decreases and glycolytic capacity increases.[123–125] This has been seen in a number of breeds. It has been suggested that this initial increase in anaerobic capacity may reflect a greater hypertrophy of the type II than type I fibers.[125]

From 6 months of age to mature size, there appears to be a reversal in this pattern, with a minor rise in oxidative capacity and a concomitant decline in glycolytic capacity.[125,126] In an early cross-sectional study,[19] no changes in fiber composition or enzyme activities were found in untrained standardbreds between 6 months and 2 years of age, alterations only occurring later in life with the commencement of training. In a longitudinal study in standardbreds, a control group was compared with a group undergoing regulated exercise between the ages of 7 and 18 months.[126] There was no difference in the changes between the two groups, both having an increase in type IIA/IIB ratio, an increase in citrate synthase (CS) activity, and a 30 to 70 percent increase in fiber area. These workers concluded that growth itself and spontaneous activity rather than any kind of controlled superimposed activity were the most important factors for development. On the other hand, a further longitudinal study in standardbreds examining changes from 7 months to 2 to 3 years of age concluded that training, not growth, was the main factor in inducing an increase in oxidative capacity and increased type IIA/IIB ratio.[127]

ADAPTATIONS WITH TRAINING

Metabolic Changes

Aerobic Enzymes. Although there appears to be a discrepancy on the influence of activity in early life, virtually all cross-sectional and longitudinal studies in a variety of breeds are in agreement that training from about 2 years of age causes an increase, up to twofold, in aerobic enzyme activity and an increase in high oxidative fibers.[19,44,82,126–140] This is reflected in an increased FTH/FT ratio and increased high oxidative type IIB fibers and possibly increased type IIA/IIB ratio. The major oxidative increases occur quite rapidly, probably within the first couple of months of training. Increased activity is most pronounced in the first year or 2 of training, with later increases being only relatively small[138,139] (Table 8–4). In parallel with this increase in aerobic enzyme activity is an increase in volume density of mitochondria.[131] Whether increased oxidative enzyme activities are matched by an increase in myoglobin content has not been investigated in horses. Associated with increased oxidative capacity is an increase in capillarization.[2] Increased aerobic capacity will lead to more efficient generation of ATP, influencing performance by increasing the speed at which V_{La_4} occurs.[134,141,142]

Although these aerobic changes have been observed routinely in experimental training studies and in investigations of standardbreds in training for racing, two studies examining conventional training of thoroughbreds in Australia and the United States, one experimental[143] and the other in a racing yard,[135] found no or little change in oxidative capacity and no change in fiber type. In the latter study, even at the end of 12 weeks of training and the commencement of racing, 90 percent of the type IIB fibers were still low oxidative. An extensive study of racehorses in Hong Kong prior to commencing training and 9 months later found no change in the proportion of FTH or type IIA fibers,[24] although there was

an increase in citrate synthase activity.[144] However, both longitudinal[130] and cross-sectional[138] studies in Sweden found that training caused an increase in citrate synthase activity. The differences between these studies may reflect different training programs used in different countries or that the first two studies examined changes over a considerably shorter time frame.

Although not as yet demonstrated in the horse, it has been well documented in other species that a beneficial effect of training is an increased utilization of free fatty acids at submaximal work loads. The ability of greater FFA utilization is dependent on increases in the enzymes responsible for their degradation and incorporation into the citric acid cycle. One of the enzymes of importance is 3-hydroxy acyl-CoA-dehydrogenase (HAD). Although an increase in this enzyme's activity would be expected to parallel the increase in citric acid cycle enzymes, studies in horses have not always reported an increase. Both increases on the order of 150 percent[129,130,132,135–138,145] and no change[40,82,126,139] in HAD activity have been reported (see Table 8–4). The reason for these differences is inexplicable, since variable effects have been found even in work load programs producing similar increases in aerobic enzyme activity.

Glycolytic Enzymes. Indicators of glycolytic [e.g., phosphofructokinase (PFK), aldolase, triose phosphate dehydrogenase and anaerobic (LDH) metabolism generally have been found to be unaltered[40,132,135,136,139,143,144] or, for LDH, decreased with training[126,130,133,134,138,139] (see Table 8–4). In contrast, in the early study by Lindholm and Piehl,[19] a marked increase in PFK was found. Using training programs with an intensive anaerobic component, increases have been reported in LDH activity.[137,146] This increase in LDH is thought to be due to a change in isoenzyme pattern, with an increase in both M (muscle) and H (heart type) subunits.[146] The general lack of

Table 8-4. *Cross-Sectional Study of Mean Citrate Synthase (CS), 3-Hydroxy-Acyl CoA Dehydrogenase (HAD), and Lactate Dehydrogenase (LDH) Activities in the Middle Gluteal Muscle of Thoroughbreds and Standardbreds of Varying Ages*

				Enzyme Activities (mmol/kg/min)					
		Thoroughbreds				Standardbreds			
Age	Sex	No	CS	HAD	LDH	No	CS	HAD	LDH
1	M	20	31	20	1793	10	29	29	1936
1	S	21	32	18	1714	15	30	23	1927
2	M	23	44	22	1558	11	35	31	1938
2	S	20	42	22	1458	14	42	25	1639
3	M	21	64	31	1549	12	55	31	1362
3	S	17	58	31	1515	15	54	33	1317
4–6	M	17	67	31	1490	15	56	33	1669
4–6	S	24	67	38	1397	15	68	34	1460
Age		XXX	XXX	XX			XXX	NS	XXX
Sex			NS	NS	NS		NS	NS	NS

Note: Significance over the four age groups: XX, $p < 0.01$; XXX, $p < 0.001$; M = mare (filly); S = stallion (colt).
Sources: Adapted from Roneus M, Lindholm A, Asheim A: Muscle characteristics in thoroughbreds of different ages and sexes. Equine Vet J 1991; 23:207 and Roneus M: Muscle characteristics in standardbred trotters of different ages and sexes. Equine Vet J (in press), with permission.

change in glycolytic activity is in accord with findings in other species. On the other hand, aerobic training usually results in a decrease in total LDH and an increase in the proportion of H subunits.

Other Enzymes. Only limited studies have been carried out investigating alterations in other enzymes with training. A marked increase in alanine aminotransferase (ALT) was considered to reflect an improved ability to metabolize pyruvate to alanine, reducing formation of lactate and increasing production of α-ketoglutarate, an intermediate of the citric acid cycle.[128] During glycolysis, extramitochondrial NADH is produced, and this is unable to enter mitochondria directly for oxidation to NAD. Therefore, a number of indirect routes, called *shuttles,* have been defined and are thought to allow electrons from NADH to enter the electron-transport chain. The best documented are the α-glycerophosphate and malate-aspartate shuttles involving the enzymes glycerol-3-phosphate dehydrogenase (GPDH) and aspartate aminotransferase (AST), respectively. In horses it would appear that the latter shuttle is the most important, since AST increases markedly with training,[128] while GPDH remains unaltered.[145] Whether hexokinase, responsible for the conversion of glucose to glucose-6-phosphate, increases with training is uncertain, since the few studies measuring this enzyme have shown either an increase[144] or no change.[145] An increase in this enzyme is likely to be beneficial, since it would increase the uptake of circulating glucose.

Nucleotides. With respect to ATP production and degradation, there have been few reports on the effects of training. The activities of the key enzymes creatine kinase (CK) and AMP deaminase even in the resting state are found to be higher in the thoroughbred than in other species.[85,101] CK increased slightly with anaerobic training in an experimental study,[128] while no change was found in a longitudinal study of thoroughbreds in race training.[144] In other species, no change occurs with aerobic training, but an increase occurs with anaerobic training. Training results in an increase in AMP deaminase and other enzymes associated with purine nucleotide degradation. It has been postulated that the increase in AMP deaminase with training is beneficial in that it should play a role in ensuring a rapid and near-maximal stimulation of glycolysis.[101] Although training may increase enzyme activities in accord with those in other species, the concentration of the phosphagen pool remains unaltered.[19,137]

Glycogen. Glycogen is found in higher quantities in equine muscle than in other species and explains the sweet taste to connoisseurs of horse steaks. The glycogen content of muscle in well-trained horses is generally on the order of 500 to 650 mmol glucosyl units per kilogram dry weight. Where investigated, training has been shown to produce an increase in glycogen.[19,40,128,143] Whether this is a training effect per se or a reflection of increased dietary intake of soluble starches resulting from a change in diet for horses in training has not been investigated. A detailed study of glycogen changes in a training program involving 2 days per week of intense exercise[61] indicated that with adequate nutrition, training does not cause a progressive reduction in glycogen content that may affect performance, as has been suggested (Fig. 8–13). However, it is possible that training programs involving frequent bouts of prolonged submaximal or high-intensity exercise may lead to a gradual lowering of glycogen content as repletion occurs rela-

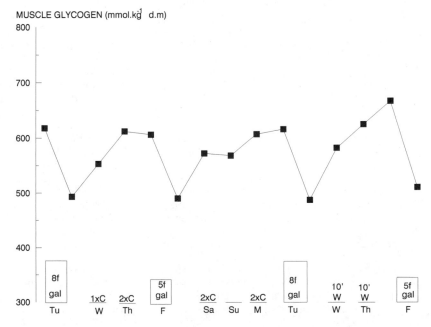

Figure 8-13. Mean changes in the glycogen content of the middle gluteal muscle during 2 weeks of training (gal = gallop; 8f = 1600 m; 5f = 1000 m; c = canter; w = walk). (Adapted, with permission, from Snow DH, Harris RC: Effects of daily exercise on muscle glycogen in the thoroughbred racehorse. In: Persson SGB, Lindholm A, Jeffcott LB (eds): Equine Exercise Physiology 3. Davis, Calif, ICEEP Publications, 1991, p 299.)

tively slowly. Such an effect has been reported during an intensive endurance training program.[133]

Repletion of glycogen to baseline values appears to occur relatively slowly in horses compared with rats and humans. In the former species, hepatic gluconeogenesis aids in rapid repletion. The slower repletion in the horse may be more related to the extent of the depletion rather than to a true difference in rate. Increasing blood glucose concentration would appear to have little influence on the rate of glycogen repletion in the adequately fed horse.[147]

Claims of increased glycogen content by dietary manipulation using either increased carbohydrate[148,149] or fat[150–152] may be more a reflection of initial low glycogen content due to inadequate nutrition.[153] Feeding isocaloric diets but with altered protein and fat content resulted in lower muscle glycogen content with either increased fat or protein.[154]

Lipid and Carnitine. In contrast to what might have been expected, an intensive training program resulting in increased citrate synthase activity did not result in increased intramuscular triglyceride content.[133] Whether increased dietary fat intake influences intramuscular lipid content has not been investigated.

Carnitine has been found to increase with age and training, which is not surprising since it is highly correlated to oxidative capacity of muscle fibers.[155,156] To try to enhance muscle carnitine content, commercial preparations have been made available. However, investigations indicate that this substance is only very poorly absorbed from the equine gastrointestinal tract,[157] and muscle content does not increase even following intravenous administration.[158]

Buffering Capacity. During intense exercise, the detrimental effects of proton formation on intracellular pH are partially offset by the buffering capacity of the cells and export via the bicarbonate system. Within muscle, buffering occurs through phosphocreatine hydrolysis (dynamic) and physicochemical (static) buffering by proteins, dipeptides, and inorganic phosphate.[159] It has been postulated that the ability of muscle to buffer protons may be a key determinant of sprint performance.[160] The thoroughbred horse has been found to have a very high buffering capacity when compared with humans.[161] This may be related to this species' myofibers containing considerably greater content of the histidine dipeptide carnosine than humans, contributing approximately 30 percent of the nonbicarbonate buffering. It has been found that carnosine content is related to fiber type, being highest in type IIB fibers and contributing up to 50 percent of their buffering capacity.[162] This helps to explain the high content in thoroughbred[163] and quarter horse[164] muscle.

A titrimetric method for the determination of buffering capacity has been described in detail.[165] When determinations are carried out on freeze-dried samples, there is an approximately 15 percent lower buffering capacity due to the loss of bicarbonate. A comparison of the three reports on buffering capacity has shown a great similarity when results were standardized to a common base, with capacity on the order of 210 μmol/kg of dry muscle in a pH range of 7.0 to 6.0.[165] An increase in buffer content with training would be of benefit to horses competing in highly anaerobic exercise. The few studies that have examined this have reported a marked increase[166] or a slight increase.[167,168] In measuring carnosine content, a decrease with age and training was found in a thoroughbred racing stable.[163] This may be related to a decrease in type IIB fibers. Therefore, the increase in buffering capacity with training is due to changes in other chemical constituents.

To try to improve maximal performance, attempts have been made to increase buffering capacity both intra- and extracellularly. The best known of these is the oral administration of a sodium bicarbonate solution several hours prior to racing. Depending on the dose administered, this can cause a marked increase in extracellular and possibly intracellular buffering capacity. In horses, because of better tolerance, considerably greater amounts have been given, sometimes in excess of 1 g/kg of body weight. As detailed in a review by Snow,[169] although there is a great deal of evidence in humans to show a beneficial effect in intense exercise lasting 1 to 2 minutes, whether this occurs in horses has been difficult to show experimentally. However, anecdotal evidence from the racetrack indicates generally a beneficial effect on racing times. Experimentally, it has been found in horses that bicarbonate administration may retard the decline in muscle ATP.[170]

Recently, it has been shown in humans that the administration of relatively high doses of creatine, 20 to 30 g/day for 5 days, results in an increased muscle creatine/phosphocreatine pool.[171] The effect was most pronounced in individuals with initially the lowest muscle content. The effects on performance in humans and horses is currently being investigated. In humans, a beneficial effect on running times over 300 and 1000 m has been reported.[172] This beneficial effect may occur by increasing the dynamic buffering pool or increasing the activity of the phosphocreatine.

Fiber Type Alterations. In humans, aerobic training has been associated with increases in oxidative enzyme activities and a marked decrease in type IIB fibers.[173] However, in horses, it would appear that although there generally is a transformation of type IIB to type IIA fibers, this is rather limited and possibly absent in conventionally trained thoroughbreds.[24,135,143] Instead, type IIB fibers with high oxidative capacity are found. Even studies in elite endurance ride horses have shown a high proportion of type IIB fibers.[39,43,65] However, as shown by White and Snow,[17] it is likely that many of these high oxidative IIB fibers are actually type IIAB fibers, since most workers classify any fiber showing any grade of gray as a type IIB fiber. An increase in type IIA fibers is associated with changes in myosin isoform patterns.[6,173]

Until recently, it has been considered that very little change, if any, occurs with training in the proportion of type I fibers of the middle gluteal muscle. However, large-scale investigations have indicated a significant increase in type I fibers with age and training. In large groups of nonintensively trained Andalusian and Arabian horses ranging in age from 10 days to 24 years, an almost 100 percent increase in the proportion of type I fibers was recorded, with most change occurring progressively between 1 and 10 years.[174] Similar changes have been found in large-scale cross-sectional studies in both thoroughbreds and standardbreds[24,138,139] (Table 8–5). The reasons for this are presently uncertain, since this increase could represent (1) splitting of type I fibers, (2) gradual transformation of type IIA to type I fibers, although the intermediate type IIC fibers are rarely recorded in adult muscle, or (3) a loss of fibers with age and being greatest in type II fibers. Against a training effect is the finding that in 70 thoroughbreds examined at the beginning and 9 months later at the end of a racing season no change or a decrease in percentage of type I fibers was found.[24]

Fiber Sizes. It is obvious that the maximal increase in muscle mass occurs during the growth stage, and it is believed that this occurs as a result of hypertrophy rather than hyperplasia. In horses, approximately 80 percent of growth has occurred by 18 months,[175] and therefore, it would be expected that the greatest change in fiber size would take place during this phase. A 30 to 70 percent increase in fiber size was found between 7 and 18 months of age.[126] However, in a cross-sectional study examining a large group of standardbreds between the ages of 1 and 6 years, there was only a tendency for about a 10 percent increase in fiber areas with age.[139] An increase in fiber area was found in thoroughbreds during the period from about 1 year until they commenced training.[24] This was essentially age-related, since no change was seen in a group of thoroughbreds during training.[40]

With respect to fiber areas, reports have indicated increases,[19,176] no change,[40,177] or decreases in the size of type IIB fibers.[39,44,132,133] It is not surprising that little, if any, increase in fiber area occurs with aerobic training of mature horses because low oxidative fibers are transformed to high oxidative fibers, which have smaller areas. A decrease in fiber size when becoming aerobic is thought to be favorable because it permits faster diffusion of oxygen through the muscle fiber and more rapid removal of waste products (e.g., CO_2). In standardbreds of a similar age, inactive animals had larger fiber areas than active horses.[132] Despite this, muscle mass appeared greater in the best-performing standardbred horses when compared with their inactive cohorts. In an extensive study of endurance-trained horses of Andalusian and Arab breeds, overall there were minimal effects of training state on myofiber size.[177] However, in contrast, in relatively untrained Andalusian and Arabian horses, a progressive increase in cross-sectional area of all fiber types was seen until 24 years of age.[43] The increase was most prominent in the type I and IIA fibers. This latter finding may be partly explained by the slower maturation of these horses and their low grade of activity. In standardbreds undergoing draught work, an increase in fiber area of type IIA fibers occurred with a trend for an increase in type IIB fibers.[82] What is certain is that with sufficient aerobic training the proportion of muscle occupied by type IIA fibers is increased due to an increase in their number.

The finding of little or no increase in fiber size is difficult to reconcile with the generally accepted opinion that gluteal mass increases with training. Although not reported in horses and generally discounted in other species, hyperplasia may occur. This has been described recently in humans.[178] Whether there is an increase in overall muscle size may not be resolved until noninvasive techniques such as ultrasound and computed tomography are used to measure muscle mass.

Table 8-5. Results from a Cross-Sectional Study of Mean Fiber Type Percentages in the Middle Gluteal of Thoroughbreds and Standardbreds of Varying Ages

			Fiber Type (%)						
			Thoroughbreds				Standardbreds		
Age	Sex	No	I	IIA	IIB	No	I	IIA	IIB
1	M	20	8	27	65	10	15	37	49
1	S	21	10	34	56	15	18	40	43
2	M	23	11	37	52	11	15	40	45
2	S	20	11	42	46	14	15	40	45
3	M	21	17	42	42	12	17	41	42
3	S	17	15	47	38	15	21	48	31
4–6	M	17	14	45	40	15	19	47	34
4–6	S	24	18	53	29	15	21	48	30
Age			XXX	XXX	XXX		X	XXX	XXX
Sex			NS	XXX	XXX		NS	X	XXX

Note. Significance over the four age groups: X, $p < 0.05$; XX, $p < 0.01$; XXX, $p < 0.001$; M = mare (filly); S = stallion (colt).
Sources: Adapted from Roneus M, Lindholm A, Asheim A: Muscle characteristics in thoroughbreds of different ages and sexes. Equine Vet J 1991; 23:207 and Roneus M: Muscle characteristics in standardbred trotters of different ages and sexes. Equine Vet J (in press), with permission.

Detraining (Relative Inactivity)

Because horses have enforced periods of rest due to injury and illness during training/racing and also are rested between racing programs, a knowledge of this effect on muscle is important. Unfortunately, our knowledge in this area is rather limited due to few studies having been carried out. A study in thoroughbreds found a decline in enzyme activities after 5 weeks of inactivity, but after 10 weeks there was an inexplicable increase.[128,146,145] However, in a further study, enzyme activities that increased with training progressively declined during inactivity.[40] Associated with this was a decline in type II high oxidative fibers. In intensively trained thoroughbreds, a 5-week period of inactivity resulted in no change in enzyme activities or fiber composition from posttraining values.[133] Thoroughbreds undergoing a conventional training program were examined 6 weeks after the cessation of training.[143] A complexity of results was obtained, with indications of fiber oxidative capacity increasing during the detraining period. In endurance-trained horses, a decline to pretraining enzyme activities had occurred by 3 months of inactivity.[136] Glycogen content also decreases with inactivity.[40,128] The influence of different periods of inactivity is an area that warrants further investigation due to the varying results so far obtained.

Summary of Training Effects

From the preceding description it can be seen that numerous changes occur within muscle during training, and these are mainly related to improvement in oxidative capacity. The major changes would appear to occur fairly rapidly. However, it would appear that for major changes to occur, especially in conversion of low to high oxidative fibers, a threshold of training intensity is required. At an intensity of 40 percent $\dot{V}_{O_2max}$, no change was noted, with only moderate changes in oxidative fibers at 80 percent $\dot{V}_{O_2max}$.[168] It is also likely that training effects will be more pronounced in previously untrained horses than in those reentering a training program. Increased aerobic capacity and increased proportion of fast-twitch high oxidative fibers results in more highly fatigue-resistant fibers and is reflected in improved performance as the speed increases at which the onset of blood lactate accumulation occurs. This improvement will be beneficial in such competitions as endurance, eventing, and possibly even harness racing, where the lower speeds compared with thoroughbred racing require a lower rate of ATP turnover. In submaximal effort, especially endurance rides, associated with this increased oxidative capacity is an increase in HAD activity, which together are responsible for increased utilization of blood-borne FFAs. Greater FFA utilization leads to a glycogen-sparing effect and prolonged endurance capacity.

Although the preceding changes are considered to be desirable, there is controversy about the adaptive requirements for horses competing in galloping races. The limited studies in thoroughbreds have provided differing findings. With conventional training methods, little change in fiber type or enzyme activities has been recorded,[24,135,143] while in Sweden, horses exhibited a marked increase in high oxidative fibers, citrate synthase, and HAD with age.[138] However, when an interval training program, as has been recommended by many proponents of modern training methods is used, changes are found.[128,137] As previously argued,[179] it is debatable whether any marked degree of aerobic enhancement involving type IIB fibers is beneficial. Extensive recruitment of these fibers, as seen with interval training involving repeated bouts of maximal effort, will result in many of the type IIB fibers becoming oxidative and smaller in size and then transforming to type IIA. Both the smaller fiber size and change in contractile properties (i.e., reduction in $\dot{V}_{max}$) will affect speed. Since force output is related to total cross-sectional area of fiber mass recruited, diminution in fiber size will reduce maximal force output. Changes in force output and contractile speed will affect acceleration and possibly also stride length. Therefore, for quarter horses, racehorses, and thoroughbreds competing over distances less than 1000 m, strength rather than aerobic increases should be aimed for. Unfortunately, at present, no work other than draught training in standardbreds[180] has been carried out on how to strength train racehorses. Techniques need to be developed so that strength/power output can be measured. For thoroughbreds racing over longer distances, it is likely that a balance between stamina and strength has to be obtained. For horses competing in national hunt races, because of their longer duration, a greater aerobic program can be utilized. This has been done with great success by a number of British trainers. The optimal training program with respect to muscle development warrants further investigation.

Once optimal fitness is attained, it is uncertain how much training between races is required to maintain muscle fitness. From detraining studies it would appear that metabolic changes can be maintained for up to several weeks. Therefore, in certain situations, for both physical and mental reasons, it would be quite advantageous to reduce training intensity.

EFFECTS OF ANABOLIC STEROIDS

In attempts to enhance the improvement seen with training, anabolic steroids have been administered at regular intervals during training and racing programs. The use and effects of anabolic steroids have been reviewed recently.[181] These steroids can lead to increased protein retention and increased muscle mass, which occurs due to hypertrophy rather than hyperplasia of fibers. Although anabolic steroids have been shown to result in increased muscle mass in female and hypogonadal animals in a number of species, their possible effects in eugonadal males are more debatable. A recent study in humans using injections of testosterone ethanoate showed increased muscle protein synthesis and muscle mass.[182] A retrospective analysis of a number of human studies has shown that these steroids may improve performance.[183] It has been shown that the effects of anabolic steroids are enhanced by training, but it is controversial whether these positive results are due to direct effects on muscle or rather are due to the capacity to undertake increased training. The central nervous system effects of these compounds, including increased aggressiveness, would appear to allow athletes to train and perform at higher levels.

Although there are many who believe that anabolic steroids, including cocktails of different esters and compounds, are beneficial, if not even essential, in the training of a successful racehorse, there are others who claim that they are of little value. There have been reports of improved performance, but these have not been backed up with detailed information. In two experimental investigations, no improvement in performance[184,185] or changes in muscle were seen.[40,186] However, the design of these studies may have precluded demonstration of a beneficial effect.

RELATIONSHIP OF FIBER TYPE COMPOSITION TO PERFORMANCE

When the same muscle is sampled at a uniform site, differences are found between individuals. In humans, this difference has been related to athletic performance ability. In the vastus lateralis, a muscle that is very active during running, elite sprinters have almost all type II fibers at the site of sampling, while successful long-distance runners have almost all type I fibers. Middle-distance runners and the general population have approximately equal proportions of both types.[187] From studies in dizygous and monozygous twins, it is generally believed that the proportions of type I and type II fibers are genetically determined.[188] This also has been supported by studies in other species, including an investigation using two inbred strains of mice.[189] The latter concluded that the heritability of fiber type percentage, total fiber number, and relative size of type I and type II fibers were highly significant. Furthermore, the results indicated a polygenic mode of inheritance. It was found that the dominant fiber in terms of fiber number is also dominant in terms of area, and this is consistent with findings in horses that in the deeper parts of the middle glu-

teal muscle the type I fibers are larger than type II fibers.[190]

In horses, differences in fiber type between individuals also support a genetic as well as a phenotypic basis. In examining the middle gluteal muscle of a number of breeds, a relationship was found between the percentage of type II fibers and the type of performance the breed was best suited for.[45,48] For example, the quarter horse had a considerably greater proportion of type II fibers than the Arabian or a Heavy Hunter type of animal (Table 8–6). In hindsight, these initial studies could be criticized because relative sample depth variations may account for some of the differences, since little account was taken of the relative size of the muscles in different breeds. However, subsequent studies by various groups of workers also have been able to show a breed difference. Essén-Gustavsson and colleagues[33] in Sweden have consistently reported the mean proportion of type II fibers lower in standardbreds than in thoroughbreds. Arabian and Andalusian horses, breeds suited for endurance performance, have a lower proportion of type II fibers than thoroughbreds.[190]

In addition to this genetically based difference between breeds, sex differences have been reported in a number of species, with males having a higher proportion of type II fibers than females.[189] In an early study, it was reported that thoroughbred stallions had significantly more type II fibers than mares.[45] This was attributed to a higher selection pressure for breeding stallions than mares. Larger-scale studies on general populations of standardbreds and thoroughbreds have found no difference between stallions and mares in the proportion of type I fibers, but stallions have a higher ratio of type IIA to type IIB fibers from 1 year of age.[138,139] A higher proportion of type I fibers in stallions was seen in Andalusians but not in Arabians.[174] Stallions also were found to have a higher type IIA/IIB ratio.

Although very difficult to accurately measure in all but the smallest muscles, the number of fibers found in a particular muscle can vary quite considerably between breeds. This has been shown in laboratory animals,[189]

Table 8-6. *Fiber Composition in the Middle Gluteal of Different Breeds of Horses, % Fiber Type (Mean ± SEM)*

	n	ST	FTH	FT
Quarter horse[45]	28[*,‡]	8.7 ± 0.8	51.0 ± 1.6	40.3 ± 1.6
Thoroughbred[45]	50[*,‡]	11.0 ± 0.7	57.1 ± 1.3	32.0 ± 1.3
Thoroughbred[45]	22[*,†]	7.3 ± 0.9	61.2 ± 1.5	28.8 ± 1.5
Arab[48]	6[*]	14.4 ± 2.5	47.8 ± 3.2	37.8 ± 2.8
Standardbred[19]	8	24.0 ± 3.6	49.0 ± 3.1	27.0 ± 3.3
Standardbred[45]	9[*,†]	18.1 ± 1.6	55.4 ± 2.2	26.6 ± 2.0
Shetland pony[48]	4[*]	21.0 ± 1.2	38.8 ± 1.9	40.2 ± 2.7
Pony [48]	8[*]	22.5 ± 2.6	40.4 ± 2.3	37.1 ± 2.8
Heavy hunter[48]	7[*]	30.8 ± 3.1	37.1 ± 3.3	37.8 ± 2.8
Donkey[48]	5[*]	24.0 ± 3.0	38.2 ± 3.0	32.1 ± 3.4

[*]Out of work.
[†]Elite stallions at stud.
[‡]Elite broodmares.
Source: Adapted from Snow DH: Skeletal muscle adaptations: A review. *In* Snow DH, Persson SGB, Rose RJ (eds): Equine Physiology. Cambridge, Granta Editions, 1983, p 160, with permission.

meat-producing species such as pigs,[191] and horses and dogs.[192] Animals bred for speed, such as the greyhound and thoroughbred racehorse, have a greater number of fibers within the semitendinosus than "slower" breeds of the species. Although the difference was present in early life, it became more pronounced in the mature animal, again raising the controversial question of whether selective hyperplasia occurs. There is no reason not to suspect that similar differences occur in other key locomotory, if not all, muscles. A greater number of fibers in the best-performing racehorses may explain the finding that the best standardbreds appear to have bulkier muscles, despite having smaller fiber areas.[132] It would appear that difference in fiber number is largely under genetic control, although, as discussed earlier, the possibility exists for training-induced hyperplasia.

These genetically based differences have raised the possibility of whether at an early age, prior to purchase and training, a muscle biopsy will allow selection of horses suited for a particular type of competition. In a study of thoroughbred racehorses with proven performance, sprinters and medium-distance horses had a significantly higher proportion of type II fibers than stayers (2400 to 3000 m).[45] Biopsy findings from the semitendinosus of 14 yearling thoroughbreds were compared to their 2- and 3-year-old racing performance.[193] Horses were divided into two groups: those having less than or more than 90 percent type II fibers. Results indicated a higher percentage of desirable performance characteristics in the horses with greater than 90 percent type II fibers. Interestingly, there was a marked difference in the distance the two groups raced over, being 1440 and 2720 m for the high and low type II groups, respectively. In quarter horses, horses that raced successfully had a significantly slightly higher proportion of type II fibers than those which were unsuccessful.[194] In a small-scale study in standardbreds, there was an indication that performance could be related to the percentage of type IIB fibers, but there was no relationship to type I.[195]

With respect to endurance performance, studies have indicated that horses with the highest proportion of type I fibers usually have the best performance.[37,39,65] In an extensive study in Arabians and Andalusians in which biopsies were collected from sites at three different depths, the most successful horses had a higher percentage and larger type I and IIA fibers and with a greater homogeneity in size across the muscle.[43] It was also concluded that the higher proportion of type I fibers was genetically determined, while other differences were due to training.

Therefore, the preceding findings do support a basis for trying to select horses using fiber composition as one criterion. However, it has to be realized that successful performance is dependent on interaction between many genetic and phenotypic factors. Thus finding a horse with the desired fiber composition is no guarantee for success; rather, it improves the chance. Assessment of fiber composition probably has more usefulness in eliminating horses with an undesirable proportion of a particular fiber type. For this purpose, it probably has its greatest application in selection for endurance events. Its use in racehorses is probably much more limited due to the following factors:

1. A relatively narrow range in the proportions of type I to type II fibers exists. For example, in thoroughbreds, the approximate range for type I fibers is 5 to 25 percent, in contrast to humans, where in the vastus lateralis the range is 5 to 95 percent.
2. There is only a relatively narrow range of race distances (e.g., thoroughbreds normally race over distances of 1000 to 3200 m).
3. Nonhomogeneity of the middle gluteal muscle is a factor, making collection of samples from a standardized site imperative if horses are to be consistently evaluated.
4. There are numerous other factors influencing racing performance.

The value of fiber composition may be increased if fiber area measurements and total muscle size (providing an indirect measurement of fiber number) also can be readily determined.

Exertional Myopathies

Muscle disorders are a common cause of poor performance in horses. Most muscle problems in horses often have been grouped together in a syndrome referred to as *tying up,* and as a result, specific subsets of muscle disease went largely unrecognized. More recently, efforts have been made to provide a better classification system for muscle disorders in horses.[196] The most commonly identified muscle disorders in horses are myopathies induced by exercise. The exertional myopathies identified in horses so far include local muscle strains, exertional rhabdomyolysis, and mitochondrial myopathy. Abnormalities of muscle membrane conduction, including myotonia, hyperkalemic periodic paralysis, and stress-induced tetany, have been identified in a number of horses. These conditions are precipitated by factors other than exercise and are reviewed elsewhere.[197]

LOCAL MUSCLE STRAIN

Local muscle strain is a common injury in performance horses. Several factors may predispose horses to muscle strains, such as an inadequate warmup, preexisting lameness, exercise to the point of fatigue, and insufficient training. Lumbar and gluteal muscles are frequently injured in jumpers and dressage and harness horses. Lameness is often mild, and horses usually are reluctant to engage their hindquarters during exercise. Deep palpation of the epaxial and gluteal muscles results in pain and dorsiflexion of the spine. Horses that show pain but resist dorsiflexion, ventroflexion, and lateral bending upon manipulation may have a myopathy secondary to an underlying disorder of the spine or sacroiliac joint.

The semimembranosus and semitendinosus muscles are more frequently damaged in working quarter horses. These muscles are usually torn at the point of a tendinous insertion. Affected muscles are painful upon deep palpation and may appear warm. In chronic cases, hardened areas within the muscle may represent fibrosis and ossification. The stride has a short anterior phase with a characteristic hoof slapping gait.

Diagnosis. Serum activities of CK and AST usually are only mildly elevated. In addition to palpation, diagnosis can be confirmed by thermography or scintigraphy.[198] Light microscopic evaluation of muscle biopsies is frequently normal unless damage is severe.

Treatment. Adequate rest and nonsteroidal anti-inflammatory medication form the basis for treatment. Hand walking once the initial stiffness has dissipated may be beneficial. In addition, massage and the intermittent application of heat may aid the healing process. Exercise should be resumed gradually, preceded by an appropriate warmup period. Adequate conditioning should be ensured before starting strenuous exercise. Saddles should be checked for proper fit. In severe cases, the semimembranosus/semitendinosus muscles may develop fibrotic, ossifying lesions that permanently shorten the anterior phase of the stride. In these cases, tenectomy may be needed to restore limb function.

REPAIR OF MUSCLE WITH DAMAGE

Muscle damage in the horse usually occurs from excessive exertion, tearing or trauma of individual muscles, or specific diseases that produce rhabdomyolysis. Skeletal muscle shows a remarkable ability to regenerate following injury. Complete repair of muscle fibers without any residual scarring is dependant on the degree of damage that occurs to the basement membrane surrounding each muscle fiber. Severe trauma or tearing of a muscle that results in destruction of the basement membrane usually results in the proliferation of connective tissue and scar formation. Rhabdomyolysis in foals and exertional myopathies in adult horses do not usually damage the basement membrane; thus complete repair of muscle tissue is possible.

Following injury, the damaged portion of a muscle fiber is sealed off by new sarcolemmal membrane within 10 to 20 hours[199] (Fig. 8–14). Macrophage infiltration and phagocytosis of necrotic elements within the damaged muscle fiber can be observed within 16 hours to 4 days of injury.[200,201] Repair of the damaged segment can only occur through the activation and multiplication of satellite cells, since myonuclei are in a postmitotic stage. Satellite cells migrate along an intact basement membrane and form myoblasts which fuse together to form myotubes within 1 week following acute damage. The high RNA content of myotubes gives them a basophilic appearance in hematoxylin-eosin stains. As myofibrils are formed, the central nucleus of the myotube is gradually displaced, and within 1 to 2 months of the injury, it takes its customary subsarcolemmal position. If damaged fibers loose their innervation, new neuromuscular junctions are established by sprouts from nearby axons.

EXERTIONAL RHABDOMYOLYSIS

Exertional rhabdomyolysis, which literally means the dissolution of striated muscle fibers following exercise, is a common problem in performance horses. A number of other terms have been used to describe this condition, including *tying up, set fast, azoturia, Monday morning disease,* and *chronic intermittent rhabdomyolysis.* It has been implied or assumed that all horses that show evidence of muscle pain and cramping following exercise have the same disease. As a result, a great deal of controversy and confusion has developed regarding the cause and approach to treatment of this condition. Exertional rhabdomyolysis likely represents a pathologic description of a number of muscle diseases that have common clinical signs. Two general syndromes are apparent from a clinical standpoint: (1) acute rhabdomyolysis following exercise in horses that have a previous history of satisfactory performance, and (2) recurrent exertional rhabdomyolysis following mild exercise in horses with a history of poor performance.

Acute Exertional Rhabdomyolysis

Clinical Signs. Signs of exertional rhabdomyolysis can range in severity from mild stiffness following exercise to recumbency.[200] During exercise, horses develop a short, stiff stride, sweat profusely, and have an elevated respiratory rate. Upon stopping, horses are reluctant to move, males frequently posture to urinate, and in severe cases, myoglobinuria may be apparent. Physical examination reveals painful muscle cramps, especially in the gluteal area. Scintigraphic evaluation of horses with rhabdomyolysis following exercise shows symmetrical damage to the gluteal, semitendinosus, and semimembranosus muscles.[198] Some horses may be extremely painful, which could be confused with colic. Muscle pain usually persists for several hours. Endurance horses often show other signs of exhaustion, including a rapid heart rate, dehydration, hyperthermia, synchronous diaphragmatic flutter, and collapse.

Diagnosis. A diagnosis of exertional rhabdomyolysis is made on the basis of a history of muscle cramping and stiffness following exercise and moderate to marked elevations in serum myoglobin, CK, LDH, and AST. Serum levels of these muscle proteins peak following acute rhabdomyolysis at about 5 minutes (myoglobin), 5 hours (CK), 12 hours (LDH), and 24 hours (AST), respectively (Fig. 8–15). Myoglobinuria may occur when the renal tubular uptake of myoglobin is overwhelmed. Small-molecular-weight proteins such as myoglobin and CK are cleared within 48 to 72 hours, mainly by the kidney. Larger-molecular-weight enzymes such as AST are cleared by the reticuloendothelial system and may take up to 2 weeks to return to baseline.

Treatment. The objective of treatment is to relieve anxiety and muscle pain, correct fluid and acid-base deficits, and prevent renal compromise. The hydration status of horses with myoglobinuria should be assessed immediately. Oral and/or intravenous fluid therapy is a first-

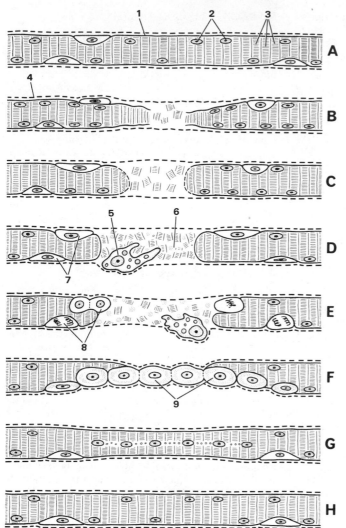

Figure 8-14. *Regeneration of a skeletal muscle fiber. A, A healthy fiber showing an intact sarcolemma (1), multiple subsarcolemmal nuclei (2), and myofibrils in register (3). B, Segmental disruption of the fiber with an intact basement membrane (4). C, Proliferation of the sarcolemmal membrane occurs to compartmentalize the damaged area. D, Macrophages (5) infiltrate and phagocytize necrotic debris (6). E, Satellite cells (7) are activated and replicate to form myoblasts (8). F, Myoblasts fuse to form myotubes (9). G, Synthesis of new myofilaments and formation of myofibrils progress, and myonuclei remain in a central position. H, A repaired fiber with peripherally displaced nuclei following complete myofibrillogenesis. (Adapted from Krstic RV: General Histology of the Mammal. New York, Springer-Verlag, 1984, p 273, with permission.)*

order priority in dehydrated horses prior to the administration of nonsteroidal anti-inflammatory drugs (NSAID). Myoglobin can be nephrotoxic, particularly in the face of dehydration and NSAID therapy. Blood urea nitrogen and serum creatinine concentrations should be monitored in horses with myoglobinuria. Since alkalosis is a common finding in horses with acute rhabdomyolysis, isotonic saline with dextrose or balanced polyionic fluids are recommended. If exhausted horses are markedly hyperthermic, the fluids can be chilled and external cooling should be initiated. In critical cases of rhabdomyolysis, plasma electrolytes should be monitored, since severe muscle necrosis can result in marked electrolyte imbalances.

Acepromazine, an alpha-adrenergic antagonist, is helpful in relieving anxiety and may increase muscle blood flow. Its use is contraindicated in dehydrated horses. In extremely painful horses, detomidine provides better sedation and analgesia. Nonsteroidal anti-inflam-

matory drugs at relatively high doses provide pain relief. Intravenous dimethyl sulfoxide (as a <20 percent solution) and corticosteroid administration also have been advocated in the acute stage. Muscle relaxants such as methocarbamol seem to produce variable results.

Rest with hand walking once the inital stiffness has abated is of prime importance. At this time, the diet should be changed to good-quality hay with little grain supplementation. The amount of rest a horse should receive is controversial. Horses with recurrent problems with rhabdomyolysis appear to benefit from an early return to a regular exercise schedule. Horses that appear to have damaged their muscles from overexertion may benefit from a longer rest period with regular access to a paddock. Training should be resumed gradually, and a regular exercise schedule, which will match the degree of exertion to the horse's underlying state of training, should be established. Endurance horses should be encouraged to drink electrolyte-supplemented water dur-

CK & AST (U/l)   Myoglobin (ug/ml)

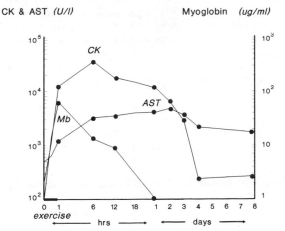

Figure 8-15. *The time course of alterations in serum creatine kinase (CK), aspartate aminotransferase (AST), and myoglobin (Mb) following an episode of exertional rhabdomyolysis.*

ing an endurance ride and should be monitored particularly closely during hot humid conditions.

Pathophysiology of Acute Rhabdomyolysis. The most common cause of exertional rhabdomyolysis is strenuous exercise that exceeds the horse's underlying state of training. This includes both exercise at speed and endurance riding. The etiopathogenesis of rhabdomyolysis following strenuous exertion likely involves a deficiency of high-energy phosphates in muscle cells following either a marked lactic acidosis (high-speed exercise) or a depletion of intracellular glycogen (prolonged slow exercise). Muscle damage following endurance rides may be accentuated by hyperthermia and electrolyte imbalances. Hyperthermia, low muscle pH, and a deficiency in ATP impair the function of essential membrane pumps such as the sodium/potassium, calcium/magnesium, and calcium/ATPase pumps. If this situation cannot be corrected, the sarcoplasmic calcium concentration rises and acts to inhibit mitochondrial respiration, to damage cellular membranes through the activation of phospholipase, to disrupt myofibrils through the activation of neutral proteases, and to disturb the cytoskeleton.[203]

The incidence of muscle stiffness and exertional rhabdomyolysis has been observed to increase during an outbreak of respiratory disease. Both equine herpes virus 1 and equine influenza virus have been implicated as causative agents.[196,204] Mild muscle stiffness with concurrent viral infections is likely to be the result of the release of endogenous pyrogens. More severe rhabdomyolysis may be due to exertion during a concurrent systemic infection and/or viral replication in muscle tissue. Severe rhabdomyolysis and death have occurred in young horses during influenza outbreaks. Vigorous exercise may not be necessary to trigger rhabdomyolysis and myoglobinuria in these horses.

Recurrent Exertional Rhabdomyolysis

In some predisposed horses, exertional rhabdomyolysis may occur repeatedly following minimal exercise. Although clinical signs are only apparent intermittently with exercise, subclinical episodes of rhabdomyolysis with 100-fold increases in serum CK are quite common.[205] Recurrent exertional rhabdomyolysis (RER) is first identified shortly after horses commence training, and the incidence appears highest in young, nervous fillies. Almost all breeds are affected.[202] The cause of RER appears to be distinct from excessive exertion; however, to date, the pathophysiology of RER is not well understood. A wide variety of factors appears to trigger recurrent episodes of rhabdomyolysis in susceptible horses.

Carbohydrates. The two most important contributing factors to RER are diet and exercise regimens. Carlström[206] first noted that in draft breeds, high-carbohydrate diets and day of rest could induce exertional rhabdomyolysis. This remains a common manner for triggering rhabdomyolysis in susceptible horses, but the mechanism responsible for rhabdomyolysis is unclear. Muscle glycogen concentrations appear to be higher in horses with RER than in healthy horses. Carlström proposed that muscle damage was due to rapid glycogen breakdown and lactic acidosis. Muscle damage, however, occurs during aerobic exercise, and lactic acid concentrations in damaged muscle are much lower than those found in healthy horses after maximal exertion.[207]

Vitamin E and Selenium. Vitamin E and selenum deficiency can cause acute rhabdomyolysis in foals and adult horses.[208] Most horses with RER, however, do not appear deficient in vitamin E and selenium,[200,209] and the incidence of RER does not appear to be greater in areas where the soil is selenium-deficient. As a general rule, serum levels of selenium or glutathione peroxidase activities should be assessed in horses from areas with low soil selenium, and dietary supplementation should be provided for horses that are deficient.

Electrolytes. Determination of electrolyte imbalances is hampered by the difficulty of assessing intramuscular stores. Techniques such as erythrocyte potassium concentrations and fractional exretion of electrolytes have been used to estimate deficits. These results are affected by exercise and diet, respectively. Potassium deficiency may produce an exertional myopathy by diminishing local capillary vasodilation. Red blood cell potassium concentrations in young thoroughbred horses with muscle soreness were found to be lower than concentrations in healthy horses.[210] In contrast, evaluation of potassium balance using renal fractional excretions has shown normal values for horses with RER.[211] Potassium deficiencies are rare in horses fed alfalfa hay.

Low renal fractional excretion of sodium has been observed in mature pleasure horses with RER in England.[212] In some cases, dietary supplementation with additional sodium (30 to 45 g NaCl in adults) results in a lower incidence of rhabdomyolysis. The favorable response of many horses to sodium bicarbonate supplementation may be due to the addition of sodium to the diet. Low fractional excretion of phosphorus also has been reported in some horses with RER. Dietary supplementation with calcium (11 to 33 g calcium in adults) may be beneficial in these cases.[211] Dietary electrolyte imbalances appear to be an uncommon cause of exertional myopathies in horses in Australia and the western United States.[213,214]

Hormones. Secondary hypothyroidism has been proposed to be a triggering factor in exertional rhabdomyolysis. Hypothyroidism results in impaired protein turnover, depressed muscle oxidative metabolism, and decreased myosin ATPase activity. Signs of muscle stiffness have been reported in a few horses with low T_4 activity but normal thyroid-stimulating hormone (TSH) stimulation. Most horses with RER, however, appear to be euthyroid. Interpretation of T_3 and T_4 should be performed with caution in horses on NSAID, since falsely low baseline values can be obtained. Recent studies of thyroxine levels in horses with exertional rhabdomyolysis did not show any difference in plasma concentrations compared with healthy horses. However, in some cases, there was a decreased thyroxine response to thyroid-releasing hormone. It was suggested that these horses may have a reduced thyroid reserve.

Because RER appears to be more common in females, a possible triggering effect of sex hormones has been suggested. A study of thoroughbreds in training did not find a correlation between plasma progesterone activity and serum CK level after exercise.[216] Some fillies, however, appear to have a lower incidence of RER while on progesterone therapy.

Metabolic Causes. Approximately 50 percent of human cases of RER are due to enzyme deficiencies in glycolysis or fatty acid metabolism. Glycogenolytic enzyme abnormalities have been investigated in horses with RER, but no specific enzyme deficiencies have been identified.[217] A glycogen storage disorder characterized by the accumulation of an abnormal polysaccharide has been described in quarter horse–related breeds.[218] Carnitine palmitoyl transferase 1 activity has been investigated in a few cases and found to be normal.[219]

Ion Channels. An initial association between malignant hyperthermic reactions to halothane anesthesia and a history of RER led to speculation that rhabdomyolysis may be due to abnormal intramuscular calcium regulation.[220] Recently, the cause of malignant hyperthermia in pigs and some humans has been identified as a cysteine/arginine transposition in the calcium release channel.[221] Evidence for abnormal membrane function in horses with RER has been suggested by a prolonged time to 50 percent relaxation of in vitro muscle twitches in horses with RER[222] and a reduced threshold for calcium-induced calcium release in sarcoplasmic reticular membrane fractions from affected horses.[223] Furthermore, in some cases of RER, treatment with drugs that affect calcium release from the sarcoplasmic reticulum (dantrolene) and affect other membrane channels (phenytoin)

appears to be effective in preventing RER. Muscle damage following exercise may be due to exessive release of calcium from the terminal cisternae, impaired uptake of calcium into the sarcoplasmic reticulum following a contraction, or increased permeability of the sarcolemma to calcium ions in horses with RER.

Clinical Evaluation of RER. Because RER is likely to have several causes, a thorough history and a complete clinical evaluation of the horse are imperative. A minimum database includes a complete blood count, serum biochemistry profile, serum vitamin E and selenium concentrations, urinalysis and determination of renal fractional excretion of electrolytes (sodium, potassium, phosphorus), and the peak serum CK response to an exercise challenge. In addition, a muscle biopsy may provide additional information in recurrent cases.

Muscle Biopsy. Deep biopsies of the gluteus medius muscle of horses with RER frequently contain pathologic features ranging from acute degeneration to varying stages of regeneration. The PAS stain for glycogen usually is very dark.[207,224] Some horses accumulate a PAS-positive polysaccharide and have vacuoles in subsarcolemmal regions of type II fibers.[217] Acute lesions include randomly scattered hypercontracted type II muscle fibers with degenerate mitochondria and segmental fiber necrosis with varying degrees of calcification.[225,226] (Fig. 8–16). Macrophage infiltration of necrotic fibers occurs within days of rhabdomyolysis, and small basophilic fibers with central nuclei are apparent within 1 to 2 weeks. Central nuclei persist in repaired fibers for 1 to 2 months following injury (Fig. 8–17).

Prophylaxis. The most important factors in prophylaxis are diet and exercise schedules. Horses susceptible to RER require a rigid, regular exercise schedule and appear to manage best without days off work. The best diet usually consists of good-quality hay, a balanced vitamin and mineral supplement, and a minimum of grain. If necessary, extra calories may be provided in the form of corn oil or powdered fat supplements. Changes in management that will reduce stress and excitement are beneficial. The incidence of RER can be dramatically reduced in many horses with management changes alone. In some individuals, however, further prophylaxis may be required.

Highly excitable horses may improve with low-dose tranquilization prior to exercise. Fillies that appear to develop rhabdomyolysis during estrus may benefit from progesterone supplementation. Oral sodium bicarbonate and dimethylglycine have been recommended on the basis that they buffer or decrease lactate production. However, since profound lactic acidosis is seldom found in association with RER, any purported beneficial effects must lie elsewhere.

If the management changes alone are insufficient, some horses may improve with daily medication to prevent muscle damage. Dantrolene at 2 mg/kg PO 1 hour prior to exercise may reduce the incidence of RER in horses with abnormal regulation of intracellular calcium

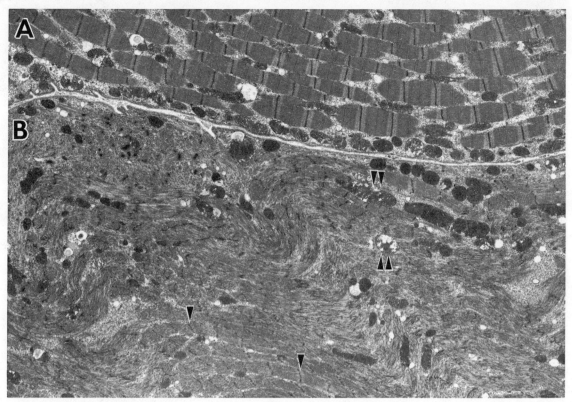

Figure 8-16. *Ultrastructural alterations in a muscle fiber following acute exertional rhabdomyolysis. The muscle fiber at the top of the figure (A) shows an orderly arrangement of myofibrils. In contrast, rhabdomyolysis is evident in the fiber at the bottom of the figure (B). Disruption of myofibrils, streaming of Z lines (single arrow), and degeneration of mitochondria (double arrow) are apparent. Note that the sarcolemma remains intact (× 4800).*

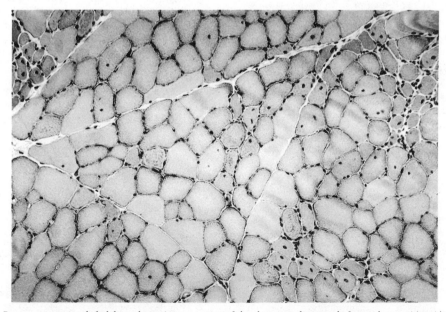

Figure 8-17. *Recurrent exertional rhabdomyolysis. A cross section of the gluteus medius muscle from a horse with evidence of several previous episodes of exertional rhabdomyolysis. The nuclei of normal muscle fibers have a characteristic subsarcolemmal position. Small, basophilic, regenerative muscle fibers with large central nuclei are scattered throughout the section. Later stages of regeneration are represented by large fibers with small centrally placed nuclei (hematoxylin and eosin stain).*

173

similar to malignant hyperthermia. This medication may be more effective in thoroughbred horses with a family history of RER because malignant hyperthermia is known to be a heritable disorder, and anesthetic-related episodes occur more commonly in thoroughbred horses.[220] A gradual reduction in the dose of dantrolene can be attempted over time. Long-term therapy has the potential for hepatotoxicity. Phenytoin at serum concentration of 6 to 8 μg/ml has been used with apparent success in some horses with prolonged muscle twitch times. The oral dosage necessary to produce this serum level must be established for each individual but usually lies between 5 and 12 mg/kg twice daily. High serum levels should be avoided because somnolence and seizure-like activity may occur.[222]

MITOCHONDRIAL MYOPATHY

A defect in a mitochondrial respiratory enzyme has been identified in an Arabian horse with severe exercise intolerance following a few minutes of light exercise. The filly had a 20-fold increase in plasma lactic acid at a trot (4 to 7 m/s) and showed little increase in oxygen uptake with increasing trotting speed. There was no evidence of rhabdomyolysis either in measurements of serum CK or in muscle biopsies following exercise. The mitochondrial staining of muscle biopsies was increased, and mitochondria were enlarged with bizarre cristae formations. A deficiency of complex 1 (NADH CoQ reductase) was determined by biochemical analysis.[227]

Conclusions

As described in this chapter, equine skeletal muscle is essentially similar to all mammalian muscles. However, through evolution and, more recently, selective breeding, the horse has developed muscle characteristics that allow breeds to have great strength (draft breeds, Shetland ponies), speed, and stamina (the Arabian) or sheer speed (quarter horse and thoroughbred).

Great advances have been made in the understanding of skeletal muscle fiber types, adaptations with training, and the cause of fatigue through the ease of taking sequential biopsies. Our knowledge in this area is almost equal to that in humans and some laboratory animals. These studies have shown that adaptations with training superimposed on genetic traits have allowed muscles to be extremely efficient in generating and maintaining high-energy turnover. Activities of key metabolic enzymes as well as glycogen are extremely high. Experimental studies have enabled a better understanding of the causes of fatigue as well as nutritional requirements, allowing the veterinarian to give scientifically based advice to trainers and owners. The extensive studies in this area also have helped to dispel many myths.

Although much has been learned, there is still a great deal more information required. Training studies, often limited because of small numbers, have often yielded conflicting results. For example, it is still uncertain whether enhanced buffering capacity, which should be of benefit, occurs with all types of training. Possibly

due to methodologic difficulties, it is still uncertain whether muscle fiber numbers decrease, increase, or remain unaltered despite obvious visible changes in muscle bulk. Little is known of the effects of short and moderate rest periods or the effect of decreasing the training load, such as may occur in a racehorse with a limb injury.

Despite there being obvious differences in fiber type composition in key locomotory muscles, early promises on the usefulness of small muscle biopsy specimens for performance prediction have largely remained unfulfilled due to heterogeneity within muscles. However, it may be that more samples at different depths of the muscle could provide more reliable information.

Fortunately, with the exception of the exertional rhabdomyolysis syndrome, which still largely remains an enigma, muscle disorders are of little importance in the horse. However, as seen in the recent development of hyperkalemic periodic paralysis, muscle disorders can appear suddenly and spread rapidly due to highly selective breeding. It is also likely that as the sophistication of detection and analysis increases, more subtle but performance-important muscle disorders will be described.

References

1. Gunn HM: Muscle, bone and fat proportions and muscle distribution of thoroughbreds and other horses. *In* Gillespie JR, Robinson NE (eds): Equine Exercise Physiology 2. Davis, Calif, ICEEP Publications, 1987, p. 253.
2. Henckel P: A histochemical assessment of the capillary blood supply of the middle gluteal muscle of thoroughbred horses. *In* Snow DH, Persson SGB, Rose RJ (eds): Equine Exercise Physiology. Cambridge, Granta Editions, 1983, p 225.
3. Karlström K, Essén-Gustavsson B, Lindholm A, et al: Capillary supply in relation to muscle metabolic profile and cardiocirculatory parameters. *In* Persson SGB, Lindholm A, Jeffcott LB (eds): Equine Exercise Physiology 3. Davis, Calif, ICEEP Publications, 1991, p 239.
4. Patou MP: Dorso-ventral axis determination of chick limb bud development. *In* Ede DA, Hinchliffe JR, Balls M (eds): Vertebrate Limb and Somite Morphogenesis. Cambridge, Cambridge University Press, 1977, p 257.
5. Whalen RG: Myosin isoenzymes as molecular markers for muscle physiology. J Exp Biol 1985; 115:43.
6. Pette D, Staron RS: Cellular and molecular diversities of mammalian skeletal muscle fibers. Rev Physiol Biochem Pharmacol 1990; 116:1.
7. Rudolph JA, Speir SJ, Byrns G, et al: Periodic paralysis in quarter horses: A sodium channel mutation disseminated by selective breeding. Nature Genet 1992; 23:241.
8. Takashima H, Nishimura S, Matsumoto T, et al: Primary structure and expression from complementary NA of skeletal muscle ryanodine receptor. Nature 1989; 339:439.
9. Hoffman EPRH, Brown LM, Kunckel LM: Dystrophin: The protein product of the Duchenne muscular dystrophy locus. Cell 1987; 51:919.
10. Lazarides E, Capetanaki YG: The striated muscle cytoskeleton: Expression and assembly in development. *In* Emerson C, Fischman DA, Nadal-Ginard B, Siddiqui MAQ (eds): Molecular Biology of Muscle Development. New York: Alan R Liss, 1985, p 756.
11. Wang K, Ramirez-Mitchell R, Palter D: Titin is an extraordinarily long, flexible, and slender myofibrillar protein. Proc Natl Acad Sci USA 1984; 81:3685.
12. Horak V, Draber P, Hanak J, et al: Fiber composition and tubulin localization in muscle of thoroughbred sprinters and stayers. *In* Persson SGB, Lindholm A, Jeffcott LB (eds): Equine Exercise Physiology 3. Davis, Calif, ICEEP Publications, 1991, p 262.

13. Kayar SR, Hoppeler H, Essén-Gustavsson E, et al: The similarity of mitochondrial distribution in equine skeletal muscles of differing oxidative capacity. J Exp Biol 1988; 137:253.

14. Kayar SR, Hoppeler H, Mermod L, et al: Mitochondrial size and shape in equine skeletal muscle: A three-dimensional reconstruction study. Anat Rec 1988; 222:333.

15. Essén B: Studies on the regulation of metabolism in human skeletal muscle using intermittent exercise as an experimental model. Acta Physiol Scand 1978; (suppl 454):1.

16. Valberg S, Essén-Gustavsson B: Metabolic response to racing determined in pools of type I, IIA, and IIB fibers. *In* Gillespie JR, Robinson NE (eds): Equine Exercise Physiology 2. Davis, Calif, ICEEP Publications, 1987, p 290.

17. White MG, Snow DH: Quantitative histochemistry of myosin ATPase activity after acid preincubation and succinate dehydrogenase activity in equine skeletal muscle. Acta Histochem Cytochem 1985; 18:483.

18. Lindholm A: Muscle Morphology and Metabolism in Standardbred Horses at Rest and During Exercise. Ph.D. thesis, Royal Veterinary College, Stockholm, 1973.

19. Lindholm A, Piehl K: Fibre composition, enzyme activity and concentration of metabolites and electrolytes in muscles of standardbred horses. Acta Vet Scand 1974; 15:287.

20. Snow DH, Guy PS: Percutaneous needle muscle biopsy in the horse. Equine Vet J 1976; 8:150.

21. Snow DH: A percutaneous muscle biopsy needle for simultaneous sampling at two sites. J Physiol (Lond) 1986; 376:12P.

22. Snow DH, Harris RC: Comparison of biochemical changes following exercise at two sites within a muscle. Proc Int Union Physiol Sci 1986;16:404.

23. Rome LC, Sosnicki AA, Goble DO: Maximum velocity of shortening of three fibre types from horse soleus muscle: Implications for scaling with body size. J Physiol (Lond) 1990; 431: 173.

24. Snow DH: Skeletal muscle adaptations: A review. *In* Snow DH, Persson SGB, Rose RJ (eds): Equine Exercise Physiology. Cambridge, Granta Editions, 1983, p 160.

25. Ranvier L: De quelques facts relates à l'histologie et à la phyiologie des muscles strés. Arch Physiol Norm Pathol 1874; 6:1.

26. Brooke MH, Kaiser KK: Three myosin ATPase systems, the nature of their pH lability and sulfhydryl dependence. J Histochem Cytochem 1970; 18:670.

27. Snow DH, Billeter R, Mascarello F, et al: No classical type IIB fibres in dog skeletal muscle. Histochemistry 1982; 75:53.

28. Billeter R, Lador J, Howald H, et al: Gel electrophoresis of proteins from single equine muscle fibres. *In* Gillespie JR, Robinson NE (eds): Equine Exercise Physiology 2. Davis, Calif, ICEEP Publications, 1987, p 359.

29. Sinha AK, Rose RJ, Pozgaj I, et al: Indirect myosin immunocytochemistry for the identification of fiber types in equine skeletal muscle. Res Vet Sci 1992; 53:25.

30. Snow DH, Billeter R, Jenny E: Myosin types in equine skeletal muscle. Res Vet Sci 1981; 30:381.

31. Stull CL, Albert WW: Comparison of muscle fiber types of two-year-old fillies of the belgian, standardbred, thoroughbred, quarter horse and welsh breeds. J Anim Sci 1980; 51:340.

32. Gunn HM: Differences in the histochemical properties of skeletal muscles of different breeds of horses and dogs. J Anat 1978; 127:615.

33. Valberg S, Essén-Gustavsson B, Skoglund Wallberg H: Oxidative capacity of skeletal muscle fibre types in racehorses: histochemical versus biochemical analysis. Equine Vet J 1988; 20: 291.

34. Lopez-Rivero JL, Aquera E, Rodriguyes-Barbudo MV, et al: Degree of correspondence between contractile and oxidative capacity in horse muscle fibre: A histochemical study. Histol Histopathol 1990; 5:49.

35. Andrews FM, Spurgeon TL: Histochemical staining characteristics of normal horse skeletal muscle. Am J Vet Res 1986; 47:1843.

36. Van den Hoven R, Meijer AEFH, Wensing TH, et al: Enzyme histochemical features of equine gluteus muscle fibres. Am J Vet Res 1985; 46:1755.

37. Snow DH, Baxter P, Rose RJ: Muscle fibre composition and glycogen depletion in horses competing in an endurance ride. Vet Rec 1981; 108:374.

38. Snow DH, Kerr MG, Nimmo MA, et al: Alterations in blood, sweat, urine and muscle composition during prolonged exercise in the horse. Vet Rec 1982; 110:377.

39. Essén-Gustavsson G, Karlstrom K, Lindholm A: Fibre type, enzyme activities and substrate utilization in skeletal muscle of horses competing in endurance rides. Equine Vet J 1984; 16:197.

40. Nimmo MA, Snow DH, Munro CD: Effects of nandrolone phenylpropionate in the horse: 3. Skeletal muscle composition in the exercising animal. Equine Vet J 1982; 14:229.

41. Lopez-Rivero JL, Aquera E, Monterde JG, et al: Fibre size and composition in the middle gluteal muscle of the Andalusian horse. Equine Vet J 1990; 22:286.

42. Lopez-Rivero JL, Serrano AL, Diz AM, et al: Variability of muscle fibre composition and fibre sizes in the horse gluteus medius: An enzyme-histochemical and morphometric study. J Anat (in press).

43. Lopez-Rivero JL, Serrano AL, Henckel P, et al: Distribution of fiber type size in the gluteus medius muscle of successfully and unsuccessfully endurance-raced horses. Personal communication, 1992.

44. Henckel P: Training and growth induced changes in the middle gluteus muscle of young standardbred trotters. Equine Vet J 1983; 15:134.

45. Snow DH, Guy PS: Fiber type and enzyme activities of the gluteus medius of different breeds of horse. *In* Poortmans J, Nisert G (eds): Biochemistry of Exercise. Baltimore, University Park Press, 1981, p 275.

46. Hoppeler H, Claassen H, Howald H, et al: Correlated histochemistry and morphometry in equine skeletal muscle. *In* Snow DH, Persson SGB, Rose RJ (eds): Equine Exercise Physiology. Cambridge, Granta Editions, 1983, p 184.

47. Hoppeler H, Jones JH, Linstedt SL, et al: Relating maximal oxygen consumption to skeletal muscle mitochondria in horses. *In* Gillespie JR, Robinson NE (eds): Equine Exercise Physiology 2. Davis, Calif, ICEEP Publications, 1987, p 278.

48. Snow DH, Guy PS: Fibre composition of a number of limb muscles in different breeds of horses. Res Vet Sci 1980; 28:137.

49. van den Hoven R, Wensing TH, Breukink HJ, et al: Variations of fiber types in the triceps brachii, longissimus dorsi, gluteus medius and biceps femoris. Am J Vet Res 1985; 46:939.

50. Lindholm A, Bjerneld H, Saltin B: Glycogen depletion patterns in muscle fibres of trotting horses. Acta Physiol Scand 1974; 90:475.

51. Lindholm A, Saltin B: The physiological and biochemical response of standardbred horses to exercise of varying speed and duration. Acta Vet Scand 1974; 15:310.

52. Kai M: Distribution of fibre types in equine middle gluteal muscle. Bull Equine Res Inst 1985; 21:46.

53. Bruce VL, Turek RJ: Muscle fiber variations in the gluteus medius of the horse. Equine Vet J 1984; 17:317.

54. Raub RH, Bechtel PJ, Lawrence LM: Variation in the distribution of muscle fiber types in equine skeletal muscles. J Equine Vet Sci 1985; 5:34.

55. Kline KH, Lawrence LM, Novakofok J, Bechtel PJ: Changes in muscle fiber type variation within the middle gluteal of young and mature horses as a function of sampling depth. *In* Gillespie JR, Robinson NE (eds): Equine Exercise Physiology 2. Davis, Calif, ICEEP Publications, 1987, p 271.

56. Lopez-Rivero JL, Diz AM, Monterde JG, et al: Intramuscular distribution of fiber types in the gluteus medius of the horse: A histochemical analysis. Anat Histol Embryol (in press).

57. Bruce VL, Schurg WA: Muscle fiber and nerve innervation in the gluetus medius of the horse. Anat Histol Embryol 1990; 19:77.

58. Bruce VL, Turek RJ, Schurg WA: Muscle fibre compartmentalization in the gluteus medius of the horse. Equine Vet J 1993; 25:69.

59. Rivero JLL, Serrano AL, Diz AM, et al: Changes in cross-sectional area and capillary supply of the muscle fiber population in equine gluteus muscle as a function of sampling depth. Am J Vet Res 1993; 54:32.

60. Kline KH, Bechtel PJ: Changes in the metabolic profile of the equine gluteus medius as a function of sampling depth. Comp Biochem Physiol 1988; 91A:815.

61. Snow DH, Harris RC: Effects of daily exercise on muscle glycogen in the thoroughbred racehorse. *In* Persson SGB, Lindholm

A, Jeffcott LB (eds): Equine Exercise Physiology 3. Davis, Calif, ICEEP Publications, 1991, p 299.

62. Wood CH, Ross TT, Armstrong JB, et al: Homogeneity of muscle fiber composition in the gluteus medius of the horse. J Equine Vet Sci 1988; 4:294.

63. Henneman E, Olsen CB: Relations between structure and function in the design of skeletal muscle. J Neurophysiol 1963; 28:581.

64. White MG, Snow DH: Quantitative histochemical study of glycogen depletion in the maximally exercised thoroughbred. Equine Vet J 1987; 19:67.

65. Hodgson D, Rose RJ, Allen J: Muscle glycogen depletion and repletion patterns in horses performing various distances of endurance exercise. In Snow DH, Persson SGB, Rose RJ (eds): Equine Exercise Physiology. Cambridge, Granta Editions, 1983, p 229.

66. Hodgson D, Rose RJ, Allen J, et al: Glycogen depletion patterns in horses performing maximal exercise. Res Vet Sci 1984; 36:169.

67. Valberg S: Glycogen depletion patterns in the muscle of standardbred trotters after exercise of varying intensities and durations. Equine Vet J 1986; 18:479.

68. Gottlieb M, Essén-Gustavsson B, Persson SGB: Muscle glycogen depletion patterns during draught work in standardbred horses. Equine Vet J 1989; 21:110.

69. Valberg S, Essén-Gustavsson B, Lindholm A, et al: Energy metabolism in relation to skeletal muscle fibre properties during treadmill exercise. Equine Vet J 1985; 17:439.

70. Lovell DK, Reid TA, Ross RJ: Effects of maximal exercise on equine muscle: Changes in metabolites, pH and temperature. In Gillespie JR, Robinson NE (eds): Equine Exercise Physiology 2. Davis, Calif, ICEEP Publications, 1987, p 312.

71. Harris RC, Marlin JD, Snow DH: Response to intermittent maximal exercise in the thoroughbred horse: Lactate kinetics and the relationship between plasma ammonia increase and performance. In Persson SGB, Lindholm A, Jeffcott LB (eds): Equine Exercise Physiology 3. Davis, Calif, ICEEP Publications, 1990, p 173.

72. Harris RC, Marlin DJ, Snow DH, et al: Muscle ATP loss and lactate accumulation at different work intensities in the exercising thoroughbred horse. Eur J Appl Physiol 1991; 62:235.

73. Rose RJ, Hodgson DR, Kelso TB, et al: Maximum O$_2$ debt deficit and muscle metabolite in thoroughbred horses. J Appl Physiol 1988; 64:781.

74. Miller-Graber PA, Lawrence LA, Kurcz E, et al: The free amino acid profile in the middle gluteal before and after fatiguing exercise. Equine Vet J 1990; 22:209.

75. Marlin DJ, Harris RC, Snow DH: Rates of blood lactate disappearance following exercise of different intensities. In Persson SGB, Lindholm A, Jeffcott LB (eds): Equine Exercise Physiology 3. Davis, Calif, ICEEP Publications, 1990, p 188.

76. Valberg S, Essén-Gustavsson B, Lindholm A, et al: Blood chemistry and skeletal muscle metabolic responses during and after different speeds and durations of trotting. Equine Vet J 1989; 21:91.

77. Gollnick PD, Bertocci LA, Kelso TB, et al: The effect of high-intensity exercise on the respiratory capacity of skeletal muscle. Pflugers Arch 1990; 415:407.

78. Nimmo MA, Snow DH: Muscle glycogen, lactate and pyruvate following maximal exercise in the thoroughbred horse. In Snow DH, Persson SGB, Rose RJ (eds): Equine Exercise Physiology. Cambridge, Granta Editions, 1983, p 160.

79. Snow DH, Harris RC, Gash S: Metabolic response of equine muscle to intermittent maximal exercise. J Appl Physiol 1985; 58:1689.

80. Harris RC, Marlin DJ, Snow DH: Metabolic response to maximal exercise of 800 and 2000 m in the thoroughbred horse. J Appl Physiol 1987; 63:12.

81. Sewell DA, Harris RC, Hanak J, et al: Muscle adenine nucleotide degradation in the thoroughbred horse as a consequence of racing. Comp Biochem Physiol 1992; 101B:375.

82. Gottlieb JR, Essén-Gustavsson B, Lindholm A, et al: Effects of a draught loaded interval training program on skeletal muscle in the horse. J Appl Physiol 1989; 67:570.

83. Gottlieb M, Essén-Gustavsson B, Lindholm A, et al: Circulatory and muscle metabolic responses to draught work compared to increasing trotting velocities. Equine Vet J 1988; 20:430.

84. Gottlieb M, Essén-Gustavsson B, Skoglund-Wallberg H: Blood and muscle metabolic responses to draught work of varying intensity and duration in horses. Res Vet Sci 1989; 47:102.

85. Snow DH, Harris RC: Thoroughbreds and greyhounds: Biochemical adaptations in creatures of nature and man. In Gilles R (ed): Circulation, Respiration and Metabolism. Berlin, Springer-Verlag, 1985, p 227.

86. Weber JM, Parkhouse WS, Dobson GP, et al: Lactate kinetics in exercising thoroughbred horses: Regulation of turnover rate in plasma. Am J Physiol 1987; 253:896.

87. Sewell DA, Harris RC: Adenine nucleotide degradation in the thoroughbred horse with increasing exercise duration. Eur J Appl Physiol 1992; 65:271.

88. Valberg S: Metabolic response to racing and fiber properties of skeletal muscle in standardbred and thoroughbred horses. J Equine Vet Sci 1987; 7:6.

89. Harris P, Snow DH: The effect of high intensity exercise on the plasma concentration of lactate, potassium and other electrolytes. Equine Vet J 1988; 20:109.

90. Lindner A, von Wittke P, Schmald M, et al: Maximal lactate concentrations in horses after exercise of different duration and intensity. J Equine Vet Sci 1992; 12:36.

91. Snow DH, Mason DK, Ricketts SW, Douglas TA: Post-race blood biochemistry in thoroughbreds. In Snow DH, Persson SGB, Rose RJ (eds): Equine Exercise Physiology. Cambridge, Granta Editions, 1983, p 389.

92. Åsheim A, Knudsen D, Lindholm A, et al: Heart rates and blood lactate concentrations of standardbred horses during training and racing. J Am Vet Med Assoc 1970; 157:304.

93. Snow DH: Unpublished data, 1992.

94. Marlin DJ, Harris RC, Harman J, et al: Influence of post-exercise activity on rates of muscle and blood lactate disappearance in the thoroughbred horse. In Gillespie JR, Robinson NE (eds): Equine Exercise Physiology 2. Davis, Calif, ICEEP Publications, 1986, p 321.

95. Bayly WM, Grant BD, Pearson RC: Lactate concentrations in thoroughbred horses following maximal exercise under field conditions. In Gillespie JR, Robinson NE (eds): Equine Exercise Physiology 2. Davis, Calif, ICEEP Publications, 1987, p 426.

96. Nimmo MA, Snow DH: Time course of ultrastructural changes in skeletal muscle after two types of exercise. J Appl Physiol 1982; 52:910.

97. McCutcheon LJ, Byrd SK, Hodgson DR, et al: Ultrastructural alterations in equine skeletal muscle associated with fatiguing exercise. In Persson SGB, Lindholm A, Jeffcott LB (eds): Equine Exercise Physiology 3. Davis, Calif, ICEEP Publications, 1991, p 269.

98. McCutcheon LJ, Byrd SK, Hodgson DR: Ultrastructural changes in skeletal muscle after fatiguing exercise. J Appl Physiol 1992; 72:1111.

99. Byrd SK, McCutcheon LJ, Hodgson DR, et al: Altered sarcoplasmic reticulum function after high intensity exercise. J Appl Physiol 1989; 67:2072.

100. Foster CVL, Harman J, Harris RC, et al: ATP distribution of single muscle fibres before and after maximal exercise in the horse. J Physiol 1986; 378:64.

101. Cutmore CM, Snow DH, Newsholme AE: Effects of training on enzyme activities involved in purine nucleotide metabolism. Equine Vet J 1986; 18:72.

102. Harris RC, Katz A, Sahlin D, et al: The effect of freeze-drying on measurements of pH in biopsy samples of the middle gluteal muscle of the horse: Comparison of sample pH to the pyruvate + lactate content. Equine Vet J 1989; 21:45.

103. Raffin JP, Thebault MT: AMP deaminase from equine muscle: Purification and determination of regulatory properties. Int J Biochem 1991; 23:1069.

104. Essén-Gustavsson B, Valberg S: Blood and muscle ammonia concentrations in horses during treadmill work and after exercise. In Gillespie JR, Robinson NE (eds): Equine Exercise Physiology 2. Davis, Calif, ICEEP Publications, 1987, p 456.

105. Keenan DM: Changes in plasma uric acid levels in horses after galloping exercise. Res Vet Sci 1978; 25:127.

106. Sjøgaard G, Adams RP, Saltin B: Water and ion shifts in skeletal

muscle of humans with intense dynamic knee extension. Am J Physiol 1985; 248:R190.

107. Harris P, Snow DH: Plasma potassium and lactate concentrations in thoroughbred horses during exercise of varying intensity. Equine Vet J 1992; 23:220.

108. Medbø JI, Sejersted OM: Plasma potassium changes with high intensity exercise. J Physiol (Lond) 1990; 421:105.

109. Sahlin K, Broberg S: Release of K^+ from muscle during prolonged dynamic exercise. Acta Physiol Scand 1989; 136: 293.

110. Jeul C: The effects of β_2-adrenoceptor activation on ion shifts and fatigue in mouse soleus muscle stimulated in vitro. Acta Physiol Scand 1988; 134:209.

111. Snow DH, Harris RC, McDonald IA, et al: Effects of high-intensity exercise on plasma catecholamines in the thoroughbred horse. Equine Vet J 1992; 24:462.

112. Snow DH, Fixter LM, Kerr MG, et al: Alterations in composition of venous plasma FFA pool during prolonged and sprint exercise in the horse. In Knuttgen HG, Vogel JA, Poortmans J (eds): Biochemistry of Exercise (Proc 5th Int Meeting), Champaign, Illinois, Human Kinetics Publishers, 1983, p 336.

113. Foster CVL, Harris RC: Changes in free and bound carnitine in muscle with maximal sprint exercise in the thoroughbred horse. In Gillespie JR, Robinson NE (eds): Equine Exercise Physiology 2. Davis, Calif, ICEEP Publications, 1987, p 332.

114. Foster CVL, Harman J, Harris RC, et al: ATP distribution of single muscle fibres before and after maximal exercise in the horse. J Physiol (Lond) 1986; 378:64.

115. Foster CVL, Harris RC: Formation of acetylcarnitine in muscle of horse during high intensity exercise. Eur J Appl Physiol 1987; 56:639.

116. Pösö AR, Essén-Gustavsson B, Lindholm A, et al: Exercise-induced changes in muscle and plasma amino acid levels in the standardbred horse. In Persson SGB, Lindholm A, Jeffcott LB (eds): Equine Exercise Physiology 3. Davis, Calif, ICEEP Publications, 1991, p 202.

117. Rose RJ: Endurance exercise in the horse: A review, part 1. Br Vet J 1986; 142:532.

118. Lindholm A: Substrate utilization and muscle fiber types in standardbred trotters during exercise. Proc Am Assoc Equine Pract 1979; 25:329.

119. Pette D (ed): Plasticity of Muscle. Berlin, Walter de Gruyter, 1980.

120. Gunn HM: Growth changes in skeletal muscle histochemistry of thoroughbreds and other horses. In Persson SGB, Lindholm A, Jeffcott LB (eds): Equine Exercise Physiology 3. Davis, Calif, ICEEP Publications, 1991, p 245.

121. Raub RH, Kline KK, Lawrence LM, et al: Distribution of muscle fiber type in fetal equine gluteus medius muscle. J Equine Vet Sci 1986; 6:148.

122. Goldspink G: Malleability of the motor system: A comparative approach. J Exp Biol 1985; 115:375.

123. Thornton JR, Taylor AW: Skeletal muscle characteristics of foals at two to four weeks and eight months of age. In Snow DH, Persson SGB, Rose RJ (eds): Equine Exercise Physiology. Cambridge, Granta Editions, 1983, p 218.

124. Bechtel PJ, Kline KH: Muscle fiber type changes in the middle gluteal of quarter and standardbred horses from birth through one year of age. In Gillespie JR, Robinson NE (eds): Equine Exercise Physiology 2. Davis, Calif, ICEEP Publications, 1987, p 265.

125. Kline KH, Bechtel PJ: Changes in the metabolic profile of equine muscle from birth through one year of age. J Appl Physiol 1990; 68:1399.

126. Essén-Gustavsson B, Lindholm A, McMiken D, et al: Skeletal muscle characteristics of young standardbreds in relation to growth and early training. In Snow DH, Persson SGB, Rose RJ (eds): Equine Exercise Physiology. Cambridge, Granta Editions, 1983, p 200.

127. Roneus M, Essén-Gustavsson B, Lindholm A, et al: Skeletal muscle characteristics in young trained and untrained standardbred trotters. Equine Vet J 1992; 24:292.

128. Guy PS, Snow DH: The effect of training and detraining on muscle composition in the horse. J Physiol (Lond) 1977; 269:33.

129. Essén-Gustavsson B, Lindholm A, Thornton J: Histochemical properties of muscle fiber types and enzyme activities in skeletal muscles of standardbred trotters of different ages. Equine Vet J 1980; 12:175.

130. Lindholm A, Essén-Gustavsson B, McMiken D, et al: Muscle histochemistry and biochemistry of thoroughbred horses during growth and training. In Snow DH, Persson SGB, Rose RJ (eds): Equine Exercise Physiology. Cambridge, Granta Editions, 1983, p 211.

131. Straub R, Dettwiler M, Hoppeler H, et al: The use of morphometry and enzyme activity measurementes in skeletal muscles for the assessment of the working capacity of horses. In Snow DH, Persson SGB, Rose RJ (eds): Equine Exercise Physiology. Cambridge, Granta Editions, 1983, p 193.

132. Essén-Gustavsson B, Lindholm A: Muscle fibre characteristics of active and inactive standardbred horses. Equine Vet J 1985; 17:434.

133. Essén-Gustavsson B, McMiken D, Karlström K, et al: Muscular adaptation of horses during intensive training and detraining. Equine Vet J 1989; 21:27.

134. Roneus M, Essén-Gustavsson B, Lindholm A, et al: A field study of circulatory response and muscle characteristics in young thoroughbreds. In Gillespie JR, Robinson NE (eds): Equine Exercise Physiology 2. Davis, Calif, ICEEP Publications, 1987, p 376.

135. Hodgson DR, Rose RJ, Dimauro J, et al: Effects of training on muscle composition in horses. Am J Vet Res 1986; 47:12.

136. Hodgson DR, Rose RJ: Effects of a nine-month endurance training programme on muscle composition in the horse. Vet Rec 1987; 121:271.

137. Lovell DK, Rose RJ: Changes in skeletal muscle composition in response to interval and high intensity training. In Persson SGB, Lindholm A, Jeffcott LB (eds): Equine Exercise Physiology 3. Davis, Calif, ICEEP Publications, 1991, p 215.

138. Roneus M, Lindholm A, Åsheim A: Muscle characteristics in thoroughbreds of different ages and sexes. Equine Vet J 1991; 23:207.

139. Roneus M: Muscle characteristics in standardbred trotters of different ages and sexes. Equine Vet J (in press).

140. Lopez-Rivero JL, Morales-Lopez JL, Galisteo AM, et al: Muscle fibre type composition in untrained and endurance-trained Andalusian and Arab horses. Equine Vet J 1991; 23:91.

141. Straub R, Hoppeler H, Dettwiler M, et al: Beurteuchung der trainierbarkeit und der momentanen leistungskapazitart mit hilfe von Muskeluntersuchungen beim pferd. Schweiz Arch Tierheilk 1982; 124:529.

142. Wilson RG, Thornton JR, Inglis S, et al: Skeletal muscle adaptation in racehorses following high intensity interval training. In Gillespie JR, Robinson NE (eds): Equine Exercise Physiology 2. Davis, Calif, ICEEP Publications, 1987, p 367.

143. Foreman JH, Bayly WM, Allen JR, et al: Muscle responses of thoroughbreds to conventional race training and detraining. Am J Vet Res 1990; 51:909.

144. Cutmore CM, Snow DH, Newsholme EA: Activities of key enzymes of aerobic and anerobic metabolism in middle gluteal muscle from trained and untrained horses. Equine Vet J 1985; 17:354.

145. Snow DH, Guy PS: The effects of training and detraining on the activity of a number of enzymes in the horse skeletal muscle. Arch Int Physiol Biochem 1979; 87:87.

146. Guy PS, Snow DH: The effects of training and detraining on LDH isoenzymes in horse skeletal muscle. Biochem Biophy Res Commun 1977; 25:863.

147. Snow DH, Harris RD, Harman J, et al: Glycogen repletion following different diets. In Gillespie JR, Robinson NE (eds): Equine Exercise Physiology 2. Davis, Calif, ICEEP Publications, 1986, p 701.

148. Topliff DR, Potter GD, Dutson JL, et al: Diet manipulation and muscle glycogen in the equine. In Proceedings of the 8th Equine Nutrition and Physiology Symposium, 1983, p 119.

149. Topliff DR, Potter GD, Kreider JL, et al: Diet manipulation, muscle glycogen metabolism and anaerobic work performance in the equine. In Proceedings of the 9th Equine Nutrition and Physiology Symposium, 1985, p 224.

150. Oldham SL, Potter JD, Evans JW, et al: Storage and mobilization of muscle glycogen in racehorses fed a control and high-fat diet.

In Proceedings of the 11th Equine Nutrition and Physiology Symposium 1989, p 57.

151. Harkins JD, Morris GS, Tulley RT, et al: Effects of added dietary fat on racing performance in thoroughbred horses. J Equine Vet Sci 1992; 12:123.

152. Scott BD, Potter GD, Greene LW, et al: Efficacy of fat-supplemented diet on muscle glycogen concentration in exercising thoroughbred horses maintained in varying body conditions. J Equine Vet Sci 1992; 12:109.

153. Snow DH: A review of nutritional aids to energy production for athletic performance. Equine Athlete 1992;5(5):1.

154. Pagan JD, Essén-Gustavsson B, Lindholm A, et al: The effect of dietary energy source on exercise performance in standardbred horses. *In* Gillespie JR, Robinson NE (eds): Equine Exercise Physiology 2. Davis, Calif, ICEEP Publications, 1987, p 686.

155. Foster CVL, Harris RC: Plasma carnitine concentration in the horse following oral supplementation using a triple dose regime. Equine Vet J 1989; 21:376.

156. Foster CVL, Harris RC: Total carnitine content of the middle gluteal muscle of thoroughbred horses: Normal values, variability and effect of acute exercise. Equine Vet J 1992; 24:52.

157. Foster CVL, Harris RC, Snow DH: The effect of oral L-carnitine supplementation on the muscle and plasma concentrations in the thoroughbred horse. Comp Biochem Physiol [A] 1988; 91:827.

158. Foster CVL: Aspects of Carnitine Metabolism and Function in the Horse. Ph.D. thesis, C.N.A.A., United Kingdom, 1989.

159. Sewell DA, Harris RC, Dunnett M: Carnosine accounts for most of the variation in physico-chemical buffering in equine muscle. *In* Persson SGB, Lindholm A, Jeffcott LB (eds): Equine Exercise Physiology 3. Davis, Calif, ICEEP Publications, 1991, p 276.

160. Parkhouse WS, McKenzie DC, Hochochka PW, et al: The relationship between carnosine levels, buffering capacity, fiber type and anaerobic capacity in elite athletes. *In* Knuttgen HG, Vogel JA, Poortmans J (eds): Biochemistry of Exercise. Champaign, Illinois, Human Kinetics Publishers, 1983, p 590.

161. Harris RC, Marlin DJ, Dunnett M, et al: Muscle buffering capacity and dipeptide content in the thoroughbred horse, greyhound dog and man. Comp Biochem Physiol [A] 1990; 97:249.

162. Sewell DA, Harris RC, Marlin DJ, et al: Estimation of the carnosine content of different fibre types in the middle gluteal muscle of the thoroughbred horse. J Physiol (Lond) 1992; 455:447.

163. Marlin DJ, Harris RC, Gash SP, et al: Carnosine content of the middle gluteal muscle in thoroughbred horses with relation to age, sex and training. Comp Biochem Physiol [A] 1989; 93:629.

164. Bump KD, Lawrence LM, Moses LR, et al: Effect of breed type on muscle carnosine. *In* Proceedings of the 11th Equine Nutrition and Physiology Symposium, 1989, p 252.

165. Marlin DJ, Harris RC: Titrimetric determination of muscle buffering capacity (βm_{titr}) in biopsy samples. Equine Vet J 1991; 23:193.

166. McCutcheon LJ, Kelso TB, Bertocci LA, et al: Buffering and aerobic capacity in equine muscle: Variation and effect of training. *In* Gillespie JR, Robinson NE (eds): Equine Exercise Physiology 2. Davis, Calif, ICEEP Publications, 1987, p 348.

167. Fox G, Henckel P, Juel C, et al: Skeletal muscle buffer capacity changes in standardbred horses: Effect of growth and training. *In* Gillespie JR, Robinson NE (eds): Equine Exercise Physiology 2. Davis, Calif, ICEEP Publications, 1987, p 341.

168. Sinha AK, Ray SP, Rose RJ: Effect of training intensity and detraining on adaptations in different skeletal muscles. *In* Persson SGB, Lindholm A, Jeffcott LB (eds): Equine Exercise Physiology 3. Davis, Calif, ICEEP Publications, 1991, p 223.

169. Snow DH: Update on the use of sodium bicarbonate in horses. Equine Athlete 1992; 5(4):1.

170. Greenhaff PL, Harris RC, Snow DH, et al: The influence of metabolic alkalosis upon exercise metabolism in the thoroughbred horse. Eur J Appl Physiol 1991; 63:129.

171. Harris RC, Soderlund K, Hultman E: Elevation of creatine in resting and exercised muscle of normal subjects by creatine supplementation. Clin Sci 1992; 83:367.

172. Harris RC, Viru M, Greenhaff PL, et al: The effect of oral creatine supplemenation on running performance during short term exercise in man (abstract). J Physiol (Lond) 1993; 467–74P.

173. Baumann H, Jaggi M, Soland F, et al: Exercise training induces transitions of myosin isoform subunits within histochemically typed human muscle fibres. Pflugers Arch 1987; 409:349.

174. Lopez-Rivero JL, Galisteo AM, Aquera E, et al: Skeletal muscle histochemistry in male and female Andalusian and Arabian horses of different ages. Res Vet Sci (in press).

175. Evans JW, Borton A, Hintz HF, et al: The Horse. San Francisco, WH Freeman and Co, 1977.

176. Taylor AW, Brassard L: Skeletal muscle fiber distribution and area in trained and stalled standardbred horses. Can J Anim Sci 1981; 61:601.

177. Lopez-Rivero JL, Aquera E, Monterde JG, et al: Skeletal muscle fiber size in untrained and endurance-trained horses. Am J Vet Res 1992; 53:847.

178. Sjostrom M, Lexell J, Eriksson A, et al: Evidence of fibre hyperplasia in human skeletal muscles from healthy young men. Eur J Appl Physiol 1991; 62:301.

179. Snow DH, Vogel CJ: Equine Fitness: The Care and Training of the Athletic Horse. North Pomfret, Vermont, David and Charles, 1987, p 102.

180. Gottlieb-Vedi M: Circulatory and Muscle Metabolic Responses to Draught Work of Varying Intensity and Duration in Standardbred Horses. Ph.D. thesis, Uppsala, Sweden, Swedish University of Agricultural Sciences, 1988.

181. Snow DH: Anabolic steroids. *In* Sams R, Hinchcliff K (eds): Drug Use in Performance Horses. Philadelphia, WB Saunders Co, in press.

182. Griggs RC, Kingston W, Jozefowcz RF, et al: Effect of testosterone on muscle mass and muscle protein synthesis. J Appl Physiol 1989; 66:498.

183. Elsahoff JD, Jacknow AD, Shain SG, et al: Effects of anabolic-androgenic steroids on muscular strength. Ann Intern Med 1991; 115:387.

184. Snow DH, Munro CD, Nimmo MA: The effect of nandrolone phenylpropionate in the horse: 2. General effects in animals undergoing training. Equine Vet J 1982; 14:224.

185. Thornton J, Dowsett KF, Mann R, et al: Influence of anabolic steroids on the response of training to 2 year old horses. *In* Persson SGB, Lindholm A, Jeffcott LB (eds): Equine Exercise Physiology 3. Davis, Calif, ICEEP Publications, 1991, p 503.

186. Snow DH, Munro CD, Nimmo MA: Effects of nandrolone phenylpropionate in the horse: 1. Resting animal. Equine Vet J 1982; 14:219.

187. Saltin B, Henriksson J, Nygaard E, et al: Fiber types and metabolic potentials of skeletal muscles in sedentary man and endurance runners. Ann NY Acad Sci 1977; 301:3.

188. Komi PV, Vitasalo J, Hasu M, et al: Skeletal muscle fibres and muscle enzyme activities in monozygous and dizygous twins of both sexes. Acta Physiol Scand 1977; 100:385.

189. Nimmo MA, Wilson RH, Snow DH: The inheritance of skeletal muscle fiber composition in mice. Comp Biochem Physiol [A] 1985; 81:109.

190. Lopez-Rivero JL, Aguera E, Monterde JG, et al: Comparative study of muscle fiber type composition in the middle gluteal muscle of Andalusian, thoroughbred and Arabian horses. J Equine Vet Sci 1989; 9:337.

191. Staun H: Various factors affecting number and size of muscle fibres in the pig. Acta Agriculture Scand 1963; 13:293.

192. Gunn HM: Total fibre numbers in cross sections of the semitendinosus in athletic and non-athletic horses and dogs. J Anat 1979; 128:821.

193. Barlow DA, Lloyd JM, Hellhake P, et al: Equine muscle fiber types: A histological and histochemical analysis of select thoroughbred yearlings. J Equine Vet Sci 1984; 4:60.

194. Wood HC, Ross TT, Armstrong JB, et al: Variations in muscle fiber composition between successfully and unsuccessfully raced quarter horses. J Equine Vet Sci 1988; 8:217.

195. Roneus M, Essén-Gustavsson B, Arnason T: Racing performance and longitudinal changes in muscle characteristics in standardbred trotters. J Equine Vet Sci 1993; 13:355.

196. Freestone JF, Carlson GP: Muscle disorders in the horse: A retrospective study. Equine Vet J 1991; 23:86.

197. Hodgson DR: Diseases of muscle. *In* Smith BP (ed): Large Animal Internal Medicine. Philadelphia, WB Saunders Co, 1988, p 1335.

198. Morris E, Seeherman HJ, O'Callaghan MW, et al: Scintigraphic

identification of skeletal muscle damage in horses 24 hours after strenuous exercise. Equine Vet J 1991; 23:347.

199. Grounds MD: Towards understanding skeletal muscle regeneration. Pathol Res Pract 1991; 187:1.

200. McEwen SA, Hulland TJ: Histochemical and morphometric evaluation of skeletal muscle from horses with exertional rhabdomyolysis (tying-up). Vet Pathol 1986; 23:400.

201. Meijer VAEFH, van den Hoven R, Wensing T, et al: Histochemical changes in skeletal muscle of racehorses susceptible to exertional rhabdomyolysis: I. Early myopathic changes. Acta Histochem 1989; 87:1.

202. Harris PA: The equine rhabdomyolysis syndrome in the United Kingdom: Epidemiological and clinical descriptive information. Br Vet J 1991; 147:373.

203. Penn AS: Myoglobinuria. In Engel AG, Brown BQ (eds): Myology. New York, McGraw-Hill, 1986, p 1785.

204. Harris PA: An outbreak of equine rhabdomyolysis syndrome in a racing yard. Vet Rec 1990; 127:468.

205. Valberg S, Jönsson L, Holmgren N: Muscle histopathology and plasma aspartate aminotransferase, creatine kinase and myoglobin changes with exercise in horses with recurrent exertional rhabdomyolysis. Equine Vet J 1993; 25:11.

206. Carlström B: Uber die atiologie und pathogenese der kreuzlahme des pferdes (Haemoglobinaemia paralytica). Scand Arch 1931; 62:1.

207. Valberg S, Häggendal J, Lindholm A: Blood chemistry and skeletal muscle metabolic responses to exercise in horses with recurrent exertional rhabdomyolysis. Equine Vet J 1993; 25:17.

208. Owens R, Moore JN, Hopkins JB, et al: Dystrophic myodegeneration in adult horses. J Am Vet Med Assoc 1977; 17:343.

209. Ronéus B, Hakkarainen J: Vitamin E in skeletal muscle tissue and blood glutathione peroxidase activity from horses with azoturia–tying-up syndrome. Acta Vet Scand 1985; 26:425.

210. Bain FT, Merritt AM: Decreased erythrocyte potassium concentration associated with exercise-related myopathy in horses. J Am Vet Med Assoc 1990; 196:1259.

211. Harris PA, Snow DH: Role of electrolyte imbalances in the pathophysiology of the equine rhabdomyolysis syndrome. In Persson SGB, Lindholm A, Jeffcott JR (eds): Equine Exercise Physiology 3. Davis, Calif, ICEEP Publications, 1991, p 435.

212. Harris PA, Colles C: The use of creatinine clearance ratios in the prevention of equine rhabdomyolysis: A report of four cases. Equine Vet J 1988; 20:459.

213. Hodgson DR: Exercise-associated myopathy: Is calcium the culprit? Equine Vet J 1993; 25:1.

214. Valberg SJ: Unpublished data, 1992.

215. Harris PA, Marlin D, Gray J: Equine thyroid function tests: A preliminary investigation. Br Vet J 1992; 148:71.

216. Frauenfelder HC, Rossdale PD, Rickets SW: Changes in serum muscle enzyme levels associated with training schedules and stages of oestrous cycle in thoroughbred racehorses. Equine Vet J 1986; 18:371.

217. Valberg SJ, Cardinet GH III: Glyco(geno)lytic capacity of skeletal muscle in horses with recurrent rhabdomyolysis. In Persson SGB, Lindholm A, Jeffcott JR (eds): Equine Exercise Physiology 3. Davis, Calif, ICEEP Publications, 1991, p 429.

218. Valberg S, Cardinet GH III, Carlson GP, et al: Polysaccharide storage myopathy associated with exertional rhabdomyolysis in the horse. Neuromuscular Disord 1992; 2:351.

219. Scholte HE, Verduin MHM, Ross JD, et al: Equine exertional rhabdomyolysis: Activity of the mitochondrial respiratory chain and carnitine system in skeletal muscle. Equine Vet J 1991; 23:142.

220. Waldron-Mease E: Correlation of post-operative and exercise-induced equine myopathy with the defect malignant hyperthermia. Proc Am Assoc Equine Pract 1978; 24:95.

221. Fujii J, Otsu K, Korato F, et al: Identification of a mutation in porcine ryanodine receptor associated with malignant hyperthermia. Science 1991; 253:448.

222. Beech J, Fletcher JE, Lizzo F, et al: Effect of phenytoin on the clinical signs and in vitro muscle twitch characteristics in horses with chronic intermittent rhabdomyolysis. Am J Vet Res 1988; 49:2130.

223. Beech J, Lindborg S, Fletcher JE, et al: Caggience contractures, twitch characteristics and the threshold for Ca^{2+}-induced Ca^{2+} release in skeletal muscle from horses with chronic intermittent rhabdomyolysis. Res Vet Sci 1993; 54:110.

224. Arighi M, Baird JD, Hulland TJ: Equine exertional rhabdomyolysis. Comp Cont Ed 1984; 6:S726.

225. Lindholm A, Johansson HF, Kjaersgaard P: Acute rhabdomyolysis (tying-up) in standardbred horses: A morphological and biochemical study. Acta Vet Scand 1974; 15:325.

226. Meijer VAEFH, van den Hoven R, Wensing T, et al: Histochemical changes in skeletal muscle of racehorses susecptible to exertional rhabdomyolysis: II. Later myopathological and regeneration phenomena. Acta Histochem 1989; 87:13.

227. Valberg SJ, Carlson GP, Cardinet GH III, et al: Skeletal muscle mitochondrial myopathy as a cause of exercise intolerance in a horse. Muscle Nerve (in press).

228. Bloom W, Fawcett DW: A Textbook of Histology. Philadelphia, WB Saunders Co, 1986, p 282.

229. Bloom W, Fawcett DW: A Textbook of Histology. Philadelphia, WB Saunders Co, 1986, p 287.

230. Krstic RV: General Histology of the Mammal. New York, Springer-Verlag, 1984, p 265.

231. Lazarides E, Capetanaki YG: The striated muscle cytoskeleton: expression and assembly in development. In Emerson C, Fischman DA, Nadal-Ginard B, Siddiqui MAQ (eds): Molecular Biology of Muscle Development. New York, Alan R Liss 1985, p 756.

232. Krstic RV: General Histology of the Mammal. New York, Springer Verlag, 1984, p 273.

9

Thermoregulation

FINOLA McCONAGHY

The athletic horse during exercise derives energy for muscular contraction from the conversion of stored chemical energy to mechanical energy. This process is relatively inefficient, and about 80 percent of the energy released from energy stores is lost as heat.[1] If this heat is not dissipated, life-threatening elevations in body temperature may develop. The physiologic mechanisms that effect heat dissipation, governed by the thermoregulatory system, are essential for the horse to function as an athletic animal.

The primary means of heat dissipation in the horse is evaporation of sweat. Evaporative cooling is an efficient mechanism enabling horses to perform a variety of athletic events with only minor elevations in body temperature. However, exercise-induced heat stress can occur when heat production during exercise exceeds heat dissipation. This is likely when animals are forced to exercise in adverse environmental conditions (i.e., high temperature and humidity), when they have been inadequately conditioned, or when they are suffering an impairment of the thermoregulatory system (anhidrosis). Careful preparation for athletic events, monitoring during events, and early recognition of impending signs of heat stress will minimize the risk of development of life-threatening hyperthermia.

Horses have coped with temperatures as variable as 58°C in Northern Australia[2] to −40°C in western Canada.[3] Despite large fluctuations in environmental temperature, horses are able to maintain their internal body temperature within a very narrow range by elaborate thermoregulatory mechanisms. The thermoregulatory system controls body temperature by altering heat flow between the animal and its environment.

Mechanisms of Heat Transfer

Heat will flow from one area to another by four basic mechanisms: radiation, convection, conduction, and evaporation. Homeothermy requires that heat produced or gained from the environment equals heat loss to the environment, as indicated by the equation[4,5]

$$\text{Gains} = \text{Losses}$$
$$M - W = \pm R \pm C \pm K + E$$

where
M = metabolic heat production
W = mechanical work
R = heat exchange by radiation
C = heat exchange by convection
K = heat exchange by conduction
E = heat exchange by evaporation

RADIATION

Radiation involves the movement of heat between objects without direct physical contact via electromagnetic radiation of two distinct types. *Short-wave,* or *solar, radiation* is received from the sun by any object exposed to sunlight. *Long-wave radiation* is emitted and absorbed by the surfaces of all organisms and relates to heat interchanges between an animal and its surroundings.

The heat load from solar radiation, both direct and reflected, can be significant in hot environments, where animals are exposed to sunlight for prolonged periods. When an animal is standing in bright sunlight, the amount of solar radiation absorbed may exceed approximately ≈800 W/m², significantly greater than its own metabolic heat production.[6]

CONVECTION

Convection occurs within all fluids due to the mixing of particles within the fluid. Temperature differences within the fluid result in a difference in the density of the fluid particles. Warm particles are less dense and will rise, whereas cold particles will fall. Free convective heat transfer takes place at the surface of a solid body within a fluid medium which is at a different temperature. This type of transfer takes place continuously between the surface of the body and the surrounding air. Forced convective heat transfer occurs if there are fluid movements induced by gross pressure differences, e.g., due to wind blowing across the body surface.[7] Free convection at the skin surface can result in significant heat losses if ambient air temperatures are low. A hair coat will entrap a layer of air close to the skin and resist convective heat transfer. Wind will increase forced convective losses by disrupting this insulating layer. The hair coat of the horse is generally fine and sleek in summer to aid heat loss,[2] whereas in winter a thick hair coat develops, with acclimatization to cold stress, resulting in increased insulation.[8]

CONDUCTION

Direct transfer of heat between surfaces that are in contact occurs as a result of *conduction.* In the standing animal, most of this transfer is to air, which has poor thermal conductivity, and thus conductive heat transfer plays a small role in the total heat balance. However, this route of heat transfer can become significant if the animal is lying on a cool or wet surface.

A number of behavioral strategies are utilized by animals to affect conductive heat exchange. Changes in posture can alter the surface area available for heat exchange. For example, by lying down and drawing the limbs close to the body, the surface area can be reduced considerably. In contrast, morphologic adaptation by burros and mules (long ears, short legs, and lean body conformation) increases available surface area for convective heat loss and may help increase heat tolerance.[2]

The extremities of animals, the limbs and head, have a high surface area to mass ratio, and thus maximal conductive heat exchange can occur at these sites. Changes in surface temperature at these sites can be affected by alterations of skin blood flow. The skin temperature of the horse, reflecting skin blood flow, varies in direct proportion to ambient temperature, with greatest temperature changes occurring at the extremities.[9-11]

At low ambient temperature, local vascular shunts direct blood away from the extremities to reduce the rate of convective heat loss, while at high temperatures, vasodilation occurs to promote heat loss.[8,10] An example of how horses utilize this mechanism is provided by noting that skin temperature will fall from 26°C at an ambient temperature of 25°C to 17°C at 15°C (ambient), and even further vasoconstriction occurs at an ambient temperature of 5°C with skin temperature decreasing to 10°C.[10]

EVAPORATION

Evaporation is the principal means by which homeotherms, such as horses, lose heat in warm environments via the physiologic processes of panting, sweating, and insensible perspiration. The conversion of water from liquid to vapor is an endothermic process. Thus evaporation of water at the surface of the body results in heat loss. The exact amount of energy involved in this process is dependent on the temperature and vapor pressure of the surrounding air.[4] The latent heat of vaporization of 1 g of water is 598 cal (2501 J) at 0°C and 575 cal (2406 J) at 40°C.[12] Evaporation of 1 liter of sweat in a human being can remove 580 kcal (2428 kJ) from the body[13] (1 calorie = 4.186 J).

The skin–ambient vapor pressure difference is the driving force for vaporization. When the vapor pressure at the skin surface reaches a maximum value, corresponding to saturation at skin temperature, sweat rate exceeds evaporation rate, and sweat drips off the skin without resulting in cooling. This corresponds to the limit of the efficiency of sweating and is usually associated with rising body temperature.[14] This limit will be reached faster if the air vapor pressure is high, as occurs in humid conditions.

During panting, inspired air is almost fully saturated with water at a temperature similar to the deep-body temperature as it passes over the wet surfaces of the upper respiratory tract. The associated heat loss is governed by the ambient air humidity and respiratory ventilation rate. Although horses do not pant routinely, there is evidence of considerable evaporative heat loss from the respiratory tract during exercise in response to normal ventilation.[15,16]

Insensible perspiration involves the passage of water through the skin by processes other than sweating. The skin is not impermeable to water, and thus water can diffuse out as a result of the skin–ambient vapor pressure gradient. In humans, approximately 10 g/m²/h of water passes through the skin in ambient conditions, increasing to 30 g/m²/h in a warm environment.[12]

Regulation of Internal Body Temperature

Thermoregulatory mechanisms maintain the body temperature of homeotherms within a narrow range by regulating heat production and heat loss. A complex neurophysiologic mechanism is present which regulates internal body temperature. The principal neuronal elements of the thermoregulatory system are peripheral thermoreceptors, the spinal cord,[17] and the hypothalamus.[18,19] Peripheral thermoreceptor organs are located in a number of locations, including the skin, the buccal cavity, skeletal muscle, the abdomen, regions of the spinal cord, the medulla oblongata, and the preoptic–anterior hypothalamic region of the midbrain.[20] These temperature-sensitive structures are responsible for detection of a disturbance and produce proportional nerve impulses. In order for information from thermosensitive receptors in several parts of the body to be translated into appropriate instructions to the effector organs, there must be convergence of the neural pathways from these temperature sensors and transmission of this information to an interpretive center. A coordinating center in the central nervous system receives afferent nerve impulses and produces efferent impulses, initiating a correction that is transmitted to the effector organs. There is considerable evidence from animal experiments that the hypothalamus may represent this interpretive center. Thermal stimulation of peripheral temperature sensors, the spinal cord,[17] and the hypothalamus[18,19] results in appropriate thermoregulatory effector activity. However, destruction of the hypothalamus affects thermoregulatory responses to local heating of all these structures. This suggests that integrity of particular hypothalamic areas is necessary for normal thermoregulation and that most of the regulation of internal temperature occurs in the hypothalamus. Effector organs are responsible for correction of the initial disturbance, which, in turn, will result in a reduction of stimulation of sensory organs.

Physiologic Thermoregulatory Mechanisms for Heat Loss

The thermoregulatory system utilizes various mechanisms of heat flow to effect heat loss from the body. Highly effective mechanisms for dissipating heat include sweating and panting, which exploit the significant heat loss associated with the evaporation of water, in addition to convective heat loss. The cardiovascular system has a role in thermoregulation, blood flow being used as a means for heat transfer from sites of heat production within the body core to areas where dissipation of heat can occur, primarily the skin and respiratory tract.

Mechanisms of Evaporative Heat Loss

The principal physiologic thermoregulatory mechanisms that utilize the vaporization of water from the body surface are panting and sweating. The Hominoidae, including humans, and the Equidae are the only families which depend on sweating as the primary mechanism for thermoregulation,[21] while the sheep, dog, and pig rely much more on respiratory heat loss.[22]

Panting has advantages over sweating in that its efficiency is not limited by the hair coat, which can insulate the animal against both radiant heat and the effects of cold, as well as reducing fluid and electrolyte losses in sweat. Disadvantages of panting exist during exercise, when there is competition between maximal gaseous exchange and maximal evaporative heat loss.

HUMANS

Sweating is the most important means of heat loss in human beings, with respiratory heat loss accounting for only 11 percent of total heat loss in a thermoneutral environment.[23] This percentage increases with rising core temperature. Minute volume, which is directly related to respiratory heat loss,[24] increases with rising core temperature by approximately 1.5 liter/min/°C.[25] Increasing minute volume increases heat loss by 0.17 W/liter at 30°C and even higher at lower ambient temperatures, to 0.69 W/liter at 10°C.[25]

HORSES

Like humans, horses rely primarily on sweating for heat loss, with the respiratory tract contributing to heat loss especially during exercise. Respiratory frequency has been reported to be dependent on environmental temperature during rest and exercise, increasing 1.9 breaths/min for every 1°C increase in ambient temperature.[26] In contrast, Honstein and Monty[27] found no significant difference in respiratory frequency between horses at rest in a cool and warm environment, but the environmental conditions were variable, since the experiment was carried out in natural conditions, but in a climate-controlled room. Investigations of the exact proportion of heat dissipated by the respiratory tract have reported different values depending on the type of horse, the ambient temperature, and the exercise level. Ponies at rest in ambient conditions (21 to 23°C) lose 14 to 22 percent of total heat production by pulmonary ventilation,[11] while horses in a cooler environment of 16°C show a respiratory heat loss of 38 percent at rest and 17 percent during maximal exercise.[28] While horses do not normally pant,[29] if evaporation of sweat is limited by high humidity or anhidrosis, they may experience tachypnea.[30] Pulse-respiratory inversion (respiratory rate in excess of heart rate), frequently shown by endurance horses during recovery from exercise in hot humid environments,[31] may represent a form of panting.

The reliance of humans and horses on sweating may relate to their need to lose heat during sustained activity. This is supported by the greater sweat rate produced in horses by epinephrine infusion than by elevation of environmental temperature.[32]

In horses, rectal temperature is reported to be significantly higher (~0.5°C greater) in hot than in thermoneutral environments.[9] Temperature variations such as these may reflect an adaptation to desert environments, similar to that in camels.[33] In order to limit the need for sweating, some species inhabiting hot arid environments have relatively labile body temperatures allowing storage of heat. Body temperatures of the camel rise to 41°C during the day and decrease to as low as 34°C during the night.[34] Such thermolability obviates the need for evaporative cooling, thus conserving water.[35]

Evaporative Heat Loss from the Respiratory Tract

Heat exchange occurs within the large surface area of the upper respiratory tract.[12] Inspired air is heated to body temperature and saturated with water vapor by the time it reaches the alveoli. During expiration, some heat passes back to the mucosa, and some condensation of water occurs. The difference between the initial heat transfer to the inspired air and the transfer back to the mucosa is the respiratory heat loss. The quantity of heat loss depends on the environmental temperature and humidity; the warmer and more humid the air, the smaller is the heat loss. In some animals, panting increases ventilation rate, resulting in greater heat loss from the respiratory tract.[36,37]

Evaporative Heat Loss from Sweating

FUNCTION OF THE SWEAT GLANDS

The glands of the general body surface of humans have a primary heat-regulatory function, whereas the glands on the palms and soles are concerned with emotional responses and are insensitive to heat. The sweat glands of the horse resemble the sweat glands of humans in their heat-regulatory function.[30] Specialized sweat glands in specific locations (e.g., perianal, inguinal) are regarded as scent glands and discharge odoriferous substances. These glands may have a role in sexual activity and have a function in the establishment of territories.

CHEMICAL COMPOSITION OF SWEAT

Humans. The ionic concentration of sweat in humans varies markedly between individuals and is strongly affected by the sweating rate and the state of heat acclimatization of the subject.[38-42] Human thermogenic sweat is hypotonic relative to plasma. Sodium chloride is the main constituent, with the chloride concentration being 30 to 50 mM[39] and sodium concentration 20 to 60 mM[39,43] (Table 9–1). The concentration of NaCl increases as sweat rate increases. Increased activity results in increased electrolyte concentration in both serum and

Table 9-1. Electrolyte Composition of Equine and Human Sweat

	Na$^+$	K$^+$	Cl$^-$
Horse			
Jirka and Kotas, 1959	382	48	432
Soliman and Nadim, 1967	593	48	—
Carlson and Ocen, 1979	132	53	174
Kerr et al., 1980	146	55	199
Rose et al., 1980	249	78	301
Kerr et al., 1983	147	57	200
Plasma composition	139	3.7	100
Man			
Costill et al., 1977	50	4.7	40
Plasma composition	140	4	101

sweat.[44] During short-term strenuous exercise, the NaCl concentration may increase by up to 50 percent above initial values, while prolonged exercise tends to result in decreases in the concentration of electrolytes in sweat.[40,42,44–46]

Potassium concentration in sweat is only slightly higher than that of plasma at low sweat rates (10 to 35 mM) and decreases to 5 mM as sweat rate increases. Potassium secretion is not affected by acclimization or dietary intake.[47] Sweat calcium concentration similarly decreases with increasing sweat rate from 3 to 10 mM to 1 to 2 mM. Bicarbonate concentration is 2 to 10 mM and tends to increase with sweat rate. Traces of magnesium, iodide, phosphorus, sulfate, iron, zinc, copper, cobalt, lead, manganese, molybdenum, tin, and mercury are also present, as well as negligible amounts of vitamins.[48]

Formation of Sweat in Humans. In humans, a highly sophisticated mechanism for electrolyte reabsorption is present in the sweat glands. An ultrafiltrate of plasma-like isotonic precursor fluid ($Na^+ = 150$ mM, $Cl^- = 124$ mM) is secreted by the secretory coil of the sweat gland. As the precursor fluid flows through the duct, much of the sodium chloride is reabsorbed in excess of water, resulting in sweat that is hyposmotic.[49]

The absorption of NaCl by the duct is due to active transport of the Na^+ by a $Na^+ - K^+$ sensitive ATPase. Na^+ diffuses passively from the lumen to the cell interior and is then actively pumped out from the cell to the interstitium at the peritubular cell membrane in exchange for K^+, with Cl^- passively following Na^+.[49]

The principal factor resulting in the reduction of NaCl in sweat that occurs with prolonged heat exposure appears to be an increase in activity of the pituitary-adrenal cortex mechanism elicited by a salt deficiency.[42]

Equine Sweat Composition. The composition of horse sweat during exercise, heat stress, and epinephrine infusion has been measured by a number of investigators.[50–58] The concentration of electrolytes reported in these studies is presented in Table 9–1. A number of methods of sweat collection have been utilized in these studies of sweat composition, including directly scraping sweat off the horse, collecting the drops that run off the horse, and collecting the sweat onto absorbent pads. Residual electrolytes from previous sweating and artificial elevation due to evaporation also will alter the sweat composition. These methodologic problems may explain the significantly higher electrolyte concentration reported by the early investigators[51,52] when compared with later studies.

Equine sweat, unlike that of humans, is hypertonic relative to plasma, with a sodium concentration similar or slightly higher than plasma, chloride significantly higher, and potassium 10 to 20 times greater than serum concentrations. High-intensity exercise in horses produces more dilute sweat than low-intensity prolonged exercise (McConaghy et al., unpublished data), a process that may be due to increased epinephrine concentrations that result during high-intensity exercise.[58,59] Epineph-

rine infusion results in production of more dilute sweat than that occurring during exercise.[53,57] Epinephrine concentrations are elevated during exercise in horses,[58,59] and sweat in this species is produced in response to both sympathetic nervous activity and circulating epinephrine.[57,60,61] There is little change in sweat electrolyte concentration with prolonged sweating in response to submaximal exercise[55–57] or in response to training (McConaghy et al., unpublished data).

Sweat produced by the horse has an unusually high concentration of a protein relative to many other species. This protein is referred to as *latherin*[62] and is responsible for producing the lather seen on horses after exercise. Latherin has a surfactant-like action, promoting spreading and evaporation of sweat and possibly aiding evaporation and cooling.[63–65]

INNERVATION OF THE SWEAT GLANDS

The primary sudomotor mechanism in humans is cholinergic,[49] whereas in the majority of other species the sudomotor mechanism is essentially an adrenergic sympathetic one.[66] Sweating appears to be under sympathetic nervous control in the cow, sheep, goat, pig, donkey, and horse.[66] This innervation involves alpha receptors in the cow, sheep, and goat, alpha and beta receptors in the dog, and $beta_2$ receptors in the horse.[67–69]

The exact action of the nervous system on sweat glands is not clear. The final stimulus to the glands must be humoral, either blood-borne or released from adjacent nerve endings.[70] For example, sweat glands in humans, horses, and the footpads of dogs and cats have a nerve supply closely associated with them.[66,71,72] However, in the majority of other species, there must be a nonneural peripheral component in the sudomotor control mechanism. The sweat glands of humans, dogs, and horses respond to both adrenergic and cholinergic drugs,[73,74] whereas those of sheep and goats,[75] donkeys,[76] and pigs[77] respond to adrenergic but not cholinergic substances.

Experimentally, sweating in horses can be stimulated by intravenous and local injection of epinephrine.[74,78–80] However norepinephrine, the usual adrenergic postganglionic neurotransmitter, results in minimal sweating.[59,61,67] During exercise, the circulating epinephrine concentration is sufficient to cause sweating.[80] Stimulation of the sympathetic chain in horses inhibits sweating,[79] while loss of sympathetic outflow stimulates sweating.

Circulatory Adjustments for Thermoregulation

The flow of blood is a highly effective avenue for heat transfer via conduction. By altering blood flow between various organs, the cardiovascular system can act as a major thermoregulatory effector mechanism. Thermoregulation via adjustments in blood flow is so efficient that thermal stability under the range of thermoneutral conditions can be maintained by the balance between peripheral vasodilation and vasoconstriction.

The principal means for the role of the cardiovascular system as a thermoregulatory effector include (1) increasing the cardiac output ($\dot{Q}$) and (2) redistributing the cardiac output, particularly blood flow to the skin.

SKIN BLOOD FLOW

On exposure to heat, an increase in blood flow to the skin occurs which results in conduction of heat to the surface of the body, thus increasing skin temperature and facilitating convective heat loss from the body to the environment. In more severe heat stress, blood flow to the skin also provides the latent heat for vaporization of sweat and supplies fluid for sweat production. In cold environments, reduced blood flow to the skin decreases skin temperature, limiting heat loss from the body.

The anatomic arrangement of the skin vasculature is designed to facilitate heat transfer. Three plexuses of vessels are present in the skin such that a large volume of blood can be redistributed to the skin to maximize heat loss. Specialized vessels, arteriovenous anastamoses (AVAs) are present in the skin which contribute to this process. AVAs are short vessels that connect arteries and veins, and opening of these vessels results in bypass of capillary beds, allowing a greatly increased blood flow through the skin.

Control of skin blood flow is primarily mediated by the sympathetic nervous system. Response to heat involves vasodilation of arterioles and AVAs, while vasoconstriction in response to cold involves both arterioles and veins.

CARDIAC OUTPUT

In response to heating, cardiac output ($\dot{Q}$) rises in order to maintain central blood pressure in the face of increased skin blood flow. In humans, cardiac output commonly increases 50 to 70 percent[81] in response to heat stress and may more than double if the increase in core temperature exceeds 2°C. The increase in sympathetic nervous activity associated with heat stress results in a rise in heart rate and an increase in myocardial contractile force and stroke volume.[82,83] The alteration in $\dot{Q}$ in the horse during heat stress is unknown.

REDISTRIBUTION OF THE CARDIAC OUTPUT

Redistribution of the $\dot{Q}$ will differ between species depending on the relative importance of the two major heat loss mechanisms, sweating and panting.[84] In panting animals, such as sheep and dogs, heat stress causes major increases in blood flow to respiratory muscles[85] and the nasobuccal regions.[86] However, animals such as humans and horses, which rely on sweating for heat loss, show an increased blood flow to the skin.[81]

Redistribution of the $\dot{Q}$ in response to heat stress has not been studied in the horse. Because of the similarities between the thermoregulatory systems of horses and humans, similar responses to heat stress may occur. Exact measurements of redistribution of the $\dot{Q}$ are not possible in humans. However, all available estimates indicate that the entire increase in $\dot{Q}$ that occurs in heat stress is directed to the skin.[82] In all the major organs in which flow has been measured (sphlanchnic, renal, and skeletal muscle), decreases in blood flow occur.[13] The decrease in renal and splanchnic blood flows are reported to be on the order of 25 to 40 percent.[81]

Thermoregulation During Exercise

During exercise, the chemical processes involved in supplying energy for muscular activity produce a significant amount of heat as a by-product. As a result, the thermal loads that the body can be exposed to during prolonged exercise can rival those which occur in the most extreme environments. For example, a hot environment can impose a thermal load of approximately 200 W, while exercise can produce one of about 1000 W.[87] Without thermoregulatory mechanisms to dissipate metabolic heat loads, body temperature could be elevated 1°C with every 5 to 8 minutes of exercise.[88]

It was observed by Nielsen in 1938[89] that a stable elevation of internal body temperature occurs during exercise in humans which is proportional to the intensity of exercise and relatively independent of environmental changes. In 1966, Saltin and Hermansen[90] further investigated this relationship in humans and discovered that body temperature elevation during exercise is related to the relative rather than the absolute work load.[91] A similar relationship is reported to exist in horses.[92] Robinson in 1949[93] first observed the linear relationship between sweating rate and internal temperature, with the elevated body core temperature during exercise triggering a heat-dissipation response that is related to the magnitude of the elevation. These observations have been instrumental in the attempt to define temperature regulation during exercise.

Under normal circumstances during exercise, a metabolic heat load is produced that is proportional to the intensity of the exercise bout. This heat load is transferred from working muscles to the body core, resulting in elevation of core temperature. Sweating is initiated at a certain core temperature, dictated also by skin temperature, and sweating continues at a rate proportional to the increase in core temperature. At some point, determined by environmental conditions, the evaporative rate will match the rate of energy production. At this point, heat production will equal heat loss, and the body temperature will become stable and constant at a higher than resting core temperature.[93]

Energy Exchanges During Exercise

Heat transfer in the horse during exercise is depicted in Figure 9–1. At the onset of exercise, the rate of heat production in muscle greatly exceeds the rate of heat dissipation, resulting in a rapid elevation of muscle temperature. Muscle temperature can increase at a rate of 1°C/min at the beginning of strenuous exercise,[94] and muscle temperatures of 45°C have been reported in exercising horses.[15,95,96] Heat flows down the temperature gradient

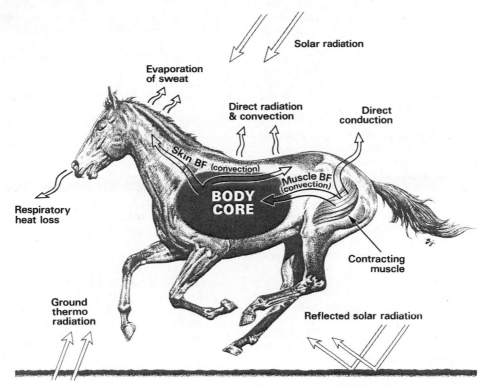

Figure 9-1. *Mechanisms for the transfer of heat within the body of a horse during exercise. Heat is gained as a by-product of muscular work and via radiation from the environment. Heat load is dissipated via evaporative, convective, and conductive mechanisms.*

from the muscle to the surrounding tissue primarily via convection. An additional small amount of heat is transferred by direct conduction. The convective transfer occurs as a result of blood flow through the muscle. Muscle blood flow is greatly increased during exercise, which both increases oxygen supply and enhances removal of metabolic wastes and heat. Increases in blood flow to the working muscles of the horse of tenfold or greater from resting levels have been recorded immediately after exercise from the iliac artery.[97]

During the early minutes of exercise, heat storage exceeds heat dissipation, and core temperature rises in proportion to the exercise intensity. The rise in core temperature during exercise has a number of advantages. It allows storage of heat, which reduces the amount of heat that must be dissipated. In addition, a moderate elevation of muscle temperature results in an improvement of muscular performance,[98] facilitates oxygen release from red blood cells,[99] and causes an increase in maximal heart rate.[100] Metabolic reactions are accelerated, and enzyme activity is enhanced by moderate increases in temperature; thus energy production is faster when core temperature is elevated.[101]

The core temperature rises slowly, reflecting the large amount of energy that can be stored within the entire body mass. As the rate of heat dissipation rises to balance the rate of heat production, core temperature reaches a plateau and remains relatively stable for the duration of exercise. The rise in core temperature stimulates centrally located thermoreceptors, causing an increase in blood flow to the skin and the initiation of sweating. The increase in skin blood flow transfers heat to the skin for dissipation. The net transfer of heat from the muscles to the skin for dissipation depends on the core to skin temperature gradient.[87] Skin temperature is initially lower than the core temperature. At the onset of exercise, skin temperature falls slightly due to increased convection resulting from the motion of the subject and then gradually rises. When skin temperature is high, as in a warm environment, heat transfer to the skin is compromised.

Heat is transferred from the skin to the environment by convection, radiation, sweat evaporation, and respiratory losses. Environmental conditions, mainly temperature, govern which of these modes is most effective. Loss of heat by convection and radiation depends on a temperature difference between the skin and the environment. When environmental temperature is low (~10°C), the mean skin temperature will be approximately 25 to 28°C, resulting in a temperature difference of 15 to 18°C. Under these conditions, convection and radiation alone would be sufficient to dissipate the entire heat load imposed by moderate exercise. As the ambient temperature increases, the skin-environmental temperature gradient falls, becoming negligible at about 36°C and actually reversing at higher environmental temperatures. Thus heat loss via convection and radiation becomes ineffective, and the body must rely on sweat evaporation for heat loss.

In moderate ambient temperatures, approximately 50 percent of the metabolic heat load is dissipated by radiation and convection and the other 50 percent by evaporation.[102] However, when skin temperature and ambient temperature are equal, evaporative cooling becomes the only avenue for dissipation of heat. The rate of heat loss by evaporation of sweat depends mainly on the water vapor pressure gradient between the skin and the environment and the fraction of the body surface area that is covered with sweat. High environmental humidity will decrease the water vapor pressure gradient and limit the ability of the body to lose heat via sweating. The environmental conditions of high ambient temperature and humidity present a serious threat to the body's mechanisms of heat loss and can result in dangerous elevations of body temperature if exercise continues.

Estimations of Heat Production During Exercise

In order to make estimations of heat production during exercise, calculations can be made using oxygen consumption as an indicator of metabolic rate. The metabolic heat load can be estimated from the following formula[91]:

$$\text{Metabolic heat} = \dot{V}_{O_2} \text{ (liters/min)} \times k \\ \times \text{ exercise duration (minutes)}$$

where $\dot{V}_{O_2}$ = oxygen consumption and k = amount of heat liberated per liter of oxygen consumed (k = 4.7 to 5.1 kcal depending on the substrates used).[101] Assuming a 20 percent metabolic efficiency, approximately 1 kcal/liter of O_2 is available for muscular work.

Horses are capable of very high work intensities, and the rate of heat production may exceed basal levels by 40 to 60-fold[29] during racing speeds. The basal metabolic rate of a resting horse has been recorded at 2.2 to 4.2 ml/kg/min.[103] This value is similar to that calculated from the metabolic body size (a function of the body weight to the 3/4 power, 3 kcal/kg$^{3/4}$/h).[101] The metabolic body size of a 450-kg horse is 97.7 kg$^{3/4}$, the basal metabolic rate is 285 kcal/h, equivalent to an oxygen uptake of 58.6 liters/h or 2.2 ml/kg/min. An elite thoroughbred racehorse during a race exercised at around 16 to 17 m/s, an intensity requiring its maximal oxygen uptake (~85 to 90 liters O_2/min). This exercise level would be associated with a heat production of 450 kcal/min (90 liters/min × 5 kcal/liter). If this metabolic heat load was not dissipated, an elevation of body temperature of 1°C for every minute of exercise could occur, assuming the heat capacity of the horse is the same as that of humans (0.83 kcal/kg/°C).[104]

An endurance horse exercising at a mean speed of 4 to 5 m/s consumes approximately 25 liters of O_2 per minute (about 40 percent of maximal oxygen uptake), producing a heat load of about 100 kcal/min. This would result in an increase in body temperature of about 0.25°C/min, or 15°C/h, if no dissipation occurred.

Despite the lower rate of heat production during endurance exercise, heat dissipation is more important than during racing because of the prolonged duration of the exercise. A thoroughbred racehorse typically races at maximal speed for 1 to 3 minutes. This would be associated with heat production of 1350 to 2250 kcal (450 kcal/min). The body is able to store a large amount of heat (0.83 kcal/kg/°C), 415 kcal/min for a 500-kg horse. If all the heat produced during a race was stored, the body temperature would rise 3.25 to 5.42°C. Measurements of exact heat production during exercise have been made.[28] At the trot and canter, heat production was 78 and 131 kcal/min, respectively. These levels of heat production would result in body temperature elevations of 0.13°C/min at the trot and 0.23°C/min at the canter. Recorded rectal temperature rises of only 0.02°C/min and 0.035°C/min occurred, indicating storage of approximately 15 percent of the heat produced.

Heat that is stored during exercise is dissipated after cessation of exercise. Core temperature continues to rise within the first few minutes of recovery from maximal exercise[28] as heat is redistributed from the muscles.

Amount of Heat Dissipated by Sweating

Evaporation of 1 liter of sweat dissipates approximately 580 kcal of heat.[101] The amount of heat loss by evaporation of 1 liter of sweat is equivalent to the heat generated by 1 to 2 minutes of maximal exercise (450 kcal/min) or 5 to 6 minutes of submaximal endurance exercise (100 kcal/min). In order to dissipate the heat produced by prolonged submaximal exercise, a large amount of sweat must be evaporated. An hour of submaximal exercise would produce 6000 kcal (60 min × 100 kcal/min), and to dissipate this heat by evaporative processes, 11 liters of sweat would be required. Anything that jeopardizes evaporation of sweat can have potentially adverse effects on performance due to increased demand on the thermoregulatory and cardiovascular systems.[105] The effectiveness of evaporative cooling is dependent on the environmental temperature, the relative humidity, wind velocity, and body surface area to body weight ratio. Horses have a relatively low surface area to body weight ratio compared with other species. A 60-kg human has a surface area of approximately 1.7 m^2 compared with a 500-kg horse with a surface area of only 5 m^2 (Hodgson et al., unpublished data). This may present a limitation to the efficacy of sweating in the horse.

Heat loss from sweating in humans results in a decrease in skin temperature of about 2°C,[82] and in horses, a temperature 2.5°C below that of core temperature has been recorded from a thermocouple measuring the temperature of blood draining primarily from the skin.[15] Thus sweating results in significant cooling of blood flowing through the skin. In order for this mechanism of heat loss to be utilized, skin blood flow must be high. In exercising humans, up to 15 percent of the cardiac output may be directed to the skin.[82] If it is assumed that a similar proportion of the $\dot{Q}$ is distributed to the skin of the horse, heat loss via sweating can be estimated Assuming that the $\dot{Q}$ of an exercising endurance horse is approximately 160 liter/min (40 percent $\dot{V}_{O_2max}$) and the specific heat capacity of blood is 0.9 kcal/liter/°C, cooling of the blood due to sweating represents a loss of 55 kcal/min (0.15×160 liters/min $\times 2.5°C \times 0.9$ kcal/liter/°C). The sweat rate necessary to result in this heat loss is 95 ml/min or 5.7 liters/h (580 kcal/liter). This heat loss represents only 55 to 60 percent of the heat load that would result from endurance exercise (100 kcal/min).

Heat loss via sweating also can be estimated by measuring the sweat volume lost during exercise. Sweating rates of horses exercising in the heat may reach 10 to 15 liters/hr.[29,106] It seems likely that sweating results in heat dissipation of greater than 60 percent of total heat produced. Heat loss via sweating may be more efficient than calculated using values from humans, since a greater proportion of the $\dot{Q}$ of the horse may be distributed to the skin during exercise. Data on distribution of $\dot{Q}$ in the horse during exercise are lacking.

Estimation of Sweat Losses During Exercise

Sweating rates have been estimated by weighing horses before and after exercise. Moderate exercise (3.5 m/s) for 6 hours resulted in a 5 to 6 percent loss of body weight (27 kg), with one horse losing 46.4 kg, 9.1 percent of body weight.[29] In another study in cool weather conditions, weight loss of 37 ± 2.6 kg (7.6 ± 0.5 percent) occurred during exercise at 18 km/h for 58 to 80 km.[57] During the first 100 km of the Tevis Cup ride, the mean weight loss was 17.5 kg,[29] with a maximal weight loss recorded from one horse of 45 kg, representing 10.5 percent of the body weight.

Thoroughbreds racing over distances of 1 to 2 miles may lose up to 10 liters during the warmup, race, and initial recovery period.[106] Direct measurements of sweat rates on the neck and back of horses exercising on a treadmill at 40 percent $\dot{V}_{O_2max}$ have been shown to be 21 to 34 ml/min/m².[15] This corresponds to 6.5 to 9 liters/h for a 450-kg horse, assuming that the total surface area of the horse can be calculated from the equation $SA = 1.09 + 0.008 \times$ body weight (kg).[15]

Amount of Heat Dissipated via the Respiratory Tract

Evaporation of water from the respiratory tract represents an important route of heat loss. Inspired air is both warmed and saturated on its passage through the lungs. Even at the elevated respiratory frequencies associated with high-intensity exercise, expired air is warmed to around 28°C[107] and is at least 85 percent saturated with water.[108] The heat loss associated with warming inspired air to near body temperature (from 16 to 33°C) contributes approximately 5 percent of total heat loss at rest and during exercise. In contrast, the evaporative heat loss as-

sociated with humidifying respired gases increases up to fivefold during exercise to remove 10 to 15 percent of total heat loss.[28]

During the gallop, biomechanical forces result in synchronization of the respiratory and stride frequencies. Thus respiratory heat loss can be modified only by altering tidal volume, blood flow to the upper respiratory tract, particularly the nasal mucosa and nasal gland secretion.[28] Despite this limitation, pulmonary ventilation doubles from moderate to maximal speed and can reach > 1400 liters/min at maximal exercise, which may increase the percentage of respiratory heat loss.[109] In addition, respiratory-locomotion coupling reduces metabolic cost of respiration.[28] Respiratory rate during low-intensity exercise in a cold environment is reduced, which may be associated with a reduced need for heat dissipation.[110]

Respiratory heat loss can be calculated by measuring pulmonary ventilation and assuming that 0.03 g of water is dissipated for every liter of air respired.[111] Utilizing this method, respiratory heat loss was calculated by Theil et al.[28] Respiratory heat loss at rest was 4.5 kcal/min (19 kJ/min), 38 percent of total heat loss, and at the walk, trot, and gallop it was 6.2 kcal/min (26 kJ/min), 12.7 kcal/min (53 kJ/min), and 20.5 kcal/min (86 kJ/min), respectively. At each exercise intensity, the respiratory tract contributed approximately 18 percent of total heat loss.[28] Heilemann et al.[112] showed similar levels of respiratory heat loss, 1.15 kcal/min (4.82 kJ/min) at rest and 12.18 kcal/min (50.98 kJ/min) during trotting (3.5 m/s).

Respiratory heat losses also can be estimated from the decrease in blood temperature that occurs as blood passes through the pulmonary circulation. Blood in the carotid artery has been measured in horses exercising on a treadmill and was found to be 0.1 to 0.3°C lower than blood in the pulmonary arteries.[15] Assuming a $\dot{Q}$ of 160 liters/min and a temperature difference of 0.2°C, respiratory heat loss represents 29 kcal/min (160 liters/min $\times 0.2°C \times 0.9$ kcal/liter/min), approximately 30 percent of the heat load produced during submaximal exercise (100 kcal/min).

Cardiovascular Function During Exercise

The cardiovascular system is vitally important during exercise to meet the increased demand of working muscle while maintaining flow to the skin in order to dissipate the heat produced. The cardiovascular system responds to this demand by increasing the total cardiac output, a greater proportion of which is redistributed to exercising muscle.

SKIN BLOOD FLOW DURING EXERCISE

Skin blood flow plays a major role in the distribution of thermal energy during exercise.[113] Skin blood flow changes in the horse in response to exercise have not been measured. Measurements in humans report an initial decrease in skin blood flow to increase blood flow to working muscle.[114] However, as core temperature rises above 38°C, the vasodilator drive for heat dissipation is stimulated, and skin blood flow begins to rise, which may lower $\dot{V}_{O_2max}$.[115,116]

CARDIAC OUTPUT DURING EXERCISE

The cardiac output increases in proportion to exercise intensity and whole-body oxygen consumption. The increase is due to increased heart rate and stroke volume.[103,117] Sixfold elevations in $\dot{Q}$ and 41 percent elevations in SV have been recorded during mild to moderate exercise.[103] However, during maximal exercise, most of the increase in cardiac output is due to the increase in heart rate.[16] In horses, the exercising muscles contribute a much larger proportion of the body mass than in humans and demand a greater activation of the cardiovascular system.[117]

Similar cardiovascular responses occur in humans in response to exercise, with increases in $\dot{Q}$ and heart rate; however, SV tends to plateau before maximal heart rate is reached and may even decrease during very severe exercise.[82] Stroke volume is maintained during prolonged exercise in horses,[118] and horses are thus better adapted than humans for the performance of endurance exercise.[118] This probably relates to postural differences between humans and quadripeds.[82]

REDISTRIBUTION OF THE CARDIAC OUTPUT DURING EXERCISE

During exercise, there is an increase in the metabolic requirements of a number of tissues. Apart from exercising muscle, blood flow is increased to the myocardium, trachea, bronchi, and respiratory muscles.[118–125] In response to these increased demands, there is a primary increase in blood flow to exercising muscles and a relative decrease in flow to skin, resting muscle, the kidneys, and the splanchnic region in proportion to exercise intensity.[120,126]

Effects of Combined Exercise and Heat Stress

When exercise is undertaken in a warm environment, the demands of muscle for increased metabolic requirements and skin blood flow for heat exchange arise concurrently.[127] The system must be carefully regulated to subserve both these functions, and problems can result when there is competition between the need for blood flow to working muscles and to the skin for heat loss, such as occurs during exercise in the heat. To avoid compromising blood flow to the skin, which would limit heat loss and result in hyperthermia, or to working muscle, which would limit aerobic metabolism, resulting in anaerobic work with its limited substrate supply, $\dot{Q}$ would have to increase continuously.

CARDIAC OUTPUT

The effect of exercise in the heat on cardiac output has not been studied in horses. The cardiovascular responses of horses to exercise differ from those of humans in a number of ways: (1) the cardiac output of horses is maintained during prolonged exercise, (2) horses do not have the problem of maintaining blood pressure associated with an upright posture, and (3) the cutaneous vasculature of horses does not show active vasodilation in response to heat stress. In the light of these differences, it seems probable that in horses the cardiac output would be maintained to a greater extent in the face of exercise in the heat.

In humans, moderate to severe exercise in the heat results in a reduction in $\dot{Q}$ below levels occurring in a thermoneutral environment.[81,128] This reduction in $\dot{Q}$ during exercise occurs as a result of (1) reduced central blood volume due to increased cutaneous venous volume in response to thermoregulatory drives, (2) decreased plasma volume due to loss of plasma water to the extravascular compartment in response to tissue hyperosmolality and increased filtration pressure in active muscles,[129] and (3) loss of body fluid in sweat.[130] The reduction in cardiac output seen in humans due to decreased plasma volume and loss of body fluid in sweat also may occur in horses during prolonged exercise in the heat.[131,132]

REDISTRIBUTION OF THE CARDIAC OUTPUT

Redistribution of the cardiac output of horses in response to exercise in the heat has not been measured. The thermoregulatory responses of horses are similar to those of humans, and blood flow redistribution in response to exercise in the heat may be similar.

The exact redistribution of the cardiac output in humans cannot be measured; only estimates can be made. As a result, there is some dispute in the literature as to whether blood flow to working muscle in humans is reduced in order to maintain skin blood flow during exercise in the heat.

The response of the cardiovascular system to exercise is somewhat modified when exercise is carried out in the heat due to the additional environmental heat load. Cutaneous vasodilation occurs at a lower level of exercise due to the earlier attainment of a critical core temperature elevation. In order to supply this volume of blood, there is an increased redistribution of blood away from splanchnic and renal vascular beds[81] as well as a heat-induced increase in $\dot{Q}$.[81,129]

However, the skin must be relatively vasoconstricted during heavier exercise in the heat because, according to Rowell, "there is simply not enough cardiac output or regional blood flow to raise skin blood flow to the levels seen at rest at equivalent levels of core temperature."[133] Thus either blood flow to skin must be reduced, which would impair heat loss, or there must be a reduction in blood flow to working muscle, which would reduce metabolic performance. There is evidence

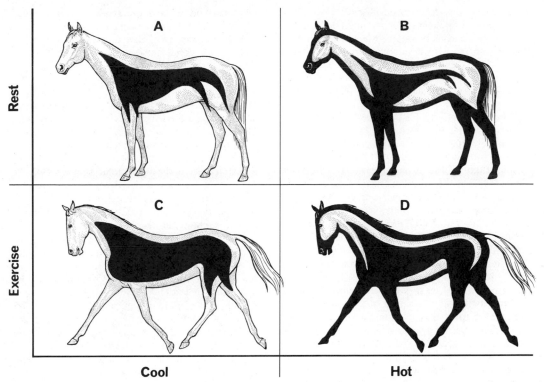

Figure 9-2. Schematic illustration of altered distribution of blood volume in response to heat stress at rest and during exercise. A, *The horse at rest in a cool environment.* B, *The horse at rest exposed to high ambient temperatures. There is a mild increase in cardiac output with a substantial proportion of this increase redistributed to the skin to aid in heat loss.* C, *The horse exercising in a cool environment. Most heat is lost without the need for sweat production. As a result, the proportion of cardiac output directed to the skin remains relatively low.* D, *Exercise in the heat. Environmental and exercise induced heat loads impose great demands on thermoregulatory function necessitating redistribution of a much larger proportion of the cardiac output to the skin for heat loss.*

in humans that blood flow to working muscle in humans is not compromised during exercise and heat stress[134,135]; thus skin blood flow must be reduced. A cutaneous vasoconstrictor response occurs when central blood volume decreases to levels regarded as critical as a mechanism for avoiding circulatory collapse.[129,130] Circulatory regulation appears to take precedence over thermoregulation. Thus a major factor limiting the ability to exercise or to tolerate heat is the threat of circulatory collapse.[136]

Experiments have been performed in sheep to measure exact blood flow redistribution during exercise in the heat. Significant decreases in blood flow to both skin and exercising muscle occurred,[137] in contrast to the findings in humans, suggesting that either physiologic responses of humans and sheep differ or that the estimations derived from studies in humans are inaccurate. The reliance of sheep on panting for thermoregulation does imply that significant differences in thermoregulatory responses between sheep and humans may exist. Documentation of redistribution of the cardiac output of horses in response to exercise in the heat may assist in clarifying this dilemma, for horses and humans man-

ifest remarkable similarities in thermoregulatory mechanisms. Distribution of the cardiac output of horses at rest and during exercise in a thermoneutral and a warm environment is depicted in Figure 9–2.

Clinical Problems Associated with Heat Stress and Exercise in Horses

A number of clinical problems, including exhaustive disease syndrome, synchronous diaphragmatic flutter, heat stress (stroke), rhabdomyolysis, and anhidrosis, can occur as a result of prolonged heat and work stress.

EXHAUSTIVE DISEASE SYNDROME

Protracted submaximal exercise is associated with production of a significant heat load. As detailed in an earlier section, approximately 11 liters of sweat would need to be evaporated to dissipate the heat produced by each hour of submaximal exercise. The substantial loss of fluid and electrolytes associated with sweating at this rate results in significant adverse effects on thermoregulatory and cardiovascular mechanisms.[138-142] Endurance horses forced to exercise for prolonged periods in hot environments can become severely dehydrated, and this may progress to development of hypovolemic shock.[29,143-150] This condition, when combined with energy depletion and profound fatigue, has been referred to as *exhausted horse syndrome*.

Effect of Sweat Loss on Body Fluid Composition

The total-body water of a normal 450 to 500-kg horse is approximately 300 liters, consisting of approximately 200 liters of intracellular fluid (ICF) and 100 liters of extracellular fluid (ECF).[151] Water moves freely between the ECF and ICF, its distribution between the compartments depending on the respective content of exchangeable cations, the principal cations being sodium in the ECF and potassium in the ICF.[152,153] Despite distinct differences in electrolyte composition, these compartments maintain similar osmolalities.[154]

The major components of the ECF are plasma, interstitial fluid, lymph, and transcellular fluid, mainly gastrointestinal fluid. Sweat is derived from interstitial fluid, with subsequent transfer of plasma and cellular fluid to the interstitial space to maintain interstitial fluid volume. Consequently, sweating during exercise depletes both the extracellular and cellular fluid compartments.[155-157] A water loss of 40 liters, such as may occur during an endurance ride, would be derived from both the ECF and ICF volumes.[29,146] This represents a loss of over 15 percent of the total-body water.

In horses, absorption of up to 20 liters of fluid from the substantial gastrointestinal tract fluid reserve can help to maintain plasma volume.[158] This may explain the minor elevations in packed cell volume (PCV) and total plasma protein concentration (TPP) shown by some endurance horses following losses of 30 to 40 kg during a ride.[29]

In addition to significant water losses, substantial losses of electrolytes occur. Electrolyte losses occurring as a result of sweat loss during prolonged exercise in horses in a warm environment involve reductions in plasma chloride, potassium, calcium, and magnesium.[143,146,147,159-161] The chloride loss in sweat is 20 percent greater than the sodium loss, and as a result, the greatest reduction is in plasma chloride,[146,162] with potassium concentration decreasing moderately[56,163] and sodium concentration decreasing only slightly.[56,143,163] Thus an ECF deficit of 25 liters would be associated with a chloride deficit of about 4000 mmol (mEq).[29] In order to maintain electrical neutrality, this hypochloremia is associated with an increase in plasma bicarbonate, inducing a metabolic alkalosis. In addition, mild metabolic alkalosis often occurs secondary to chloride ion depletion via sweat loss.[145,149]

When endurance rides are conducted in cool climates, sweat losses may be minimal, and changes in PCV, TPP, and electrolyte concentration are insignificant.[56,159,160,163] Many endurance horses develop transient fluid and electrolyte imbalances but are able to recover and replace losses via feed and water consumption. Alterations tend to be more severe in very competitive horses which are being pushed at a fast pace, resulting in a greater degree of dehydration, higher heart rates, and a more significant degree of metabolic alkalosis at the end of the ride.[149,163]

Pathogenesis

Major alterations of fluid and electrolyte balance adversely affect athletic performance[164] and may result in a life-threatening metabolic state. Electrolytes are essential for control of membrane potential, muscle contraction, nerve conduction, and enzyme reactions, and they play a central role in the physiologic processes of exercise. The sodium deficit associated with sweat loss results in a reduction of plasma volume, for ECF sodium is the principal determinant of ECF volume.[151] Sodium depletion in combination with dehydration results in decreased plasma volume, increased blood viscosity, inadequate tissue perfusion, and inefficient oxygen and substrate transport.[150] This may contribute to impaired renal function and partial renal shutdown.[146] Hyponatremia also can lead to intermittent muscular cramping, possibly due to inhibition of Na^+,Ca^{2+}-ATPase.[165] Severe hyponatremia results in fatigue, diarrhea, central nervous system signs, and muscular spasms in humans, and similar effects are likely to develop in horses.[166]

Potassium depletion modifies membrane potentials and may reduce the response of vascular smooth muscle to catecholamines, resulting in peripheral vasodilation and reduced central blood volume.[165,167] This imposes an additional burden on the heart, already affected by hypokalemia and increased oxygen demand associated with hyperpyrexia.[166] Hypokalemia also can have a direct pathologic effect on renal nephrons,[165] which can contribute to the development of renal failure.

Metabolic alkalosis associated with depletion of K, Cl, Ca, and Mg during exercise may alter membrane potential and neuromuscular transmission and contribute to gastrointestinal stasis, cardiac arrhythmias, muscle cramps, and synchronous diaphragmatic flutter.[145,147,149,168,169]

Dehydration results in a significant impairment in the efficiency of evaporative cooling by reducing skin blood flow and sweating with resultant elevations in core temperature. Dehydration is the most important single predisposing factor for the development of heat illness.[47] In humans, dehydration affects both thermoregulatory mechanisms, reducing skin blood flow and the sweat response and energy utilization via accelerated depletion of glycogen stores and resulting in an excessive rise in body temperature and heart rate.[140,170-175] Dehydration is likely to have similar effects in horses, resulting in hyperthermia and the potential for damage to the central nervous system.

The combined effects of energy depletion, electrolyte loss, acid-base imbalance, and dehydration may alter both gastrointestinal and central nervous system function, reducing the ability to voluntarily replace fluid losses. Medical intervention is necessary if untoward sequelae resulting from these changes are to be avoided.

Clinical Signs

Affected horses become severely depressed and are un-interested in feed and water. Dehydration is expressed clinically as decreased skin turgor, sunken eyes, dry mucous membranes, firm, dry feces, and decreased urine output.[147,148,168] Rectal temperature is often markedly elevated (40 to 42°C). Respiratory rate is elevated, possibly in an attempt to increase respiratory heat loss, as is heart rate to help maintain cardiac output. Cardiovascular compromise results in increased capillary refill time, decreased pulse pressure and jugular distensibility, and cardiac irregularities. Intestinal stasis commonly occurs with reduced borborygmi and a loss of anal tone. Muscle spasms and cramps are frequently present, and synchronous diaphragmatic flutter ("thumps") may develop in some cases.

A number of serious complications may develop one to several days following exhaustion. The complications are most likely to occur if horses fail to receive immediate and thorough treatment at the time of development of clinical signs. Exertional rhabdomyolysis, renal failure, hepatic dysfunction, gastrointestinal dysfunction, laminitis, central nervous system disorders, and even death have been reported. Intensive and immediate treatment at the time exhaustion develops will reduce the risk of occurrence of these problems.

Clinicopathological Alterations

Exhausted endurance horses have clinicopathologic alterations indicative of severe dehydration, with hematocrit elevations to 0.45 to 0.60 liter/liter. Plasma protein concentrations are generally in the range 72 to 82 g/liter but may reach 100 to 120 g/liter.[147] Hematology reveals a stress neutrophilia with a left shift, increased immature neutrophils, lymphopenia, and a marked eosinopenia.[176]

Electrolyte alterations include primarily hypochloremia, with plasma chloride concentrations often in the range 80 to 90 mmol/liter, and moderate hypokalemia and hyper- or hyponatremia may be present. Calcium and magnesium concentrations tend to decline, which are proposed to contribute to the risk of the development of synchronous diaphragmatic flutter.

The plasma activities of creatinine phosphokinase (CK), lactate dehydrogenase (LDH), alkaline phosphatase (ALP), and aspartate amino transferase (AST) may be elevated. Marked elevations of CK, AST, and LDH will be present if exertional rhabdomyolysis has developed.[177] Plasma creatinine, urea, and bilirubin may be transiently elevated during endurance rides and will be persistently elevated if renal damage develops.

Treatment

Early recognition and treatment will greatly reduce the severity of the exhaustive disease syndrome. During the course of an endurance ride, signs of a problem developing may first be noticed during veterinary examination at check points or in the course of the ride. Affected horses may show signs of distress, fatigue, significant dehydration, and sustained elevation of heart rate, respiratory rate, and rectal temperature. In well-condi-tioned horses who retain good thermoregulatory function, the heart rate should fall to less than 55 beats/min, the respiratory rate to less than 25 breaths/min, and the rectal temperature to below 39.5°C after about 30 minutes.[168,178] Any horse showing a significant and persistent elevation of heart rate, respiratory rate, or rectal temperature should not be allowed to continue exercise.[179]

Horses suffering mild signs will usually respond to rest and simple therapy, including cold hosing, standing the horse in shade, and voluntary rehydration. The horse should be offered small amounts of cool water at frequent intervals and be given access to palatable feed. These animals should be watched closely until recovery is complete. Once homeostasis is restored, the animal can replenish accumulated deficits by voluntary consumption.

Horses with marked elevations of rectal temperature (greater than 40.5°C) should be cooled as quickly as possible. Hosing down with cold water and ventilation via natural breeze in an open space or fanning will encourage heat loss via convection and evaporation. Particular attention should be given to cooling the head, neck, and large subcutaneous vessels between the hind legs. Shade, cool airflow, and cool water will dramatically increase radiant, evaporative, and convective heat losses. Cold water enemas and fluids via nasogastric tube will help lower the core temperature.

Fluid therapy is an essential component of therapy. Horses affected by dehydration following prolonged exercise may only replace 62 percent of their water deficit voluntarily by water consumption.[180] The principal drives for voluntary water consumption are volume depletion and sodium concentration. Plasma sodium concentrations are often within normal limits, which may reduce the drive for voluntary rehydration. Active fluid therapy may be required to fully replenish fluid deficits. Rehydration fluid should be of similar composition to plasma, since hyponatremia and hypochloremia can be exacerbated if the entire deficit associated with sweat loss is replaced with water.[158]

Fluid therapy should be instituted immediately in any horse showing severe signs or failing to respond to conservative treatment within 30 minutes. Fluid can be administered by nasogastric tube, giving 8 liters of isotonic fluid continued at 30 to 60-minute intervals as required. In severe, acute cases, if colic is present or if there is ileus, intravenous administration is preferable.

The exact volume, rate, and route of fluid administration necessary depends on the severity of the presenting signs. Volumes required may be up to 50 liters, which can be administered at flow rates of 5 to 10 liters/h. A severely affected horse may have a sodium deficit of around 4000 mmol, which will require 30 liters of Ringer's solution for replacement. Horses which develop synchronous diaphragmatic flutter and gastrointestinal atony will benefit from intravenous calcium therapy (see Treatment for SDF).

Response to therapy includes improved mucous membrane color and capillary refill time and increased pulse pressure. There should be an improvement in the animal's attitude and desire to eat, with return of gastrointestinal motility.

Horses affected by exhaustive horse syndrome should not be transported for 12 to 24 hours because a high degree of muscular activity is associated with prolonged transport, which puts the horse at further risk of postexhaustive problems.[161] These include exertional rhabdomyolysis, laminitis, and renal failure.

Treatment for exertional rhabdomyolysis, a severe complication that may be associated with the exhaustive horse syndrome, consists of strict rest, nonsteroidal anti-inflammatory drugs, and fluid therapy.

Prevention

The risk of this problem developing will be reduced by adequate preparation and careful management at competitions, with consideration of the effect of the ambient weather conditions at the time of the event.

Preparation for the Event

Physical Training. Physical training in humans results in a number of physiologic alterations that result in improved heat tolerance and thus performance in the heat. Training acts as a form of heat acclimation by imposing a heat load on the body, repeatedly stimulating heat-loss mechanisms.[181–184]

There is a lowered threshold for the initiation of sweating and peripheral vasodilation,[185–190] with earlier activation of heat-loss mechanisms. The sensitivity of both these responses is also enhanced, so there is greater sweat production and increased skin blood flow for the same elevation of body temperature.[186,188] These adaptations result in enhanced transfer of heat from the core to the periphery and increased efficiency of evaporative cooling. As a consequence, less heat is stored, a steady thermal state is reached sooner, and a lower internal temperature is maintained. A lower core temperature increases the core-skin temperature gradient so that a smaller skin blood flow is needed for transfer of metabolic heat to the skin. Thus a small fraction of the $\dot{Q}$ need go to the skin, cardiac demand is reduced, and the capacity for continued skeletal muscle perfusion is improved.[190]

Training also results in an expansion of plasma volume, which improves thermoregulatory function by enhancing sweat production and assisting conductance of heat, as well as reducing cardiovascular demand associated with working in the heat.[191–197] Increased blood volume decreases competition between working muscles and skin; thus blood flow to the skin can be maintained during exercise. In addition, there is an increase in work capacity resulting from a decreased rate of glycogen utilization in response to training.[198]

Although studies of training effects on thermoregulatory mechanisms are lacking in horses, it is likely that similar responses occur. Adequate training for endurance rides should help reduce the risk of exhaustive horse syndrome, as well as exertional rhabdomyolysis.[177]

Training in humans also results in a decreased salt concentration in sweat in response to salt depletion due to losses in sweat.[199–201] Aldosterone released in response to fluid and electrolyte losses acts at the level of the sweat duct to reduce the salt concentration of sweat.[202] Unfortunately, this response appears to be lacking in the horse (McConaghy et al., unpublished data).

Training also decreases the levels of subcutaneous fat, which can improve heat dissipation because this adipose tissue layer acts as an insulator, limiting the rate of heat loss from the body and also reducing the body surface area to mass ratio.

Heat Acclimatization. Heat acclimatization by training in humid heat further improves heat tolerance during exercise, as well as improving cardiovascular function for work performance.[190] Similarly, endurance horses may benefit from repeated work in the heat if they are going to be competing in hot environments.

It was recommended that human athletes training for the Barcelona Olympics commence their heat acclimation 2 weeks prior to leaving for Barcelona. Between 10 and 14 days of work in the heat are sufficient to induce many of the physiologic improvements associated with heat acclimatization in humans. Athletes were instructed to arrive 3 weeks before the competition in order to train under the specific weather conditions of Barcelona.[47]

A similar training regimen may benefit horses. If an important competition is being held in potentially hot and humid conditions, animals may benefit from traveling to the area a number of weeks early and performing the final training under the exact environmental conditions of the event.

Electrolyte Supplementation. Electrolyte supplements are recommended during training if horses are sweating heavily. Free-choice salt should be available, and supplementation can occur via addition to the feed. Supplements should contain equal amounts of sodium and chloride, with half as much potassium.[29] A suitable commercial salt preparation is Lite-salt.

Weather Conditions at the Event

Attention should be paid to weather conditions at the time of the event, and race speed should be adjusted accordingly. High levels of humidity will reduce sweat evaporation, severely limiting this important mechanism for heat dissipation. During competitions in adverse environmental conditions, horses should be carefully monitored for signs of heat stress. Riders should monitor their horses, the heart rate and respiratory rates can be measured at frequent intervals, and the general attitude and willingness of the horse should be observed. If a marked or sudden elevation of heart rate and respiratory rate occurs or the horse appears distressed or unwilling to maintain speed, cessation of exercise and careful examination should be carried out. Exercise should be continued at a reduced speed only if the horse recovers immediately. If the horse remains distressed, it should be walked quietly to a rest stop for veterinary attention.

Cancellation of the competition should be considered if weather conditions are sufficiently severe. The sum of the ambient temperature (in degrees Fahrenheit) and relative humidity (percent) is a simple index of the relative risk of the development of heat exhaustion.[31] Heat loss via evaporation is compromised when this sum is greater than 150, especially if humidity contributes more than 50 percent of the total. If the sum exceeds 180, mechanisms of heat loss become ineffectual, and competitions should be postponed.

Management at the Event

Watering the Horse During the Ride. In humans, exercise in the heat without water intake results in rising rectal temperature and heart rate with a sudden drop in skin blood flow, falling heart rate, and advancing heat exhaustion.[204] This is due to dehydration resulting in partial breakdown of homeothermy during exercise in the heat. Similar effects probably occur in horses.

Dehydration can be reduced by careful attention to voluntary intake of water, electrolytes, and energy sources.[204,205] Electrolyte and energy replacements are recommended for human athletes during prolonged exercise.[47] Addition of electrolytes to administered fluids replaces electrolyte losses and can aid fluid absorption from the gastrointestinal tract.[206] Addition of carbohydrates in themselves may benefit certain types of athletic performance[207] and is likely to assist in the uptake of water and electrolytes from the small intestine. In humans, small amounts of glucose or glucose polymers may assist performance of prolonged exercise by delaying glycogen depletion and exhaustion.[204,208]

Consumption of plain water during exercise is not as beneficial as consumption of isotonic fluid, because water will decrease plasma sodium concentration, resulting in removal of this mechanism as a stimulus for continued water consumption.[209] Hyperhydration prior to commencement of exercise, e.g., by consumption of fluids including glycerol, may aid in decreasing thermoregulatory strain during exercise.[210] Similarly, forced hydration during the early stages of prolonged events may help reduce the speed with which dehydration develops.[47]

Similar principles for fluid administration during exercise can be applied to horses. During the course of the ride, horses should be offered water and electrolyte-spiked water at frequent intervals. Electrolyte supplements also may be administered directly as a slurry paste in horses not showing clinical dehydration. The horse should be well hydrated at the commencement of the competition. Nasogastric administration of isotonic fluid before the competition may benefit horses that do not drink well during rides.

Cooling the Horse During the Ride. The hyperthermia of exercise promotes glycogen depletion and blood lactate accumulation, which may contribute to fatigue and early exhaustion. Kozlowski et al.[211] found that cooling exercising dogs significantly reduced core temperature, decreased the rate of glycogen depletion, and increased exercise duration. Cooling the body during competitions by pouring water over the head and neck at regular intervals is recommended for human athletes. The head

and neck are most appropriate, since these areas have a large blood supply and minimal vasoconstriction occurs during exercise.[47] Many investigators have shown that cooling the head and neck during hyperthermia reduces the rise in core temperature.[212–218] Horses can be cooled during the ride by pouring cool water over the head, neck, and legs. Avoiding "packs" of other horses will help maximize convective heat losses.

SYNCHRONOUS DIAPHRAGMATIC FLUTTER

Synchronous diaphragmatic flutter (SDF) is a spasmodic contraction of the diaphragm synchronous with the heart beat.[169] This condition is seen most commonly in endurance horses performing in hot, humid weather. However, SDF also has been reported in horses with transit tetany, lactation tetany, and electrolyte imbalances secondary to digestive disturbances.[150]

Clinical Signs

The primary sign is a spasmodic twitch in the flank area unassociated with normal respiratory movements. This movement may be strong enough to produce an audible thump, which has lead to the condition being known as "thumps." This twitch is palpable when a hand is placed at the flank, and synchrony with the heart beat will be noted if the heart is auscultated simultaneously. Gastrointestinal atony also may be present, probably due to hypocalcemia and associated electrolyte losses.

Pathogenesis

It has been proposed that alterations in electrolyte levels and acid-base balance alter the membrane potential of the phrenic nerve, allowing it to discharge in response to the electrical impulse produced by atrial depolarization. Hypocalcemia, hypokalemia, and alkalosis may all contribute to the development of the condition. Hypocalcemia lowers the depolarization threshold of nerves to electrical stimulation, whereas hypokalemia can cause hyperirritability of long nerves. Alkalosis can result in a decrease in both total and ionized serum calcium. All these conditions can contribute to phrenic nerve hypersensitivity, allowing it to discharge in response to the electrical impulse generated during atrial depolarization.[150]

Treatment

SDF is not life-threatening but may indicate metabolic alterations that should be treated promptly. The problem will often resolve spontaneously with rest. Enteral or parenteral administration of balanced electrolyte solutions will assist resolution. If necessary, intravenous calcium can be administered. Calcium borogluconate (20 percent) is readily available for the treatment of hypocalcemia ("milk fever") in cattle. The solution commonly is supplied in 500-ml bags which should be diluted 1:4 in isotonic saline and administered slowly to effect. Auscultation of the heart should be carried out during administration, and the infusion should be stopped if any irregularities in heart rate or rhythm develop.

Chronic SDF

SDF can be a recurrent problem in some horses. Administration of electrolytes during prolonged exercise should help to reduce the risk of recurrence, since volume depletion and metabolic alkalosis are predisposing factors. Chronic recurrent SDF may be due to an alteration in the anatomic structures surrounding the phrenic nerve, such as adhesions and fibrosis secondary to pleuropneumonia.

HEAT STRESS (STROKE)

Heat stress occurs when the heat load exceeds the capacity of the thermoregulatory system to effect heat dissipation.

Predisposing Factors in Humans

A number of factors are associated with an increased risk of heat stress in humans, and it is likely that similar conditions also will adversely affect the thermoregulatory system of the horse. Any factors that reduce heat loss or increase heat gain will predispose to heat stroke in humans.[105] High exercise intensities and ambient temperatures in excess of 37°C (99°F) result in high levels of thermal stress.[219,220] High relative humidity limits the process of evaporative cooling.[47]

Individuals who are not exposed to repetitive heat stress because they live in temperate climates or who do not regularly exercise at a rate sufficient to induce sweating will be more at risk.[6] High levels of subcutaneous fat in unfit individuals act as an insulator, decreasing heat loss from the body and decreasing the body surface area to mass ratio.[203,221] Infectious disease results in the production of endogenous pyrogens which cause an elevation of the thermoregulatory setpoint, resulting in heat intolerance. Other stressors include hypoglycemia, fatigue, abrupt changes in daily routine, psychological stress, and transcontinental flights leading to changes in circadian rhythms.[222] Horses are likely to be adversely affected by similar factors (see below).

Pathogenesis

The pathogenesis of heat stress in humans has been studied in detail. Failure of the temperature regulatory system at a critical level seems to be the cause of heat stroke.[223] During exercise and heat stress there are competing demands for blood flow between exercising muscles, myocardium (to perform work), fat (to provide substrates), and skin (to dissipate heat).[13,81,82] These demands, together with sweat losses and fluid redistribution to the interstitial fluid space of active muscles, result in a falling central venous volume and pressure.[13,82,224,225] Subsequently, low-pressure baroreceptors are activated,[13,82,225,226] and vasoconstrictor stimuli for blood pressure regulation overcome thermoregulatory drives for cutaneous vasodilation.[82] In addition, sweat output declines with severe heat stress due to decreasing blood volume and increasing osmotic pressure.[6,224] The combination of reduced skin blood flow and sweating results in a progressive elevation in core temperature. Falling central venous pressure elicits a reduction in blood flow

to fat, reducing substrate availability as well as blood flow to working muscles and the central nervous system.[226] A further decline in central venous pressure enforces further reductions in skin blood flow, uncontrollable elevation of core temperature, and collapse due to central nervous system dysfunction or the other effects of severe hyperthermia detailed below. High body temperature appears to be the cause of collapse, since there is good evidence that heat has deleterious effects on body tissues.

The principal damaging effects of heat are liquification of membrane lipids, damage to cellular mitochondria and nuclei, increases in cellular energy requirements, and impairment of blood supply.[227] Animal tissues can be destroyed by acute exposure to temperatures of 44 to 46°C or prolonged exposure to lower temperatures, e.g., 42 to 45°C.[227] Specific tissues affected by heat are the brain, skin, heart, kidney, liver, gastrointestinal tract, adrenal gland, lung, blood vessels, and blood.[228–230] Red blood cells are damaged, resulting in erythrocyte sphering, increased blood viscosity, formation of microemboli, and the development of disseminated intravascular coagulation. Vascular lesions, damage to electrolytes, and circulatory alterations due to heat stroke result in impairment of blood supply to most organs, and tissues with a high metabolic rate are most affected.[231]

Horses at Risk of Developing Heat Stress

Heat stress occurs most commonly in poorly trained horses forced to exercise for prolonged periods in hot, humid weather, but it can occur after short-duration, high-intensity events such as racing. Horses transported in hot, humid conditions in poorly ventilated transport vehicles also may be affected. Horses kept in cool stalls and exercised in the hottest part of the day may be at risk. Exercising horses in weather conditions that have abruptly become excessively hot and humid will increase the risk of heat stress.

Excessive warmup in bright sun before a competition can result in rapid elevations of core temperature and shorten the time to reaching critical levels of hyperthermia.[232] Hyperthermia can develop rapidly in young, inexperienced horses that may become overly excited, there being high levels of catecholamines and an increased metabolic rate.

Racehorses receiving furosemide prophylactically to control exercise-induced pulmonary hemorrhage may be mildly dehydrated. In humans, dehydration is a very significant factor predisposing to the development of heat stroke. Excessive elevations in body temperature during exercise occur in dehydrated subjects.[140,170–175] With reduced efficiency of sweating,[170,233,234] there is a decrease in stroke volume and cardiac output, resulting in a reduction in peripheral blood flow and thus inefficient conduction of heat from the body core to the periphery.[140,194,204]

It seems probable that dehydration would have similar effects on the thermoregulatory capacity of horses. Furosemide has been shown to decrease heat transfer from the body core to the periphery.[131] It would seem prudent to monitor horses receiving furosemide for signs of impending heat stress during exercise in the heat.

Clinical Signs

Horses affected by heat stress frequently show depression and weakness and refuse to continue to exercise. Heart rate, respiratory rate, and rectal temperature are elevated, with rectal temperatures of up to 43°C. Peripheral vasodilation, in an attempt to increase heat loss, results in congestion of mucous membranes and increased capillary refill time. The sweating response is often inadequate, with hot, dry skin. Muscular disorders such as exertional rhabdomyolysis also may develop. The condition may progress to ataxia, collapse, convulsions, coma, and death.

Treatment

Treatment is directed toward immediate reduction of body temperature. The horse should be moved to a well-ventilated area and should be fanned, if possible, to increase convective heat loss from the skin. Large volumes of cool water should be showered over the horse, with particular attention to the large superficial vessels of the head, neck, and legs. Ice packs can be placed over large subcutaneous vessels to assist cooling. This also may promote cooling of deeper tissues as the venous blood flows toward the heart.

Pouring iced water over the entire body is not recommended because it can result in peripheral vasoconstriction, reducing heat transfer to the periphery and thus preventing heat loss. Cold water administered via nasogastric intubation and/or as an enema may be useful in assisting cooling of the body core. Intravenous fluid therapy is not as important as for treatment of exhausted horses, but plasma volume expansion will assist heat dissipation and is indicated where horses fail to respond to cooling down or if the horse is dehydrated.

Antipyretic agents such as NSAIDs should be used carefully and only in conjunction with fluid therapy. High doses should be avoided in dehydrated animals because the risk of NSAID toxicity is greatly increased if perfusion to vital organs is compromised.

Prevention

Assessment should be made of the factors that contributed to the condition developing, and if necessary, adjustments to the training and management of horses should be instituted. If adverse weather conditions played a significant role in the pathogenesis, exercise in the heat should be avoided. Horses should be exercised only in the cooler times of the day, such as the morning and evening.

If a competition is to be held during extreme heat or humidity, organizers of the event should be advised of the risk to animals, and thought should be given to postponing the event. Competitors should monitor their horses carefully and not force them to exercise at a high intensity for prolonged periods. If a horse has suffered from heat stress previously, it is at a higher risk and possibly should be withdrawn from the competition.

Animals should be transported in well-ventilated trucks and, if possible, only during the cooler periods of the day. Sick, febrile animals should be kept quiet in a thermoneutral environment (~18 to 25°C). Horses moved from temperate to tropical climates should be allowed to acclimatize before being exercised at high intensities.

ANHIDROSIS

This condition is manifested as an inability to sweat in response to an appropriate stimulus.[235] The disorder occurs mainly in horses in hot, humid climates, particularly in horses bred in temperate areas and transported to the tropics. It has been estimated that 20 percent of horses in tropical climates (e.g., Florida) may develop partial or complete anhidrosis.[236,237] The loss of the ability to sweat affects a major avenue for heat dissipation, may result in a severe limitation to exercise performance, and may lead to the development of severe exercise hyperthermia.[238]

Clinical Signs

Affected horses are unable to sweat normally, resulting in heat intolerance and possibly reduced exercise capacity, particularly during exercise lasting more than a few minutes. Following exercise, horses show excessive elevations in rectal temperature and respiratory rate. Fatigue, depression, anorexia, and weight loss also may occur. The skin may be affected, becoming dry and flaky, and alopecia may occur, particularly on the face. Most horses retain some ability to sweat under the mane and saddle area and between the hind legs.[30] Affected horses develop the problem in summer and often recommence sweating in the winter months.[236]

Diagnosis

Diagnosis is based primarily on clinical signs. Intradermal skin testing is also available. Intradermal injection of 0.5 ml of 1:1000 epinephrine will produce a marked sweat response in normal horses and is delayed, decreased, or absent in anhidrotic horses.[30] Histologic examination of skin samples may be unrewarding, although some ultrastructural changes in the sweat glands, including contraction of the duct lumen and obstruction with cellular debris, may be found.[239] However, this is thought to be an effect rather than a cause of the condition.[239] Histologic examination also may help predict the severity of the condition and the potential for recovery.[240]

Pathogenesis

The exact etiology of this condition is unknown. Hypothyroidism, hypochloremia, elevated blood epinephrine levels, and exhaustion of the sweat glands have all been suggested. Heat stress is associated with the development of the disease.[237] Prolonged stimulation of the sweat glands by heat exposure is thought to induce a gradual decrease in sweat production.[30] Prolonged high sweat output may alter sweat gland receptor responsiveness to adrenergic stimulation.[241]

Treatment

There is no effective treatment apart from removal of the horse to a more temperate area. Subsequently, a return to normal sweating may occur, but the condition will often recur if the horses return to a hot, humid environment. Provision of air-conditioned stalls, stall fans, and exercise only in the coolest part of the day may help. Some owners have reported an improvement with electrolyte supplementation.[236]

Conclusions

The horse has an exceptional capacity for the performance of exercise, of both maximal intensity and duration. The thermoregulatory system of the horse is capable of maintaining homeothermy in the face of the substantial heat loads generated during all types of exercise.

Heat generated within exercising muscles is redistributed to the rest of the body via the circulation and then dissipated from the respiratory tract and the body surface by the number of mechanisms. Heat is transferred from the body surfaces to the environment by conduction, radiation, and evaporation, with evaporation of sweat the principal method utilized.

In order to maintain heat loss during prolonged exercise, sweat losses may be significant, up 40 liters, equivalent to 10 percent of the body weight. Failure to recognize the potential for fluid losses of this magnitude can have serious consequences for the animal. Prolonged exercise in combination with fluid and electrolyte imbalances can result in the development of a number of pathologic conditions. An understanding of thermoregulatory mechanisms will both reduce the risks associated with strenuous exercise and aid in development of strategies to enhance athletic performance.

References

1. Brody S: Bioenergetics and Growth. New York, Reinhold, 1945, p 3.
2. Hafez ESE: Principles of animal adaptation. *In* Hafez ESE (ed): Adaptation of Domestic Animals. Philadelphia, Lea & Febiger, 1986, p 3.
3. Cymbaluk NF, Christison GI: Environmental effects on thermoregulation and nutrition of horses. Vet Clin North Am 1990, p 355.
4. Monteith JL: Specification of the environment for thermal physiology. *In* Monteith JL, Mount LE (eds): Heat Loss from Animals and Man. London, Butterworths, 1973, p 1.
5. Yousef MK: Thermoneutral zone. *In* Yousef MK (ed): Stress Physiology in Livestock, vol 1. Boca Raton, Fla, CRC Press, 1985, p 67.
6. Robertshaw D: Contributing factors to heat stroke. *In* Khogali M, Hales JRS (eds): Heat Stroke and Temperature Regulation. Sydney, Australia, Academic Press, 1983, p 13.
7. Mitchell D: Convective heat transfer from man and other animals. *In* Monteith JL, Mount LE (eds): Heat Loss from Animals and Man. London, Butterworths, 1973, p 59.
8. Young BA, Coote J: Some effects of cold on horses. University of Alberta Feeders' Day Report, 1973, p 21.
9. Honstein RN, Monty DE: Physiologic responses of the horse to a hot, arid environment. Am J Vet Res 1977; 38:1041.
10. Palmer SE: Effect of ambient temperature upon the surface temperature of the equine limb. Am J Vet Res 1983; 44:1098.
11. Kaminski RP, Forster HV, Bisgard GE, et al: Effect of altered ambient temperature on breathing in ponies. J Appl Physiol 1985; 58:1585.
12. Ingram DL, Mount LE: Man and Animals in Hot Environments. Berlin, Springer-Verlag, 1975.
13. Rowell LB: Human Circulation: Regulation During Physical Stress. New York, Oxford University Press, 1986.
14. McLean JA: Loss of heat by evaporation. *In* Monteith JL, Mount LE (eds): Heat Loss from Animals and Man. London, Butterworths, 1973, p 19.
15. Hodgson DR, McCutcheon LJ, Byrd SK, et al: Dissipation of metabolic heat in the horse during exercise. J Appl Physiol 1993; 74:116.
16. Evans DL, Rose RJ: Cardiovascular and respiratory responses to exercise in thoroughbred horses. J Exp Biol 1988; 134:397.
17. Thauer R: Thermosensitivity of the spinal cord. *In* Hardy JD, Gagge AP, Stolwijk JAJ (eds): Physiological and Behavioral Temperature Regulation. Springfield, Ill, Charles C Thomas, 1970, p 472.
18. Bligh J: The thermosensitivity of the hypothalamus and thermoregulation in mammals. Biol Rev 1966; 41:317.
19. Bligh J: Temperature Regulation in Mammals and Other Vertebrates. Amsterdam, North-Holland Publishing Co, 1973.
20. Jessen C: Thermal afferents in the control of body temperature. Pharmacol Ther 1985; 28:107.
21. Fowler M: Restraint and Handling of Wild and Domestic Animals. Ames, Iowa, Iowa State University Press, 1978.
22. Jenkinson DM: Evaporative temperature regulation in domestic animals. Symp Zool Soc Lond 1972; 31:345.
23. Burch GE: Study of water and heat loss from the respiratory tract of man. Arch Intern Med 1945; 76:308.
24. Burch GE: Rate of water and heat loss from the respiratory tract of normal subjects in a subtropical climate. Arch Intern Med 1945; 76:315.
25. Hanson RG: Respiratory heat loss at increased core temperature. J Appl Physiol 1974; 37:103.
26. Pollmann U, Hörnicke H: Characteristics of respiratory air flow during exercise in horses with reduced performance due to pulmonary emphysema or bronchitis. *In* Gillespie JR, Robinson NE (eds): Equine Exercise Physiology 2. Davis, Calif, ICEEP Publications, 1987, p 760.
27. Honstein RN, Monty DE: Physiologic responses of the horse to a hot, arid environment. Am J Vet Res 1977; 38:1041.
28. Thiel M, Tolkmitt G, Hörnicke H: Body temperature changes in horses during riding: time course and effects on heart rate and respiratory frequency. *In* Gillespie JR, Robinson NE (eds): Equine Exercise Physiology 2. Davis, Calif, ICEEP Publications, 1987, p 183.
29. Carlson GP: Thermoregulation, fluid and electrolyte balance. *In* Snow DH, Persson SGB, Rose RJ (eds): Equine Exercise Physiology. Cambridge, Granta Editions, 1983, p 291.
30. Evans CL, Smith DFG, Ross KA, et al: Physiological factors in the condition of "dry-coat" in horses. Vet Rec 1957; 69:1.
31. Mackay-Smith M, Cohen M: Exercise physiology and diseases of exhaustion. *In* Mansmann RA, McAllister ES (eds): Equine Medicine and Surgery, vol 2 (ed 3). Santa Barbara, Calif, American Veterinary Publishers, 1982, p 117.
32. Allen TE, Bligh J: A comparative study of the temporal patterns of cutaneous water vapour from some domesticated mammals with epitrichial sweat glands. Comp Biochem Physiol 1969; 31:347.
33. Macfarlane WV: Terrestrial animals in dry heat: Ungulates. *In* Dill DB, Adolph EF, Wilber CG (eds): Handbook of Physiology: Adaptation to the Environment. Washington, American Physiological Society, 1964, p 509.
34. Schmidt-Nielsen K: Desert Animals: Physiological Problems of Heat and Water. London, Oxford University Press, 1964.
35. Jenkinson DM: Evaporative temperature regulation in hot arid environments. Symp Zool Soc Lond 1972; 31:357.
36. Hales JRS, Webster MED: Respiratory function during thermal tachypnoea in sheep. J Physiol (Lond) 1967; 190:241.
37. Brockway JM, McDonald JD, Pullar JD: Evaporative heat loss mechanisms in sheep. J Physiol (Lond) 1965; 179:554.
38. Amatruda TT, Welt LG: Secretion of electrolytes in thermal sweat. J Appl Physiol 1953; 5:759.
39. Costill DL: The marathon: physiological, medical, epidemiolog-

ical and psychological studies. Sweating: Its composition and effects on body fluids. Ann NY Acad Sci 1977; 301:160.

40. Nowak S, Zazgornik J: Electrolyte secretion in sweat in the initial phase of sweat glands activity. Acta Physiol Pol 1966; 17:395.

41. Robinson S, Kincaid RK, Rhamy RK: Effect of salt deficiency on the salt concentration in sweat. J Appl Physiol 1950; 3:55.

42. Robinson S, Robinson AH: Chemical composition of sweat. J Appl Physiol 1954; 34:202.

43. Gordon RS, Cage GW: Mechanism of water and electrolyte secretion by the eccrine sweat gland. Lancet 1966; 1:1246.

44. Kunstlinger U, Ludwig H, Stegemann J: Metabolic changes during volleyball matches. Int J Sports Med 1987; 8:315.

45. Dill DB, Hall FG, Beaumont WV: Sweat chloride concentration: sweat rate, metabolic rate, skin temperature, and age. J Appl Physiol 1966; 21:99.

46. Ohara K: Chloride concentration in sweat: Its individual, regional, seasonal and some other variations, and interrelations between them. Jpn J Physiol 1966; 16:274.

47. Cedaro RL: Report to the Australian Olympic Committee of Environmental Considerations and Related Matters for Australian Athletes Competing in the 1992 Barcelona Games, 1991.

48. Ladell WSS: Thermal sweating. Br Med Bull 1945; 3:175.

49. Sato K: The physiology, pharmology and biochemistry of the eccrine sweat gland. Rev Physiol Biochem Pharmacol 1977; 79:52.

50. Smith F: Note on composition of the sweat of the horse. J Physiol (Lond) 1890; 11:497.

51. Jirka M, Kotas J: Some observations on the chemical composition of horse sweat. J Physiol (Lond) 1959; 147:74.

52. Soliman MK, Nadim MA: Calcium, sodium and potassium level in the serum and sweat of healthy horses after strenuous exercise. Zentralbl Veterinarmed 1967; 14:53.

53. Carlson GP, Ocen PO: Composition of equine sweat following exercise in high environmental temperatures and in response to intravenous epinephrine administration. J Equine Med Surg 1979; 3:27.

54. Kerr MG, Munro CD, Snow DH: Equine sweat composition during prolonged heat exposure. J Physiol (Lond) 1980; 307: 52P.

55. Rose RJ, Arnold KS, Church S, et al: Plasma and sweat electrolyte concentrations in the horse during long-distance exercise. Equine Vet J 1980; 12:19.

56. Snow DH, Kerr MG, Nimmo MA, et al: Alterations in blood, sweat, urine and muscle composition during prolonged exercise in the horse. Vet Rec 1982; 110:377.

57. Kerr MG, Snow DH: Composition of sweat of the horse during prolonged epinephrine (adrenaline) infusion, heat exposure, and exercise. Am J Vet Res 1983; 44:1571.

58. Evans CL, Smith DFG, Weil-Malherbe H: The adrenaline and noradrenaline of venous blood of the horse before and after exercise. J Physiol (Lond) 1955; 128:50P.

59. Evans CL: Physiological mechanisms that underlie sweating in the horse. Br Vet J 1966; 122:117.

60. Evans CL: Sweating in relation to sympathetic innervation. Br Med Bull 1955; 13:197.

61. Anderson MG, Aitken MM: Biochemical and physiological effects of catecholamine administration in the horse. Res Vet Sci 1977; 22:357.

62. Jenkinson DM, Mahon RM, Manson W: Sweat proteins. Br J Dermatol 1974; 90:175.

63. Eckersall PD, Kerr MG, Snow DH: An investigation into the proteins of horse sweat (Equus caballus). Comp Biochem Physiol [B] 1982; 73:375.

64. Eckersall PD, Snow DH: Characterization of glycoproteins in the sweat of the horse (Equus caballus). Res Vet Sci 1984; 36:231.

65. Beeley JG, Eason R, Snow DH: Isolation and characterization of latherin, a surface-active protein from horse sweat. Biochem J 1986; 235:645.

66. Jenkinson DM: Comparative physiology of sweating. Br J Dermatol 1973; 88:397.

67. Johnson K: Sweat gland function in isolated perfused skin. J Physiol (Lond) 1975; 250:633.

68. Smith J, Mayhew I: Horner's syndrome in large animals. Cornell Vet 1977; 67:529.

69. Snow D: Identification of the mediator involved in adrenaline-mediated sweating in the horse. Res Vet Sci 1977; 23:246.

70. Weiner JS, Hellmann K: The sweat glands. Biol Rev 1960; 35:141.

71. Takagi S, Tagawa M: Nerve fibers supplying the horse sweat gland. Jpn J Physiol 1961; 11:158.

72. Jenkinson DM, Blackburn PS: The distribution of nerves, monoamine oxidase and cholinesterase in the skin of the horse. Res Vet Sci 1968; 6:165.

73. Aoki T: Stimulation of the sweat glands in the hairy skin of the dog by adrenaline, noradrenaline, acetylcholine, mecholyl and pilocarpine. J Invest Dermatol 1955; 24:545.

74. Evans CL, Smith DFG: Sweating responses in the horse. Proc R Soc Lond Biol 1956; 145:61.

75. Robertshaw D: The pattern and control of sweating in the sheep and the goat. J Physiol (Lond) 1968; 198:531.

76. Robertshaw D, Taylor CR: Sweat gland function of the donkey (Equus asinus). J Physiol (Lond) 1969; 205:79.

77. Ingram DL: Stimulation of cutaneous glands in the pig. J Compr Pathol 1967; 77:93.

78. Evans CL, Smith DFG: On sweating in the horse. J Physiol (Lond) 1954); 126:45P.

79. Bell FR, Evans CL: Sweating responses in the horse. J Physiol (Lond) 1956; 134:421.

80. Evans CL, Smith DFG, Weil-Marherbe H: The relationship between sweating and the catechol content of the blood in the horse. J Physiol (Lond) 1956; 132:542.

81. Rowell LB: Human cardiovascular adjustments to exercise and thermal stress. Physiol Rev 1974; 54:75.

82. Rowell LB: Cardiovascular adjustments to thermal stress. In Shepherd JT, Abboud FM (eds): Handbook of Physiology, vol 3 Bethesda, MD, American Physiological Society, 1983, p 967.

83. Koroxenidis GT, Shepherd JT, Marshall RJ: Cardiovascular response to acute heat stress. J Appl Physiol 1961; 16:869.

84. Hales JRS: Effects of exposure to hot environments on the regional distribution of blood flow and on cardiorespiratory function in sheep. Pflügers Arch 1973; 344:133.

85. Hales JRS: Effects of heat stress on blood flow on respiratory and non-respiratory muscles in sheep, Pflügers Arch 1973;345:123.

86. Pleschka K: Control of tongue blood flow in regulation of heat loss in mammals. Rev Physiol Biochem Pharmacol 1984; 100:75.

87. Nadel ER: Control of sweating rate while exercising in the heat. Med Sci Sports 1979; 11:31.

88. Nadel ER: Problems with Temperature Regulation During Exercise. New York, Academic Press, 1977.

89. Nielsen M: Die regulation der korpertemperatur bei musckelarbeit. Scand Arch Physiol 1939; 79:193.

90. Saltin B, Hermansen L: Esophageal, rectal, and muscle temperature during exercise. J Appl Physiol 1966; 21:1757.

91. Åstrand PO, Rodahl K: Textbook of Work Physiology: Physiological Bases of Exercise. New York, McGraw-Hill, 1979, p 295.

92. Snow DH, Mackenzie G: Effect of training on some metabolic changes associated with submaximal endurance exercise in the horse. Equine Vet J 1977; 9:226.

93. Robinson S: Physiological adjustments to heat. In Newburg CH (ed): Physiology of Heat Regulation and the Science of Clothing. Philadelphia, WB Saunders Co, 1949, p 193.

94. Saltin B, Gagge AP, Stolwijk JAJ: Muscle temperature during submaximal exercise in man. J Appl Physiol 1968; 25:679.

95. Lindholm A, Saltin B: The physiological and biochemical response of standardbred horses to exercise of varying speed and duration. Acta Vet Scand 1974; 15:310.

96. Jones JH, Taylor CR, Lindholm A: Blood gas measurements during exercise: Errors due to temperature correction. J Appl Physiol 1989; 67:879.

97. Fregin GF, Thomas DP: Cardiovascular response to exercise in the horse: A review. In Snow DH, Persson SGB, Rose RJ (eds): Equine Exercise Physiology. Cambridge, Granta Editions, 1982, p 76.

98. Asmussen E, Boje O: Body temperature and the capacity for work. Acta Physiol Scand 1945; 10:1.

99. Gollnick PD: Biochemical correlates of fatigue in skeletal muscle. In Hales JRS, Richards DAB (eds): Heat Stress: Physical Exertion and Environment. Amsterdam, Elsevier, 1987, p 161.

100. Goetz TE, Manohar M: Isoproterenol-induced maximal heart rate in normothermic and hyperthermic horses. Am J Vet Res 1990; 51:743.

101. Kleiber M: The Fire of Life. New York, Wiley, 1961.
102. Adams WC, Fox RH, Fry AJ, et al: Thermoregulation during marathon running in cool, moderate and hot environments. J Appl Physiol 1975; 38:1030.
103. Thomas DP, Fregin GF: Cardiorespiratory and metabolic responses to treadmill exercise in the horse. J Appl Physiol 1981; 50:864.
104. Burton AC, Edholm OG: Man in a Cold Environment. London, Edward Arnold, 1955.
105. Robertson J: Preventing heat stress in sports. Physiol Sports Med 1991; 19:31.
106. Carlson GP: Hematology and body fluids in the equine athlete: A review. In Gillespie JR, Robinson JR (eds): Equine Exercise Physiology 2. Davis, Calif, ICEEP Publications, 1987, p 393.
107. Cain JB, Livingstone SD, Nolan RW, et al: Respiratory heat loss during work at various ambient temperatures. Respir Physiol 1990; 79:145.
108. Schroter RC, Watkins NV: Respiratory heat exchange in mammals. Respir Physiol 1989; 78:357.
109. Hörnicke H, Weber M, Schweiker W: Pulmonary ventilation in thoroughbred horses at maximum performance. In Gillespie JR, Robinson, NE (eds): Equine Exercise Physiology 2. Davis, Calif, ICEEP Publications, 1987, p 216.
110. Dahl LG, Gillespie JR, Kallings P, et al: Effects of a cold environment on exercise tolerance in the horse. In Gillespie JR, Robinson, NE (eds): Equine Exercise Physiology 2. Davis, Calif, ICEEP Publications, 1987, p 235.
111. Kaminski RP, Forster HV, Bisgard GE, et al: Effect of altered ambient temperature on metabolic rate during CO_2 inhalation. J Appl Physiol 1985; 58:1592.
112. Heilemann M, Woakes AJ, Snow DH: Investigations on the respiratory water loss in horses at rest and during exercise. In Meyer H (ed): Contributions to Water and Mineral Metabolism of the Horse. Berlin, Verlag Paul Parey, 1990, p 52.
113. Mitchell JW: Energy exchanges during work. In Nadel ER (ed): Problems with Temperature Regulation during Exercise. New York, Academic Press, 1977, p 11.
114. Johnson JM, Rowell LB, Brengelmann GL: Modification of the skin blood flow–body temperature relationship by upright exercise. J Appl Physiol 1974; 37:880.
115. Saltin B, Gagge AP, Bergh U, et al: Body temperatures and sweating during exhaustive exercise. J Appl Physiol 1972; 32:635.
116. Brengelmann GL, Johnson JM, Hermansen L, et al: Altered control of skin blood flow during exercise at high internal temperatures. J Appl Physiol 1977; 43:790.
117. Engelhardt WV: Cardiovascular effects of exercise and training in horses. Adv Vet Sci 1977; 21:173.
118. Manohar M: Respiratory muscle perfusion during strenuous exercise. In Persson SGB, Lindolm A, Jeffcott LB (eds): Equine Exercise Physiology 3. Davis, Calif, ICEEP Publications, 1991, p 1.
119. Fixler DE, Atkins JM, Mitchell JH, et al: Blood flow to respiratory, cardiac and limb muscles in dogs during graded exercise. Am J Physiol 1976; 231:1515.
120. Parks CM, Manohar M: Distribution of blood flow during moderate and strenuous exercise in ponies (Equus caballus) Am J Vet Res 1983; 44:1861.
121. Armstrong RB, Delp MD, Goljan EF, et al: Distribution of blood flow in muscles of miniature swine during exercise. J Appl Physiol 1987; 62:1285.
122. Armstrong RB, Delp MD, Goljan EF, et al: Progressive elevations in muscle blood flow during prolonged exercise in swine. J Appl Physiol 1987; 63:285.
123. Manohar M: Inspiratory and expiratory muscle perfusion in maximally exercised ponies. J Appl Physiol 1990; 68:544.
124. Manohar M: Tracheobronchial perfusion during exercise in ponies. J Appl Physiol 1990; 68:2182.
125. Manohar M: Bronchial circulation during prolonged exercise in ponies. Am J Vet Res 1992; 53:925.
126. Manohar M: Furosemide and systemic circulation during severe exercise. In Gillespie JR, Robinson NE (eds): Equine Exercise Physiology 2. Davis, Calif, ICEEP Publications, 1987, p 132.
127. Bell AW, Hales JRS: Circulatory implications of exercise and heat stress. Pharmacol Ther 1985; 31:103.
128. Rowell LB, Marx HJ, Bruce RA, et al: Reductions in cardiac output, central blood volume, and stroke volume with thermal

stress in normal men during exercise. J Clin Invest 1966; 5:1801.
129. Nadel ER, Caferelli E, Roberts ME, et al: Circulatory regulation during exercise in different ambient temperatures. J Appl Physiol 1979; 46:430.
130. Nadel ER: Circulatory and thermal regulations during exercise. Fed Proc 1980; 39:1491.
131. Naylor JRJ, Bayly WM, Gollnick PD, et al: Effects of dehydration on thermoregulatory responses of horses during low intensity exercise. J Appl Physiol 1993; 75:994.
132. Naylor JRJ, Bayly WM, Gollnick PD, et al: Equine plasma and blood volumes decrease with dehydration but subsequently increase with exercise. J Appl Physiol 1993; 75:1062.
133. Rowell LB: Competition between skin and muscle for blood flow during exercise. In Nadel ER (ed): Problems with Temperature Regulation during Exercise. New York, Academic Press, 1977, p 49.
134. Savard GK, Nielsen B, Laszyznska J, et al: Muscle blood flow is not reduced in humans during moderate exercise and heat stress. J Appl Physiol 1988; 64:649.
135. Nielsen M, Herrington LP, Winslow C-EA: The effect of posture on peripheral circulation. Am J Physiol 1990; 127:573.
136. Bell AW, Hales JRS: Cardiac output and its distribution during exercise and heat stress. In Schonbaum E, Lomax P (eds): Thermoregulation: Pathology, Pharmacology and Therapy. New York, Pergamon Press, 1991, p 105.
137. Bell AW, Hales JRS, King RB, et al: Influence of heat stress on exercise-induced changes in regional blood flow in sheep. J Appl Physiol 1983; 55:1983.
138. Costill DL, Fink W: Plasma volume changes following exercise and thermal dehydration. J Appl Physiol 1979; 37:521.
139. Nielsen B: Effect of changes in plasma volume and osmolarity on thermoregulation during exercise. Acta Physiol Scand 1974; 90:725.
140. Nadel ER, Fortney SM, Wenger CB: Effect of hydration state on circulatory and thermal regulations. J Appl Physiol 1980; 49:715.
141. Fortney SM, Nadel ER, Wenger CB, et al: Effect of blood volume on sweating rate and body fluids in exercising humans. J Appl Physiol 1981; 51:1594.
142. Fortney SM, Wenger CB, Bove JR, et al: Effect of hyperosmolality on control of blood flow and sweating. J Appl Physiol 1984; 57:1688.
143. Carlson GP, Mansmann RA: Serum electrolyte and plasma protein alterations in horses used in endurance rides. J Am Vet Med Assoc 1974; 165:262.
144. Carlson GP: Hematologic alterations in endurance-trained horses. In Proceedings of the International Symposium on Equine Hematology, 1975, p 444.
145. Carlson GP: Fluid and electrolyte alterations in endurance-trained horses. In Proceedings of the International Symposium on Equine Hematology, 1975, p 473.
146. Rose RJ, Purdue RA, Hensley W: Plasma biochemical alterations in horses during an endurance ride. Equine Vet J 1977; 9: 122.
147. Carlson GP: Physiologic responses to endurance exercise. Am Assoc Equine Pract 1979; 25:459.
148. Fowler ME: Veterinary problems during endurance rides. Am Assoc Equine Pract 1979; 25:469.
149. Rose RJ, Ilkiw JE, Martin ICA: Blood-gas, acid-base and hematological values in horses during an endurance ride. Equine Vet J 1979; 11:56.
150. Carlson GP: Medical problems associated with protracted heat and work stress in horses. Comp Cont Ed Pract Vet 1985; 7:S542.
151. Rose RJ: A physiological approach to fluid therapy in the horse. Equine Vet J 1981; 13:7.
152. Edelman IS, Leibman J, O'Meara MP, et al: Interrelationships between serum sodium concentration, serum osmolality and total exchangeable sodium, total exchangeable potassium and total body water. J Clin Invest 1958; 37:256.
153. Edelman IS, Leibman J: Anatomy of body water and electrolytes. Am J Med 1959; 27:256.
154. Rose RJ: Electrolyte and acid-base balance: Applications in equine practice. Equine International Medicine, Proc 206 Univ Syd Postgrad Committee in Vet Sci, 1993, p 21.

155. Kozlowski S, Saltin B: Effect of sweat loss on body fluids. J Appl Physiol 1964; 19.1119.
156. Beaumont WJ, Strand JC, Petrofsky JS, et al: Changes in total plasma content of electrolytes and proteins with maximal exercise. J Appl Physiol 1973; 34:102.
157. Maughan RJ, Whiting PH, Davidson JL: Estimation of plasma volume changes during marathon running. Br J Sports Med 1985; 19:138.
158. Carlson GP: Hematology and body fluids. In Gillespie JR, Robinson NE (eds): Equine Exercise Physiology 2. Davis, Calif, ICEEP Publications, 1987, p 393.
159. Fregin GF: General discussion of physiologic observations recorded on 117 horses during 100-mile endurance rides. Am Assoc Equine Pract 1979; 25:315.
160. Lucke JN, Hall GN: Biochemical changes in horses during a 50-mile endurance ride. Vet Rec 1978; 102:356.
161. Lucke JN, Hall GN: Further studies on the metabolic effects of long distance riding: Golden Horseshoe Ride 1979. Equine Vet J 1980; 12:189.
162. Rose RJ, Hodgson DR: Hematological and plasma biochemical parameters in endurance horses during training. Equine Vet J 1982; 14:144.
163. Rose RJ: Hematological changes associated with endurance exercise. Vet Rec 1982; 110:175.
164. Williamson HM: Normal and abnormal electrolytic levels in the racing horses and their effect on performance. J S Afr Vet Assoc 1974; 45:335.
165. Fettman MJ: Fluid and electrolyte metabolism during heat stress. Comp Cont Ed Pract Vet 1986; 8:391.
166. Knochel JP: Clinical physiology of heat exposure. In Maxwell MH, Kleeman CR (eds): Clinical Disorders of Fluid and Electrolyte Metabolism. New York, McGraw-Hill 1980, p 1519.
167. Knochel JP, Dotin LN, Hamburger RJ: Pathophysiology of intense physical conditioning in a hot climate. J Clin Invest 1972; 51:242.
168. Fowler ME: The exhausted horse syndrome. Am Assoc Equine Pract 1979; 25:479.
169. Hinton MH, Yeats JJ, Hastie PS, et al: Synchronous diaphragmatic flutter in horses. Vet Rec 1976; 99:402.
170. Horstman DH, Horvath SM: Cardiovascular and temperature regulatory changes during progressive dehydration and euhydration. J Appl Physiol 1972; 33:446.
171. Senay LC: Temperature regulation and hypohydration: A singular view. J Appl Physiol 1979; 47:1.
172. Buskirk ER, Iampietro PF, Bass DE: Work performance after dehydration: Effects of physical conditioning and heat acclimatization. J Appl Physiol 1958; 12:189.
173. Moroff SV, Bass DE: Effects of overhydration on man's physiological responses to work in the heat. J Appl Physiol 1965; 20:267.
174. Pitts GC, Johnson RE, Consolazio FC: Work in the heat as affected by intake of water, salt and glucose. Am J Physiol 1944; 142:253.
175. Armstrong L: The impact of hyperthermia and hypohydration on circulation, strength, endurance and health. J Appl Sports Sci Res 1988; 2:60.
176. Carlson GP, Ocen PO, Harrold D: Clinicopathological alterations in normal and exhausted endurance horses. Theriogenology 1976; 6:93.
177. Hodgson DR: Myopathies in the athletic horse. Comp Cont Ed Pract Vet 1985; 7:S551.
178. Hinton MH: The biochemical and clinical aspects of exhaustion in the horse. Vet Ann 1978; 18:169.
179. Hall-Patch PK, Orton RG, Sampson JH: Competitive trail and endurance riding in the UK. Vet Rec 1977; 100:192.
180. Carlson GP, Rumbaugh GE, Harrold D: Physiologic alterations in the horse produced by food and water deprivation during periods of high environmental temperatures. Am J Vet Res 1979; 40:982.
181. Pandolf KB: Effects of physical training and cardiorespiratory physical fitness on exercise-heat tolerance: Recent observations. Med Sci Sports Exerc 1979; 11:60.
182. Gisolfi CV, Wilson NC, Claxton B: Work-heat tolerance of distance runners. Ann NY Acad Sci 1977; 301:139.
183. Piwonka RW, Robinson S, Gay VL, et al: Preacclimatization of men to heat by training. J Appl Physiol 1965; 20:379.
184. Piwonka RW, Robinson S: Acclimatization of highly trained men to work in severe heat. J Appl Physiol 1967; 22:9.
185. Wyndham CH: Effect of acclimatization on the sweat rate/rectal temperature relationship. J Appl Physiol 1967; 22:27.
186. Nadel ER, Pandolf KB, Roberts MF, et al: Mechanisms of thermal acclimation to exercise in heat. J Appl Physiol 1974; 37:515.
187. Baum E, Brück K, Schwennicke JP: Adaptive modifications in the thermoregulatory system of long-distance runners. J Appl Physiol 1976; 40:404.
188. Roberts MF, Wenger CB, Stolwijk JAJ, et al: Skin blood flow and sweating changes following exercise training and heat acclimation. J Appl Physiol 1977; 43:133.
189. Taylor NAS: Eccrine sweat gland adaptations to physical training and heat acclimation. Sports Med 1986; 3:387.
190. Wells CL, Constable SH, Haan AL: Training and acclimatization: Effects on responses to exercise in a desert environment. Aviat Space Environ Med 1980; 51:105.
191. Appenzeller O: Influences of physical training, heat acclimation and diet on temperature regulation in man. In Khogali M, Hales JRS (eds): Heat Stroke and Temperature Regulation. Sydney, Australia, Academic Press, 1983, p 283.
192. Brotherhood J, Brozovic B, Pugh LGC: Haematological status of middle- and long-distance runners. Clin Sci Mol Med 1975; 48:139.
193. Holmgren A, Massfeldt T, Sjostrand T, et al: Effect of training on the work capacity, total haemoglobin, blood volume, heart volume and heart rate in the recumbent and upright position. Acta Physiol Scand 1960; 43:822.
194. Nadel ER, Mack GW, Nose H, et al: Tolerance to severe heat and exercise: Peripheral vascular responses to body fluid changes. In Hales JRS, Richards DAB (eds): Heat Stress: Physical Exertion and Environment. Amsterdam, Elsevier, 1987, p 117.
195. Senay LC, Mitchell D, Wyndham CH: Acclimatization in a hot, humid environment: Body fluid adjustments. J Appl Physiol 1976; 40:786.
196. Wyndham CH, Benade AJA, Williams CG, et al: Changes in central circulation and body fluid spaces during acclimatization to heat. J Appl Physiol 1968; 25:586.
197. Libert J, Amoros C, Nisi J, et al: Thermoregulatory adjustments during continuous heat exposure. Eur J Appl Physiol 1988; 57:499.
198. Kirwan J, Costill D, Kuipers H: Substrate utilization in leg muscles of men after heat acclimation. J Appl Physiol 1987; 63:31.
199. Daly C, Dill DB: Salt economy in humid heat. Am J Physiol 1937; 118:285.
200. Dill DB, Hall FG, Edwards HT: Changes in composition of sweat during acclimatization to heat. Am J Physiol 1938; 123:412.
201. Dill DB: Life, Heat and Altitude. Cambridge, Mass, Harvard University Press, 1938.
202. Robinson S, Gerking SD, Turrell ES, et al: Effect of skin temperature on salt concentration of sweat. J Appl Physiol 1950; 2:654.
203. Shapiro Y: Pathophysiology of hyperthermia and heat intolerance. In Hales JRS, Richards DAB (eds): Heat Stress: Physical Exertion and Environment. Amsterdam, Elsevier, 1987, p 263.
204. Nielsen B: Effects of fluid ingestion on heat tolerance and exercise performance. In Hales JRS, Richards DAB (eds): Heat Stress: Physical Exertion and Environment. Amsterdam, Elsevier, 1987, p 133.
205. Lamb DR, Brodowicz GR: Optimal use of fluids of varying formulations to minimize exercise-induced disturbances in homeostasis. Sports Med 1986; 3:247.
206. Carter J, Gisolfi C: Fluid replacement during and after exercise in the heat. Med Sci Sports Exerc 1989; 21:532.
207. Felig P, Wahren J: Fuel homeostasis in exercise. N Engl J Med 1975; 293:1078.
208. Fielding RA, Costill DL, Fink WJ, et al: Effect of carbohydrate feeding frequencies and dosage on muscle glycogen use during exercise. Med Sci Sports Exer 1985; 17:472.
209. Nadel ER: New ideas for rehydration during and after exercise in hot weather. Sports Nutr 1988; 1:1.
210. Lyons T, Riedesel M, Meuli L, et al: Effects of glycerol-induced hyperhydration prior to exercise in the heat on sweating and core temperature. Med Sci Sports Exerc 1990; 22:477.
211. Kozlowski S, Brezezinska Z, Kruk B, et al: Exercise hyperthermia

as a factor limiting physical performance: Temperature effect on muscle metabolism. J Appl Physiol 1986; 59:766.

212. Shavartz E: Effect of a cooling hood on physiological responses to work in a hot environment. J Appl Physiol 1970; 29:36.

213. Kissen A, Hall J, Kleem F: Physiological responses to cooling the head and neck versus the trunk and leg areas in severe hyperthermic exposure. Aerospace Med 1971; 42:882.

214. Nunneley S, Troutman S, Webb P: Head cooling in work and heat stress. Aerospace Med 1971; 42:64.

215. Marcus P: Some effects of cooling and heating areas of the head and neck on body temperature measurements at the ear. Aerospace Med 1973; 44:397.

216. Brown G, Williams G: The effect of head cooling on deep body temperature and thermal comfort in man. Aviat Space Environ Med 1982; 53:583.

217. Williams C, Shitzer A: Modular liquid cooled helmet for thermal comfort. Aerospace Med 1974; 45:1030.

218. Gordon N, Bogdanffy G, Wilkinson J: Effect of a practical neck cooling device on core temperature during exercise. Med Sci Sports Exerc 1990; 22:245.

219. Lind A: A physiological criteria for setting thermal environmental limits for everyday work. J Appl Physiol 1963; 18:51.

220. Adams WC: Influence of exercise mode and selected ambient conditions on skin temperature. Ann NY Acad Sci 1977; 301:110.

221. Robinson S: The effect of body size upon energy exchange in work. Am J Physiol 1942; 136:363.

222. Armstrong L, De luca J, Hubbard R: Time course of recovery and heat acclimation ability of prior exertional heatstroke patients. Med Sci Sports Exer 1990; 22:36.

223. Kholagi M, Elkhatib G, Attia M, et al: Induced heat stroke: model in sheep. *In* Hales JRS, Richards DAB (eds): Heat Stroke and Temperature Regulation. Sydney, Australia, Academic Press, 1983, p 253.

224. Nadel ER: Body fluid and electrolyte balance during exercise: Competing demands with temperature regulation. *In* Hales JRS (ed): Thermal Physiol. New York, Raven Press, 1984, p 365.

225. Nadel ER: Recent advances in temperature regulation during exercise in humans. Fed Proc 1985; 44:2286.

226. Hales JRS: Proposed mechanisms underlying heat stroke. *In* Hales JRS, Richards DAB (eds): Heat Stress: Physical Exertion and Environment. Amsterdam, Elsevier, 1987, p 85.

227. Brinnel H, Cabanac M, Hales JRS: Critical upper levels of body temperature, tissue thermosensitivity, and selective brain cooling in hyperthermia. *In Hales JRS, Richards DAB (eds): Heat Stress: Physical Exertion and Environment. Amsterdam, Elsevier, 1987, p 209.*

228. Khogali M: Heat stroke: An overview. *In* Khogali M, Hales JRS (eds): Heat Stroke and Temperature Regulation. Sydney, Australia, Academic Press, 1983, p 1.

229. Britt RH, Lyons BE, Ryan T, et al: Effect of whole-body hyperthermia on auditory brainstem and somatosensory and visual-evoked potentials. *In* Hales JRS (ed): Thermal Physiology. New York, Raven Press, 1984, p 519.

230. Mustafa MKY, Khogali M, Gumaa K: Central nervous system, blood clotting and respiratory functions associated with heat stroke. *In* Hales JRS, Richards DAB: Heat Stress: Physical Exertion and Environment. Amsterdam, Elsevier, 1987, p 277.

231. Shibolet S, Lancaster MC, Danon Y: Heat stroke: A review. Aviat Space Environ Med 1976; 47:280.

232. Jessen C: Hyperthermia and its effect on exercise performance. *In* Hales JRS, Richards DAB (eds): Heat Stress: Physical Exertion and Environment. Amsterdam, Elsevier, 1987, p 241.

233. Greenleaf JE, Castle BL: Exercise temperature regulation in man during hypohydration and hyperhydration. J Appl Physiol 1971; 30:847.

234. Candas V, Libert JP, Brandenberg G, et al: Hydration during exercise: Effects on thermal and cardiovascular adjustments. Eur J Appl Physiol 1986; 55:113.

235. Quinton PM: Sweating and its disorders. Annu Rev Med 1983; 34:429.

236. Warner AE: Equine anhidrosis. Comp Cont Ed Pract Vet 1982; 4:S434.

237. Warner AE, Mayhew IG: Equine anhidrosis: A survey of affected horses in Florida. J Am Vet Med Assoc 1982; 180:627.

238. Barnes J: "Dry sweating" in horses. Vet Rec 1938; 50:977.

239. Jenkinson DM, Montgomery I, Elder HY, et al: Ultrastructural variations in the sweat glands of anhidrotic horses. Equine Vet J 1985; 17:287.

240. Jenkinson DM, Loney C, Elder HY, et al: Effects of season and lower ambient temperature on the structure of the sweat glands in anhidrotic horses. Equine Vet J 1989; 21:59.

241. Warner AE, Mayhew IG: Equine anhidrosis: a review of pathophysiological mechanisms. Vet Res Commun 1983; 6:249.0

II

Practical Considerations in Equine Sports Medicine

10

Nutrition and the Athletic Horse

LAURIE LAWRENCE

Nutrient Digestion and Absorption

In order for nutrients in the feed to be utilized by horses, they must first be digested and absorbed. The purpose of digestion is to break large, complex molecules into smaller molecules that can be absorbed from the intestines into the blood. As nonruminant herbivores, horses digest and absorb some feeds like monogastrics but handle other feeds in a manner similar to ruminants. Most digestion begins in the small intestine, where enzymes produced by the intestinal mucosa and the pancreas are responsible for breaking down proteins, fats, and the soluble carbohydrates such as starch and sucrose. Proteins or soluble carbohydrates that escape digestion in the small intestine, as well as fiber, may be digested in the large intestine by the microbial populations in the cecum and colon.

In the small intestine, dietary proteins are broken down and absorbed as their constituent amino acids. The amino acids are transported in the blood to tissues for use in protein synthesis or energy metabolism. Despite the fact that equine diets are relatively low in fat, horses appear to be able to digest most fats efficiently.[1] Dietary triglycerides are absorbed as fatty acids and glycerol but may be resynthesized into triglycerides for transport to sites of storage or metabolism. Starch is digested to glucose in the small intestine, and other soluble carbohydrates are digested to their component sugars. Glucose or the other simple sugars (usually fructose) are transported in the blood to tissues for energy metabolism or storage.

Fiber digestion occurs in the large intestine and results in the production of volatile fatty acids, primarily acetate, propionate, and butyrate. The volatile fatty acids (VFAs) may be used by the horse for immediate energy production or for the synthesis of glucose or fat. Any soluble carbohydrate (starch or glucose) that reaches the large intestine also will be subjected to the microbial fermentation, resulting in VFA production. Depending on the composition of the diet, a significant amount of the dietary protein may be digested in the large intestine. Gibbs and coworkers[2] demonstrated that while the protein in hay may be 74 percent digestible, less than 30 percent of the digestion occurs in the small intestine. When horses consume mixed diets (hay and concentrate), a greater proportion of protein digestion may occur in the small intestine.[3] Whereas small intestinal digestion results in the absorption of protein as amino acids, ammonia is an important product of the digestion of protein in the large intestine. The absorbed ammonia can be used to synthesize nonessential amino acids in horses, or it can be excreted as urea in the urine. It is possible that some amino acids may be absorbed intact from the large intestine of the horse,[4,5] but the quantitative significance of this process has not been established.

The large intestine has other digestive/absorptive roles and is an important site of phosphorus absorption in horses.[6] In addition, large amounts of water and electrolytes are absorbed from the large intestine, and the ability of the large intestine to store water may be one of its most important functions.[7] A considerable amount of B vitamin synthesis occurs in the large intestine,[8] and absorption from the large intestine has been demonstrated for several B vitamins.[8,9]

Nutrient Metabolism

AT REST

Following a meal, the process of digestion and absorption will result in an increase in circulating levels of several nutrients. The effects of diet and feeding schedule on glucose metabolism have received the most attention from researchers because of the relationship between glucose and insulin. When a horse receives a meal consisting of a concentrate feed (such as corn), blood glucose levels will rise from a prefeeding concentration of approximately 4 to 5.5 mmol/liter to a concentration of 6.5 to 7.5 mmol/liter within 2 hours of feeding.[10,11] The extent of the increase in blood glucose concentration will depend on meal size and composition. When a high-roughage meal is consumed, the increase in blood glucose is much smaller,[10–12] but mixed meals (hay plus concentrate or complete pellet) also elicit a significant increase in blood glucose concentration.[10,13] Plasma insulin concentration increases in response to the rise in blood glucose and facilitates the transport of glucose into peripheral tissues. By 5 to 6 hours after a meal, blood glucose concentrations will have returned to prefeeding levels.[10] Once inside the cell, glucose may be used for energy production, glycogen synthesis, or fat synthesis. Little is actually known about the regulation of these processes in the various tissues of the horse, but it is generally believed that glucose metabolism at the cellular level is the same in horses as in other monogastrics.

Following a meal, plasma concentrations of amino acids also will increase. Peak levels of most amino acids in the plasma will occur 2 to 5 hours after a meal depending on the size of the meal,[14,15] and more stable plasma amino acid concentrations are observed when horses consume several small meals rather than a few larger meals.[15] Insulin promotes the uptake of amino acids by muscle and other tissues, and as a result, plasma amino acid concentrations decline in the postabsorptive period.

Although several studies have demonstrated that horses can digest and utilize different types of dietary fat, there is very little information on postabsorptive lipid metabolism. In humans, triglycerides of dietary origin are transported in the blood by chylomicrons to sites of metabolism or storage. Uptake of lipid into cells is then facilitated by lipoprotein lipase, which hydrolyzes the triglyceride and allows fatty acids to move into the cell. Once inside the cell, the fatty acids may be oxidized for energy, or they may be used to resynthesize triglycerides. Similar processes have been presumed to occur in the horse, but there are few studies that have comprehensively evaluated the fate of dietary fat in resting horses. It appears that there are differences in the lipoprotein profile of horses and other animals[16] and that the composition of the lipoproteins may be altered in horses receiving additional dietary fat.[17]

Although the acetate, propionate, and butyrate produced by microbial fermentation in the large intestine are technically fatty acids, their transport and metabolism differ significantly from the scheme described above. Short-chain fatty acids are not transported by chylomicrons or other lipoproteins and appear to be taken up rapidly and transported in the blood. When VFAs were infused into the cecum, plasma concentrations peaked at 30 minutes after infusion.[18] At tissue sites, the VFA may be used for energy or for synthesis of glucose or fat. All the major VFAs are taken up by the liver, which has gluconeogenic and lipogenic capability.[18]

Acetate is quantitatively the most important VFA. On an all-roughage ration, the molar percentage of VFAs in cecal or colon fluid is about 70 percent acetate, 17 percent propionate, 8 percent butyrate, and 5 percent others (isobutyrate, isovalerate, and valerate).[19] The percentage of acetate will decrease and the percentage of propionate will increase as grain replaces hay in the ration.[19] Plasma acetate levels have been reported to be lower in lactating mares fed a high-concentrate ration than in mares receiving a ration high in roughage.[20] Acetate can be used for energy or for fatty acid synthesis. Propionate can be used for energy but may be of particular interest because of its glucogenic properties. Infusing propionate into fasted ponies results in an increase in blood glucose levels.[21] Using radioactive tracers, Simmons and Ford[22] recently estimated that propionate production by the cecum and colon could account for 50 to 61 percent of plasma glucose in resting ponies receiving high-fiber diets. Butyrate also may be used for energy by horses and has been reported to cause an increase in plasma insulin levels when infused in ponies.[23]

Volatile fatty acids probably play an extremely important role in energy metabolism in horses on high-roughage rations. As was noted previously, hay diets produce a small increase in blood glucose levels, probably because of the relatively low level of soluble carbohydrates in many roughages. Because hays are also low in ether extract, they provide little energy in the form of long-chain triglyceride. In addition, more than two-thirds of the digestible dry matter of an all-roughage ration is digested in the large intestine, where VFAs are produced.[3] It has been suggested that VFA production in the cecum could meet 30 percent of a horse's energy requirement at maintenance.[24] However, based on the considerations above, this estimate could be low. In addition, this estimate considered only digestion and VFA production by the cecum and did not include any contribution of the colon, which also contributes to fiber digestion.[25]

It is clear that following a meal, the availability of many substrates is increased. Insulin appears to play an important role in regulating the fate of the various nutrients in resting animals. Under the influence of insulin, anabolic processes are favored and catabolic processes are suppressed. Insulin is a positive regulator of glucose transport into the cell. Glucose transport in muscle and adipose tissue appears to be regulated by the glucose transporter (GLUT-4), which is translocated from an intracellular storage compartment to the plasma membrane under the influence of insulin.[26] Insulin increases the activity of glycogen synthase and thus promotes the storage of glucose as glycogen. Increased availability of glucose in the cell also increases the flux of glucose into the tricarboxylic acid (TCA) cycle and results in increased availability of acetyl-CoA for fatty acid synthesis. In adipose tissue, insulin is a positive regulator of lipoprotein lipase, which allows the removal of triglycerides from circulating lipoproteins and chylomicrons and thus promotes the storage of fat. Insulin also has a positive effect on amino acid uptake and may enhance protein synthesis. Insulin has a negative effect on phosphorylase, the enzyme responsible for glycogen breakdown. Insulin also has a negative effect on gluconeogenesis, amino acid catabolism, and lipolysis.

The response of plasma insulin to a meal closely follows the glucose response, and after a few hours, plasma insulin levels will decline.[10] If another meal is not consumed, the individual will eventually enter a fasting state. A fasting state is typically characterized by low concentrations of insulin and elevated levels of glucagon. The glucagon responses of horses have not been studied extensively, but in other animals, glucagon acts to enhance processes that stabilize plasma glucose concentrations. Glucagon is a positive modifier of phosphorylase activity in liver, thus stimulating glycogen breakdown and release of glucose into the circulation. Even a brief fast (16 to 24 hours) can result in markedly diminished liver glycogen stores in humans.[27] In other animals, glucagon also affects lipid metabolism by decreasing lipogenesis and enhancing lipolysis. As a result of lipolysis in adipose tissue, triglycerides are broken down and free fatty acids and glycerol are released into the blood. Free fatty acids are then available for oxidation to provide energy. Mobilization of fatty acids allows a greater proportion of the body's energy needs to be met by fat oxidation, thus sparing glucose utilization. The respiratory quotient (R or RQ) in fasting animals will approach 0.7, whereas in fed animals, the RQ will be closer to 1.0, indicating that carbohydrate is a more important fuel in fed animals.

If a fast is extended beyond 16 to 24 hours, further metabolic adaptations will occur. As liver glycogen stores become depleted, gluconeogenesis will become more important. The glycerol liberated from triglyceride hydrolysis is an important gluconeogenic precursor. There also will be an increased catabolism of amino acids, which can provide carbon skeletons for oxidation or glucose synthesis. Most of the amino acids are considered to be glucogenic, except leucine and lysine, which can only be metabolized for energy through conversion to acetyl-CoA or acetoacetyl-CoA. When amino acids are catabolized, the amino group must be removed. Typically, the amino group is transferred to another carbohydrate compound in a transamination reaction. Pyruvate, α-ketoglutarate, and glutamate can be aminated to form alanine, glutamate, and glutamine, respectively. When amino acid catabolism occurs in the muscle, alanine and glutamine serve to transport the amino group to the liver, where urea synthesis can occur. In the liver, the carbon skeletons from alanine and glutamine can be used for gluconeogenesis. The exact contribution of amino acids to energy metabolism in the fasting horse is not known, but in growing horses, the plasma concentrations of alanine, glutamine, and glutamate increased during a 48-hour fast, indicating that some amino acid catabolism was occurring.[15]

In many animals subjected to a prolonged fast, the increased mobilization of fatty acids and decreased availability of carbohydrate can lead to a ketotic condition. Some equids, however, appear to develop a hyperlipidemia in response to prolonged fasting that is characterized by elevated plasma triglyceride levels.[28] In severe cases, when plasma triglyceride concentrations rise above 500 mg/dl, the affected animals (usually ponies) often die.[28] A divergence of opinion exists as to whether the problem is attributable to a defect in triglyceride clearance[29,30] or to overproduction.[31] Either way, the response to prolonged fasting suggests that lipid metabolism in horses may not be identical to lipid metabolism in humans and that further research will be necessary before fat metabolism in the equine athlete is fully understood.

DURING EXERCISE

The fuels that are catabolized during exercise to supply ATP for muscle contraction ultimately originate from the diet. When exercise is undertaken within a few hours of a meal, the nutrients from that meal are available for catabolism. However, more commonly, fuel will be provided from the mobilization of nutrients that were stored after previous meals. During exercise, the most common fuels for muscle contraction are carbohydrate and fat. It has not been determined whether protein is an important fuel in horses, but in other species the contribution of protein catabolism has been estimated at 5 to 15 percent of oxidative energy production.[32]

A number of factors will influence the choice of substrate for energy production by working muscle. These factors include (but are not limited to) intensity of the exercise, duration of the exercise, fitness of the individual, and nutritional status. At rest and during low-intensity exercise, the oxidation of fat will commonly account for more than 50 percent of total energy production in humans.[33] The contribution of fat increases as the duration of the exercise bout increases so that after several hours of submaximal work, more than 75 percent of energy production in humans may come from fat catabolism.[34] Training also increases the contribution of fat to energy production during exercise, as evidenced by a lower RQ in trained individuals during an exercise bout and a reduced rate of glycogen utilization.[35] The importance of fat as a fuel during exercise decreases as exercise intensity increases. However, even during very high intensity exercise, some fat is being catabolized.

The fatty acids catabolized by muscle may be derived from endogenous triglycerides, circulating triglyc-

erides, or circulating free fatty acids (FFAs). Plasma FFAs are believed to be quantitatively the most important fat source for exercising muscle.[33] FFAs in the plasma originate from triglyceride hydrolysis in adipose tissue and thus represent a virtually endless supply of substrate in normal individuals. The contribution of plasma FFAs to energy production appears to be related to the supply of FFAs available to the muscle cell. During submaximal exercise, plasma FFA concentrations may initially decrease but will eventually increase as a result of accelerated release from adipose tissue under the influence of elevated catecholamines and decreased insulin. Increased availability of plasma FFAs during long-term exercise may permit the increased reliance on fat that occurs in the later stages of exercise. Some studies have shown that conditions that elevate plasma FFA concentrations prior to exercise can increase the proportion of energy derived from fat and spare muscle glycogen use.[36,37]

Endogenous (intramuscular) triglycerides also may be an important source of fatty acids for energy production during exercise.[38,39] Training appears to increase the ability to utilize intramuscular triglyceride during exercise.[40] Because training appears to blunt the catecholamine response and result in lower plasma FFA concentrations during exercise, increased dependence on intramuscular triglyceride could still allow greater fat use, even in the face of reduced plasma FFA availability.[39]

Studies with other species have suggested that circulating triglycerides may be a minor source of fat for exercising muscle,[41] but their contribution to muscle metabolism in horses has not been described. Similarly, the role of volatile fatty acids in energy production in exercising horses has not been well studied. However, it seems likely that acetate absorbed from the large intestine would be an available energy source for exercising muscle and that propionate could be an important glucogenic substance during long-term exercise.

As the intensity of exercise increases, the relative contribution of fat to total energy production decreases. During very high intensity exercise, the catabolism of carbohydrate may account for the majority of energy used,[42] and most of the carbohydrate will be derived from muscle glycogen.[43,44] Because the duration of exercise is short, total glycogen depletion during very intense exercise is not large. Several studies have reported that muscle glycogen stores are depleted 20 to 35 percent by short-term intense exercise.[45–47] Conversely, although the rate of glycogen utilization is low during submaximal long-term exercise, total glycogen depletion may be quite significant. It would not be uncommon for the muscle glycogen stores of endurance horses to be depleted by more than 50 to 75 percent after an 80- or 160-km ride.[48,49]

Adequate muscle glycogen stores appear to be important for peak performance in both short, intense work bouts and long-term exercise. A negative effect of reduced muscle glycogen stores on work performance has been demonstrated in the horse.[50] Studies with humans have demonstrated the importance of muscle glycogen content to human work performance, especially during long-term exercise.[27]

Although muscle glycogen is the primary source of carbohydrate during high-intensity exercise, blood glucose may contribute 10 to 40 percent of the total energy for submaximal exercise.[51] In the latter stages of a long-term submaximal exercise bout when muscle glycogen stores have been reduced, blood glucose may be the major source of carbohydrate for exercising muscle.[52,53] The uptake of glucose by muscle increases during long-term exercise even though plasma insulin concentrations are depressed. Muscle contraction appears to allow glucose uptake by activating the glucose transporter (GLUT-4), although the exact mechanism is not fully understood.[26]

Except in the period immediately following a meal, most of the circulating blood glucose will originate from the liver. During the initial stages of exercise, hepatic glucose is derived from glycogenolysis; however, gluconeogenesis becomes increasingly important as the availability of glucogenic precursors (glycerol, lactate, and alanine) increases and liver glycogen stores decrease. When liver glycogen stores are depleted, hepatic gluconeogenesis does not appear to be capable of maintaining glucose homeostasis in exercising humans.[42] The fall in blood glucose concentration that coincides with the depletion of muscle and liver glycogen has been associated with the onset of fatigue in long-term exercise.[52] Studies with human athletes have demonstrated that fatigue can be delayed if normal blood glucose levels are maintained by intravenous glucose infusion or oral supplementation with glucose or other carbohydrates.[54,55]

As mentioned previously, the extent of amino acid oxidation during exercise has not been determined in the horse. However, an increase in plasma alanine and glutamine concentrations during short-term exercise and an increase in plasma urea concentration during long-term exercise suggest that some protein catabolism does occur in the exercising horse.[49,56] In other animals, muscle has the capacity to oxidize only a few amino acids. Oxidation of the branched-chain amino acids (leucine, valine, and isoleucine) has received the most attention, but alanine, glutamate, and aspartate also may be utilized to some extent.[57] Of the three branched-chain amino acids, leucine appears to be quantitatively the most important. Estimates of the contribution of leucine to energy production during exercise vary from less than 5 percent[58] up to 20 percent,[59] but total energy production from protein use during exercise frequently is suggested to be less than 10 percent.[32,57,60,61] Carbohydrate availability may increase the use of protein as an energy source. When humans exercised in a glycogen-depleted state or after a long-term fast (3.5 days), protein catabolism was increased.[58,62] Other factors such as training and diet manipulation also may affect the amount of protein catabolized during exercise.

DURING RECOVERY

Once the exercise bout is over, some metabolic processes adjust rapidly, while others return to normal fairly slowly. After high-intensity exercise, plasma lactate concentrations may initially increase but will usually begin to decrease within a few minutes of the end of exercise. Lactate is taken up by liver or extrahepatic tissues for glycogen resynthesis or for oxidation.[52,63] Plasma glucose concentrations increase in horses following intense exercise such as racing,[64] probably from increased hepatic glycogenolysis as well as increased gluconeogenesis. Because the breakdown of muscle glycogen provides a great proportion of the energy for high-intensity exercise, increased availability of plasma glucose will allow repletion of depleted muscle glycogen stores. Plasma FFA concentrations may not rise following intense exercise, possibly because mobilization is balanced by uptake.[64] However, mobilization of fatty acids from adipose tissue does appear to occur in the recovery period from intense exercise because glycerol concentrations are elevated by about 10-fold.[47,65] Thus, in the period following intense exercise, fatty acids are made available to meet energy needs, and glycerol is available for hepatic gluconeogenesis. In horses, some fatty acids also must be reesterified in the liver because plasma triglyceride levels rise after exercise.[65]

Following long-term submaximal exercise, there is a different pattern of recovery responses. After long-term exercise, plasma lactate levels are not very high because little lactate is produced. In addition, plasma glucose concentrations are often depressed, and carbohydrate stores will be markedly reduced. In one study, long-term exercise in the horse was reported to deplete 60 percent of the glycogen stored in the muscle and 85 percent of the glycogen stored in the liver.[45] Thus the restoration of glucose homeostasis and glycogen stores is important in the recovery period. If no carbohydrate is consumed in the postexercise period, restoration of glycogen stores will rely on gluconeogenesis. Following long-term exercise, insulin concentration will be low, while the levels of glucagon and other catabolic hormones such as cortisol and catecholamines will be elevated, allowing continued mobilization of fatty acids and glycerol. In addition to glycerol, some alanine will be available as a glucogenic precursor. When carbohydrate is not consumed in the postexercise period, glycerol and alanine will be the primary sources of carbon for glucose synthesis, and the restoration of glycogen stores will be slow.[66–68] Consumption of carbohydrate is necessary to replete muscle and liver glycogen stores following severe glycogen depletion. In humans, the amount and timing of carbohydrate consumption in the postexercise period will affect the rate of glycogen repletion. In one study, glycogen synthesis was increased when the amount of carbohydrate ingested was increased from 0.35 g glucose per kilogram of body weight to 0.70 g/kg, but not when the amount was further increased to 1.4 g/kg.[69] In another study, the rate of glycogen synthesis was improved when carbohydrate was consumed immediately after exercise rather than 2 hours after exercise.[70]

Glycogen resynthesis appears to be controlled by several factors. The consumption of carbohydrate provides substrate and elicits an increase in insulin. Although non-insulin-dependent glucose transport is still increased immediately following an exhaustive exercise bout, the presence of insulin may further accelerate glucose uptake. It has been suggested that it is the ability to transport glucose into the cell that limits the rate of glycogen synthesis.[71] The activity of glycogen synthase is also an important regulator of glycogen synthesis and may be enhanced by insulin. Therefore, it has been suggested that the best strategies for rapid repletion of glycogen stores include consumption of carbohydrate immediately after exercise and at frequent intervals (2 hours) for 6 to 24 hours.[70,72] The rate of glycogen synthesis will decline as glycogen stores are replenished, even if glucose is available. When muscle glycogen levels are low, more glycogen synthase is present in the active form; as glycogen levels rise, more glycogen synthase will be present in the inactive form.

Nutrient Requirements of Performance Horses

ENERGY

In 1989, the National Research Council Subcommittee on Horse Nutrition (NRC) recommended that daily energy be increased 25, 50, and 100 percent above maintenance for light, medium, and intense work, respectively.[73] *Light work* was described as pleasure and equitation work; medium work was ranch work, barrel racing, jumping, etc.; and *intense work* was described as race training and polo. These recommendations are useful estimates for some horses but may not be specific enough for others.

Several studies have attempted to develop more accurate estimates for the energy requirements of performance horses. One method for determining the energy cost of exercise is to measure the amount of oxygen consumed and carbon dioxide produced during exercise.[74,75] This method is currently only practical in laboratory situations where horses exercise on a treadmill, but it can provide useful information that can be extrapolated to other situations. The results of one study suggested that the energy cost of exercise could be predicted by the following equation:

$$\text{Energy expenditure (cal/kg/min)} = e^{3.02 + .0065x}$$

where x is the velocity (m/min).[74] This equation is useful for horses exercising on level ground and a normal track surface, but it is not easily applied to situations where velocity is not the sole determinant of intensity. Another option would be to relate energy expenditure to another measurement of exercise intensity such as oxygen uptake. In field situations, heart rate measurements may be used to estimate the intensity of a given work bout as a percentage of $\dot{V}_{O_2max}$.[76] Figure 10–1 illustrates the energy cost of exercise performed at different intensities. It is apparent from Figure 10–1 that high-intensity exercise is energetically much more expensive on a per-minute basis than low-intensity exercise. However, most horses will be capable of high-intensity exercise (>100 percent $\dot{V}_{O_2max}$) for relatively short periods of time (<5 minutes), while low- or moderate-intensity exercise can be sustained for several hours. Thus, when the total cost of exercise is determined, duration of the exercise also must be considered. The approximate digestible energy (DE) costs of horses performing different activities are shown in Figure 10–2. The amount of DE was arrived at using an efficiency of DE use for exercise of 57 percent.[74]

Although collection of respiratory gases during exercise allows an accurate measurement of energy production during an individual exercise bout, it does not reflect the daily energy requirement. The daily energy

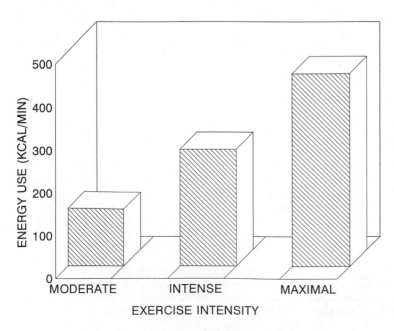

Figure 10-1. Estimated energy use (kcal/ min) of a 500-kg horse performing different types of exercise. Moderate, intense, and maximal exercise in this figure represent work efforts of approximately 60, 90, and 120 percent of $\dot{V}_{O_2max}$.

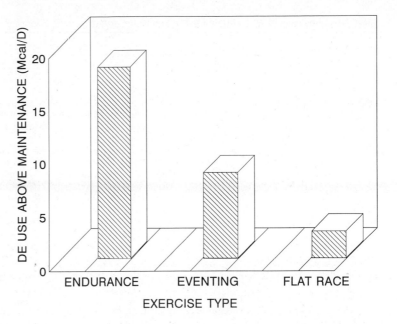

Figure 10-2. *Estimated digestible energy use (above maintenance) of a 500-kg horse during a 50- to 80-km endurance race, the second day of an advanced 3-day event, or a 1600-m flat race.*

requirement is the sum of the energy expended in exercise and the maintenance requirement. As is apparent in Figure 10–2, the amount of energy expended by a horse during a race is not very great, and thus the total daily requirement (including maintenance) for many racehorses might be calculated at less than 24 Mcal/d. Surveys of feeding practices at racetracks indicate that most thoroughbred and standardbred racehorses will be receiving more than 30 Mcal/d. The discrepancy between the calculated requirement and actual practice probably relates to the inability of the calculated requirement to account for extra exercise such as warming up, cooling out, and stall activity. Therefore, some researchers have estimated the daily energy requirements of exercising horses by determining the amount of DE necessary to maintain body weight when horses perform different activities.[77,78] This method is the most practical in normal environments but assumes that maintenance of a particular body weight is desirable.

The importance of body weight and body condition to athletic performance has received considerable attention in humans but not in horses. In humans, body composition is often characterized with a two-compartment model composed of lean body mass and body fat. As a non-force-generating component of the body, excess fat is considered a detriment in many activities, especially those which include running.[79] The negative correlation between running speed and body fat appears to be stronger in men than in women, but significant correlations have been reported for both sexes.[80] In an effort to quantify the effect of excess fat on running performance, researchers have tested human athletes when they were carrying added weight around the trunk.[81] In one study, the addition of weight equivalent to 15 percent of body weight resulted in an 8.6 percent decrease in running performance, while addition of weight equivalent to 5 percent of body weight caused a 4 percent

decrease in performance. While carrying excess weight, individuals perform submaximal exercise at a higher percentage of $\dot{V}_{O_2max}$, which may result in earlier fatigue.[81] Although the relationship between body fatness and running performance has not been studied in horses, the effect of weight carrying on oxygen uptake has been evaluated. The addition of a 10 percent load to horses exercising on a horizontal treadmill increased oxygen consumption by 15 percent.[82] These results, and the fact that thoroughbred racehorses are handicapped with small amounts of lead weight, suggest that even small changes in body fat could affect performance of certain athletic horses.

Unfortunately, it is difficult to accurately assess body fat in horses. Indirect techniques such as hydrostatic (underwater) weighing and whole-body counting of potassium-40 are not applicable to horses. In 1976, workers at Cornell University determined that the thickness of subcutaneous fat over the rump was significantly correlated with whole-body fat.[83] Rump fat thickness can be determined noninvasively using ultrasound technology and percentage of body fat then predicted from experimentally derived equations.[83,84] Unfortunately, the correlations between rump fat thickness and percentage of body fat are derived from very small sample numbers, so application of this technique to practical situations must be approached with caution. Another technique that may have application to evaluation of body fatness in horses is condition scoring. Condition scoring is a subjective system, but it requires no equipment. Several condition scoring systems exist, and a version of the system devised at Texas A&M University is shown in Table 10–1.[85] The combination of condition scoring and regular body weight measurements could be useful in evaluating energy balance in performance horses. Whether horses should be fed to a specific level of body fatness is not known.

Table 10-1. Summary of a Condition Scoring System for Horses

Condition	Score	Description
Poor	1	Horse very emaciated; bone structure very apparent, including cervical and lumbar vertabrae
Very thin	2	Horse emaciated; bone structure still visible in shoulder and pelvis; cervical vertabrae barely visible
Thin	3	Neck thin; junction of neck, withers, and shoulder accentuated; pelvic structure still accentuated; transverse processes of lumbar vertabrae cannot be felt
Moderately thin	4	Neck, withers, and shoulder not obviously thin; spine still apparent but not individual vertabrae; outline of ribs still visible
Moderate	5	Neck blends smoothly into withers and shoulder; back (loin) is relatively flat; ribs are not visible but are easily felt
Moderately fleshy	6	Neck, shoulder, and withers appear more filled and rounded; loin area may have slight depression along spine (crease); tailhead and ribs are starting to feel soft or spongy
Fleshy	7	Fat deposited along withers and neck; tailhead soft; ribs filling with fat; crease along spine may be more visible
Fat	8	Neck thickened; fat accumulating in buttocks; definite crease along spine; ribs are hard to feel
Extremely fat	9	Bulging fat in neck, withers, and shoulder; prominant crease down back; patchy fat over ribs

Adapted from Henneke DR, Potter GD, Krieder JL: A condition score relationship to body fat content of mares during gestation and lactation. *In* Proceedings of the 7th Equine Nutrition and Physiology Symposium. Warrenton, VA, 1981, p 105.

In human athletics, considerable effort has been expended in profiling the body composition characteristics of athletes in different sports.[79] For example, while marathoners and distance runners are fairly lean, athletes involved in strength activities may tolerate higher levels of body fat.[86] Currently, there are few studies that have investigated the desirable body composition for horses involved in different activities. In one study, the body condition of horses competing in an endurance ride was studied.[87] Average condition score for the horses in the race was 4.67 (1 to 9 scale), and percentage of body fat, predicted from rump fat thickness, averaged 7.8 percent, which compares well with reported body fat percentages in human long-distance runners.[88] Gallagher and coworkers reported that standardbred horses in race training had an average condition score of 5.7, while thoroughbreds at a nearby track had an average condition score of 5.0[89,90] These are very preliminary observations, and further studies on horses of different athletic types are necessary before recommendations concerning optimal end points for body condition are made.

Because the amount of body fat carried by an individual may affect performance, it might be tempting to restrict calories in an attempt to produce a very lean body condition. However, fat is not the only body component of importance to athletic performance. Aerobic capacity (expressed as maximum oxygen uptake in liters per minute) and total strength are more closely related to lean body mass than to body fat.[91] This observation is important because of the relationship between lean body mass and body fat during weight change. It is a common, but probably erroneous, perception that weight change in adult animals involves only fat tissue. Weight gain or loss can involve changes in lean tissue as well as fat. In humans, weight change in lean individuals may be up to 50 percent lean. In fatter individuals, a greater proportion of the weight change will be fat, but even in obese people, lean tissue may still account for 25 percent of the change.[92,93] If the same relationships

hold true for horses, then loss of body weight by an equine athlete could reduce lean body mass and adversely affect performance. Fortunately, regular exercise favors fat loss and may spare lean tissue loss,[94,95] particularly if the individual is in positive energy balance. Thus the most desirable program for weight control would combine dietary management and exercise to maximize lean body mass and minimize body fat. Although some horses may appear overfat when they begin a training program, severe caloric restriction that results in significant weight loss may not be desirable because of concomitant loss of lean body mass.

PROTEIN

The importance of protein to athletic performance has been pondered for decades, it not centuries. Even ancient Greek athletes may have believed that the addition of meat to their diets would improve performance.[96] More recently, the importance of protein as a fuel for exercise has been discounted. In 1978, the NRC stated that exercise does not increase the protein requirement of horses.[97] Fat and carbohydrate are the most important fuels for exercise, but it now appears that under certain situations, protein may contribute 5 to 15 percent of the total energy used.

In other species, the evidence for the catabolism of protein during exercise comes from the observation of metabolic changes during exercise and from studies using radioisotope-labeled amino acids. In horses, several studies have documented that plasma alanine concentrations increase during moderate exercise.[56,98,99] In addition, plasma urea concentrations increase following long-term exercise.[49] No studies with labeled amino acids have been used to determine whether certain amino acids are preferentially catabolized by horses, but it can be inferred from studies with other species that the branched-chain amino acids, especially leucine, are most important. Most amino acids in the body are contained in structural proteins and are therefore not readily available for energy production. However, there are some amino acids free in the plasma and some labile proteins in the liver that could provide amino acids for energy production. In addition, exercise may make amino acids available by altering protein turnover either by increasing protein degradation or by decreasing protein synthesis.[100]

Some athletes consume high-protein diets in order to support changes in body composition: increased muscle or lean body mass. This practice is based on the assumption that individuals in training actually do increase lean body mass. In some cases, the amount of lean body mass is not affected by training, although the percentage of the body that is lean body mass may be increased. That is, training may result in a decrease in body fat, but not necessarily an increase muscle mass. In humans, an increase in lean body mass will occur most commonly as a consequence of strength training. For example, weight lifters have been reported to experience periods of negative nitrogen balance even when protein intakes are relatively high.[86] Effects of training on lean body mass are more likely to occur in the early phases of training and in young athletes who are growing and training simultaneously. Dietary protein intake also may play a role in ameliorating the effects of weight loss on lean body mass loss in certain situations.[101]

In 1978, the NRC indicated that a 500-kg horse in heavy work had the same protein requirement as a 500-kg horse at maintenance—about 630 g crude protein.[97] This recommendation was somewhat impractical because of the difficulty in formulating palatable diets that would meet the energy requirement without greatly exceeding the protein requirement. In 1989, the crude protein recommendations for working horses were increased (Table 10–2). There are several reasons for increasing the crude protein level above the 1978 recommendation. Horses may lose 1 to 1.5 g nitrogen per kilogram of sweat; thus exercising horses could easily lose 5 to 7 g nitrogen per day.[102] Increased nitrogen retention has been reported in horses in training,[103] and changes in plasma urea and alanine concentrations suggest that some protein catabolism occurs during exercise. In addition, an increased protein intake may be necessary to offset the increased endogenous fecal nitrogen losses associated with higher dry matter intakes of hard-working horses.[102]

While there is little controversy over the suggestion that regular exercise can elevate the protein requirement of horses, there is debate regarding the magnitude of the increase. The 1989 recommendations for hard-working horses are more than double the 1978 recommendations. The 1989 recommendations were arrived at by maintaining the same protein/calorie ratio in the diets of working horses as in the diets of horses at maintenance.[73] While these recommendations provide a practical way to adjust protein intake for working horses, they are not necessarily accurate estimates of need. Studies that accurately estimate protein and amino acid requirements of horses have not been performed. In one study, horses performing hard or medium work had similar indices of protein status when they received 0.8 or 1.2 g crude protein per kilogram of body weight.[104] However, in that study, the horses on the higher-protein diet recovered from a 1.6-km track test faster than the horses on the low-protein diet. In addition, all horses in the study lost weight, indicating that the diets used may not have been adequate in energy.[104]

Some estimate of the appropriateness of the current recommendations for horses may be gained by comparing these recommendations with those made for human athletes. Several sources suggest that 1.2 to 1.5 g protein per kilogram of body weight is sufficient for most human athletes.[105–107] Only weight lifters in rigorous strength training may have a requirement above 2 g/kg.[86] If these recommendations are applied to 500-kg horses, the requirement will be between 600 g (at 1.2 g/kg) and 1000 g (at 2 g/kg) per day. These values can be compared with the current recommendations for working horses in Table 10–2. While it appears that the NRC recommendations for moderate and intense work greatly exceed the values that are estimated from human recommendations, the types of protein consumed by horses and humans are considerably different. While horses frequently consume low-quality proteins from roughages and cereal grains, humans consume high-quality protein from animal sources. Once the differences in protein digestibility and quality (amino acid balance) between the different foods are considered, the recommendations for human and equine athletes become more comparable. No studies have examined the importance of protein quality for athletic horses, but it has been suggested that the total amount of protein consumed by human athletes can be reduced when protein quality is increased.[86,96] Therefore, it is possible that fewer grams of total protein may be required when horses are fed higher-quality protein sources such as soybean meal or milk protein.

Protein supplementation above 1.5 g/kg of body weight has little observable benefit on human athletic performance.[57,59,86,96,107] Similarly, studies with horses have found no positive effects of high dietary protein.[56,99,108,109] Conversely, it has been suggested that diets containing excessive levels of protein may be detrimental to equine performance. Meyer[102] suggested that digestible protein intakes above 2g/kg of body weight per day should be avoided in endurance horses because of effects on water intake and urea and ammonia metabolism. Exercising horses consuming 1741 g crude protein

Table 10-2. Daily Crude Protein Requirements of Exercising Horses

	Body Weight		
	400 kg	500 kg	600 kg
Maintenance	536 g	656 g	776 g
Light work	670 g	820 g	970 g
Moderate work	804 g	984 g	1164 g
Intense work	1072 g	1312 g	1552 g

From National Research Council: Nutrient Requirements of Horses, 5th ed. Washington, National Academy Press, 1989.

per day (> 3 g/kg of body weight) excreted more urea in sweat and had higher plasma urea levels than horses consuming 836 g crude protein per day.[99] In addition, an increase in postexercise orotic acid excretion in the horses receiving the high-protein diet was interpreted to suggest that an intake of 1741 g crude protein per day might exceed the capacity of the urea cycle.[99] If protein replaces carbohydrate in the diet, then glycogen storage may be affected. In one study with horses, muscle glycogen concentrations were lower on a high-protein diet,[109] but in another study, no effect was observed.[108] Feeding very high protein diets to rats reduced muscle and liver glycogen concentrations before exercise and slowed muscle glycogen repletion after exercise.[110,111] Another potentially deleterious effect of excessive protein intake is increased urinary nitrogen excretion. Increased urinary nitrogen excretion may contribute to increased inspired ammonia levels, which could adversely affect respiratory health.

CALCIUM AND PHOSPHORUS

Because skeletal integrity is of such importance to performance horses, calcium and phosphorus nutrition are of prime concern. Calcium and phosphorus are the major minerals in bone, accounting for about 50 percent of the equine skeleton.[73] In addition, calcium has an integral role in muscle contraction, and phosphorus is essential in energy production. Dietary calcium and phosphorus requirements are highest in growing horses that are depositing new bone at a rapid rate. However, even adult horses require calcium and phosphorus to maintain bone integrity. Repeated bouts of exercise can cause bone remodeling and increased bone density,[112,113] and thus exercise may increase the calcium and phosphorus requirements. The current calcium and phosphorus recommendations for mature horses at maintenance and heavy work are shown in Table 10–3. As with the protein recommendations, the nutrient/calorie ratios were maintained in the diet, resulting in a large increase in the recommended total daily calcium and phosphorus consumption by working horses. How well these recommendations compare with the actual needs of working horses is not known. Meyer[102] suggests that the calcium and phosphorus requirements of working horses are only slightly higher than maintenance. Using a small number of yearling standardbred horses, Schryver and coworkers found a trend for increased bone calcium deposition with exercise but could not define an increase in the dietary calcium requirement.[113a] While sweat contains some calcium (about 200 mg/liter), even heavily sweating horses (10 to 20 liters/day) would be expected to lose less than 5 g Ca per day.[102] Although calcium and phosphorus requirements may not be affected greatly by exercise, attention to calcium and phosphorus nutrition in working horses is extremely important. Diets containing inadequate levels of these nutrients or an imbalanced Ca/P ratio can result in abnormal bone physiology. Diets that are low in calcium and high in phosphorus can cause demineralization of bone and, in extreme cases, lameness.[114] A high level of

Table 10-3. Estimated Daily Mineral Requirements of 500-kg Horses*

Mineral	Maintenance	Work
Ca (g)	20	40
P (g)	14	29
Mg (g)	7.5	15.1
K (g)	25	49.9
Na (g)	8.2	34.5
S (g)	12.3	17.3
Fe (mg)	328	460
Mn (mg)	328	460
Cu (mg)	82	115
Zn (mg)	328	460
Se (mg)	0.8	1.15
I (mg)	0.8	1.15
Co (mg)	0.8	1.15

*Assuming a dry matter intake of 8.2 kg/day for maintenance and 11.5 for intense work.
From National Research Council: Nutrient Requirements of Horses, 5th ed. Washington, National Academy Press, 1989.

phosphorus in the diet can decrease calcium absorption.[115] Thus, even when diets appear adequate in calcium, a high phosphorus intake may result in a calcium deficiency. Diets for all classes of horses should have a Ca/P ratio of at least 1:1.

In practical feeding situations, deficiencies, excesses, or an imbalance in calcium and phosphorus can occur easily. Many owners and trainers are unaware of the importance of a correct Ca/P ratio,[116] and the combination of certain common feeds can result in improper calcium or phosphorus nutrition. Grass hays tend to be low to moderate in calcium and phosphorus, while legume hays are usually quite high in calcium. Most cereal grains are very low in calcium and fairly high in phosphorus. It is not uncommon for a hard-working horse to receive a large amount of concentrate and a limited amount of hay. If the hay is a grass variety and the concentrate is plain oats (or another cereal grain), then it would be possible for dietary phosphorus to exceed dietary calcium. This situation appears to be quite common in many parts of the world, including Asia and Australia.[117] In the United States, diets may contain more legume roughage, and the situation may be less prevalent. Rations that contain a large amount of alfalfa or clover may contain levels of calcium well in excess of the required amount. The Ca/P ratio of diets containing a large amount of legume hay may be greater than 3:1. High-calcium diets appear to be well tolerated by mature horses, possibly because the efficacy of calcium absorption from the small intestine is decreased when calcium is abundant.

Evaluating the calcium and phosphorus adequacy of a diet is somewhat clouded by the issue of calcium and phosphorus availability. The availability of these nutrients in the various feeds is not 100 percent. The NRC recommendations for working horses use absorption efficiencies of 50 percent for calcium and 35 percent for phosphorus. The presence of oxalate or phytate in feeds can affect calcium and phosphorus availability and result in true digestibility values much lower than those used by the NRC for estimating requirements. Some tropical grasses are very high in oxalate, while cereal grains and cereal hays are high in phytate. A calculated phosphorus digestibility of 20 percent has been reported for pelleted oat hay, but it was suggested that the true value might actually be lower.[118] It is possible to ensure calcium and phosphorus adequacy by incorporating inorganic sources into rations. Some common inorganic sources of calcium and phosphorus are listed in Table 10–4. The availability of calcium and phosphorus from inorganic sources is high, and most commercial feeds will use one or more of these sources to balance the calcium and phosphorus ratio and ensure adequate levels of each nutrient.

Young horses in training will undergo more bone remodeling than older horses and thus will be most sensitive to calcium and phosphorus nutrition. However, the nutrition received by horses during their early growth period may be of more importance to overall soundness than the nutrition received as adults. Improper nutrition has been suggested as a predisposing cause of developmental orthopedic disease (DOD), but other factors such as genetics and activity level also may be involved.[119] Many theories exist as to the primary nutritional agent responsible for DOD, but two recent reviews of the topic indicate that there is little consensus in this area.[119,120] Excess calories, excess soluble carbohydrate, excess protein, excess calcium, excess phosphorus, excess vitamin A, deficient calcium, and deficient copper have each been implicated as causal factors.[73,119,121–124] As noted earlier, rations using grass hay and cereal grains may be high in phosphorus and deficient in calcium, while the widespread use of alfalfa in the United States frequently results in rations that are high in calcium. A relationship between high-calcium intakes during early growth and eventual bone pathology has been proposed but not substantiated.[124] It has been recommended that diets for young horses should not exceed the calcium requirement by more than 25 to 50 percent.[120] The NRC recommendations for growth

emphasize the importance of using balanced rations. Diets that are excessive in any nutrient or deficient in any nutrient should not be fed to young horses.

ELECTROLYTES

The role of electrolytes in thermoregulation, fluid balance, and acid-base balance of performance horses has been discussed previously (see Chaps. 5 and 9). On a daily basis, the majority of electrolyte loss occurs through the urine, feces, and, in performance horses, through sweat. Meyer[102] reviewed the literature on electrolyte losses during exercise and concluded that 125 g Na, 75 g K, and 175 g Cl per day are necessary to replace the electrolyte losses of hard-working horses. Horses that are treated with diuretic drugs prior to racing will have additional electrolyte losses. Failure to replace electrolyte losses may have a detrimental effect on the equine athlete. After 2 to 3 weeks on an exercise program, ponies receiving a very low sodium diet began to sweat less than ponies on a higher-sodium diet.[125] In addition, feed and water intake was reduced by the very low sodium diet. Very low potassium intakes can cause similar effects on sweating rates and feed intake.[126] Electrolytes may be provided to horses in the ration or as a separate supplement. Although horses may not regulate their own sodium balance precisely, sodium-depleted horses will voluntarily increase their salt intake if a salt block (lick) is available.[127] Because many common horse feeds are relatively low in sodium content, it is recommended that salt be provided free choice to horses of all classes. Salt can be offered loose or as a block. In the United States, white salt usually contains only sodium and chloride, although some products may be iodized. Trace mineralized salt is usually brown or reddish brown in color and contains some additional trace minerals such as copper, zinc, and iron. It should be noted that salt supplements typically do not contain potassium. Fortunately, roughages are relatively high in potassium, and many rations will therefore contain adequate potassium for most horses. If very low roughage rations are being fed, then potassium supplementation may be necessary. The addition of electrolytes to horse feeds should be approached conservatively because high levels of salt may decrease feed intake. Similarly, the addition of electrolytes to drinking water may reduce water consumption. Electrolytes that are consumed in excess of the horse's requirement are usually excreted and are not stored for future use.

During an extended workout, especially in a hot environment (such as endurance rides or combined training events), some horses may require additional electrolytes. These can be provided to the horse at rest periods during the exercise bout. It also may be possible to create a reservoir of electrolytes in the large intestine through manipulation of the pre-event feeding practices.[102] It has been suggested that horses receiving a high-fiber meal containing electrolytes prior to exercise will have more electrolytes and water available to replace exercise-induced losses than horses that receive a lower-fiber, lower-electrolyte meal.[102]

Table 10-4. Composition of Common Calcium and Phosphorus Supplements*

Supplement	% Ca	% P
Steamed bone meal	30.7	12.9
Calcium carbonate	39.4	.04
Dicalcium phosphate	22.0	19.0
Limestone	34.0	.02
Ground oystershell	38.0	.07
Deflourinated phosphate	32.0	18.0
Monosodium phosphate	—	22.5

*Based on a dry matter content of 97 to 100%. These ingredients also may contain significant quantities of other minerals.
From National Research Council: Nutrient Requirements of Horses, 5th ed. Washington, National Academy Press, 1989.

TRACE MINERALS

Very few studies have investigated the trace mineral requirements of performance horses. Recommendations for daily intakes (see Table 10–3) have been based on studies of horses in other physiologic states (maintenance, growth, lactation), on extrapolation from studies with other animals, and the absence of clinical deficiency signs when horses are fed typical diets. Therefore, whether the recommendations for trace mineral intakes are sufficient for optimal performance in horses is not known. Conversely, there is little information to suggest that supplementation of trace minerals above the current recommended levels is necessary or beneficial for performance.

The trace minerals of most interest in performance horses are those associated with red blood cell formation or metabolism, such as iron, copper, and zinc. In human athletes, especially women, it appears that daily iron losses can frequently exceed daily intakes, resulting in a decline in iron status.[128] In these athletes, iron deficiency will progress through three stages: (1) depletion of iron stores, (2) diminished erythropoiesis, and (3) reduced hemoglobin production resulting in anemia.[128] Reduced hemoglobin levels are associated with impaired exercise performance, including a reduction in $\dot{V}_{O_2max}$.[129] It should be noted that decreased hemoglobin concentration is not apparent until the later stages of iron deficiency. Thus, even when human athletes have other signs of poor iron status, iron supplementation may not affect performance,[130,131] suggesting that iron status must be markedly depressed to affect performance. Conversely, some researchers have reported a non-hemoglobin-related effect of iron supplementation on performance. Performance was improved in iron-deficient rats within 15 hours of receiving an injection of iron dextran.[132] Hemoglobin concentration was not affected, and the authors postulated that ionic iron may play a metabolically active role during exercise.

In human athletes, iron status declines during training, when iron intakes fail to meet iron losses, which may be higher than 2 mg/day.[128] If horses sustain similar losses (they have not been measured), a 500-kg horse might lose about 15 mg Fe per day. Even considering that the availability of iron in horse feeds may be less than 15 percent,[73] these losses would predict a dietary requirement of no more than 300 mg/day (based on an estimate of loss of 30 mg/day and 10 percent availability). Forages fed to horses usually contain at least 100 mg Fe per kilogram, and grains will contain at least 50 mg Fe per kilogram. Thus a hard-working 500-kg horse consuming 5 kg hay and 5 kg grain would be receiving approximately 750 mg Fe.

Iron, alone or in combination with copper, zinc, and several vitamins, is often supplemented to horses in an effort to increase the oxygen-carrying capacity of the blood. Benefits of this practice have not been documented. In controlled studies, the use of iron supplements has failed to produce increases in hemoglobin or packed cell volume in horses.[133,134] In addition, this practice is based on the assumption that the oxygen-carrying capacity of the blood is a limiting factor in equine performance. Pate[135] has suggested that hemoglobin concentrations above 150 to 160 g/liter are necessary for maximal oxygen delivery in human athletes. The significance of resting hemoglobin concentration to oxygen transport in exercising horses is probably not as great as in humans. Because of splenic contraction, hemoglobin concentration in horses will usually rise above 200 g/liter during intense exercise, and oxygen transport will be augmented by 40 to 60 percent.[136]

Many other trace minerals are necessary for exercising horses, but very little is known about requirements. A deficiency of any trace mineral is likely to affect exercise performance, and the diets of performance horses should be evaluated for trace mineral status using the NRC recommendations. It is not uncommon for feeds from specific areas to be deficient in one or more trace minerals. For example, feeds from certain parts of the United States may be low in selenium, necessitating some supplementation. In addition, the presence of a high concentration of one mineral may interfere with the absorption of other minerals. Indiscriminate use of trace mineral supplements should be avoided because of the potential for toxicity.

VITAMINS

Many common horse feeds are good sources of vitamins. In addition, some vitamins are synthesized and absorbed in the large intestine. However, the requirements of performance horses for most vitamins have not been studied, and the adequacy of typical diets for optimal performance is unknown.

The NRC recommends that hard-working horses (500 kg) receive 22,000 IU of vitamin A per day. In horses, dietary beta-carotene can be converted to vitamin A such that 1 mg beta-carotene is equivalent to 400 IU vitamin A.[137] Fresh growing pasture will usually contain more than 50,000 IU vitamin A activity per kilogram of dry matter (DM) and may contain more than 150,000 IU/kg DM.[137] Plasma vitamin A levels are usually highest in horses on pasture.[138] Once the green plants are harvested and stored as hay, carotene content and vitamin A activity will decline. Good-quality forage that is green in color and has been stored for a short time may have 10,000 to 20,000 IU vitamin A activity per kilogram of dry matter. Cereal grains are relatively poor sources of vitamin A, but if performance horses are receiving a good-quality roughage, then their vitamin A intake should be adequate.

Vitamin E (alpha-tocopherol) functions as a biologic antioxidant that protects membranes against damage from free radicals. This function may be particularly important during exercise, when the formation of damaging compounds such as peroxide and hydroxyl radicals may be increased.[139] In vitamin E–deficient rats, exercise performance is impaired,[140] but studies in horses have failed to show a clear relationship between vitamin E intake and performance. Petersson and coworkers[141] could not demonstrate differences in any indicators of membrane integrity between exercised and nonexercised horses receiving a diet low in vitamin E (<10 mg/kg) for 4 months. In addition, there did not appear to be any effect of dietary vitamin E level on the horses' response to a standardized exercise test. These authors concluded that horses could consume low levels of vitamin E for at least 4 months without showing any signs of deficiency.

When the NRC revised the *Nutrient Requirements of Horses* in 1989, it increased the previous recommendation[97] for vitamin E more than fivefold from 15 to 80 mg/kg DM. This increase may seem excessive when the results of Petersson and coworkers are considered; however, vitamin E has other functions that may justify a higher dietary intake. Studies with many species have demonstrated a positive effect of vitamin E supplementation on immune function.[142] Any improvement in immune function could have potential benefit to performance horses, which have an increased risk of respiratory disease.

Most common equine feeds (hay and cereal grains) will contain less than 50 mg vitamin E per kilogram of dry matter. Therefore, supplemental vitamin E must be added to many rations to meet the current NRC recommendation. Vitamin E is available as a dietary supplement in various forms (including D,L-alpha-tocopheryl acetate, D,L-alpha-tocopheryl succinate, D,L-alpha-tocopheryl nicotinate, D-alpha-tocopheryl acetate, and D-alpha-tocopheryl succinate) which may have different biologic potencies.[143] Alcohol forms of vitamin E are also available but may be less stable during processing and storage. Little is known about the relative potency of the forms of vitamin E in horses. The NRC suggests that D,L-alpha-tocopheryl acetate has a potency of 1.0, compared with 1.36 for the D form of the acetate ester.[73]

B VITAMINS

As discussed earlier in this chapter, B vitamins may be obtained from the diet or from microbial synthesis in the large intestine. Whether horses are capable of synthesizing adequate quantities of B vitamins to meet the needs of high performance has been questioned.[144] The B vitamins play important roles in red blood cell physiology and in energy metabolism and are therefore key nu-

trients for exercising horses. In other species, deficiencies of folacin or vitamin B_{12} can result in megaloblastic anemia, but this situation has not been documented in the horse. Studies that have examined the effect of vitamin B_{12} or folacin supplementation on red blood cell numbers in performance horses have not been conducted. Alterations in blood levels of these vitamins in performance horses have been reported, but the significance of such changes to performance is not known. The NRC currently makes no recommendation for desirable dietary folacin or vitamin B_{12} levels.

Thiamin (vitamin B_1), riboflavin (vitamin B_2), niacin, pyridoxine (vitamin B_6), pantothenic acid, and biotin are involved in energy metabolism usually as cofactors in enzymatic reactions (Table 10–5). Because exercise increases energy expenditure, the requirements for these vitamins may be increased. When exercising horses were fed diets containing 2, 4, or 28 mg thiamin per kilogram of dry matter, the diets containing the two lower thiamin levels resulted in negative thiamin balance, while the high diet resulted in very positive thiamin balance, suggesting that much of the thiamin in the high diet was being excreted.[145] During a submaximal exercise test, blood lactate levels were lowest in the horses receiving 28 mg/kg. The results of this study may be interpreted to suggest that the thiamin requirement of working horses is between 4 and 28 mg/kg. The current NRC recommendations for dietary thiamin are 3 mg/kg for horses at maintenance and 5 mg/kg for working horses.[73]

The riboflavin requirement for exercise has not been studied in horses. Some studies with humans suggest that regular exercise may increase the amount of riboflavin necessary to maintain riboflavin status,[146,147] but the current Recommended Dietary Allowances (RDAs) for humans do not include an increment for activity.[148] The current recommendation for riboflavin intake in humans is less than 2 mg/day. The NRC recommendation for working horses of 2 mg riboflavin per kilogram of dry matter is actually higher than the recommendation for humans when differences in body weight are considered. The NRC does not make recommendations for any other B vitamins or for vitamin C. Biotin supplementation (up to 30 mg/day) has been re-

Table 10-5. The Role of B Vitamins in Energy Metabolism

Vitamin	Cofactor	Role
Thiamin	Cocarboxylase or thiamin pyrophosphate	Decarboxylation reactions; pyruvate to acetyl-CoA; TCA cycle, etc.
Riboflavin	Flavin mononucleotide (FMN) and flavin adenine nucleotide (FAD)	Transfer of electrons in oxidation reactions
Niacin	Nicotinamide adenine dinucleotide (NAD)	Transfer of hydrogen ions in oxidation-reduction reactions
Pyridoxine	Pyridoxal phosphate	Transamination and deamination
Pantothenic acid	Coenzyme A; acyl	Oxidation of carbohydrates and fats; carrier protein synthesis of fatty acids
B_{12}	Various	Conversion of propionate to succinate
Biotin	Various	Carboxylation and decarboxylation; reactions in TCA cycle, lipogenesis, gluconeogensis, etc.

ported to improve hoof condition in some horses.[149] Recently, the effect of biotin supplementation (50 mg/day) on the response to exercise was tested in thoroughbred racehorses. Biotin supplementation increased plasma biotin concentrations but did not affect V_{LA4}.[150] More research is needed to determine the effect of exercise on the vitamin requirements of horses. For example, low plasma ascorbic acid concentrations in horses compared with other species have caused speculation that horses may require supplementation of this vitamin.[151]

MEETING NUTRIENT REQUIREMENTS

Rations fed to horses frequently represent a compromise between the need to provide a balanced ration that meets nutrient requirements and the availability and cost of certain feeds. In almost all cases, the nutrient needs of performance horses will be met with a combination of roughage and concentrate feeds. Most performance horses will be unable to consume enough feed to meet their energy needs from roughage only, necessitating the use of some concentrate. Conversely, rations that contain a large percentage of concentrate may cause gastrointestinal problems, so at least some roughage must be fed. Meyer[102] recommends that the minimum forage consumption for a performance horse be 0.5 kg per 100 kg of body weight. Jackson and Pagan[152] state that feeding at least 1.0 kg forage per 100 kg of body weight is an important management practice to reduce the incidence of colic.[152] The NRC suggests that hard-working horses receive 0.75 to 1.5 kg roughage per 100 kg of body weight.[73] It is possible that an important criterion is the level of fiber in the diet, although a requirement for dietary fiber has not been determined.

Roughage is usually provided to the horse as hay, chaffed hay, or pasture, although other sources such as soybean hulls and beet pulp are sometimes used. Beet pulp is often included as the fiber source in feeds for horses with chronic obstructive pulmonary disease. At racetracks and in other urban or suburban environments, hay is the usual roughage source. The plant types used for hay generally may be classified as legumes, grasses, or cereals (Table 10–6). In the United States, hay from cereal sources (usually oats) is least common.

Grass and legume hays are the most common roughages. It is apparent in Table 10–6 that there are distinct nutrient differences in grasses and legumes that may affect their desirability or usefulness as feeds for performance horses. These differences pertain primarily to protein and mineral content. The energy content of hays can be more markedly affected by the stage of maturity at the time of harvest than by plant type. Figure 10–3 illustrates the effect of plant maturity on energy content of forages.[153] Fiber content of the plants increases with increasing maturity, while protein content and palatability decrease. Using forages harvested at an early stage of maturity will make it easier to meet the nutrient needs of hard-working horses because nutrient content and palatability are maximized. Another factor that must be considered in selecting roughages for performance horses is the wholesomeness or cleanliness of the feed. Baling hay at correct moisture levels is essential to the preservation of nutrient content. When hay is baled at a very low moisture content, leaf shattering is increased, and many nutrients will be lost. Baling hay at too high a moisture content will usually be much more detrimental to quality than baling at a low moisture content. Hay baled at a high moisture content will often contain mold that can cause respiratory irritation. In addition, the heating that occurs during the molding process can affect the digestibility of some nutrients. In climates that prevent adequate drying of the forage prior to baling, preservatives may be applied to the hay to prevent molding. A common preservative is propionic acid. When used at appropriate concentrations, propionic acid application can allow hay to be baled at relatively high moisture levels without molding. Horses may prefer untreated hay to treated hay, but they readily consume treated hay when an alternative is not offered.[154] Propionic acid is a normal product of digestion and is not detrimental to horses at the levels used to preserve hay. Forages also may be stored at a high moisture content by ensiling. Ensiled hay ("haylage") has been fed successfully to horses; however, it is possible for haylage to contain mold, and its use has been discouraged.[155] If ensiled forage is used for horses, it should be examined carefully for the presence of mold or other contaminants before feeding.

Table 10-6. Nutrient Compositions of Common Forages*

Legumes		Grasses	Cereals
Alfalfa		Timothy	Oat (hay)
Clover		Orchardgrass	Barley (hay)
Lespedeza		Bromegrass	Wheat (hay)
Birdsfoot trefoil		Fescue	
		Bermuda grass	
		Bluegrass (usually pasture)	
DE	1.9 to 2.5 Mcal/kg	1.8 to 2.4 Mcal/kg	1.9 to 2.0 Mcal/kg
CP	13 to 20%	7 to 13%	8 to 9%
Ca	0.9 to 1.8%	0.2 to .5%	0.15 to 0.3%
P	0.2 to 0.4%	0.2 to .4%	0.2 to 0.3%

*100% dry matter basis; the values presented represent average ranges; some samples may be outside the range given.

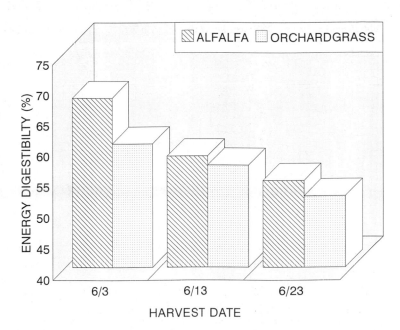

Figure 10-3. Effect of stage of maturity of a forage at harvesting on energy digestibility. When harvested in the early bloom stage (6/3), the forage is more digestible than when harvested in late bloom (6/23). (Data from Darlington JM, Hershberger TV: Effect of forage maturity on digestibility, intake, and nutritive value of alfalfa, timothy, and orchardgrass by equine. J Anim Sci 1968; 27:1521.)

Hay may be fed long or processed. Processed hay (pelleted or cubed) may have some advantages in terms of convenience and reduced wastage. However, processing increases cost and does not usually increase digestibility. When long-stem hay is fed, horses will spend more time eating, which may be of consequence in certain situations. If horses are confined to stalls for most of the day, long-stem hay may provide them with a way to constructively occupy their time. If horses are working many hours a day, then processed hay may be more desirable.

When hay is used as the forage source, it is easy to monitor consumption. When horses have access to pasture, it is much more difficult to estimate nutrient intake. The nutrient content of pasture may be estimated from the type and maturity of the plants that are being consumed by the horse. Pasture intake of horses during a 3-hour tethered grazing session was estimated at 1.75 kg of dry matter.[156] Pasture consumption may be influenced by the type of forage, the length of the grazing period, and the availability of other feed.

The combination of roughage and concentrates should provide a balanced ration. For example, if a legume hay is being used, then the protein content of the concentrate can be lower than if a grass hay is being used. A concentrate that is to be used with a grass hay may have a different mineral content than a concentrate to be used with a legume hay. Concentrate feeds may be composed of single grains (oats, barley, corn, etc.) or a combination of grains and other ingredients. Commercial concentrate feeds usually include a variety of ingredients that are combined to form a pellet or a sweet feed. Pelleting prevents the horse from sorting the ingredients. The nutrient compositions of several feeds commonly included in concentrate mixes are shown in Table 10–7. The contribution of each ingredient to a concentrate feed

will depend on the nutrient composition and cost of each ingredient and the desired composition of the final mix. Some commercial feeds are formulated with specific amounts of each ingredient, while others are formulated to provide the desired nutrient composition for the lowest price. Examples of how several different combinations can result in concentrate feeds with similar nutrient values are shown in Table 10–8.

Dietary Manipulations of Potential Benefit to Performance Horses

Once a horse's nutrient requirements have been met, can dietary factors affect performance? Are some feeds more ergogenic than others, and are there feeding practices that do not relate to nutrient composition that are important to performance? While many trainers agree that

Table 10-7. Nutrient Composition of Some Feeds Commonly Used in Concentrate Mixes*

Feed	DE (Mcal/kg)	CP (%)	Ca (%)	P (%)
Dehydrated alfalfa	2.3	18	1.5	0.25
Barley grain	3.6	12	0.05	0.35
Beet pulp	2.8	9	0.6	0.1
Corn grain	3.8	10	0.05	0.3
Molasses	3.4	7	0.2	0.1
Oats	3.2	13	0.1	0.3
Soybean meal	3.6	49	0.35	0.7
Wheat bran	3.3	17	0.14	1.27

*100% dry matter basis; some values represent approximate averages across different varieties or processing methods.
From National Research Council: Nutrient Requirements of Horses, 5th ed. Washington, National Academy Press, 1989.

*Table 10-8. Examples of Different Feeds that Can Be Used to Produce Concentrate Feeds with Similar Nutrient Compositions**

Mix 1	**Mix 2**
60.0% oats	60.0% corn
30.0% corn	25.0% oats
5.0% molasses	5.0% molasses
3.0% dehydrated alfalfa meal	4.0% dehydrated alfalfa meal
0.25% dicalcium phosphate	4.0% soybean meal
0.75% calcium carbonate	0.25% dicalcium phosphate
1.0% other[†]	0.75% calcium carbonate
	1.0% other
Mix 3	**Mix 4**
63.00% oats	60.00% oats
10.00% barley	10.00% barley
20.00% corn	10.00% corn
5.00% molasses	10.00% vegetable oil
0.25% dicalcium phosphate	5.00% molasses
0.75% calcium carbonate	3.00% soybean meal
1.00% other	0.25% dicalcium phosphate
	0.75% calcium carbonate
	1.00% other

*All rations contain approximately 12 percent crude protein, 0.4 percent calcium, and 0.35 to 0.39 percent phophorus (dry matter basis); mix 1 and mix 3 contain approximately 3.3 Mcal DE/kg DM; increased use of corn in mix 2 increases the DE content by about 6 percent, while the inclusion of vegetable oil in mix 4 increases the DE content by about 15 percent.
†Other ingredients such as salt, trace mineralized salt, vitamins, etc. may be added to meet sodium, chloride, or micronutrient needs.

the answer to these questions is "yes," few will agree as to what the performance-enhancing feeds or practices might be.

PRE-EVENT FEEDING PRACTICES

Surveys of feeding practices associated with performance horses indicate that most trainers/riders alter the horse's diet on the day of the competition.[116,157] The diet may be changed by withholding all feed, reducing feed (usually roughage), increasing feed (usually concentrate), or adding a supplement of specific nutrients (frequently electrolytes). Some of these alterations may have more potential to affect performance than others. In addition, some practices may be more beneficial for one type of athletic event than another.

The consumption of a meal can cause a number of hemodynamic changes that may be related to the movement of fluid into the gastrointestinal tract. Horses secrete large amounts of saliva during chewing, and gastric and intestinal secretions are released into the intestine during digestion. These fluids originate from the extracellular fluid, and thus eating may result in a degree of hypovolemia in horses. Total protein (TP) concentration and packed cell volume (PCV) were elevated at about 1 hour after feeding in horses receiving 5.5 kg of hay and 2.7 kg of a complete cubed diet. Feeding hay alone (5.5 kg) produced the same response, whereas a small meal of the cubed feed (1.8 kg) did not affect TP and PCV.[158] Clarke and coworkers[159] found that a large meal of a complete pelleted ration could induce an average reduction in plasma volume of about 15 percent in ponies. They also noted that in some ponies (described as

"greedy eaters"), the reduction in plasma volume was as high as 24 percent.[160]

In addition to affecting plasma volume, the presence of a large meal in the digestive tract may result in alterations of blood flow. Consuming a meal in the 2 hours prior to an exercise bout increased cardiac output in miniature swine during the exercise.[161] In this study, the total splanchnic blood flow was increased at rest and during exercise by feeding, while flow to certain hindlimb muscles was decreased during exercise. Cardiac output during exercise also was increased in ponies that had received a large meal 1.4 hours before exercise compared with ponies that exercised after a 24-hour fast.[162] In addition, blood flow to the digestive tract was increased by feeding, but a decrease in blood flow to the locomotor muscles did not occur. In fact, blood flow to the locomotor muscles was higher in the fed ponies compared with the fasted ponies. The authors suggested that greater blood flow in the fed ponies was achieved by elevating the cardiac output. The ponies in this study exercised at approximately 75 percent of $\dot{V}_{O_2max}$; differences in blood flow to the locomotor muscles might have been altered by feeding state if the ponies had exercised at or above 100 percent of $\dot{V}_{O_2max}$.

The results of the studies described above may suggest that at least during submaximal effort, horses are capable of maintaining adequate muscle blood flow despite any hemodynamic perturbations caused by the consumption of a relatively large meal just prior to exercise. However, whether fed horses can maintain blood flow to muscles during more intense exercise is unknown.

In any case, some of the effects of consuming a

meal are short-lived (<3 hours) and appear to be reduced if smaller amounts of food are consumed.[160] Allowing horses to consume feed, particularly roughage, in the 4 to 6 hours before an event may actually be of benefit in certain situations. Meyer[102] suggests that feeding prior to exercise will increase the amount of fluid in the digestive tract, which could provide an effective reservoir of water and electrolytes to replace sweat loss during exercise. Voluntary water consumption is highly correlated with dry matter intake, and high-fiber feeds may stimulate greater water consumption than low-fiber feeds.[163] Water consumption is affected by other factors, such as ambient temperature and hydration status, but horses will consume about 2.5 to 3.5 kg water per kilogram of dry matter.[163] Dry matter digestibility is negatively correlated with fecal water content and total fecal water excretion.[163] Thus it appears that high-fiber feeds do have potential to hold more fluid in the gastrointestinal tract, but whether that water is available to replace the fluids lost through sweating is not known. In fact, Cuddeford and coworkers[164] recently suggested that the hydrophilic polysaccharides in high-fiber feeds may adsorb water and electrolytes, making them unavailable for absorption by the horse. Consuming a high-roughage meal within a few hours of competition would probably have no benefit to racehorses. If a racehorse consumed 3 kg of hay, the added effects of hay and water (about 3 kg water per kilogram of dry matter) would result in an extra 10 to 12 kg of weight to be carried during the race. In addition, the potential contribution of nutrients absorbed from the hay would not be expected to have a major impact on energy production during a short, intense exercise bout.

The consumption of a high-concentrate meal prior to exercise can influence the availability of several fuels to exercising muscle. Following a meal, glucose levels will increase. Insulin concentration also will rise, and the uptake of glucose by peripheral tissues will occur. Exercise and insulin both facilitate the uptake of glucose by muscle through the GLUT-4 transporter, but they may affect the transporter by different mechanisms because their effects on glucose uptake are additive.[165] The rapid uptake of glucose from the plasma in fed, exercising individuals may result in a fall in plasma glucose levels. Costill[37] noted that blood glucose during a 30-minute exercise bout fell below fasting concentrations when men consumed 75 g glucose approximately 45 minutes before the exercise. A similar response was noted in standardbreds that were exercised about 2.5 hours after a meal of corn grain.[166] Although a fall in blood glucose in fed, exercising individuals might be expected to have a negative effect on performance, the drop in blood glucose may be transient and does not necessarily impair performance.[167] Nonetheless, when submaximal exercise is performed shortly after a carbohydrate meal, the oxidation of circulating glucose is increased, and the respiratory quotient (RQ) may be elevated, at least during the early stages of exercise, indicating that fat is a less important fuel during exercise in this situation.[37,167,168] Concentrations of plasma free fatty acids are lower in fed conditions in both humans and

horses,[166,169] presumably because insulin suppresses the mobilization of free fatty acids from adipose.

Consumption of a meal prior to maximal exercise could impair performance if the increased uptake of glucose by muscle fibers increased flux through the glycolytic cycle and increased the amount of lactate produced. In one study, plasma lactate concentrations were higher in human athletes performing an intense exercise test after consuming a meal; however, in this test, the exercise time following the pre-exercise meal was slightly longer than the exercise bout following fasting.[169] In this study and at least one other, ingestion of carbohydrate actually appeared to enhance high-intensity performance.[167,169] In the second study, plasma lactate concentrations were similar in fed and fasted individuals performing intense exercise. Plasma lactate concentrations were not affected by feeding state in horses performing a brief high-speed test that was preceded by a warmup.[166] At this time, there is no evidence to suggest that a small or moderate-sized concentrate meal ingested 2 to 3 hours prior to exercise is detrimental to performance in horses; however, there are also no data to suggest a beneficial effect.

Because of the effects on carbohydrate utilization, the consumption of a carbohydrate meal by human athletes within 1 hour of long-term submaximal exercise has been discouraged by some authors.[170,171] Fatigue during endurance-type exercise may be associated with the depletion of glycogen stores, while an increased utilization of fat during exercise may spare glycogen utilization and delay the onset of fatigue. If consuming a carbohydrate meal suppresses the availability of fatty acids and enhances carbohydrate utilization (as indicated by an increased RQ), then it may accelerate the rate of glycogen depletion and facilitate the development of fatigue. Some studies have reported that consuming a meal or a glucose beverage within 1 hour of exercise can reduce endurance.[172] However, other studies have found that carbohydrate intake before exercise actually can improve performance, particularly if the meal is consumed 3 to 6 hours before exercise.[173-175] Coggan and Swanson[176] suggest that any beneficial effects might be related to "topping off" of glycogen stores or the just the presence of additional fuel. Differences in results may be related to the type of exercise, the training status of the individuals, or the amount, form, and timing of the carbohydrate ingested.

Because some of the potentially negative effects of consuming a high-carbohydrate meal are manifested through the effects of insulin, foods that provide some additional fuel without eliciting a large glucose or insulin response have been studied. The *glycemic index* describes the ability of foods to raise blood glucose levels. In one study, a low-glycemic-index food (lentils) was found to be superior to high-glycemic-index foods (glucose or potato) as a pre-exercise meal.[168] In horses, corn grain has a relatively high glycemic index, while forages will have a lower glycemic index.[10] The effect of feeding horses low- or high-glycemic-index feeds just prior to exercise has been tested during limited exercise bouts but not during endurance exercise.[177,178] Lower insulin concentrations[177] and higher plasma free fatty acid concentrations[178] when horses received the low-glycemic-index feed may indicate that roughage feeding prior to long-term submaximal exercise may have some metabolic benefits to horses.

Although fasting will elevate plasma free fatty acid concentrations and lower the RQ, endurance horses probably should not be fasted before a competition. In humans, even a short fast (16 hours) can reduce liver glycogen, which is needed to maintain plasma glucose levels during long-term exercise. Fasting would be expected to have the same effect on horses. In addition, horses that have had roughage within the last 12 hours would be expected to have some absorption of volatile fatty acids from the large intestine, which could provide a source of energy and substrate for gluconeogenesis. Finally, fasting might decrease water intake and affect hydration in horses.

One of the most useful nutritional manipulations for human endurance athletes is the consumption of carbohydrate during exercise.[53–55,179] It appears that carbohydrate supplementation can delay fatigue by 30 to 60 minutes when it is administered throughout a long-term exercise bout or toward the end of the bout but prior to the onset of fatigue.[53,176] Consumption of carbohydrate during the later stages of endurance exercise appears to delay the fall in blood glucose by providing additional carbohydrate for oxidation.[53] When carbohydrate is consumed throughout exercise, it does not appear to reduce the rate of muscle glycogen depletion[53] but may spare hepatic glycogenolysis, possibly by affecting the glucagon/insulin ratio or cortisol concentration.[180] The ability of carbohydrate supplements to enhance endurance in humans suggests that this may be a practice that could be of potential benefit to some horses.

Coyle[53] suggests that a carbohydrate supplement for a human athlete exercising at about 70 percent of $\dot{V}_{O_2max}$ should provide at least 1 g glucose per minute. A number of compounds have been tested in humans as potential sources of carbohydrate, including sucrose, maltose, glucose polymers, soluble starch, fructose, and glucose.[181–185] These supplements are usually provided as a beverage and thus offer a source of fluid as well. However, in order to provide an adequate amount of glucose, the beverages may be somewhat concentrated with regard to carbohydrate content, and concentrated beverages may be emptied more slowly from the stomach.[72] There is little information regarding the factors that affect gastric emptying in horses or on the levels of supplemental carbohydrate necessary to achieve appropriate rates of glucose availability in exercising horses.

ACID-BASE BALANCE

One of the greatest challenges faced by the exercising horse is the maintenance of acid-base balance. Maximal and near-maximal exercise can result in a systemic acidosis and a local acidosis in the working muscle. Intramuscular acidosis may result in fatigue by impairing the activity of glycolytic enzymes or by affecting the contractile apparatus. The development of the local acidosis

can be delayed or reduced by at least three potential mechanisms: (1) reduced production of lactate and H^+, (2) increased buffering of the H^+ by intracellular buffers, and (3) increased movement of H^+ out of the muscle and into the systemic circulation. It is believed that the movement of lactate and H^+ out of cell is influenced by the pH of the perfusing medium,[186,187] which in the case of the exercising horse would be the systemic circulation. The effects of ingesting buffers, such as sodium bicarbonate, on systemic pH, lactate, and H^+ movement and performance have been studied extensively in humans. When sodium bicarbonate is ingested at a rate of at least 300 mg/kg prior to exercise, elevations in blood pH and blood bicarbonate level occur.[188,189] During intense exercise, treated individuals will maintain a higher blood pH and frequently have higher blood lactate levels.[188,190] It is believed that the higher blood pH promotes the movement of lactate out of the muscle and into the blood, thus reducing or delaying the accumulation of lactate and H^+ in the active muscle fibers.[191] Improvements in performance have been reported frequently but not consistently.[188–194] Improvement in performance appears to be most common in events where a high-intensity effort is maintained for at least 1 to 7 minutes.[195] Increased systemic buffering does not appear to affect very short-term maximal activity[196] or long-term submaximal activity.

In the late 1980s and early 1990s, the prerace administration of sodium bicarbonate to horses became a widely used practice, especially in standardbreds.[197] Its use is now prohibited by many racing jurisdictions, and compliance is enforced by prerace acid-base testing. It is not clear whether the banning of sodium bicarbonate is based on its potential to affect performance or a concern for the horse's health.[198] When administered in conjunction with other treatments that can affect blood pH or electrolyte balance (such as furosemide), a large dose of sodium bicarbonate can negatively affect the horse.[199] Studies that have examined the effects of sodium bicarbonate on performance have produced equivocal results.[200–205] However, from a metabolic standpoint, the effects of sodium bicarbonate on horses have been very comparable with the effects on humans,[201,204,205] suggesting that there may be an opportunity to affect performance in horses by manipulating acid-base balance.

Electrolytes have important roles in acid-base balance, and thus a dietary factor that appears to be of importance to systemic acid-base status is dietary cation-anion balance (DCAB). Although several other ions may be included in the equation, DCAB is most frequently defined as follows:

$$DCAB = mEq\ [(Na + K) - Cl]/kg\ diet\ DM$$

Other minerals that may be included are Ca, Mg, P, and S. In other species, DCAB affects such processes as milk production and growth, possibly through effects on acid-base balance.[206,207] When diets containing DCABs of 21, 125, 231, and 350 were fed to sedentary horses, the lowest DCAB resulted in decreased arterial and venous pH and urine pH compared with the two highest DCAB diets.[208] In a subsequent experiment, when trained horses were fed diets containing DCABs of 10, 131, 206, and 323, lactate levels following a high-intensity exercise test were higher in horses receiving the highest DCAB compared with the lowest DCAB.[209] In this study, sulfur was included in the equation to calculate DCAB. In addition to altering systemic acid-base balance, DCAB may affect other physiologic processes of importance to the horse. Wall and coworkers[210] reported that lowering DCAB to 5 resulted in increased calcium excretion and suggested that this could result in negative calcium balance in horses receiving low levels of dietary calcium.

Thus far, the available data suggest that diets containing low DCABs should be avoided. Fortunately, many common horse rations will have at least a moderate DCAB, particularly if they contain at least 50 percent hay. For example, a ration consisting of 5 kg timothy hay, 5 kg oat grain, and 50 g salt would have a DCAB of about 200 (using Na, K, and Cl in the equation). The amount of hay in the ration will affect DCAB because most hays are fairly high in potassium. Diets with low DCABs might be more common in situations where hay intake is limited. Beet pulp is much lower in potassium content than most hays, and therefore, a diet that depends on beet pulp as the roughage source might have a lower DCAB.

DIETARY ENERGY SOURCE

Fat and carbohydrate are the primary sources of energy used by the muscle; similarly, fat and carbohydrate are the two primary energy sources in the diet. Carbohydrate, either from grains or from hay, is quantitatively the most important energy source in horse diets. Unless a specific source of fat (such as vegetable oil or animal fat) is added to a diet, most horse rations will contain less than 3 percent fat (dry matter basis). An exception could occur when a product such as full-fat soybeans is included in a ration. The addition of fat to horse diets has become more common in recent years, but it is still extremely unusual for dietary fat to contribute more than 35 percent of the total digestible energy. When mixed concentrate feeds that are described as "high-fat horse feeds" are used in combination with roughage, the contribution of fat to total digestible energy intake usually will be less than 20 percent and may be as low as 10 percent depending on the amount of fat in the concentrate and the roughage/concentrate ratio of the total ration.

Fat is a more energy-dense feedstuff than carbohydrate. On the basis of gross energy content, fat contains about 2.25 times as much energy per gram as carbohydrate. Once digested and absorbed, fat is used efficiently by the body for energy production and storage. Kane and coworkers[211] reported that ponies could convert the digestible energy in corn oil to net energy at an efficiency of about 85 percent. The comparative efficiency for a conventional hay/grain diet is less than 60 percent. Consequently, the incorporation of fat into horse diets can have a marked effect on the amount of energy available to the horse. In fact, one of the most common reasons for adding fat to horse diets is to increase total energy intake. When consuming some conventional diets, many hard-working horses will not consume enough food to meet their energy needs and will lose weight. Once dry matter intake has been maximized, energy intake can be increased by replacing some roughage with concentrate, but digestive disturbances may arise if insufficient roughage is available. Inclusion of fat in a diet results in an increased energy intake without the threat of side effects related to excessive soluble carbohydrate intake. Table 10–8 shows an example of how fat can be included in a concentrate feed to increase total energy. When vegetable oil replaces corn as 10 percent of the mix, digestible energy content is increased by about 15 percent. By feeding the fat-added diet instead of a more typical mix at a rate of 5 kg/day, total energy intake would be increased by about 2.5 Mcal/day. As mentioned above, fat is used very efficiently in the body, so the true effect of adding fat on energy balance may be more than is predicted just by digestible energy content.

Many studies have endeavored to determine whether supplemental dietary fat can affect the metabolism or performance of horses. It has been postulated that feeding dietary fat could increase the utilization of fat at the cellular level and have a sparing effect on carbohydrate utilization. Consequently, the effects of supplemental dietary fat on blood glucose concentrations, lactate concentrations, muscle glycogen concentrations, muscle glycogen utilization, and respiratory quotient have been studied in horses performing various types of exercise.[98,109,212–217] The results have often been conflicting, and there has been variability in the type and amount of fat, length of feeding period, and conditioning status of the horses. One group of authors suggests that there may be a level of dietary fat that produces desirable effects, whereas higher or lower levels are not effective.[217] They also suggest that the amount of carbohydrate in the diet and the training program are important determinants of the response to fat feeding.[217] It is difficult to make comparisons between horses and other species with regard to the effect of fat supplementation on exercise metabolism because the amount of fat in a "high-fat" horse diet (usually less than 20 percent of calories as fat) is not at all comparable with levels in high-fat diets for rats (usually more than 70 percent of the calories as fat) or humans. There is evidence that long-term adaptation of rats to a very high-fat diet can result in enzymatic changes that favor fat oxidation during endurance exercise,[218,219] but whether similar changes occur in horses fed much lower levels of fat is not known. In addition, muscle glycogen concentration appears to be decreased by fat feeding in rats,[220] whereas some studies have suggested that one of the metabolic effects that can benefit equine performance is an increase in muscle glycogen in response to fat feeding.[217]

NUTRITIONAL ERGOGENIC AIDS

An *ergogenic aid* is a substance that can increase or improve work production. Improved work effort may occur as a result of increased speed, increased endurance, or increased strength. Some nutritional supplements are purported to have ergogenic effects in horses. Within the scope of this discussion, nutritional ergogenic aids will include compounds or elements that can be administered orally and have a nutritionally oriented function.

In order for something to have an ergogenic effect, it must be able to affect some aspect of exercise physiology, preferably an aspect that is limiting to the athlete of interest. Coyle[221] suggests that ergogenic aids can function in the following general ways:

1. They may act as a supplementary fuel source for energy production.
2. They may affect the flux of fuels through the energy pathways.
3. They may delay or minimize the effects of end-product accumulation, such as heat or lactic acid.
4. They can affect the nervous system by affecting coordination, recruitment of muscle fibers, etc.

Many substances are marketed without any factual evidence to substantiate their function, or the descriptions of their functions are too vague to provide useful information. An understanding of the function of each compound and an understanding of the metabolism and physiology of each type of athlete are important because compounds that may be helpful to some types of athletes could actually be detrimental to other types of athletes. Once the function of a specific substance is determined, its usefulness as an ergogenic aid can be evaluated.

Ideally, each ergogenic aid should be tested in a laboratory situation to identify metabolic and physiologic functions, potential side effects, ideal dose rate, and adaptation period, and then each should be field tested to identify actual performance effects. However, this type of comprehensive evaluation is rarely performed, and conclusions about efficacy often must be drawn from a few studies or case reports. In addition, some of the information available may come from studies that have used inappropriate designs to test treated and untreated individuals. It is not uncommon to find studies where all subjects were tested in the untreated condition 1 week, placed on the treatment, and then all tested under the treated condition several days or weeks later. With this type of design, it is not possible to separate effects that might result from the treatment and effects that occur due to training and differences in the testing conditions (temperature, time of day, etc.). Better-designed studies balance or randomize treatment order and ensure that controls and treated individuals are tested under the same conditions. In addition, studies should be conducted in a "blind" manner so that the participants are unaware of which treatment is being administered. This requirement is especially important in situations where the rider/driver/handler can greatly influence the performance of the horse.

Conclusions regarding the efficacy of a particular treatment should be based on sound statistical methods. However, in many performance situations, this practice is problematic. First, it is often difficult to accurately measure "performance." Second, some differences that are detected as being statistically significant may not be biologically significant (most common with metabolic/physiologic effects). Third, and perhaps most important, the biologic effect may not be statistically detectable without using very large numbers of subjects. Rose and Lloyd[222] have recently pointed out that for some performance criteria, an ergogenic aid would have to produce a 10 percent improvement to be statistically detectable. Smaller improvements may be measurable when the external sources of variation are strictly controlled and the performance criteria are objective and highly repeatable.

Table 10–9 lists a number of compounds that are used as ergogenic aids in human and equine athletics with a brief description of their proposed metabolic role. In some cases, the roles of compounds listed in this table are not known. A brief overview of the relative merits of several compounds is included below. Because hematinics, buffers, and B vitamins were reviewed previously, they have not been included in the following discussion.

ANTIOXIDANTS

Vitamin E may be the most common antioxidant, but vitamin C, beta-carotene, and coenzyme Q10 also have antioxidant properties. Vitamin E is a common therapy or prophylactic for horses with exertional myopathies, but its effectiveness is questioned. While vitamin E deficiency can impair performance in other species, vitamin E deficiency in horses is rare, and evidence for a positive effect of supplementation above the requirement is lacking. Shelle and coworkers[223] fed supplemental vitamin E to horses and did not find any effect on glutathione peroxidase, their indicator of oxidative damage/protection. Witt and coauthors[224] did not find evidence to support an effect of supplemental vitamin E on maximal aerobic or performance capacity in humans or other animals. Similarly, supplementation with coenzyme Q10 has failed to improve measures of physical performance or fitness in horses and humans.[225,226]

Table 10-9. Partial List of Substances that Are Used as Nutritional Ergogenic Aids in Horses

Substance	Metabolic/physiologic function
Vitamin E	Antioxidant
Coenzyme Q_{10}	Antioxidant, electron transport
Vitamin C	Antioxidant, carnitine synthesis
Carnitine	Fatty acid transport into mitochondria
Branched-chain amino acids	Energy metabolism, regulation of tryptophan uptake by brain
Tryptophan	Synthesis of 5-hydroxytryptamine, which may be important in fatigue or pain
Dimethyl glycine	Methyl donor, other?
Bee pollen	Source of nutrients
Ginseng	?

*Not all substances have a proven ergogenic effect (see text); for information on B vitamins, see Table 10–5.

Snow and Harris[151] point out that ascorbic acid concentrations are lower in horses than in other species and suggest that supplementation may have a place in the exercising horse, but no studies on the effect of vitamin C on equine performance appear to have been conducted.

CARNITINE

Carnitine has several biologic functions of importance in energy metabolism. Carnitine palmitoyltransferase is the enzyme necessary for the transport of fatty acids into the mitochondria for oxidation. Thus carnitine is an essential component of fat metabolism. In addition, carnitine acyltransferase may play a role in regulating the mitochondrial ratio of free coenzyme A to acetyl-CoA, which can affect the conversion of pyruvate to acetyl-CoA, thus influencing the flux of glucose through the TCA cycle.[227]

In humans, carnitine may be obtained from dietary sources of animal origin or synthesized in the body. In horses, carnitine must be synthesized because feeds from plant sources have a low carnitine content.[228] The capacity of horses for carnitine synthesis is not known, but it may be fairly high, since horses appear to have a higher concentration of carnitine in their muscle than many other species, including humans.[227] Most of the carnitine in the body is found in the muscle, and muscle concentration may be affected by fiber type and athletic background.[229]

The effects of oral carnitine supplementation on humans and animals have been varied. Foster and coworkers[230] administered L-carnitine to horses for 58 days and noted an increase in plasma carnitine but not muscle carnitine.[230] Oral supplementation has increased muscle carnitine in rats and humans, but these changes have not always been associated with improvements in performance or alterations in metabolism. Although supplementation increased muscle carnitine concentration in rats, no differences occurred in palmitate oxidation, glycogen metabolism, or maximal exercise capacity.[231,232] Cerritelli and Marconi[227] reviewed the literature regarding the effect of oral carnitine supplementation on humans and concluded that the metabolic impact was minor. Two reports of an effect of carnitine on RQ were found,[233,234] but only one study reported a positive effect on $\dot{V}_{O_2max}$.[235]

AMINO ACIDS

Several amino acids are of interest to exercising individuals. As discussed earlier, the branched-chain amino acids (BCAAs), especially leucine, are possible sources of energy to muscle, even though their contribution may be minor. A branched-chain amino acid supplement was reported to improve the performance of some "slower" human marathon runners but had no effect on "faster" runners.[236] One study provided supplemental BCAA to horses and reported a decrease in blood lactate concentration, but the exercise test was very mild, so the biologic significance of the results is questionable.[237]

The interaction of BCAAs with another amino acid, tryptophan, also has been proposed as a factor in exercise performance. Tryptophan is used for the synthesis of 5-hydroxytryptamine in the brain. Because an increase in 5-hydroxytryptamine in the brain can induce sleep, it has been suggested that increased 5-hydroxytryptamine during exercise may be involved in central fatigue.[236] It also has been suggested that uptake of tryptophan by the brain may be altered by the ratio of BCAAs to free tryptophan such that increased BCAAs will reduce tryptophan uptake, decrease synthesis of 5-hydroxytryptamine, and delay fatigue. Conversely, it has been suggested that increased 5-hydroxytryptamine may result in a feeling of analgesia[238] and therefore an increased tolerance for the pain associated with maximal exercise.[239] At this time, any potential advantages of manipulating tryptophan metabolism in the brain of the horse are entirely speculative, and studies with humans have produced conflicting results.[236,239,240]

Glycine, as a part of dimethyl glycine (DMG), is another amino acid with proposed ergogenic effects, including a reduction in lactate production. Rose and coworkers[241] studied the effect of DMG supplementation on horses completing a standardized exercise test on a treadmill. At work intensities up to 100 percent of $\dot{V}_{O_2max}$, there were no effects on plasma lactate levels or any of the cardiorespiratory parameters measured.

References

1. Rich VB, Fontenot JP, Meacham TN: Digestibility of animal, vegetable, and blended fats by the equine. *In* Proceedings of the 7th Equine Nutrition and Physiology Symposium, Warrenton, Va, 1981, p 30.
2. Gibbs PG, Potter GD, Schelling GT, et al: Digestion of hay protein in different segments of the equine digestive tract. J Anim Sci 1988; 66:400.
3. Hintz HF, Hogue DE, Walker EF Jr, et al: Apparent digestion in various segments of the digestive tract of ponies fed diets with varying roughage-grain ratios. J Anim Sci 1971; 32(2):245.
4. Robinson DW, Slade LM: The current status of knowledge on the nutrition of equines. J Anim Sci 1974; 39(6):1045.
5. Godbee RG, Slade LM: Nitrogen absorption from the cecum of a mature horse. *In* Proceedings of the 6th Equine Nutritional and Physiology Symposium, College Station, Texas, 1979, p 75.
6. Schryver HF, Hintz HE, Craig PH, et al: Site of phosphorus absorption in the horse. J Nutr 1972; 102:143.
7. Argenzio RA: Functions of the equine large intestine and their interrelationship to disease. Cornell Vet 1975; 65:303.
8. Linerode PA: Studies on the synthesis and absorption of B-complex vitamins in the horse. Am Assoc Equine Pract 1967; 13:283.
9. Stillions MC, Teeter SM, Nelson WE: Utilization of dietary B_{12} and cobalt by mature horses. J Anim Sci 1971; 32:252.
10. Stull C, Rodiek A: Responses of blood glucose, insulin and cortisol concentrations to common equine diets. J Nutr 1988; 118:206.
11. Arana M, Rodiek A, Stull C: Blood glucose and insulin responses to four different grains and four different forms of alfalfa hay fed to horses. *In* Proceedings of the 11th Equine Nutrition and Physiology Symposium, Stillwater, Okla, 1989, p 160.
12. Bonvicin SE, Rodiek AV, Arana MJ, et al: Glycemic and hormonal effects of common feeds in exercising horses. *In* Proceedings of the 11th Equine Nutrition and Physiology Symposium, Stillwater, Okla, 1989, p 162.
13. Youket RJ, Carnevale JM, Houpt KA, et al: Humoral, hormonal and behavioral correlates of feeding in ponies: The effects of meal frequency. J Anim Sci 1985; 61(5):1103.

14. Johnson RJ, Hart JW: Influence of feeding and fasting on plasma free amino acids in the equine. J Anim Sci 1974; 38:790.
15. Russell MA, Rodiek AV, Lawrence LM: Effect of meal schedules and fasting on selected plasma free amino acids in horses. J Anim Sci 1986; 63:1428.
16. Hollanders B, Mougin A, Diaye FN, et al: Comparison of lipoprotein profiles obtained from rat, bovine, horse, dog, rabbit, and pig serum by a new two-step ultracentrifugal gradient procedure. Comp Biochem Physiol [B] 1986; 84:83.
17. Kurcz EV, Schurg WA, Marchello JA, et al: Post-prandial changes in plasma lipoprotein components in horses fed either a control or a fat-added diet. In Proceedings of the 13th Equine Nutritional Physiology Symposium, Gainesville, Fla, 1993, p 37.
18. Lieb S, Baker JP, Crawford BH Jr: Energy absorption and utilization in the equine. J Anim Sci 1970; 31:207.
19. Hintz HF, Argenzio RA, Schryver HF: Digestion coefficients, blood glucose levels and molar percentage of volatile acids in intestinal fluid of ponies fed varying forage-grain ratios. J Anim Sci 1971; 33:992.
20. Doreau M, Boulot S, Bauchart D, et al: Voluntary intake, milk production and plasma metabolites in nursing mares fed two different diets. J Nutr 1992; 122:992.
21. Argenzio RA, Hintz HF: Glucose tolerance and effect of volatile fatty acid on plasma glucose concentration in ponies. J Anim Sci 1970; 30:514.
22. Simmons HA, Ford EJH: Gluconeogenesis from propionate produced in the colon of the horse. Br Vet J 1991; 147:340.
23. Argenzio RA, Hintz HF: Volatile fatty acid tolerance and effect of glucose and VFA on plasma insulin levels in ponies. J Nutr 1971; 101:723.
24. Glinsky MJ, Smith RM, Spires HR, et al: Measurement of volatile fatty acid production rates in the cecum of the pony. J Anim Sci 1976; 42(6):1465.
25. Sauer WS, Devlin TJ, Parker RJ, et al: Effect of cecectomy on digestibility coefficients and nitrogen balance in ponies. Can J Anim Sci 1979; 59:145.
26. Barnard RJ, Youngren JF: Regulation of glucose transport in skeletal muscle. FASEB J 1992; 6:3238.
27. Hultman E: Nutritional effects on work performance. Am J Clin Nutr 1989; 49:949.
28. Jeffcott LB, Field JR: Current concepts of hyperlipaemia in horses and ponies. Vet Rec 1985; 116:461.
29. Morris MD, Zilversmit DB, Hintz HF: Hyperlipoproteinemia in fasting ponies. J Lipid Res 1972; 13:383.
30. Moser LR, Lawrence LM, Novakofski J, et al: Clearance of infused triglyceride by resting horses. Comp Biochem Physiol 1993; 104A:361.
31. Watson TDG, Burns L, Love S, et al: Plasma lipids, lipoproteins and postheparin lipases in ponies with hyperlipaemia. Equine Vet J 1992; 24(5):341.
32. Goodman MN, Ruderman NB: Influence of muscle use on amino acid metabolism. In Terjung RL (ed): Exercise and Sport Science Reviews. Philadelphia, Franklin Institute Press, 1982, p 1.
33. Gollnick PD, Saltin B: Fuel for muscular exercise: Role of fat. In Horton ES, Terjung RL (eds): Exercise, Nutrition and Energy Metabolism. New York, Macmillan, 1988, p 72.
34. Edwards HT, Margaria R, Dill DB: Metabolic rate, blood sugar and the utilization of carbohydrate. Am J Physiol 1934; 108:203.
35. Gollnick PD: Metabolism of substrates: Energy substrate metabolism during exercise and as modified by training. Fed Proc 1985; 44:353.
36. Rennie M, Winder WM, Holloszy JO: A sparing effect of increased free fatty acids on muscle glycogen content in exercising rat. Biochem J 1976; 156:647.
37. Costill DL, Coyle E, Dalsky G, et al: Effects of elevated plasma FFA and insulin on muscle glycogen usage during exercise. J Appl Physiol Respir Environ Exerc Physiol 1977; 43(4):695.
38. Issekutz B Jr, Paul P: Intramuscular energy sources in exercising normal and pancreatectomized dogs. Am J Physiol 1968; 215(1):197.
39. Holloszy JO: Utilization of fatty acids during exercise. In Biochemistry of Exercise. Champaign, Ill, Human Kinetics Publishers, 1990, p 319.
40. Hurley BF, Nemeth PM, Martin III WH, et al: Muscle triglyceride utilization during exercise: Effect of training. J Appl Physiol 1986; 60(2):562.
41. Terjung R, Mackie B, Dudley G, et al: Influence of exercise on chylomicron triacylglycerol metabolism, plasma turnover, and muscle uptake. Med Sci Sports Exerc 1983; 15:340.
42. Saltin B, Gollnick PD: Fuel for muscular exercise: Role of carbohydrate. In Horton ES, Terjung RL (eds): Exercise, Nutrition and Energy Metabolism. New York, Macmillan, 1988, p 45.
43. Wahren J: Human forearm muscle metabolism during exercise. Scand J Clin Lab Invest 1970; 25:129.
44. Katz A, Broberg S, Sahlin K, et al: Leg glucose uptake during maximal dynamic exercise in humans. Am J Physiol 1986; 251(Endocrinol Metab 14):E65.
45. Lindholm A, Bjerneld H, Saltin B: Glycogen depletion pattern in muscle fibres of trotting horses. Acta Physiol Scand 1974; 90:475.
46. Nimmo MA, Snow DH: Changes in muscle glycogen, lactate and pyruvate concentrations in the thoroughbred horse following maximal exercise. In Snow DH, Persson SGB, Rose RJ (eds): Equine Exercise Physiology. Cambridge, Granta Editions, 1983, p 237.
47. Harris RC, Marlin DJ, Snow DH: Metabolic response to maximal exercise of 800 and 2000 m in the thoroughbred horse. J Appl Physiol 1987; 63(1):12.
48. Snow DH, Baxter P: Muscle fiber composition and glycogen depletion in horses competing in an endurance ride. Vet Rec 1981; 108:374.
49. Snow DH, Kerr MG, Nimmo MA, et al: Alterations in blood, sweat, urine, and muscle composition during prolonged exercise in the horse. Vet Rec 1982; 110:377.
50. Topliff DR, Potter GD, Dutson TR, et al: Diet manipulation and muscle glycogen in the equine. In Proceedings of the 8th Equine Nutrition and Physiology Symposium, Lexington, Ky, 1985, p 167.
51. Wahren J, Felig P, Ahlborg G, et al: Glucose metabolism during leg exercise in man. J Clin Invest 1971; 50:2715.
52. Bjorkman O, Wahren J: Glucose homeostasis during and after exercise. In Horton ES, Terjung RL (eds): Exercise, Nutrition and Energy Metabolism. New York, Macmillan, 1988, p 100.
53. Coyle EF: Carbohydrate supplementation during exercise. J Nutr 1992; 122:788.
54. Coggan AR, Coyle EF: Metabolism and performance following carbohydrate ingestion late in exercise. Med Sci Sports Exerc 1989; 21(1):59.
55. Wright DA, Sherman WM, Dernbach AR: Carbohydrate feedings before, during, or in combination improve cycling endurance performance. J Appl Physiol 1991; 71(3):1082.
56. Miller PA, Lawrence LM: The effect of dietary protein level on exercising horses. J Anim Sci 1988; 66:2185.
57. Hood DA, Terjung RL: Amino acid metabolism during exercise and following endurance training. Sports Med 1990; 9(1):23.
58. Knapik J, Meredith C, Jones B, et al: Leucine metabolism during fasting and exercise. J Appl Physiol 1991; 70(1):43.
59. Dohm GL, Kasperek GJ, Tapscott EB, et al: Protein metabolism during endurance exercise. Fed Proc 1985; 44:348.
60. Kaufmann DA: Protein as an energy substrate during intense exercise. Ann Sports Med 1990; 5:142.
61. Young VR: Protein and amino acid metabolism in relation to physical exercise. In Winnick M (ed): Nutrition and Exercise. New York, Wiley, 1986, p 9.
62. Lemon PWR, Mullin JP: Effect of initial muscle glycogen levels on protein catabolism during exercise. J Appl Physiol Respir Environ Exerc Physiol 1980; 48(4):624.
63. Lindinger MI, Heigenhauser GJF, McKelvie RS, et al: Role of nonworking muscle on blood metabolites and ions with intense intermittent exercise. Am J Physiol 1990; 258(Reg Integr Comp Physiol 27):R1486.
64. Snow DH, Fixter LM, Kerr MG, et al: Alterations in composition of venous plasma FFA pool during prolonged and sprint exercises in the horse. In Knuttgen H, Vogel J, Poortmans J (eds): Biochemistry of Exercise. Champaign, Ill, Human Kinetics Publishing, 1983, p 336.
65. Poso AR, Viljanen-Tarifa E, Soveri T, et al: Exercise-induced transient hyperlipidemia in the racehorse. J Vet Med Assoc 1989; 36:603.

66. Fell RD, McLane JA, Winder WW, et al: Preferential resynthesis of muscle glycogen in fasting rats after exhausting exercise. Am J Physiol 1980; 238(Reg Integr Comp Physiol 7):R328.
67. Terblanche SE, Fell RD, Juhlin-Dannfelt BW, et al: Effect of glycerol feeding before and after exhausting exercise in rats. J Appl Physiol 1980; 50:94.
68. Favier RJ, Koubi HE, Mayet MH, et al: Effects of gluconeogenic precursor flux alterations on glycogen resynthesis after prolonged exercise. J Appl Physiol 1987; 63(5):1733.
69. Blom PCS, Hostmark AT, Vaage O, et al: Effect of different post exercise sugar diets on the rate of muscle glycogen synthesis. Med Sci Sports Exerc 1987; 19:491.
70. Ivy JL: Muscle glycogen synthesis before and after exercise. Sports Med 1991; 11(1):6.
71. Friedman JE, Neufer PD, Dohm GL: Regulation of glycogen resynthesis following exercise. Sports Med 1991; 11(4):232.
72. Costill DL, Hargreaves M: Carbohydrate nutrition and fatigue. Sports Med 1992; 13(2):86.
73. National Research Council (NRC): Nutrient Requirements of Horses, 5th ed. Washington, National Academy Press, 1989.
74. Pagan JD, Hintz HF: Equine energetics: II. Energy expenditure in horses during submaximal exercise. J Anim Sci 1986; 63: 822.
75. Rose RJ, Knight PK, Bryden WL: Energy use and cardiorespiratory responses to prolonged submaximal exercise. In, Persson SGB, Lindholm A, Jeffcott LB (eds): Equine Exerise Physiology 3. Davis, Calif, ICEEP Publications, 1991, p 281.
76. Evans DL, Rose RJ: Maximal oxygen uptake in racehorses: Changes with training state and prediction from cardiorespiratory measurements. Equine Exerc Physiol 1987; 3:52.
77. Hintz HF, Roberts SJ, Sabin SW, et al: Energy requirements of light horses for various activities. J Anim Sci 1971; 32:100.
78. Anderson CE, Potter GD, Kreider JL, et al: Digestible energy requirements for exercising horses. J Anim Sci 1983; 56(1):91.
79. Wilmore JH: Body composition in sport and exercise: Directions for future research. Med Sci Sports Exerc 1983; 15(1):21.
80. Harman EA, Frykman PN: The relationship of body size and composition to the performance of physically demanding milary tasks. In Marriot BM, Grumstrup-Scott J (eds): Body Composition and Physical Performance. Washington, National Academy Press, 1992, p 105.
81. Cureton KJ: Effects of experimental alterations in excess weight on physiological responses to exercise and physical performance. In Marriot BM, Grumstrup-Scott J (eds): Body Composition and Physical Performance. Washington, National Academy Press, 1992, p 71.
82. Thornton J, Pagan J, Persson S: The oxygen cost of weight loading and inclined treadmill exercise in the horse. In Gillespie JR, Robinson NE (eds): Equine Exercise Physiology 2. Davis, Calif, ICEEP Publications, 1987, p 206.
83. Westervelt RG, Stauffer JR, Hintz HF, et al: Estimating fat in horses. J Anim Sci 1976; 43:7.
84. Kane RA, Fisher M, Parrett D, et al: Estimating fatness in horses. In Proceedings of the 10th Equine Nutrition and Physiology Symposium, Ft. Collins, Colo, 1987, p 127.
85. Henneke DR, Potter GD, Krieder JL: A condition score relationship to body fat content of mares during gestation and lactation. In Proceedings of 7th Equine Nutrition and Physiology Symposium, Warrenton, Va, 1981, p 105.
86. Wilmore JR, Freund BJ: Nutritional enhancement of athletic performance (abstract). Nutr Rev 1984; 54:1.
87. Lawrence LM, Jackson S, Kline K, et al: Observations on body weight and condition of horses in a 150-mile endurance ride. J Equine Vet Sci 1992; 12:320.
88. Parizkova J, Bunc V, Sprynarova S, et al: Body composition, aerobic capacity, ventilatory threshold, and food intake in different sports. Ann Sports Med 1987; 3:171.
89. Gallagher K, Leech J, Stowe H: Protein, energy and dry matter consumption by racing thoroughbreds: A field survey. J Equine Vet Sci 1992; 12(1):43.
90. Gallagher K, Leech J, Stowe H: Protein, energy and dry matter consumption by racing standardbreds: A field survey. J Equine Vet Sci 1992; 12:382.
91. Vogel JA, Friedl KE: Army data: Body composition and physical capacity. In Marriot BM, Grumstrup-Scott J (eds): Body Composition and Physical Performance. Washington, National Academy Press, 1992, p 89.
92. Forbes GB: Do obese individuals gain weight more easily than nonobese individuals? Am J Clin Nutr 1990; 52:224.
93. Forbes GB: Exercise and body composition. J Appl Physiol 1991; 70(3):994.
94. Pavlou KN, Steffee WP, Lerman RH, et al: Effects of dieting and exercise on lean body mass, oxygen uptake, and strength. Med Sci Sports Exerc 1985; 17(4):466.
95. Oscai LB, Holloszy JO: Effects of weight changes produced by exercise, food restriction, or overeating on body composition. J Clin Invest 1969; 48:2124.
96. Hickson JF, Wolinski I: Human protein intake and metabolism in exercise and sport. In Hickson JF, Wolinski I (eds): Nutrition in Exercise and Sport. Boca Raton, Fla, CRC Press, 1989, p 5.
97. National Research Council (NRC): Nutrient Requirements of Horses, 4th ed. Washington, National Academy Press, 1978.
98. Essen-Gustavsson B, Blomstrand E, Karlstrom K, et al: Influence on diet on substrate metabolism during exercise. In Persson SGB, Lindholm A, Jeffcott LB (eds), Equine Exercise Physiology 3, Davis, Calif, ICEEP Publications, 1991, p 288.
99. Miller-Graber P, Lawrence L, Foreman J, et al: Effect of dietary protein level on nitrogen metabolites in exercised quarter horses. In Persson SGB, Lindholm A, Jeffcott LB (eds), Equine Exercise Physiology 3, Davis, Calif, ICEEP Publications, 1991, p 305.
100. Booth FW, Watson PA: Control of adaptations in protein levels in response to exercise. Fed Proc 1985; 44:2293.
101. Phinney SD: Exercise during and after very-low-calorie dieting. Am J Clin Nutr 1992; 56:190S
102. Meyer H: Nutrition and the equine athlete. In Gillespie JR, Robinson NE (eds), Equine Exercise Physiology 2. Davis, Calif, ICEEP Publications, 1987, p 644.
103. Freeman DW, Potter GD, Schelling GT, et al: Nitrogen metabolism in mature horses at varying levels of work. J Anim Sci 1988; 66:407.
104. Patterson PH, Coon CN, Hughes IM: Protein requirements of mature working horses. J Anim Sci 1985; 61(1):187.
105. Friedman JE, Lemon PWR: Effect of chronic endurance exercise on retention of dietary protein. Int J Sports Med 1989; 10(2):118.
106. Lemon PWR, Proctor DN: Protein intake and athletic performance. Sports Med 1991; 12(5):313.
107. Lemon PWR, Tarnopolsky MA, MacDougall JD, et al: Protein requirements and muscle mass/strength changes during intensive training in novice bodybuilders. J Appl Physiol 1992; 73(2):767.
108. Miller-Graber PA, Lawrence LM, Foreman JH, et al: Dietary protein level and energy metabolism during treadmill exercise in horses. J Nutr 1991; 121:1462.
109. Pagan JD, Essen-Gustavsson B, Lindholm A, et al: The effect of energy source on exercise performance in Standardbred horses. In Gillespie JR, Robinson NE (eds), Equine Exercise Physiology 2. Davis, Calif, ICEEP Publications, 1987, p 686.
110. Satabin P, Bois-Joyeux B, Chanez M, et al: Effects of long-term feeding of high-protein or high-fat diets on the response to exercise in the rat. Eur J Appl Physiol 1989; 58:583.
111. Satabin P, Bois-Joyeux B, Chanez M, et al: Post-exercise glycogen resynthesis in trained high-protein or high-fat-fed rats after glucose feeding. Eur J Appl Physiol 1989; 58:591.
112. Raub RH, Jackson SG, Baker JP: The effect of exercise on bone growth and development in weanling horses. J Anim Sci 1989; 67:2508.
113. McCarthy RN, Jeffcott LB: Treadmill exercise intensity and its effects on cortial bone in horses of various ages. Equine Exerc Physiol 1991; 3:419.
113a. Schryver HF, Hintz HF, Lowe JE: Calcium metabolism, body composition and sweat losses of exercised horses. Am J Vet Res 1978; 39:245.
114. Hintz HF: Nutrients. In Evans JW, Borton A, Hintz HF, Van Vleck LD (eds): The Horse, 2d ed. New York, Freeman, 1990, p 208.
115. Schryver HF, Hintz HF, Lowe JE: Calcium and phosphorus in the nutrition of the horse. Cornell Vet 1974; 64:493.
116. Schils S, Jordan RM: Nutrition practices and philosophies of race

horse trainers. *In* Proceedings of the 11th Equine Nutrition and Physiology Symposium, Stillwater, Okla, 1989, p 238.

117. Caple IW, Bourke JM, Ellis PG: An examination of the calcium and phosphorus nutrition of thoroughbred racehorses. Austr Vet J 1982; 58:132.

118. Cymbaluk NF, Christensen DA: Nutrient utilization of pelleted forages by ponies. Can J Anim Sci 1986; 66:237.

119. Jeffcott LB: Osteochondrosis in the horse: Searching for the key to pathogenesis. Equine Vet J 1991; 23(5):331.

120. Kronfeld DS, Meacham TN, Donahue S: Dietary aspects of developmental orthopedic disease. Vet Clin North Am Equine Pract 1990; 6:467.

121. Lewis LD: Care and Feeding of the Horse. Philadelphia, Lea & Febiger, 1982.

122. Knight DA, Gabel AA, Reed SM, et al: Correlation of dietary mineral to incidence and severity of metabolic bone disease in Ohio and Kentucky. *In* Proceedings of the Annual Meeting of the American Association of Equine Practitioners, 1985, p 445.

123. Glade MJ: The role of endocrine factors in developmental orthopedic disease. *In* Proceedings of the Annual Meeting of the American Association of Equine Practitioners, 1987, p 171.

124. Krook L, Maylin GA: Fractures in Thoroughbred racehorses. Cornell Vet 1988; 78(suppl 11):1.

125. Lindner A, Schmidt M, Meyer H. Investigations on sodium metabolism in exercised Shetland ponies fed a diet marginal in sodium. *In* Snow DH, Persson SGB, Rose RJ (eds): Equine Exercise Physiology. Cambridge, Granta Editions, 1983, p 310.

126. Meyer H, Gurer C, Lindner A: Effects of a low-K diet on K-metabolism sweat production and sweat composition in horses. *In* Proceedings of the 9th Equine Nutrition and Physiology Symposium, East Lansing, Mich., 1985, p 130.

127. Houpt KA, Northrup N, Wheatley T, et al: Thirst and salt appetite in horses treated with furosemide. J Appl Physiol 1991; 71:2380.

128. Weaver CM, Rajaram S: Exercise and iron status. J Nutr 1992; 122:782.

129. Woodson RD: Hemoglobin concentration and exercise capacity. Am Rev Respir Dis 1984; 129:S72.

130. Powell PD, Tucker A: Iron supplementation and running performance in female cross-country runners. Int J Sports Med 1991; 12(5):462.

131. Klingshirm LA, Pate RR, Bourque SP, et al: Effect of iron supplementation on endurance capacity in iron-depleted female runners. Med Sci Sports Exerc 1992; 24(7):819.

132. Willis WT, Gohil K, Brooks GA, et al: Iron deficiency: Improved exercise performance within 15 hours of iron treatment in rats. J Nutr 1990; 120:909.

133. Kirkham WW, Guttridge H, Bowden J, et al: Hematopoietic responses to hematinics in horses. J Am Vet Med Assoc 1971; 159:1316.

134. Lawrence LA, Ott EA, Asquith RL, et al: Influence of dietary iron on growth, tissue mineral composition, apparent phosphorus absorption, and chemical properties of bone. *In* Proceedings of the 10th Equine Nutrition and Physiology Symposium, Ft. Collins, Colo, 1987, p 563.

135. Pate RR: Sports anemia: A review of current research. Phys Sports Med 1983; 11:115.

136. McMiken DF: An energetic basis of equine performance. Equine Vet J 1983; 15(2):123.

137. National Research Council (NRC): United States–Canadian Tables of Feed Composition, 3d rev. Washington, National Academy Press, 1982.

138. Maenpaa PH, Pirhonen A, Koskinen E: Vitamin A, E and D nutrition in mares and foals during the winter season: Effect of feeding two different vitamin-mineral concentrates. J Anim Sci 1988; 66:1424.

139. Witt EH, Reznick AZ, Viguie CA, et al: Exercise oxidative damage and effects of antioxidant manipulation. J Nutr 1992; 122:766.

140. Gohil K, Packer L, DeLumen B, et al: Vitamin E deficiency and vitamin C supplements: Exercise and mitochondrial oxidation. J Appl Physiol 1986; 60:1986.

141. Petersson KH, Hintz HF, Schryver HF, et al: The effect of vitamin E on membrane integrity during submaximal exercise. *In* Persson SGB, Lindholm A, Jeffcott LB (eds), Equine Exercise Physiology 3, Davis, Calif, ICEEP Publications, 1991, p 288.

142. Tengerdy RP: The role of vitamin E on immune response and disease resistance. Ann NY Acad Sci 1990; 587:24.

143. Hidiroglou N, McDowell LR, Papas AM et al: Bioavailability of vitamin E compounds in lambs. J Anim Sci 1992; 70:2556.

144. Frape DL: Nutrition and the growth and racing performance of thoroughbred horses. Proc Nutr Soc 1989; 48:141.

145. Topliff DR, Potter GD, Kreider JL, et al: Thiamin supplementation for exercising horses. *In* Proceedings of the 9th Equine Nutrition and Physiology Symposium, East Lansing, Mich, 1985; p 167.

146. Belko AZ, Obarzawek E, Kalkwarf HJ, et al: Effects of exercise on riboflavin requirements of young women. Am J Clin Nutr 1983; 37:509.

147. Winters LRT, Yoon JS, Kalkwarf HJ, et al: Riboflavin requirements and exercise adaptation in older women. Am J Clin Nutr 1992; 56:526.

148. National Research Council (NRC): Recommended Dietary Allowances, 10th ed. Washington, National Academy Press, 1989.

149. Comben N, Clark RJ, Sutherland DJB: Clinical observations on the response of equine hoof defects to dietary supplementation with biotin. Vet Rec 1984; 115:642.

150. Lindner A, von Wittke P, Frigg M: Effect of biotin supplementation on the V_{LA4} of thoroughbred horses. J Equine Vet Sci 1992; 12(3):149.

151. Snow DH, Harris RC: The use of conventional and unconventional supplements in the thoroughbred horse. Proc Nutr Soc 1989; 48:135.

152. Jackson SG, Pagan JD: Control colic through management. J Equine Vet Sci 1992; 12(6):341.

153. Darlington JM, Hershberger TV: Effect of forage maturity on digestibility, intake and nutritive value of alfalfa, timothy and orchardgrass by equine. J Anim Sci 1968; 27:1521.

154. Lawrence LM, Moore KJ, Hintz HF, et al: Acceptability of alfalfa hay treated with an organic acid preservative for horses. Can J Anim Sci 1987; 67:217.

155. Whitlock RH: Feed additives and contaminants as a cause of equine disease. Vet Clin North Am Equine Pract 1990; 6:467.

156. Duren SE, Dougherty CT, Jackson SG, et al: Modification of ingestive behavior due to exercise in yearling horses grazing orchardgrass. Appl Anim Behav Sci 1989; 22:335.

157. Ralston SL: Nutritional management of horses competing in 160 km races. Cornell Vet 1988; 78:53.

158. Kerr MG, Snow DH: Alterations in hematocrit, plasma proteins and electrolytes in horses following the feeding of hay. Vet Rec 1982; 110:538.

159. Clarke LL, Argenzio RA, Roberts MC: Effect of meal feeding on plasma volume and urinary electrolyte clearance in ponies. Am J Vet Res 1990; 51:571.

160. Clark LL, Roberts MC, Argenzio RA: Feeding and digestive problems in horses: Physiological responses to a concentrated meal. Vet Clin North Am Equine Pract 1990; 6:433.

161. McKirnan MD, Gray CG, White FC: Effects of feeding on muscle blood flow during prolonged exercise in miniature swine. J Appl Physiol 1991; 70(3):1097.

162. Duren SE, Manohar M, Sikkes B, et al: Influence of feeding and exercise on the distribution of intestinal and muscle blood flow in ponies. Pferdeheilkunde 1992; 24.

163. Fonnesbeck PV: Consumption and excretion of water by horses receiving all hay and hay-grain diets. J Anim Sci 1968; 27:1350.

164. Cuddeford D, Woodhead A, Muirhead R: A comparison between the nutritive value of short-cutting cycle, high temperature–dried alfalfa and timothy hay for horses. Equine Vet J 1992; 24(2):84.

165. Bonen A, McDermott JC, Tan MH: Glucose transport in skeletal muscle. Biochem Exerc 1990; 21:295.

166. Lawrence LM, Soderholm V, Roberts A, et al: Metabolic changes in exercised horses fed various amounts of carbohydrate. *In* Proceedings of the 1990 Cornell Nutrition Conference, Rochester, NY, 1991, p 133.

167. Sherman WM, Peden MC, Wright DA: Carbohydrate feedings 1 h before exercise improves cycling performance. Am J Clin Nutr 1991; 54:866.

168. Thomas DE, Brotherhood JR, Brand JC: Carbohydrate feeding before exercise: Effect of glycemic index. Int J Sports Med 1991; 12(2):180.

169. Gleeson M, Greenhaff PL, Maughan RJ: Influence of a 24 h fast on high intensity cycle exercise performance in man. Eur J Appl Physiol 1988; 57:653.

170. Costill DL: Carbohydrate nutrition before, during, and after exercise. Fed Proc 1985; 44:364.

171. Williams C: Diet and endurance fitness. Am J Clin Nutr 1989; 49:1077.

172. Foster C, Costill D, Fink WJ: Effects of pre-exercise feedings on endurance performance. Med Sci Sports Exer 1979; 11:1.

173. Neufer PD, Costill DL, Flynn MG, et al: Improvements in exercise performance: Effects of carbohydrate feedings and diet. J Appl Physiol 1987; 62:983.

174. Sherman WM, Brodowicz G, Wright DA, et al: Effects of 4 h pre-exercise carbohydrate feedings on cycling performance. Med Sci Sports Exerc 1989; 21:598.

175. Wright DA, Sherman WM, Dernbach AR: Carbohydrate feedings before, during, or in combination improve cycling endurance performance. J Appl Physiol 1991; 71(3):1082.

176. Coggan AR, Swanson SC: Nutritional manipulations before and during endurance exercise: Effects on performance. Med Sci Sports Exerc 1992; 24(9):S331.

177. Rodiek A, Bonvicin S, Stull C, et al: Glycemic and endocrine responses to corn or alfalfa feed prior to exercise. *In* Persson SGB, Lindholm A, Jeffcott LB (eds): Equine Exercise Physiology 3, Davis, Calif, ICEEP Publications, 1991, p 323.

178. Zimmerman NI, Wickler SJ, Rodiek AV, et al: Free fatty acids in exercising Arabian horses fed two common diets. J Nutr 1991; 122:145.

179. Coyle EF, Hagberg JM, Hurley BF, et al: Carbohydrate feedings during prolonged strenuous exercise can delay fatigue. J Appl Physiol 1983; 55:230.

180. Mitchell JB, Costill DL, Houmard JA, et al: Influence of carbohydrate ingestion on counterregulatory hormones during prolonged exercise. Int J Sports Med 1990; 11(1):33.

181. Massicotte D, Peronnet F, Allah C, et al: Metabolic responses to [^{13}C]glucose and [^{13}C]fructose ingestion during exercise. J Appl Physiol 1986; 61(3):1180.

182. Massicotte D, Peronnet F, Brisson G, et al: Oxidation of exogenous carbohydrate during prolonged exercise in fed and fasted conditions. Int J Sports Med 1990; 11(4):253.

183. Hawley JA, Dennis SC, Laidler BJ, et al: High rates of exogenous carbohydrate oxidation from starch ingested during prolonged exercise. J Appl Physiol 1991; 71(5):1801.

184. Hawley JA, Dennis SC, Nowitz A, et al: Exogenous carbohydrate oxidation from maltose and glucose ingested during prolonged exercise. Eur J Appl Physiol 1992; 64:523.

185. Moodley D, Noakes TD, Bosch AN, et al: Oxidation of exogenous carbohydrate during prolonged exercise: The effects of the carbohydrate type and its concentration. Eur J Appl Physiol 1992; 64:328.

186. Mainwood GW, Worsley-Brown P: The effects of extracellular pH and buffer concentration on the efflux of lactate from frog sartorius muscle. J Physiol (Lond) 1975; 250:1.

187. Spriet LL, Lindinger MI, Heigenhauser GJF, et al: Effects of alkalosis on skeletal muscle metabolism and performance during exercise. Am J Physiol 1986; 251(Reg Integr Comp Physiol 20):R833.

188. Jones NL, Sutton JR, Taylor R, et al: Effect of pH on cardiorespiratory and metabolic responses to exercise. J Appl Physiol Respir Environ Exerc Physiol 1977; 43(6):959.

189. Costill DL, Verstappen F, Kuipers H, et al: Acid-base balance during repeated bouts of exercise: Influence of HCO$_3$. Int J Sports Med 1984; 5(5):228.

190. Inbar O, Rotstein A, Jacobs I, et al: The effects of alkaline treatment on short-term maximal exercise. J Sports Sci 1983; 1:95.

191. Wilkes D, Gledhill N, Smyth R: Effect of acute induced metabolic alkalosis on 800-m racing time. Med Sci Sports Exerc 1983; 15(4):277.

192. Gledhill N: Bicarbonate ingestion and anaerobic performance. Sports Med 1984; 1:177.

193. Wijnen S, Verstappen F, Kuipers H: The influence of intravenous NaHCO$_3$₋ administration on interval exercise: Acid-base balance and endurance. Int J Sports Med 1984; 5:130.

194. George KP, MacLaren DPM: The effect of induced alkalosis and acidosis on endurance running at an intensity corresponding to 4 mM blood lactate. Ergonomics 1988; 31(11):1639.

195. Linderman J, Fahey TD: Sodium bicarbonate ingestion and exercise performance. Sports Med 1991; 11(2):71.

196. McCartney N, Heigenhauser GJF, Jones NL: Effects of pH on maximal power output and fatigue during short-term dynamic exercise. J Appl Physiol Respir Environ Exerc Physiol 1983; 55(1):225.

197. Bergstein S: "Milkshakes": A bad idea the sport can do without. Harness Horse 1989; 54(36):6.

198. Milbert N: Illinois horsemen say "No, Thanks" to milkshakes. Hoof Beats, July 1991, p 33.

199. Freestone JF, Carlson GP, Harrold DR, et al: Furosemide and sodium bicarbonate-induced alkalosis in the horse and response to oral KCl and NaCl therapy. Am J Vet Res 1989; 50(8):1334.

200. Kelso TB, Hodgson DR, Witt EH, et al: Bicarbonate administration and muscle metabolism during high-intensity exercise. *In* Gillespie JR, Robinson NE (eds): Equine Exercise Physiology 2, Davis, Calif, ICEEP Publications, 1987, p 438.

201. Lawrence LM, Miller PA, Bechtel PJ, et al: The effect of sodium bicarbonate ingestion on blood parameters in exercising horses. *In* Gillespie JR, Robinson NE (eds): Equine Exercise Physiology 2, Davis, Calif, ICEEP Publications, 1987, p 448.

202. Lawrence L, Kline K, Miller-Graber P, et al: Effect of sodium bicarbonate on racing standardbreds. J Anim Sci 1990; 68:673.

203. Greenhaff PL, Hanak J, Harris RC, et al: Metabolic alkalosis and exercise performance in the thoroughbred horse. *In* Persson SGB, Lindholm A, Jeffcott LB (eds): Equine Exercise Physiology 3, Davis, Calif, ICEEP Publications, 1991, p 353.

204. Greenhaff PL, Harris RC, Snow DH, et al: The influence of metabolic alkalosis upon exercise metabolism in the thoroughbred horse. Eur J Appl Physiol 1991; 63:129.

205. Harkins JD, Kamerling SG: Effects of induced alkalosis on performance in thoroughbreds during a 1600-m race. Equine Vet J 1992; 24(2):94.

206. Patience JF, Austic RE, Boyd RD: Effect of dietary electrolyte balance on growth and acid-base status in swine. J Anim Sci 1987; 64:457.

207. Tucker WB, Harrison GA, Hemken RW: Influence of dietary cation-anion balance on milk, blood, urine and rumen fluid in lactating dairy cattle. J Dairy Sci 1988; 71:346.

208. Baker LA, Topliff DR, Freeman DW, et al: Effect of dietary cation-anion balance on acid-base status in horses. J Equine Vet Sci 1992; 12:160.

209. Popplewell JC, Topliff DR, Freeman DW: Effects of dietary cation-anion balance on acid base balance and blood parameters in anaerobically exercised horses. *In* Proceedings of the 13th Equine Nutrition and Physiology Symposium, Gainesville, Fla, 1993, p 191.

210. Wall DL, Topliff DR, Freeman DW, et al: Effect of dietary cation-anion balance on urinary mineral excretion in exercised horses. J Equine Vet Sci 1992; 12:168.

211. Kane E, Baker JP, Bull LS: Utilization of a corn oil supplemented diet by the pony. J Anim Sci 1979; 48(6):1379.

212. Hintz HF, Ross M, Lesser F, et al: Dietary fat for working horses. *In* Proceedings of the Cornell Nutrition Conference, Ithaca, NY, 1977, p 87.

213. Hambleton PL, Slade LM, Hamar DW, et al: Dietary fat and exercise conditioning effect on metabolic parameters in the horse. J Anim Sci 1980; 51:1330.

214. Duren SE, Jackson SG, Baker JP, et al: Effect of dietary fat on blood parameters in exercised Thoroughbred horses. *In* Gillespie JR, Robinson NE (eds): Equine Exercise Physiology, 2, Davis, Calif, ICEEP Publications, 1987, p 674.

215. Webb SP, Potter GD, Evans JW: Physiologic and metabolic response of race and cutting horses to added dietary fat. *In* Proceedings of the 10th Equine Nutrition and Physiology Symposium, Ft Collins, Colo, 1987, p 115.

216. Griewe KM, Meacham TN, Fregin GF, et al: Effect of added dietary fat on exercising horses. *In* Proceedings of the 11th Equine Nutrition and Physiology Symposium, Stillwater, Okla, 1989, p 101.

217. Oldham SL, Potter GD, Evans JW, et al: Storage and mobilization of muscle glycogen in exercising horses fed a fat supplemented diet. J Equine Vet Sci 1990; 10:353.

218. Miller WC, Bryce GR, Conlee RK: Adaptations to a high fat diet that increase exercise endurance in male rats. J Appl Physiol 1986; 56:78.

219. Simi B, Sempore B, Mayet MH, et al: Additive effects of training and high-fat diet on energy metabolism during exercise. J Appl Physiol 1991; 71(1):197.

220. Saitoh S, Shimomura Y, Tasaki Y, et al: Effect of short-term exercise training on muscle glycogen in resting conditions in rats fed a high fat diet. Eur J Appl Physiol 1992; 64:62.

221. Coyle EF: Ergogenic aids. Clin Sports Med 1984; 3(3):731.

222. Rose RJ, Lloyd DR: Sodium bicarbonate: More than just a "milk-shake"? Equine Vet J 1992; 24(2):75.

223. Shelle J, Van Huss W, Rook JS, et al: Relationship between selenium and vitamin E nutrition and exercise in the horse. *In* Proceedings of the 9th Equine Nutrition and Physiology Symposium, East Lansing, Mich, 1985.

224. Witt EH, Reznick AZ, Figuie CA, et al: Exercise, oxidative damage and effects of antioxidant manipulation. J Nutr 1992; 122:766.

225. Braun B, Clarkson PM, Freedson PS, et al: Effects of coenzyme Q10 on exercise performance, maximal oxygen consumption and lipid peroxidation (abstract). Med Sci Sport Exerc 1991; 23(4):S78.

226. Rathgeber-Lawrence R, Ratzlaff M, Grant BD, et al: The effects of coenzyme Q10 as a nutritional supplement on musculoskeletal fitness in the exercising horse. Equine Athlete 1991; 4(3):1.

227. Cerretelli P, Marconi C: L-Carnitine supplementation in humans: The effects on physical performance. Int J Sports Med 1990; 11(1):1.

228. Feller AG, Rudman D: Role of carnitine in human nutrition. J Nutr 1988; 118:541.

229. Arenas J, Ricoy JR, Encinas AR, et al: Carnitine in muscle, serum, and urine of nonprofessional athletes: Effects of physical exercise, training, and L-carnitine administration. Muscle Nerve 1991; 14:598.

230. Foster CVL, Harris RC, Snow DH: The effect of oral L-carnitine supplementation on the muscle and plasma concentrations in the thoroughbred horse. Comp Biochem Physiol [A] 1988; 91(4):827.

231. Simi B, Mayet MH, Sempore B, et al: Large variations in skeletal muscle carnitine levels fail to modify energy metabolism in exercising rats. Comp Biochem Physiol A 1990; 97:543.

232. Heinonen OJ, Takala J, Kvist MH: Effect of carnitine loading on long-chain fatty acid oxidation, maximal exercise capacity, and nitrogen balance. Eur J Appl Physiol 1992; 65:13.

233. Gorostiaga EM, Maurer CA, Eclache JP: Decrease in respiratory quotient during exercise following L-carnitine supplementation. Int J Sports Med 1989; 10(3):169.

234. Wyss V, Ganzit GP, Rienzi A: Effects of L-carnitine administration on $\dot{V}_{O_2max}$ and the aerobic-anaerobic threshold in normoxia and acute hypoxia. Eur J Appl Physiol 1990; 60:1.

235. Vecchiet L, DiLisa F, Pieralisi G, et al: Influence of L-carnitine administration on maximal physical exercise. Eur J Appl Physiol 1990; 61:486.

236. Blomstrand E, Hassmen P, Ekblom B, et al: Administration of branched-chain amino acids during sustained exercise: Effects on performance and on plasma concentration of some amino acids. Eur J Appl Physiol 1991; 63:83.

237. Glade MJ: Effects of specific amino acid supplementation on lactic acid production by horses exercised on a treadmill. *In* Proceedings of the 11th Equine Nutrition and Physiology Symposium, Stillwater, Okla, 1989, p 244.

238. Seltzer S, Stoch R, Marcus R, et al: Alterations on human pain thresholds by nutritional manipulation of L-tryptophan supplementation. Pain 1982; 13:385.

239. Stensrud T, Ingjer F, Holm H, et al: L-Tryptophan supplementation does not improve running performance. Int J Sports Med 1992; 13(6):481.

240. Sequra R, Ventura JL: Effect of L-tryptophan supplementation on exercise performance. Int J Sports Med 1988; 9:301.

241. Rose RJ, Schlierf HA, Knight PK, et al: Effects of *N,N*-dimethylglycine on cardiorespiratory function and lactate production in thoroughbred horses performing incremental treadmill exercise. Vet Rec 1989; 125:268.

11

Evaluation of Performance Potential

D. R. HODGSON AND R. J. ROSE

Successful athletic performance requires a complex interaction of physiologic mechanisms involving the musculoskeletal, nervous, respiratory, and cardiovascular systems. From a simplistic point of view, exercise demands the imposition of increased loads on the respiratory and cardiovascular systems in order to support the dramatic increases in metabolic rate occurring in contracting muscles during exercise. It is essential that the responses of each of these systems are appropriately integrated to ensure optimal physiologic performance. There are dramatic increases in ventilation and cardiac output with increasing metabolic rate, and not surprisingly, the capacity and health of these systems will play a substantial role in determining the performance potential of a horse. Since superior athletic performance depends on tight integration of a number of body functions, it is to be expected that many elite equine athletes have metabolic characteristics indicating this potential for superior performance. For example, top-class thoroughbred and standardbred racehorses usually have values for maximal oxygen consumption ($\dot{V}_{O_2max}$) in the range of 150 to 200 ml/kg per minute.[1,2] Conversely, although a high $\dot{V}_{O_2max}$ indicates substantial cardiorespiratory capacity, it does not ensure superior athletic performance. This is demonstrated in the horse that has a large cardiorespiratory capacity yet is endowed with a conformation that does now allow the musculoskeletal system to withstand the rigors of training and racing. However, we also have conducted exercise tests on horses in which the cardiorespiratory capacity or conformation may not be considered ideal, yet these horses performed at a level above that predicted. Parallels for this latter observation exist in human athletes, and the reasons are likely to be related to (1) our inability to measure the metabolic determinants critical to performance, (2) physiologic integration, whereby the sum of all the components contributing to exercise capacity is greater than those indicated by measurement of the parts, and (3) intangible factors such as desire, or the "*will to win.*"

Evaluation of performance potential requires an understanding of the physiologic mechanisms involved in the energetics of exercise. Muscular work requires that the physiologic systems of the horse are integrated in order to minimize stress imposed on the component mechanisms supporting the energetics. Muscular respiration depends on complex interactive systems that allow gas exchange between the muscle cells and atmosphere. Optimal gas exchange between muscle cells and the atmosphere requires (1) efficient lung function, (2) effective pulmonary circulation which is able to match the requirements of ventilation, (3) blood with an adequate hemoglobin concentration, (4) a cardiovascular system that can deliver an appropriate quantity of oxygenated blood to the periphery to match tissue respiratory requirements, and (5) control mechanisms capable of regulating arterial blood gas tensions and pH.[3]

Energy for muscular contraction is obtained predominantly by the oxidation of fuels in the mitochondria, with an additional portion delivered via biochemical mechanisms in the cell cytoplasm. This energy is used to form high-energy compounds, predominantly phosphocreatine (CP) and adenosine triphosphate (ATP). The energy from the terminal phosphate bond can be made available for cellular reactions involved in synthesis, active transport, and muscular contraction. These processes are discussed in detail in Chapter 4.

Oxygen-Transport Chain

During exercise, there are dramatically increased loads placed on muscle bioenergetics, with the need for the respiratory and cardiovascular systems to respond to support the increased gas-exchange requirements. Transfer of O_2 and CO_2 between the mitochondria and air requires a finely coordinated interaction between the cardiovascular and respiratory mechanisms which is integrated with the cellular metabolic activity (Fig. 11–1). The large increase in muscle O_2 requirements during ex-

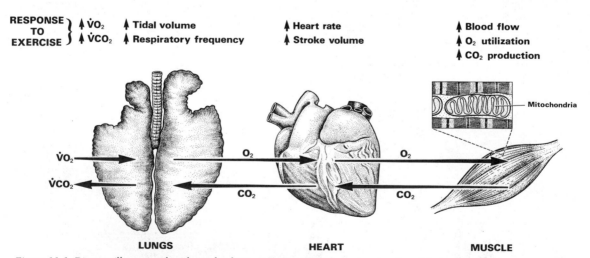

RESPONSE TO EXERCISE ⎰ ↑ $\dot{V}O_2$ ↑ Tidal volume ↑ Heart rate ↑ Blood flow
⎱ ↑ $\dot{V}CO_2$ ↑ Respiratory frequency ↑ Stroke volume ↑ O_2 utilization
  ↑ CO_2 production

Mitochondria

$\dot{V}O_2$ O_2 O_2

$\dot{V}CO_2$ CO_2 CO_2

LUNGS   **HEART**   **MUSCLE**

Figure 11-1. *Diagram illustrating the relationship between function of the lungs, heart, and working muscle and increases in oxygen uptake ($\dot{V}_{O_2}$) and carbon dioxide production ($\dot{V}_{CO_2}$) during exercise.*

ercise demands that O_2 flow to muscle increases. There is a simultaneous increase in CO_2 production which must be removed from the tissues to ensure that acidosis is avoided, since this can have profound adverse effects on muscular contractile activity.[4] Components of the oxygen-transport chain that are integral to superior athletic performance include the airways and lungs, the cardiovascular system, blood volume and hemoglobin concentration, and the musculoskeletal system.

AIRWAYS AND LUNGS

Following the onset of exercise, there is an increased respiratory drive which is thought to be due mainly to increased neural stimuli. In elite athletic horses, this may involve an increase in minute ventilation from about 100 liters/min at rest to greater than 1800 liters/min during strenuous exercise.[5,6] The increase in ventilation occurs as a result of a small increase in tidal volume and a large increase in respiratory frequency of up to 150 breaths/min. Entrainment of stride and respiratory frequencies restrict any greater increase in respiratory rate. As a result, peak airflows will be more than 6000 liters/min. Achievement of flows of this magnitude will require production of transpulmonary pressures of more than 60 cmH_2O. For such enormous flows to occur, it is important that the upper respiratory tract be optimally dilated during exercise. This active dilatation allows a reduction in upper airway resistance during exercise. Not surprisingly, restrictions to the upper airway, e.g., idiopathic laryngeal hemiplegia, may substantially alter airflow dynamics and therefore gas exchange,[7,8] thereby resulting in reduced exercise capacity. Similarly, disorders that may alter elasticity of the lung or gas exchange in the alveolus (e.g., chronic obstructive pulmonary disease) also will reduce gas exchange and therefore restrict performance.

CARDIOVASCULAR SYSTEM

Integration of cardiovascular and respiratory function during exercise is essential if superior athletic performance is to be achieved. In the transition from rest to exercise, there are dramatic alterations in the vascular system in order to accommodate the large increases in cardiac output. Initially, there is metabolic vasodilation in the vascular beds of working muscle, resulting in an increase in $\dot{V}_{O_2}$ and stimulation of heart rate and cardiac output.[9] There will be almost simultaneous dilatation of capillary beds in the pulmonary vasculature in order to support the increased gas-exchange requirements imposed by the exercise. During intense exercise, heart rate increases to greater than 230 beats/min,[10] which in elite racehorses is associated with increases in cardiac output to more than 350 liters/min.[11] Blood flow to working muscle has been shown to increase by more than 75-fold in ponies in response to intense exercise.[12] These blood flows exceeded 160 ml/kg per minute, which is almost twice the values reported to occur in humans.[13]

BLOOD VOLUME

Blood is the conduit for transport of O_2 to and CO_2 away from working muscle. Oxygen is carried by hemoglobin, and the volume of O_2 that can be carried in the circulation is related to the total blood volume and total hemoglobin concentration. Horses possess a substantial splenic reserve of erythrocytes, which are released into the circulation in response to exercise. This reserve is such that the blood oxygen concentration can increase from values of about 180 ml/liter at rest up to 280 ml/liter[14] in response to maximal exercise. This is associated with an increase in hematocrit from about 0.40 liter/liter at rest to more than 0.60 liter/liter during maximal exercise. There is also an increase in total blood volume from about 65 ml/kg at rest to more than 130 ml/kg with intense exercise.[15]

MUSCULOSKELETAL SYSTEM

During exercise, the major endpoint of the oxygen-transport chain is the contracting skeletal muscle. In its simplest form, skeletal muscle can be regarded as the apparatus which is fueled by the chemical energy sources derived from ingestion of food. As described above (and in Chap. 4), most energy for muscular contraction is derived from the oxidation of fuel in the mitochondria. In horses, skeletal muscle has an intrinsically high oxidative capacity when compared with humans and most other domestic species, and this may be enhanced by training.[16–18]

For the oxidative metabolic pathways to be able to meet the energy demands imposed by exercise, there must be adequate delivery of oxygen to the working muscle via the pulmonary and cardiovascular systems. Working muscle consumes the O_2 and in response to the increased extraction of O_2 and addition of CO_2 to capillary blood by muscle, there is an almost immediate increase in muscle blood flow. The initial vasodilation is thought to be centrally induced, with subsequent dilation occurring under the influence of local humoral control.[9] This process is selective, allowing vasodilation in the muscle units with the highest metabolic rates.[9]

Anaerobic Energy Delivery

Although the majority of energy during most intensities of exercise is provided by aerobic means, maximal exercise requires a substantial contribution from the anaerobic bioenergetic pathways. For this purpose, horses are endowed with intrinsically high activities of the enzymes involved in anaerobic energy production,[18,20,21] with horses with the higest proportion of fast-twitch (type II) muscle fibers also having the greatest glycolytic potential.[22]

From an energy point of view, it is important to consider that induction of energy production by the anaerobic pathways does not signal the down-regulation of energy supply by the aerobic pathways. Lactate is a byproduct of anaerobic energy production, and at low exercise intensities, there is little or no change in blood lactate concentration.[23] As exercise intensity increases, there is a consequent formation of lactate, with increases in the concentration of this metabolic by-product in muscle and blood. The higher the intensity of exercise, the greater is the concentration of lactate accumulating in these tissues (see Chap. 8 for further discussion).

MUSCLE POWER

Superior athletic performance requires that locomotor muscles be able to generate sufficient force for an appropriate time during the competition. To do this, equine muscle is divided into muscle fibers that may have widely variable metabolic and contractile characteristics (see Chap. 8). On the basis of contractile properties, there are two major muscle fiber types, I and II, with type II fibers often being further subdivided into subtypes IIa and IIb. Type II fibers are the most powerful, having the fastest speeds of contraction and relaxation. The speed of contraction for type IIb fibers is up to 10-fold greater than those recorded for type I fibers.[24] The horse has adapted such that fast-twitch fibers are endowed with great muscle power, a characteristic that exists at the expense of energetic efficiency. As a result, activities requiring great muscle power are normally associated with production of large proton (acid) and lactate loads by the anaerobic pathways. Therefore, although induction of the anaerobic pathways allows large amounts of energy to be produced rapidly, the associated acidosis may have detrimental effects on the muscle contractile apparatus, which, in turn, directly contributes to fatigue.[4]

The possession of substantial muscle power in horses is likely to result from the need for horses in the wild to possess the capacity for rapid bursts of high-intensity exercise when attempting to escape from predators. Domestic breeds have been selected mainly for short-term, intense exercise and therefore possess high proportions of fast-twitch fibers in key locomotor muscles. For example, thoroughbred, standardbred, and quarter horses have more than 80 percent fast-twitch fibers in the major muscles of locomotion. In contrast, horses selectively bred for endurance capacity, such as Arabian horses, often have up to 50 percent slow-twitch fibers in the locomotor muscles.[20,25,26]

BUFFERING CAPACITY

The proton load produced during intense exercise will exert detrimental effects on the contractile apparatus via a reduction in local pH. Horses possessing the capacity of superior athletic performance are able to offset these deleterious effects at least to some degree because they possess local intracellular and circulating buffer systems.[27] Local buffering systems are the result of hydrolysis of CP or occur via physiochemical means.[28] Additional buffering, in particular that occurring outside the muscle cell, is related to the bicarbonate buffering system. The high buffering capacity of muscle in horses is thought to be related to the high concentration of carnosine in muscle fibers. Carnosine contributes approxi-

mately 30 percent of the nonbicarbonate buffering, with the greatest concentrations of this dipeptide being found in type IIb fibers.[29] Buffering capacity has been hypothesized to be a key determinant in the potential for sprint performance in humans,[30] an association likely to translate to the horse, and this would, in part, explain the predominance of type II fibers and high buffering capacity in the muscles of thoroughbreds[31] and quarter horses.[32]

Conformation

Successful athletic performance is not possible unless the relationships between the functional capacities of the metabolic systems described here are combined with appropriate conformational characteristics of the locomotor system to allow effective propulsion of the horse. This interrelationship is summarized by Rooney,[33] who states, "the proper functioning of the locomotor system depends on precise synchronization of the movement of each part on every other part and in relation to the body as a whole. Pathological changes may occur whenever improper synchronization occurs."

Many volumes exist on what constitutes appropriate conformation for the athletic horse and indeed which factors are most likely to result in musculoskeletal infirmities. Some of the important factors in conformation were discussed in Chapter 3, but ideal conformation may vary considerably depending on the breed and expected use of the horse. However, Lambert[34] regards excessive loading forces on limbs of horses attempting to maintain racing speed as the major cause of breakdowns in racehorses. Lambert suggests that appropriate conformation for an elite horse, when performing at racing speeds, involves the animal having a skeletal shape that allows it to have body support on the lead hindlimb as the nonlead forelimb makes contact with the ground. The load of the body weight is then pushed smoothly over the forelimb. In addition, he suggests that appropriate conformation of the shoulder is essential to ensure dampening of the loading forces. In contrast, horses that do not have this "appropriate" skeletal shape are forced to dissociate their hindlimbs and forelimbs when attempting to maintain near-maximal speed. Lambert[34] attests that this dissociation is the factor that results in breakdown, since the horse is forced to "almost leap from hindlimb support to forelimb support," thereby dramatically increasing the stresses imposed on the forelimbs. This may explain why some horses that possess this coupling between fore and hindlimbs are able to perform at high levels despite the presence of other musculoskeletal *conformational defects*, e.g., backward deviation of the carpal joints (calf knees) or upright pasterns.

The "Will to Win"

Elite athletes demonstrate great competitiveness, or "will to win." In all probability, this characteristic is inherited, and although bad management will undoubtedly diminish the competitive spirit of a horse, there is some question as to whether this characteristic can be enhanced.

Many highly regarded trainers see this intangible quality as being integral to successful athletic performance. Horses possessing a strong "will to win" have an intrinsic desire to dominate other horses during a race and are able to continue exercise when physiologic and psychological inputs should signal a reduction in performance.

Diminution of the "will to win" may occur as a result of infirmities, such as occurs with chronic pain, boredom, or overwork ("overtraining"). Trainers have a profound influence on this aspect of competitiveness, and good trainers somehow find the correct balance between appropriate physical and psychological training for the horses under their care.

Concepts of Fatigue

Elite athletic performance is the result not only of optimal function of the key body systems, as discussed previously, but also of the capacity to develop resistance to fatigue. In most competitive athletic events, horses become fatigued and either have to stop exercise or reduce the intensity. Thus a discussion of some of the factors responsible for fatigue in both high- and low-intensity events is important for understanding the limitations to performance and performance potential. One of the important training adaptations is a delay in the onset of fatigue.

Fatigue is manifest by an inability of the horse to continue exercise at the intensity required. Superior athletes possess the capacity to offset these processes and maintain exercise intensity for longer than less capable athletes. Fatigue is a complex process that appears to involve central (psychological/neurologic) and peripheral (muscular) contributions. Peripheral aspects of the process have been afforded greatest interest, possibly because they are easier to define when compared with central contributions to reductions in performance.

In humans, there is evidence of neurophysiologic contributions to fatigue, involving an activating and an inhibitory system.[35] However, further confirmation of this mechanism is required. Central fatigue also may have a psychological component. In humans, factors such as lack of motivation have been described as causes of fatigue.[36] Since horses undergoing intense training will sometimes lose their competitive edge (referred to as becoming "sour" or "overtrained") without evidence of organic disease, it is likely that central or psychological components are responsible for the apparent fatigue. Doubtless "mental freshness" and a positive psychological approach are vital contributors to elite performance in humans, and similar factors are probably critical for optimal performance in horses.

Studies investigating the effects of peripheral fatigue demonstrate that it is task-specific and that its causes are multifactorial. Processes implicated in the cause of fatigue include impairment of excitation-contraction coupling, impaired energy production, and limitations to fuel supply. The processes involved in fatigue are related to the intensity and duration of the exercise that the horse is required to perform. As outlined in Chapter 8, a number of factors have been associated with muscular fatigue, including

1. Depletion of substrates for energy production
2. Interference in energy (ATP) production as a result of alterations in the internal milieu of the muscle fiber
3. Changes in neuromuscular irritability due to changes in electrolyte gradients
4. Interference with the contractile process which is the result of alterations in Ca^{2+} uptake or release by the sarcoplasmic reticulum
5. Decreased blood flow and/or excessive increase in muscle temperature

In many cases, a combination of these factors is likely to operate. In horses, much of the current understanding on the likely contributing factors to muscle fatigue comes from analysis of muscle biopsy samples following different intensities and durations of exercise.

FATIGUE IN RESPONSE TO HIGH-INTENSITY EXERCISE

Intense exercise results in fatigue within seconds to minutes. Depletion of the phosphagen pool (ATP and CP), reductions in intracellular pH, and possibly accumulation of lactate appear to be important factors contributing to fatigue. Cellular homeostatic mechanisms are designed to maintain intracellular ATP concentrations within a reasonably tight range. However, with short-term intense exercise, there is an initial depletion of muscular CP followed by reduction in ATP concentrations.[37–42] The greatest reductions in the concentration of ATP occur in fast-twitch fibers.[37] Whether reduction in the phosphagen pool directly induces fatigue remains to be clarified, but intense exercise which produces ATP depletion is also associated with significant reductions in intramuscular pH from around 7.0 to 7.1 at rest to 6.4 or below at fatigue. Reduced pH is known to reduce the respiratory capacity of muscle[43] and have direct effects on the contractile apparatus.[4,44–46] Acidosis and the substantial increases in muscle temperature that occur are likely to be associated with impaired sarcoplasmic reticulum function.[47] Loss of potassium from the contracting muscle and accumulation in the plasma also may be a contributory factor to fatigue.[48] Intense exercise induces increases in plasma potassium concentration to greater than 10 mmol/liter.[49] This change in potassium homeostasis also may alter sarcoplasmic reticulum function and thereby influence calcium handling within the cell.[50–52] Whether acting singly or in combination, decreased pH, a decreased nucleotide pool, increased temperature, and altered electrolyte gradients are likely to exert deleterious effects on a number of metabolic processes in muscle, resulting in fatigue.

FATIGUE DURING PROLONGED SUBMAXIMAL EXERCISE

A number of factors, including altered fluid and ion balance, hyperthermia, and depletion of muscular fuel stores, have been implicated singularly and collectively as causes of fatigue during this type of exercise. During exercise, about 80 percent of the energy produced is liberated as heat. The horse possesses a finely tuned thermoregulatory system which, under most situations, allows dissipation of this metabolic heat load. However, as ambient temperature and humidity increase, the demands placed on thermoregulation become progressively greater. Heat stress results in diversion of blood flow away from working muscle to the skin in order to dissipate heat.[9] This reduction in blood flow is proposed to contribute to fatigue. In addition to the cardiovascular demands produced by heat stress, significant volumes of fluids (more than 10 liters/h) may be lost as sweat during exercise.[53,54] If this is not replaced, these losses produce reductions in total-body water. Equine sweat is hypertonic, and thus substantial electrolyte losses accompany the fluid losses. These alterations in fluid and electrolyte balance are related directly to reductions in thermoregulatory efficency[55] and performance capacity.[53]

Depletion of the intramuscular glycogen stores is a frequently reported cause of fatigue during prolonged exercise of moderate intensity.[56] Glycogen depletion occurs in a selective manner in particular fiber types as a function of the duration or intensity of the exercise. Depletion of glycogen from within a muscle fiber is associated with decreased capacity for force production in that fiber. Although muscle fibers are selectively recruited during submaximal exercise, with additional fibers being recruited as others become exhausted, eventually a sufficient number of fibers is depleted of their carbohydrate stores that the overall force-producing capacity of the muscle falls below that required to maintain exercise intensity.[26,56–58]

The various factors responsible for fatigue in both low- and high-intensity events should be considered when assessing performance potential. Aspects of energy supply (see Chap. 4) are also important. Because successful athletic performance is multifactorial, no single measurement will accurately predict exercise capacity. However, there are a number of measurements, which range in complexity and sophistication, that are useful for providing an indication of the capacity or function of key body systems in the oxygen-transport chain.

Measurements for Evaluation of Performance Potential

ESTIMATION OF HEART SIZE

Heart size is a major determinant of maximal cardiac output and maximal aerobic capacity. Given this relationship, a number of techniques have been described which are designed to assist in determination of heart size and therefore predict cardiac output and performance capacity. For horses, initial techniques were based on measurements derived from electrocardiographic recordings and are the basis of the *heart score* concept. More recently, echocardiographic variables have been measured in resting horses in an attempt to predict performance potential. Measurement of $\dot{V}_{O_2max}$ also provides an index of cardiorespiratory function, while maximal oxygen pulse ($\dot{V}_{O_2max}/HR_{max}$) is a valuable indicator of maximal stroke volume (see Chap. 12).

Heart Score. The concept of heart score, an electrocardiographic measurement of heart size, was developed by Steel[59] in Australia in the late 1950s. The concept was based on the idea that heart size would be reflected by ventricular depolarization time. Steel proposed that the heart size could be determined by measurement of the QRS duration, in milliseconds, in electrocardiographic leads I, II, and III and then averaging the values. The recommendation for averaging values for QRS duration rather than using the longest QRS duration in the limb leads of the electrocardiogram (ECG) was based on the slightly higher correlation coefficient for heart score and heart weight ($r = .089$) when using the averaged QRS values rather than the longest QRS duration ($r = 0.86$). The heart score technique has been adopted and remains quite popular in Australia, New Zealand, South Africa, and France.

The ECG is recorded with the horse in a quiet place where there is minimal electrical interference. One of the best places for recording an ECG is the horse's box stall, since the horse is usually quiet and relaxed in this environment. Care must be taken to ensure that the horse is standing on a dry area when the recording is made. Avoiding areas where there is likely to be environmental sources of electrical interference, e.g., electric motors, is also advisable. ECG machines with filters to dampen excess electical activity are considered to provide the best result. The ECG machine should be portable and ideally should have the capacity for recordings to be made without an immediate mains power supply by using rechargeable batteries. For determination of heart score, recordings are usually made at a paper speed of 25 mm/s and a sensitivity of 1 cm = 1 mV. Faster paper speeds do not increase precision of measurement because start and end points of QRS complexes become more difficult to determine. Paper speed should be regularly calibrated using stop watch, since correct paper speed is integral to accurate measurement of the heart score. Pen heat should be adjusted to give the thinnest possible but still readable tracing of the most rapid signal on the trace.

The configurations of both QRS and T-wave complexes are affected by limb position and heart rate. Therefore, to allow standardized interpretation when attempting to determine the heart score, the ECG should always be recorded with the left forelimb slighly in front of the right forelimb and the heart rate less than 40 beats/min. Care should be taken not to handle the horse too much during recording of the ECG, since this may induce alterations in electrical activity.

The recording system used is one where metal electrodes are connected to the legs by rubber straps. Alternatively, soft-nosed "alligator" clips may be used to attach the electrodes to the skin. If clips are used, the sharp points on the teeth of the clips should be filed down to avoid unnecessary discomfort for the horse. To permit good conductivity, an electrode paste is applied under the electrodes. The usual electrode placement on the forelimb is on the caudal aspect of the distal radius, just proximal to the accessory carpal bone, while the electrodes are applied to the cranial aspect of the distal tibia, just above the point of the hock, in the hindlimbs. If the electrodes are applied directly to the skin by clips, this can be performed by attachment to the skin over the olecranon in the forelimbs and just below the stifle in the hindlimbs. For heart score determination, the machine should be able to record leads I, II, and III.

At least 25 artifact-free complexes should be recorded in leads I, II, and III. Following this, the QRS duration in each of these leads is determined. Areas of the trace without baseline wander should be selected, and complexes with characteristic waveforms should be chosen. Readings are easier when the beginning or end points of a complex can be lined up accurately against a perpendicular time line. A 10 to 15X magnifier is used, and it is important to ensure that the trace is well illuminated. Readings are made so that a double thickness of the tracing lines is not included in the duration. Measurements are made to the nearest ¼ mm or 10 points (each small square is divided into quarters). Intervals should only be calculated from areas of the trace where the heart rate is less than 40 beats/min.

Heart score is determined by measuring the duration of the QRS interval in each of the standard limb leads and then calculating the arithmetic mean of the values observed. Results are expressed in milliseconds. Because each square is divided into quarters, the results in each lead will end in zero, and average values (the heart score) will end in either 0, 3, or 6. As demonstrated in Figure 11–2, values of 100, 120, and 130 ms occur in leads I, II, and III, respectively, of a 3-year-old thoroughbred gelding. Thus the horse has a heart score of 116.

Average heart score values in mature thoroughbred horses are 113 to 116. Values over 120 are considered by some to be indicative of above-average heart size. This claim is made on the basis of the good correlation ($r = 0.89$) noted by Steel[59] between heart score and heart weight. There also was an association between heart score and prize money won by thoroughbred horses, although the correlation coefficient was lower.[60,61] Other studies have shown correlations with performance in standardbreds[62] and endurance horses.[63] However, debate persists as to the value of the heart score concept in predicting performance potential. Leadon et al.[64] performed a prospective study involving 125 thoroughbred yearlings which had heart scores and subsequent racing performance recorded. This study did not demonstrate a strong correlation between heart score and racing performance in English horses during 2- and 3-year-old seasons when based on Timeform rating. The applicability of heart score determinations in assessing performance potential also has been questioned by Physick-Sheard and Hendron,[65] who suggested the statistical analyses performed by Steel in his original work may have been inappropriate. Similarly, concern has been expressed about the repeatability of the ECG recording and measurement techniques described by

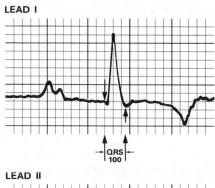

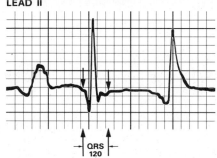

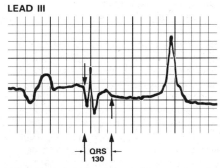

Figure 11-2. Typical electrocardiographic traces from leads I, II, and III using a standard orthogonal lead system to measure the QRS durations to obtain heart score. The arrows show the beginning and end points of the QRS complexes, and the durations are given in milliseconds. The heart score in this horse is 116.

Steel[66] and the fact that no allowance is made for variations in individual horse's body weights when heart score is determined. However, we have performed several thousand ECG analyses on athletic horses and think that if *great care* is taken in collection of the ECG recording and interpretation of the trace, useful predictive information can be obtained. In particular, we have found that elite racehorses are frequently found to have heart scores of greater than 130, whereas those with limited ability have scores below 100. Of course, exceptions to this generalization exist, but we believe that heart score may be a useful adjunct in the assessment of performance potential in horses, particularly in horses that fall into the lower or higher ranges of heart scores. Naturally, it is important not to overemphasize the heart score concept, because it cannot be assumed that heart size, even if accurate, is the only factor of importance in determining athletic performance. It is one element, and other factors, including respiratory and muscle function, conformation and biomechanics, and oxygen-carrying capacity, all play important roles in performance. However, it is apparent that for many athletic horses, those with the largest hearts are often the best performed, whereas those with small heart sizes perform poorly.

Echocardiography. Initial interest in the use of echocardiography for determination of cardiac dimensions to indicate performance potential was aroused following the first report of its use in a horse in 1977.[67] This report outlined M-mode echocardiography, where an "ice pick" image of the heart was displayed over time. These images were obtained with the operator being blind to the portion of the heart being imaged, with intracardiac structures being identified by their characteristic waveforms.[67-69] This is the technique often used for measurement of various chamber dimensions as well as assessment of valve movement.

By the mid-1980s, reports of the use of two-dimensional echocardiography in horses began to appear.[70,71] With two-dimensional echocardiography, the images are displayed in real time, with width and depth of the imaged tissue being displayed. The advent of two-dimensional echocardiography and phased-array systems enabled guided M-mode echocardiograms to be obtained by placing a cursor across the two-dimensional real-time image at the desired position. This allows determination of cardiac structure and, to some degree, function. Phased-array systems allow simultaneous display of two echocardiographic images, since the transducers contain different elements with the firing of each of the elements controlled electronically. These multiple-element transducers also can be focused. Many of the machines that have phased-array heads also contain sophisticated software that allows rapid determination of cardiac dimensions. Not surprisingly, the advantages provided by these machines come at a cost, with this form of apparatus considerably more expensive than mechanical sector scanners.

Since two-dimensional echocardiographic images are spatially correct, the combination of M-mode and two-dimensional echocardiography provides a superior technique for reproducible measurements of various intracardiac structures. The examination is performed by guiding the M-mode cursor across the desired intracardiac structures, which are visualized on the two-dimensional echocardiographic image. The plane of the M-mode beam is determined by the orientation of the two-dimensional beam. Movement of the heart is displayed on the x axis, with the depth of cardiac structures displayed on the y axis. An ECG is normally displayed for timing reference. Therefore, the combination of M-mode and two-dimensional echocardiographic examinations allows more accurate evaluation of ventricular wall and septal thicknesses and chamber dimensions. M-mode echocardiography tends to provide superior images of valvular and cardiac wall motion and thickness because

of the large number of images collected per second using this form of echocardiography.[71]

In adult horses, a 2.25- or 2.5-mHz probe is necessary to penetrate to sufficient depths (27 to 30 cm) to visualize all structures in the heart. Left and right parasternal views are normally used, with the probe head located in either the left or right cardiac windows. A long-axis plane transects the heart parallel to its long axis and perpendicular to the dorsal and ventral surfaces of the body. The short-axis plane is perpendicular to the long axis of the heart and relatively parallel to the dorsal and ventral surfaces of the horse's body.[69] Simultaneous electrocardiography is performed to time the cardiac events, since measurements are made at end systole and end diastole. This is important to ensure reproducibility of the data collected. An excellent review of the techniques employed in performing a thorough echocardiographic examination of the horse's heart is provided by Reef.[69]

Measurements of left ventricular chamber size, wall thicknesses, and ventricular septum thickness can be made by placing the M-mode cursor perpendicular to the ventricular septum and free wall echo bisecting the left ventricle.[71] Measurements also may be made from video playback of two-dimensional echocardiographic images by freezing the video images at end systole and end diastole. Although this is a useful way to store the images for later analysis, there is the potential for considerable loss of image quality (referred to as *echo dropout*) from two-dimensional images. Improved digital scan converters and video recording equipment will gradually eliminate this problem and improve the efficacy of two-dimensional echocardiography for determination of cardiac dimensions.

Positive relationships between body mass and left ventricular size measured at necropsy have been made in the horse.[68] Similarly, it has been shown that fit thoroughbred horses have larger left ventricular internal dimensions than other warm-blooded breeds of horse. From this it can be presumed that estimates of cardiac size could be made using echocardiography, and from these, some appraisal of performance capacity could be made. However, to date, there is no clear evidence of an association of echocardiographic variables measured in the resting horse and that horse's performance potential. Leadon and colleagues[64] undertook a study where they performed echocardiographic examinations in 630 thoroughbred yearlings in an attempt to correlate cardiac dimensions with subsequent performance. Measurements included left ventricular posterior wall thickness, left ventricular internal dimension, and intraventricular septal thickness in diastole and systole in M-mode. An indication of mean heart weight, as evidenced by mean wall thickness at systole and diastole, also was determined. Left ventricular area in diastole and systole was measured in two-dimensional mode. An estimate of left ventricular mass also was made. This study was unable to show a relationship between any of the values measured on echocardiography and subsequent performance, as judged by Timeform ratings.

Although there is not a large volume of information available relating the findings of echocardiographic measurements to performance capacity, it is difficult to be confident that estimations of exercise capacity can be made on the basis of echocardiographic determinations of cardiac dimensions.

TOTAL RED CELL VOLUME

Because the total volume of red cells in circulation is a major determinant of oxygen-carrying capacity in horses, measurement of the total red cell volume (CV) may provide some index of the exercise capacity. Measurement of CV is most frequently based on the use of Evans blue, a dye that enables measurement of plasma volume using the technique of dye dilution.[72] From determination of the plasma volume and hematocrit following intense exercise, the CV is determined as described (see Chap. 5).

Persson[72-75] has reported a good correlation between exercise capacity of standardbred trotters and total hemoglobin or red cell volume. Normal values for CV vary according to age. Persson recorded values as low as 44 ml/kg in yearlings, increasing up to mean values of 63 ml/kg at 3 years of age and 74 ml/kg at 4 years of age for standardbred trotters.[76] Persson found values of 89 ± 9 ml/kg in mature thoroughbred racehorses, whereas Rose[77] reported values in the range of 78 to 102 ml/kg for thoroughbred racehorses in training. Recently, studies in our laboratory have not demonstrated significant relationships between CV and cardiorespiratory variables or treadmill exercise capacity. We consider that some caution should be exercised when attempting to estimate performance potential on the basis of CV measurements.

MUSCLE BIOPSY

Fiber-type proportions within muscle are genetically determined, with type II fibers being powerful, rapidly contracting fibers, whereas type I fibers are more slowly contracting, with high aerobic capacity and are therefore most suited to endurance activities. Based on these characteristics, it is logical to suggest that horses with the best sprinting capacities will have the greatest number of type II fibers in the muscles of locomotion, whereas successful endurance horses will possess increased numbers of type I fibers. A number of studies have been performed to test this hypothesis.[20,26,56,58,78,79] Although trends within the different athletic groups could be identified (e.g., successful racing quarter horses were found to have a higher proportion of type II fibers when compared with unsuccessful cohorts), the differences were rather small. Similarly, successful endurance horses have been shown to have greater numbers of type I fibers in the muscles of locomotion than less well performed horses.[26] However, as outlined in Chapter 8, the fiber-type characteristics in many horse breeds are quite homogeneous, often making this type of predictive assessment difficult, particulary within highly selected

breeds. Added problems can arise from variations in fiber type depending on the depth from which the sample is collected. Therefore, use of muscle biopsy for evaluation of performance potential is likely to be best in endurance horses, where a high proportion of type I fibers are often correlated with the greatest athletic capacity.

MEASUREMENT OF INTERMANDIBULAR WIDTH

It has been proposed by Cook[80] that measurement of the intermandibular width may provide useful information on the performance potential of racehorses. Cook surveyed more than 48 bood mares in which laryngeal palpation was performed and the intermandibular width determined. Cook noted a direct correlation between the width of the intermandiblar space and the mares' racing performance as 3-year-olds and thought that the intermandibular width correlated with the width of the nasopharyngeal and laryngeal airways. In a number of different groups of thoroughbreds, Cook found the average intermandibular width to range from 7.2 to 8.0 cm. He proposed that an intermandibular width of less than 7.5 cm constituted a conformational defect, which he refers to as *mandibula angusta,* or "narrow mandible." A more limited study comparing 10 winning and 10 unplaced mares also showed that the winning mares had significantly greater intermandibular width.[81] Cook also suggests that there is an inverse correlation between the intermandibular width and the degree of laryngeal neuropathy experienced by horses.

In contrast, Lindsay and colleagues[82] measured the intermandibular space of 457 thoroughbred horses and related this to the incidence of idiopathic laryngeal neuropathy. These authors found the mean intermandibular width to be 8.1 cm and found no relationship between endoscopically apparent laryngeal dysfunction and intermandibular width. In addition, there was no relationship between intermandibular width, laryngeal height, or laryngeal cross-sectional area in 15 thoroughbreds.

TREADMILL TESTING

Evaluation of athletic performance using treadmills has gained popularity in recent years and may provide potentially useful information in the selection of horses. As is described in the next chapter, a number of measurements may be undertaken in the evaluation of performance. This section will not repeat the information provided in that chapter, but it will outline some of the measurements that may be useful when attempting to define a "performance profile" for a horse. As with any test or group of tests, care must always be exercised when interpreting information, since several of the variables assessed may change in response to a horse's training status and level of fitness.

In general, information related to the functional capacities of the cardiorespiratory and musculoskeletal systems is the most valuable when attempting to evaluate performance potential. To be useful to practicing veterinarians and horse owners, measurements must be relatively easy to perform, with the information easily understood and applied. Variables that can be easily measured during exercise and are potentially valuable include heart rate, blood lactate concentration, oxygen uptake, and stride length.

Heart Rate. Heart rate is simple to determine during exercise and gives some indication of cardiovascular function. Heart rate provides a reasonably good indication of cardiac output in response to exercise, since there are only modest increases in stroke volume in response to increasing work rate.[14,83] A number of different heart rate meters are available. For a more detailed description, refer to Chapter 12. The speed at which a horse reaches maximal heart rate (HR_{max}) provides an indication of cardiovascular capacity. The HR_{max} is identified when there is no further increase in heart rate despite increases in work effort. Although the HR_{max} does not increase in response to training, the speed at which this value is achieved increases as fitness improves. Thus the level of fitness must be considered when evaluating horses on the basis of measurements of heart rate responses to exercise. However, when comparisons are made between horses at the same level of training, it is usual that individuals with the greatest athletic capacity will reach HR_{max} at the highest speeds during the exercise test. In addition, Marsland[84] was able to demonstrate high correlation coefficients for the relationship between low heart rates during submaximal exercise and winning times in standardbred horses.

Values derived from the relationship between running speed and heart rate have been suggested to be useful for assessing cardiovascular capacity. Persson[75] attests that the speed at which a heart rate of 200 (V_{200}) is achieved provides a valuable reference point when assessing responses to exercise. Persson chose this value because it commonly represents a workload at which blood lactate begins to accumulate. The V_{200} is determined by measuring heart rate in response to a rapid incremental exercise test at submaximal speeds, with the final step of the test resulting in a heart rate of greater than 200 beats/min. Rose and colleagues[1] demonstrated a good correlation between V_{200} and $\dot{V}_{O_2max}$, but caution must be taken when using this variable to evaluate performance potential. An advantage of determining V_{200} is that unlike determination of HR_{max}, which requires that the horse exercise at maximal effort, V_{200} can be determined on the basis of data recorded at three or four submaximal speeds.

Recovery of heart rate following exercise may be used as an index of performance capacity in endurance horses. This is useful when assessing responses to training, with improvements in fitness translating into a more rapid reduction in heart rate following a repeatable exercise stimulus. Heart rate recovery is also used in the assessment of endurance horses at mandatory rest stops in endurance competitions. The fittest horses and those with the fewest metabolic derangements in response to the exercise experience the most rapid recoveries.[85]

Blood or Plasma Lactate Determinations. Lactate is produced by the glycolytic pathways within the working muscles and diffuses down a concentration gradient into the blood. Elevations in the rate of lactate production reflect an increased contribution of the anaerobic pathways to energy production. As a result, increases in blood or plasma lactate concentrations in response to exercise may be used to indicate metabolic capacity of horses. In most racehorses, lactate concentration in blood increases at speeds above about 6 m/s when the treadmill is set at a 10 percent slope. Blood lactate concentrations may provide a means for assessing anaerobic capacity, with those horses possessing the greatest anaerobic capacities generating the highest plasma lactate concentrations in response to a maximal exercise test.[86] Peak lactate concentration is therefore likely to be a reflection of the capacity for sprint performance.

Lactate concentration can be determined on whole blood or plasma, with the concentrations in whole blood being about 30 percent higher than those of plasma. Samples can be collected into tubes containing fluoride oxalate, the anticoagulant which prevents glycolysis in red blood cells. Alternatively, if the samples are to be kept cool and analyzed within 24 to 48 hours, lithium heparin may be used. Insertion of an intravenous catheter with connection tube attached prior to the test will allow collection of samples during the exercise test.

We subject horses to an incremental exercise test that involves four submaximal speeds (4, 6, 8, and 10 m/s) and determine plasma lactate concentration at the conclusion of each speed (see Chap. 12). Results from a number of studies indicate that horses with the highest aerobic capacities, i.e., the highest cardiac output and $\dot{V}_{O_2max}$, usually have lower lactate concentrations in response to exercise at submaximal intensities. Comparisons between horses have been based on a number of absolute and derived values. Relationships can be drawn by determining the speed at which a plasma lactate concentration of 4 mmol/liter is achieved. This is referred to as the V_{LA4},[75] and in general, horses with the greatest exercise capacities have the highest values for V_{LA4}. Training may influence the values achieved for V_{LA4}, and therefore, care must be taken to consider the fitness levels of horses when making comparisons between animals. We also have found that the blood lactate concentration attained after completion of the 10-m/s step of the incremental exercise test is a valuable tool in providing some indication of performance potential. Well-trained, superior athletic horses tend to have blood and plasma lactate concentrations of less than 7 and 5 mmol/liter, respectively, at the end of the 10-m/s exercise test.

Oxygen Uptake. As outlined in Chapter 12, the measurement of $\dot{V}_{O_2max}$ is critical in the assessment of performance capacity. Oxygen consumption increases linearly with increasing speed, with $\dot{V}_{O_2max}$ defined as the point where increases in speed do not result in further increases in $\dot{V}_{O_2}$. In some cases, this plateau is not achieved because the horse is unable to undertake a sufficient number of additional steps to allow clear definition of the plateau. In these cases, the peak $\dot{V}_{O_2}$ ($\dot{V}_{O_2peak}$) is the value ascribed for that animal.[2]

In humans, determination of $\dot{V}_{O_2max}$ is the single most commonly used test when assessing athletic performance. It is a test that many athletes "implicitly believe is the single best predictor of athletic potential."[87] Methods for assessment of $\dot{V}_{O_2}$ in response to exercise are described in Chapter 12. When compared with many other species, horses have a high aerobic capacity, which is the combination of a large red cell volume (and therefore, oxygen-carrying capacity), high maximal heart rate, and a large arteriovenous oxygen content difference. A number of reports now exist demonstrating that, as with humans, the best-performed equine athletes have the highest values for $\dot{V}_{O_2max}$ or $\dot{V}_{O_2peak}$. A positive correlation between $\dot{V}_{O_2max}$ and running speed was demonstrated by Harkins and colleagues,[88] indicating that there is some potential value in determining maximal aerobic capacity in horses. We have found that values for $\dot{V}_{O_2max}$ or $\dot{V}_{O_2peak}$ of greater than 150 ml/kg per minute are common in well-performed horses, with the best performers having values greater than 170 ml/kg per minute. These values are consistent with those reported by Seeherman and Morris.[2] However, since so many factors in addition to maximal aerobic capacity contribute to elite athletic performance, measurement of $\dot{V}_{O_2max}$ alone will not necessarily provide an accurate estimate of the potential to perform at the highest levels.

Conclusions

Prediction of performance potential is one of the elusive ideals of the science of exercise. Currently, none of the available measurements provides an accurate assessment of performance potential, but some of the indicators discussed provide a guide. It seems likely that refinement of treadmill exercise testing, with the capacity to measure physiologic indices important to athletic performance, offers the best possibility for performance prediction. However, until further prospective studies are performed with large numbers of horses allowing relative weighting of the various indices, performance prediction will remain elusive.

References

1. Rose RJ, Hendrickson DK, Knight PK: Clinical exercise testing in the normal thoroughbred racehorse. Aust Vet J 1990; 67:345.
2. Seeherman HJ, Morris EA: Application of a standardised treadmill exercise test for evaluation of fitness in 10 thoroughbred racehorses. Equine Vet J 1991; (suppl 9):26.
3. Wasserman K, Hansen JE, Sue DY, et al: Principles of Exercise Testing and Interpretation. Philadelphia, Lea & Febiger, 1987.
4. Mainwood GW, Renaud JM: The effect of acid-base balance on fatigue of skeletal muscle. Can J Physiol Pharmacol 1985; 63:403.
5. Derksen FJ: Upper airway evaluation of horses during treadmill exercise. In Proceedings of the 11th Annual Forum of the American College of Veterinary Internal Medicine, 1993, p 607.
6. Hörnicke H, Weber M, Schweiker W: Pulmonary ventilation in throughbred horses at maximum performance. In Gillespie JR, Robinson NE (eds): Equine Exercise Physiology 2. Davis, Calif, ICEEP Publications, 1987, p 216.
7. King CM: Clinical exercise testing in racehorses. Master of Veterinary Clinical Studies Thesis, University of Sydney, 1993.
8. Fulton IC, Derksen FJ, Stick JA, et al: Treatment of left laryngeal hemiplegia in standardbreds using a nerve pedicle graft. Am J Vet Res 1991; 52:1461.
9. Rowell LB: Cardiovascular adjustments to thermal stress. In Shepherd JT, Abboud FM (eds): Handbook of Physiology. The Cardiovascular System: Peripheral and Organ Blood Flow, vol 3, part 2. Bethesda, American Physiological Society, 1983, p 967.
10. Kubo K, Takagi S, Murakami M, et al: Heart rate and blood lactate concentration of horses during maximal work. Bull Equine Res Inst 1984; 21:39.
11. Evans DL, Rose RJ: Cardiovascular and respiratory responses to submaximal exercise training in the thoroughbred horse. Pflügers Arch 1988; 411:316.
12. Parks CM, Manohar M: Distribution of blood flow during moderate and strenuous exercise in ponies (Equus caballus). Am J Vet Res 1983; 44:1861.
13. Saltin B: Hemodynamic adaptations to exercise. Am J Cardiol 1985; 44:42D.
14. Evans DL, Rose RJ: Cardiovascular and respiratory responses in thoroughbred horses during treadmill exercise. J Exp Biol 1988; 134:397.
15. Persson SGB: On blood volume and working capacity in horses. Acta Physiol Scand 1967; (suppl 19):1.
16. Snow DH, Guy PS: The effects of training and detraining on the activity of a number of enzymes in the horse skeletal muscle. Arch Int Physiol Biochem 1979; 87:87.
17. Guy PS, Snow DH: The effects of training and detraining on LDH isoenzymes in horse skeletal muscle. Biochem Biophys Res Commun 1977; 25:863.
18. Hodgson DR, Rose RJ, Dimauro J, et al: Effects of training on muscle composition in horses. Am J Vet Res 1986; 47:12.
19. Hodgson DR, Rose RJ: Effects of a nine-month endurance training program on muscle composition in the horse. Vet Rec 1987; 121:271.
20. Snow DH, Guy PS: Fiber type and enzyme activities of the gluteus medius of different breeds of horse. In Poortmans J, Nisert G (eds): Biochemistry of Exercise. Baltimore, University Park Press, 1981, p 275.
21. Essén-Gustavsson B, Lindholm A: Muscle fiber characteristics of active and inactive standardbred horses. Equine Vet J 1985; 17:434.
22. Roneus M, Essén-Gustavsson B, Lindholm A, et al: Skeletal muscle characteristics in young trained and untrained standardbred trotters. Equine Vet J 1992; 24:292.
23. Weber JM, Parkhouse WS, Dobson GP, et al: Lactate kinetics in exercising thoroughbred horses: Regulation of turnover rate in plasma. Am J Physiol 1987; 253:896.
24. Rome LC, Sosnicki AA, Goble DO: Maximum velocity of shortening of three fiber types from horse soleus muscle: Implications for scaling with body size. J Physiol 1990; 431:173.
25. Snow DH, Guy PS: Fiber composition of a number of limb muscles in different breeds of horses. Res Vet Sci 1980; 28:137.
26. Hodgson DR, Rose RJ, Allen J: Muscle glycogen depletion and repletion patterns in horses performing various distances of endurance exercise. In Snow DH, Persson SGB, Rose RJ (eds): Equine Exercise Physiology. Cambridge, Granta Editions, 1983, p 229.
27. Harris RC, Marlin DJ, Dunnett M, et al: Muscle buffering capacity and dipeptide content in the thoroughbred, greyhound dog and man. Comp Biochem Physiol [A] 1990; 97:249.
28. Sewell DA, Harris RC, Dunnett M: Carnosine accounts for most of the variation in physio-chemical buffering in equine muscle. In Persson SGB, Lindholm A, Jeffcott LB (eds): Equine Exercise Physiology 3. Davis, Calif, ICEEP Publications, 1991, p 276.
29. Sewell DA, Harris RC, Marlin DJ, et al: Estimation of the carnosine content of different fibre types in the middle gluteal muscle of the thoroughbred horse. J Physiol (Lond) 1992; 455:447.
30. Parkhouse WS, McKenzie DC, Hochochka PW, et al: The relationship between carnosine levels, buffering capacity, fiber type and anaerobic capacity in elite athletes. In Knuttgen HG, Vogel JA, Poortmans J (eds): Biochemistry of Exercise. Champaign, Ill, Human Kinetics Publishers, 1983, p 590.
31. Marlin DJ, Harris RC, Gash SP, et al: Carnosine content of the

middle gluteal muscle in thoroughbred horses with relation to age, sex and training. Comp Biochem Physiol [A] 1989; 93:629.

32. Bump KD, Lawrence LM, Moses LR, et al: Effect of breed type on muscle carnosine. *In* Proceedings of the 11th Equine Nutrition Physiology Symposium, 1989, p 252.

33. Rooney JR: Biomechanics of Lameness in Horses. Baltimore, Williams & Wilkins, 1969.

34. Lambert DH: Practical experiences in the application of sports medicine. *In* Proceedings of the Annual Convention of the American Association of Equine Practitioners, 1990, p 477.

35. Grandjean E: Fatigue in industry. Br J Indust Med 1979; 36:175.

36. Åstrand P-O, Rodahl K: Textbook of Work Physiology. New York, McGraw-Hill, 1986, p 512.

37. Valberg S, Essén-Gustavsson B: Metabolic response to racing determined in pools of type I, IIA and IIB fibers. *In* Gillespie JR, Robinson NE (eds): Equine Exercise Physiology 2. Davis, Calif, ICEEP Publications, 1987, p 290.

38. Lindholm A, Bjerneld H, Saltin B: Glycogen depletion patterns in muscle fibres of trotting horses. Acta Physiol Scand 1974; 90:475.

39. Valberg S: Metabolic response to racing and fibre properties of skeletal muscle in standardbred and thoroughbred horses. J Equine Vet Sci 1987; 7:6.

40. Sewell DA, Harris RC, Hanak J, et al: Muscle adenine nucleotide degradation in the thoroughbred horse as a consequence of racing. Comp Biochem Physiol [B] 1992; 101:375.

41. Harris RC, Marlin DJ, Snow DH, et al: Muscle ATP loss and lactate accumulation at different work intensities in the exercising thoroughbred horse. Eur J Appl Physiol 1991; 62:235.

42. Sewell DA, Harris RC: Adenine nucleotide degradation in the thoroughbred horse with increasing exercise duration. Eur J Appl Physiol 1992; 65:271.

43. Gollnick PD, Bertocci LA, Kelso TB, et al: The effect of high-intensity exercise on the respiratory capacity of skeletal muscle. Pflügers Arch 1990; 415:407.

44. Nimmo MA, Snow DH: Time course of ultrastructural changes in skeletal muscle after two types of exercise. J Appl Physiol 1982; 52:910.

45. McCutcheon LJ, Byrd SK, Hodgson DR, et al: Ultrastructural alterations in equine skeletal muscle associated with fatiguing exercise. *In* Persson SGB, Lindholm A, Jeffcott LB (eds): Equine Exercise Physiology 3. Davis, Calif, ICEEP Publications, 1991, p 269.

46. McCutcheon LJ, Byrd SK, Hodgson DR: Ultrastructural changes in skeletal muscle after fatiguing exercise. J Appl Phyiol 1992; 72:1111.

47. Byrd SK, McCutcheon LJ, Hodgson DR, et al: Altered sarcoplasmic reticulum function after high intensity exercise. J Appl Physiol 1989; 67:2072.

48. Sjøgaard G, Adams RP, Saltin B: Water and ion shifts in skeletal muscle of humans with intense dynamic knee extension. Am J Physiol 1985; 248:R190.

49. Harris P, Snow DH: The effect of high intensity exercise on the plasma concentration of lactate, potassium and other electrolytes. Equine Vet J 1988; 20:109.

50. Harris P, Snow DH: Plasma potassium and lactate concentrations in thoroughbred horses during exercise of varying intensity. Equine Vet J 1992; 23:220.

51. Sahlin K, Broberg S: Release of K^+ from muscle during prolonged dynamic exercise. Acta Physiol Scand 1989; 136:293.

52. Jeul C: The effects of β_2-adrenoceptor activation on ion shifts and fatigue in mouse soleus muscle stimulated in vitro. Acta Physiol Scand 1988; 134:209.

53. Carlson GP: Hematology and body fluids in the equine athlete: a review. *In* Gillespie JR, Robinson NE (eds): Equine Exercise Physiology 2. Davis, Calif, ICEEP Publications, 1987, p 393.

54. Hodgson DR, Brown WS, McCutcheon LJ, et al: Dissipation of metabolic heat load during exercise in the horse. J Appl Physiol 1993; 74:1161.

55. Naylor JRJ, Bayly WM, Gollnick PD, et al: Effects of dehydration on thermoregulatory responses of horses during low intensity exercise. J Appl Physiol 1993; 75:994.

56. Snow DH, Baxter P, Rose RJ: Muscle fiber composition and glycogen depletion in horses competing in an endurance ride. Vet Rec 1981; 108:374.

57. Snow DH, Kerr MG, Nimmo MA, et al: Alterations in blood,

sweat, urine and muscle composition during prolonged exercise in the horse. Vet Rec 1982; 110:377.

58. Essén-Gustavsson G, Karlström K, Lindholm A: Fiber type, enzyme activities and substrate utilization in skeletal muscle of horses competing in endurance rides. Equine Vet J 1984; 16:197.

59. Steel JD: Studies on the Electrocardiogram of the Racehorse. Sydney, Australasian Medical Publishing, 1963.

60. Steel JD, Stewart GA: Electrocardiography and the heart score concept. *In* Proceedings of the Annual Convention of the American Association of Equine Practitioners, 1970, p 363.

61. Steel JD, Stewart GA: Electrocardiography of the horse and potential performance ability. J S Afr Vet Assoc 1974; 45:263.

62. Nielsen K, Vibe-Petersen G: Relationship between QRS duration (heart score) and racing performance in trotters. Equine Vet J 1980; 12:81.

63. Rose RJ, Ilkiw JE, Hodgson D: Electrocardiography, heart score and haematology in horses competing in an endurance ride. Aust Vet J 1979; 55:247.

64. Leadon D, McAllister H, Mullins E, et al: Electrocardiographic and echocardiographic measurements and their relationships in thoroughbred yearlings to subsequent performance. *In* Persson SGB, Lindholm A, Jeffcott LB (eds): Equine Exercise Physiology 3. Davis, Calif, ICEEP Publications, 1991, p 22.

65. Physick-Sheard PW, Hendron CM: Heart score: physiological basis and confounding variables. *In* Snow DH, Persson SGB, Rose RJ (eds): Equine Exercise Physiology. Cambridge, Granta Editions, 1983, p 121.

66. Bonagura JD, Herring DS, Walker F: Echocardiography. Vet Clin North Am Equine Pract 1985; 1:311.

67. Pipers FS, Hamlin RL: Echocardiography in the horse. J Am Vet Med Assoc 1977; 170:815.

68. O'Callaghan MW: Comparison of echocardiographic and autopsy measurements of cardiac dimensions in the horse. Equine Vet J 1985; 17:361.

69. Reef VB: Echocardiographic examination in the horse: The basics. Comp Cont Ed Pract Vet 1990; 12:1312.

70. Carlsten JC: Two-dimensional, real time echocardiography in the horse. Vet Radiol 1987; 28:76.

71. Reef VB: Advances in echocardiography. Vet Clin North Am Equine Pract 1991; 7:435.

72. Persson SGB: The circulatory significance of the splenic red cell pool. *In* Proceedings of the 1st International Symposium on Equine Hematology, 1975, p 303.

73. Persson SGB, Lydin G: Circulatory effects of splenectomy in the horse: III. Effect on pulse-work relationship. Zentralbl Vet Med 1973; A20:521.

74. Persson SGB: Blood volume and work performance. *In* Proceedings of the 1st International Symposium on Equine Hematology, 1975, p 321.

75. Persson SGB: Evaluation of exercise tolerance and fitness in the performance horse. *In* Snow DH, Persson SGB, Rose RJ (eds): Equine Exercise Physiology. Cambridge, Granta Editions, 1983, p 441.

76. Persson SGB: Practical aspects of blood volume measurement: procedure for determination of total red cell volume (CV) in the horse. *In* Proceedings of the International Conference on Equine Sports Medicine, 1986, p 51.

77. Rose RJ: Exercise and performance testing in the racehorse: Problems, limitations, and potential. *In* Proceedings of the Annual Convention of the American Association of Equine Practitioners, 1990, p 491.

78. Wood HC, Ross TT, Armstrong JB, et al: Variations in muscle fiber composition between successfully and unsuccessfully raced quarterhorses. J Equine Vet Sci 1988; 8:217.

79. Roneus M, Essén-Gustavsson B, Arnason T: Racing performance and longitudinal changes in muscle characteristics in standardbred trotters. J Equine Vet Sci 1993; 13:355.

80. Cook RW: Recent observations on recurrent laryngeal neuropathy in the horse: Applications to practice. *In* Proceedings of the Annual Convention of the American Association of Equine Practitioners, 1988, p 427.

81. Delahunty D, Webb S, Kelly EP, et al: Intermandibular width and cannon bone length in "winners" versus "others." J Equine Vet Sci 1991; 11:258.

82. Lindsay WA, Harrison G, Duncan ID: Is the width of the inter-

mandibular space in thoroughbreds related to equine recurrent laryngeal neuropathy. *In* Proceedings of the Annual Convention of the American Association of Equine Practitioners, 1990, p 429.

83. Fregin GF, Thomas DP: Cardiovascular response to exercise in the horse: a review. *In* Snow DH, Persson SGB, Rose RJ (eds): Equine Exercise Physiology. Cambridge, Granta Editions, 1983, p 76.

84. Marsland WP: Heart rate response to submaximal exercise in the standardbred horse. J Appl Physiol 1968; 24:98.

85. Rose RJ: An evaluation of heart rate and respiratory rate recovery for assessment of fitness during endurance rides. *In* Snow DH,

Persson SGB, Rose RJ (eds): Equine Exercise Physiology. Cambridge, Granta Editions, 1983, p 505.

86. Eaton MD, Rose RJ, Evans DL, et al: The assessment of anaerobic capacity of thoroughbred horses using maximal accumulated oxygen deficit. Aust Equine Vet 1992; 10:86.

87. Noakes TD: Implications of exercise testing for prediction of athletic performance: a contemporary perspective. Med Sci Sports Exerc 1988; 40:319.

88. Harkins JD, Beadle RE, Kamerling SG: The correlation of running ability and physiological variables in thoroughbred racehorses. Equine Vet J 1993; 25:53.

Clinical Exercise Testing

R. J. ROSE AND D. R. HODGSON

Exercise testing has been used routinely for the past 30 years in human medicine[1,2] to evaluate fitness and the significance of a range of diseases on exercise capacity. Testing usually has been performed in laboratories equipped to perform cardiovascular and respiratory measurements using either bicycle ergometers or treadmills to vary the intensity of exercise.

Exercise testing to evaluate the physiologic responses of athletic horses to exercise is a more recent event in the assessment of equine performance. Persson[3] was the first to describe standardized protocols for investigation of exercise capacity, with research performed both on the track and using a treadmill, in Swedish standardbred trotters. Persson's research established normal responses of heart rate, oxygen uptake, blood lactate, and total red cell volume in Swedish trotters. However, in the exercise tests performed on a treadmill in Persson's studies, horses were not exercised at maximal exercise intensities. In other studies using track testing, horses with lower airway disease were studied by Maier-Bock and Ehrlein[4] and Littlejohn and others[5] at submaximal intensities.

Over the past 10 years, a number of studies have been published investigating cardiorespiratory and metabolic findings in athletic horses using exercise tests undertaken either on the track or treadmill. Such studies have provided important information on expected normal physiologic responses to exercise and data on the effects of some diseases. However, measurements are still lacking on the physiologic responses of elite athletic horses to exercise. The majority of studies have been performed using experimental horses of moderate to poor athletic ability. Despite these limitations, exercise testing is at a stage of development where important conclusions can now be drawn. This chapter will consider published material on exercise testing and relate

experiences from several hundred horses tested on a treadmill at the Equine Performance Laboratory of the University of Sydney (Fig. 12–1).

Indications for Exercise Testing

Exercise testing provides a mechanism for evaluating a range of body systems under standard exercise conditions. Measurements of cardiorespiratory and metabolic function during an exercise test provide information about the capacity and efficiency of key body systems involved in energy production. Thus some conclusions may be drawn about the athletic potential of the horse (see Chap. 11) based on measurements of oxygen transport or estimates of anaerobic capacity, depending on the duration and intensity of the competitive event (see Chap. 4). Additionally, changes in levels of fitness may be evaluated using exercise testing (see Chap. 12), because resting measurements of hematology or biochemistry provide little or no indication of improvements in fitness (see Chap. 5). Exercise testing is probably of most use from a clinical point of view to assess the effect on performance of abnormalities found on physical examination or to determine the reason(s) for reduced athletic capacity in horses that have no abnormalities on resting examinations. Whatever the reason for the testing, it is important that standardized procedures are followed so that the data derived from each test can be compared against subsequent tests for the same horse or with measurements from other horses of similar age and fitness level.

TRACK VERSUS TREADMILL EXERCISE TESTS

Measurements from horses at the track are obviously much simpler and can be performed more readily with-

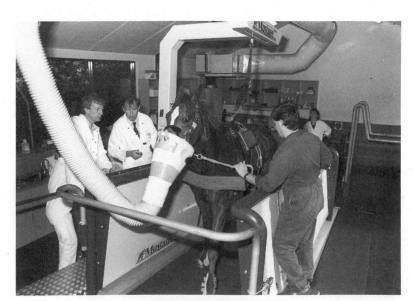

Figure 12-1. *Treadmill at the Equine Performance Laboratory of The University of Sydney.*

out access to sophisticated equipment than investigations using treadmills. Track testing is not only more easily performed than treadmill testing but also has the advantage of being undertaken in an environment similar to that in which the horse has to perform.[6,7] These advantages are outweighed by the disadvantages of track testing, which include the limited range of measurements that can be performed (usually before and after exercise), variations in track and environmental conditions, and the influence of the rider or driver. The treadmill, if situated in a room that can be climate-controlled, provides standardized conditions for testing and the opportunity to perform a range of measurements during exercise, as well as before and after. These advantages outweigh the disadvantages of the artificial nature of the treadmill environment and the fact that energy expenditure during exercise on the treadmill is quantitatively different from that during exercise on the track. Treadmill exercise testing, therefore, allows more precise identification of disturbances to particular body systems if a wide range of measurements of the function of key body systems is undertaken.

Track Exercise Testing

Track exercise tests involve various measurements undertaken during or after a standardized bout of exercise. The simplest track test is assessment of exercise capacity by timing the horse over the competition distance. A fast track time and good recovery are good evidence that the horse is fit for a particular race or event distance. This approach has the advantage of simplicity, the only piece of equipment required being a stop watch. However, in most cases where exercise testing is considered, more information is required than can be gained simply from a stop watch.

Track testing protocols have included gradually increasing increments of speed, with samples collected after each increment, submaximal tests at speeds around three-quarters pace, and maximal speed tests. Measurements that can be made easily during or following track tests include heart rate (HR) measured using an "onboard" heart rate meter and various hematologic and plasma/serum biochemical values taken after exercise.[6] Using Evans blue dye (see Chap. 5), total red cell volume, a measurement given considerable importance by Persson,[3] also can be assessed. In various experimental studies, telemetric measurements of minute ventilation, tidal volume, and oxygen uptake have been made,[8,9] as well as collection of arterial blood to measure arterial blood gases.[10,11] However, most of the latter measurements require sophisticated equipment or considerable ingenuity and are techniques restricted to experimental studies. Recovery of heart and respiratory rates has been valuable after exercise, mainly to assess the fitness of endurance horses.[12,13] Heart rate recovery appears to be less useful to assess the fitness of standardbred and thoroughbred racehorses, although a significant correlation with race performance has been reported.[14]

Treadmill Exercise Tests

WHAT TYPE OF TREADMILL SHOULD BE CHOSEN?

Early treadmills used a system of rollers under a rubber belt and were set at a fixed and often steep incline. These machines were designed for walking and slow trotting, finding most use on horse stud farms for the conditioning of yearlings. The machines were noisy, had the potential to cause concussive injuries to the limbs, and could not be used at higher speeds. The Säto treadmill, originally designed and built in Sweden, was the first commercial high-speed treadmill that allowed horses to be exercised at speeds similar to those encountered during racing. Since then, a number of companies have developed high-speed treadmills for use with horses, there being two machines currently available in the United States. The Säto treadmill* is now manufactured in Missouri and is used by a number of veterinary schools and some equine clinics. Two versions of the machine are available, depending on particular needs. The larger unit (around $60,000) is most suitable for research laboratories, whereas the smaller machine (around $36,000) is adequate for clinical exercise testing in a practice setting. The most sophisticated machine available is the Mustang,[†] which is manufactured in Switzerland. Its design includes computer software that allows direct display of heart rate and oxygen uptake ($\dot{V}_{O_2}$) during exercise, together with video input for gait analysis. A smaller version of the Mustang, similar in price to the Säto, is also available for use by trainers or veterinary clinics. Because equine practitioners do not need the complicated equipment that may be required by researchers, the main requirements of a suitable treadmill are:

1. *That the machine be capable of inclination to a maximum of 10 percent slope.* Exercise tests on a treadmill inclined at a 10 percent slope (6 degrees) enable horses to reach maximal intensities at speeds of 10 to 13 m/s, depending on age and fitness. Exercise on the slope allows horses to be exercised at speeds well below those on the track, yet maximum capacity can be assessed.
2. *That the speed be adjustable up to 14 m/s and that rapid acceleration be possible.* Some tests require acceleration to galloping speed in 5 or 6 seconds, and thus rapid acceleration is required. While safety harnesses are not essential, we have found them useful to prevent injuries, particularly in those horses which become excited or temperamental on the treadmill. It is important that an emergency stop be available which will bring the belt to an immediate stop. During treadmill exercise, because horses have no momentum, they can be brought to an instantaneous halt, even while galloping.

---

*Equispeed Technologies, 329 N. Madison, Raymore, Mo. 64085.
†Kagra AG, Saremnstorferstrasse 388, CH-5616 Fahrwangen, Switzerland.

After experimenting with various treadmill angles, we have found that a 10 percent slope provides a compromise between a steep slope that would be unrepresentative of track exercise and speeds that may be too fast for horse safety. At a slope of 6 degrees, all racehorses will reach maximal oxygen uptake ($\dot{V}_{O_2max}$) at speeds between 10 and 12 m/s. However, untrained horses may reach $\dot{V}_{O_2max}$ at treadmill speeds as low as 8 m/s. Different laboratories use different treadmill slopes, generally ranging from 6.25 percent in Swedish studies to 10 percent in investigations in Australia, the United States, and Europe.[15-20] The effect of slope on energy use can be observed by examination of the graph of slope on $\dot{V}_{O_2}$ in Chapter 4.

Protocol for the Exercise Test

INCREMENTAL VERSUS HIGH-SPEED TESTS

The majority of studies on exercise testing in athletic horses have used rapid incremental tests.[15-18,21-26] In these tests, the speed of the machine usually is increased every 60 to 120 seconds until the horse can no longer keep pace with the speed of the machine or until a predetermined heart rate has been obtained. This type of test has proven most popular because data can be gathered during both submaximal and maximal exercise. However, criticism of such a test has been made on the basis that for racehorses, exercising over sprint distances (less than 1600 m or 1 mi), tests where the speed is gradually increased may not be the most appropriate. In these cases, a "run to fatigue" test can be used, where horses are exercised at a near-maximal speed or intensity until they can no longer maintain this intensity of exercise. However, such testing requires that the horse is fully acclimatized to treadmill exercise so that rapid acceleration (5 to 6 s) to a galloping speed is possible. This type of test has been used in an attempt to measure anaerobic capacity[27] (see Chap. 4) in human athletes by determination of maximal accumulated oxygen deficit (MAOD). This type of test can be adapted for horses, with anaerobic capacity assessed by exercising the horse at 115 to 120 percent of $\dot{V}_{O_2max}$, and the accumulated $\dot{V}_{O_2}$ measured during exercise and subtracted from the total oxygen demand. For measurement of MAOD, submaximal V_{O_2} measurements have to be made so that the oxygen demand can be extrapolated above the point of $\dot{V}_{O_2max}$.

ACCLIMATIZATION TO THE TREADMILL

An acclimatization period is necessary to introduce horses to exercise on a treadmill. While the majority of horses adjust readily to treadmill exercise, many of the measurements made during treadmill exercise testing can be affected by excitement or apprehension. Heart rates and plasma or blood lactate values are higher during initial acclimatizing runs on the treadmill. We have found that for reproducible results, at least four acclimatizing runs are required in most horses, and some horses require more exposures to the treadmill.

Our protocol for acclimatization is 4 minutes of walking at 1.5 to 2.0 m/s so that the horse becomes used to the belt moving. It is important that from the beginning of exercise the horse is encouraged to move toward the front of the treadmill. The treadmill speed then is increased to 4 m/s, which is a comfortable trotting speed for most horses. After 3 minutes at 4 m/s, the speed is increased to 6 m/s, the speed at which most horses will start to canter. After 2 minutes at 6 m/s, we increase the speed to 8 m/s for 1 minute. Most horses adjust readily to treadmill exercise, with only 1 to 2 percent showing initial reluctance to exercise. Usually we give the horses two acclimatizing runs per day for 2 days, after which they undertake the exercise test. However, if the horses are not comfortable on the treadmill or are reluctant to exercise to the front of the machine, we may give a further two acclimatizing runs.

SPECIFIC PROTOCOL FOR EXERCISE TESTING

After trying a number of incremental exercise tests, we have found the following test to be practical and informative in most athletic horses: The test involves four submaximal steps (4, 6, 8, and 10 m/s) so that derived data can be obtained from linear regression analysis. A warmup period of 3 minutes at 4 m/s is followed by 90 seconds at 6 m/s and then 1-minute steps at 8, 10, 11, 12, and 13 m/s. Few horses will complete all steps, with most racehorses in training showing fatigue during or after the 12-m/s step. In contrast, endurance horses will find it difficult to exercise at speeds above 10 m/s. Fatigue can be judged easily, since horses no longer keep pace with the speed of the treadmill despite encouragement to move forward. The number of steps completed and the total run time provide an index of performance capacity and degree of fitness. Measurements of cardiorespiratory function are performed over the last 5 to 10 seconds of each exercise step, but blood lactate information is useful only at speeds greater than 6 m/s because of the variability in values, which are affected by excitement at lower speeds. The lower speeds are of longer duration because there is an initial overshoot of heart rate,[3] and the time to steady state is more prolonged than for later steps in an incremental test.[25] Although steady state cannot be ensured after 60 seconds of exercise, we find that most cardiorespiratory variables are close to steady state at the conclusion of each step in the exercise test described. However, plasma or blood lactate values do not reach steady state, and it is important that lactate values be compared on tests where each step is of the same duration and intensity.

Measurements During a Clinical Exercise Test

While treadmill exercise testing can provide a range of information, the most important relates to function of the cardiopulmonary and musculoskeletal systems. These body systems are the ones that are most intimately involved in determination of successful athletic perfor-

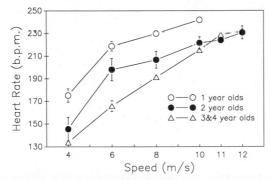

Figure 12-2. *Normal heart rate (HR) response to exercise in yearling (○), 2-year-old (●), and 3-year-old (△) thoroughbred horses. The 2- and 3-year old horses were in racing condition, but the yearlings were untrained. Values were obtained with treadmill set at 10 percent slope. (From Rose and colleagues. Aust Vet J 1990; 67:345.)*

mance. However, the central nervous system is important in exercise fatigue, and there are no measurements that can quantify the "will to win." A number of measurements are possible during treadmill exercise tests, but it is important that the measurements be useful and practical. To be useful in a clinical setting, the measurements must be easy to perform and provide information that is relevant to performance. Such measurements include heart rate, blood lactate concentrations, arterial blood gases, blood volume, stride length, and oxygen uptake. Additionally, endoscopic examination of the upper respiratory tract during exercise may be valuable in certain cases.

HEART RATE DURING EXERCISE

Heart rate is one of the easiest measurements to undertake during exercise and provides an indirect index of cardiovascular capacity and function. A number of heart rate meters are available to measure exercising heart

rate,[28,29] with the two most reliable being the EQB[*] and the Hippocard.[†] Both heart rate meters have inbuilt memories, and the Hippocard has the capacity for a subsequent printout of the heart rate. Reliable results are not always possible because of shifting electrodes or poor electrode contact with the skin. Care should be taken to ensure good electrode contact with the skin, which is possible through the use of salt solutions or electrode paste. Since stroke volume does not change greatly with increasing exercise speed,[30] the heart rate provides a guide to changes in cardiac output. The normal heart rate response to exercise in various age groups of horses is shown in Figure 12–2. In general, there is a linear increase in heart rate with increasing exercise speed up to the point at which the maximal heart rate (HR_{max}) is reached. The HR_{max} is identified when there is no further increase in heart rate despite an increase in treadmill speed. The HR_{max} does not change with training state,[31] although the speed at which HR_{max} is reached increases with increasing fitness. The increase in heart rate as speed increases is greatest in young horses, with HR_{max} being reached at relatively low exercise intensities (see Fig. 12–2). Persson[21] has suggested that a useful reference point for comparison of cardiovascular capacity is the treadmill speed at a heart rate of 200 beats/min (V_{200}). At a heart rate of 200 beats/min, most horses are close to the point of onset of blood lactate accumulation (OBLA, blood lactate concentration of 4 mmol/liter) or what has been called incorrectly the "anaerobic threshold." The V_{200} can be determined by linear regression analysis using a programmable calculator or computer spreadsheet program or by plotting the heart rate values (y axis) at treadmill speeds of 4, 6, 8, and 10 m/s (x axis) on graph paper. After drawing a straight line through the four heart rates, the speed in meters per second at a heart rate of 200 beats/min can be determined (Fig. 12–3). In

[*]EQB, Unionville, Pa. 19375.
[†]Hippocard PEH 100, Ingenieurburo Isler, CH-8034, Zurich, Switzerland.

Figure 12-3. *Determination of V_{200} from measurement of heart rates at treadmill speeds of 4, 6, 8, and 10 m/s with the treadmill set at a 10 percent slope. The $V_{HR_{max}}$ is the speed at which maximum heart rate is reached.*

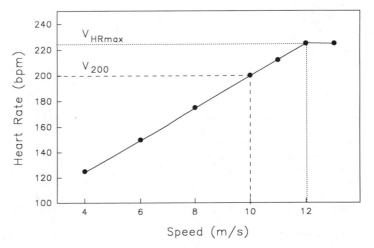

general, horses with the highest cardiovascular and metabolic capacities will have the highest V_{200} values. Measurement of V_{200} also may be useful for evaluation of improvements in fitness, since V_{200} values should increase as training progresses. However, some studies have shown little change in V_{200} values despite large increases in $\dot{V}_{O_2max}$. A high correlation ($r = 0.75$) between V_{200} and $\dot{V}_{O_2max}$ has been found in thoroughbred racehorses.[20] In standardbred trotters, Persson and Ullberg[32] reported significant correlations with total red cell volume and maximum velocity, there being correlation coefficients of around 0.6. Using the treadmill protocol described with the treadmill set at a slope of 10 percent, we have found that better-quality thoroughbred horses in training have V_{200} values in the range of 8.0 to 9.0 m/s.

However, care should be taken in using V_{200} to assess exercise capacity. At a heart rate of 200 beats/min, horses can be exercising at quite different proportions of their HR_{max} and, therefore, their $\dot{V}_{O_2max}$.[33] For example, in a horse with a maximal heart rate of 215 beats/min, a heart rate of 200 beats/min represents 93 percent of HR_{max}, whereas in a horse with an HR_{max} of 240 beats/min, a heart rate of 200 beats/min would be only 83 percent of HR_{max}. In these two cases, the former horse would be exercising close to its maximal cardiovascular capacity at a heart rate of 200 beats/min, whereas in the latter there is substantial cardiovascular reserve and different metabolic requirements. Additionally, V_{200} values may be affected by excitement and apprehension because of variability in heart rate at speeds involving trotting and slow cantering, where heart rate values may be elevated. In determinations of submaximal heart rate in horses presented for exercise testing, we have found variations in V_{200} of more than 1 m/s in individual animals during repeated tests on sequential days.

Another measurement of cardiovascular capacity is the speed at which the horse reaches HR_{max} ($V_{HR_{max}}$) (see Fig. 12–3). The $V_{HR_{max}}$ is correlated with $\dot{V}_{O_2max}$ and exercise capacity and is a better indicator of cardiovascular capacity than the V_{200} because $V_{HR_{max}}$ is not a relative measurement. The disadvantage with $V_{HR_{max}}$ is that unlike determination of V_{200}, the exercise test used must involve horses exercising up to their maximal speeds so that a plateau in heart rate can be identified. Measurement of V_{200} requires only four submaximal exercise speeds, with the maximum intensity of exercise being equivalent only to three-quarters pace on the track.

Cardiovascular Disease

We have found heart rate measurements during exercise to be useful in assessment of the functional significance of some heart murmurs, as well as electrocardiographic conduction abnormalities. Horses with functional cardiac disease will have elevations in submaximal heart rates because of reductions in stroke volume (Fig. 12–4). Values for V_{200} less than 7 m/s are abnormal and, if found in a fit horse, indicate decreased cardiac capacity. Another measurement that can be helpful in indicating reduced stroke volume is the oxygen pulse ($\dot{V}_{O_2}$/HR), which is discussed later.

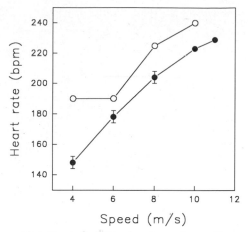

Figure 12-4. *Heart rate (HR) values from a 3-year-old racehorse with a functional systolic murmur ($\bigcirc$) compared with normal fit horses ($\bullet$).*

TELEMETRIC ELECTROCARDIOGRAPHY

An alternative to using a heart rate meter for measuring the exercising heart rate is telemetry electrocardiography. We use disposable adhesive electrodes (Red Dot, 3M Company), applied to the left chest wall, as shown in Figure 12–5. The electrodes are maintained in position by the use of foam rubber over the electrodes, held in position by a girth that holds the telemetry transmitter (Fig. 12–6). The quality of the tracing obtained using this system is excellent, and the display on the telemetry receiver* is shown in Figure 12–7. This may provide additional information to simple heart rate measurements, because dysrhythmias can occur during exercise. However, because there is a low incidence of dysrhythmias during exercise, we have found it more useful to monitor the electrocardiogram for the first 60 seconds after exercise, when conduction disturbances may be more easily recognized.

BLOOD (PLASMA) LACTATE MEASUREMENT

Lactate is produced in exercising muscle during all intensities of exercise. However, above half pace (speeds above 6 m/s on a treadmill set at a 10 percent slope), lactate production will increase as the aerobic energy contribution becomes insufficient to meet total energy requirements. Additionally, the increased energy demands of exercise result in rapid glycogenolysis, with large amounts of pyruvate production. The result is an increase in lactate production, simply by a mass action effect. Because lactate diffuses from muscle to blood, measurements of blood or plasma lactate concentrations will reflect muscle lactate concentrations. The rate of increase of lactate in the blood therefore may be used as an indirect indicator of cardiovascular and metabolic ca-

*Danika, Copenhagen, Denmark.

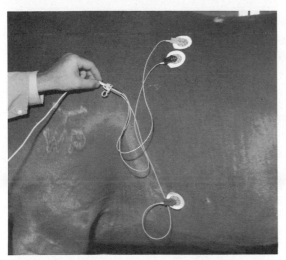

Figure 12-5. *Position of electrodes for recording the electrocardiogram by telemetry during exercise. Adhesive electrodes (Red Dot, 3M Company) are applied to the left chest wall.*

pacity. Horses with the highest aerobic capacities due to a high maximal cardiac output will tend to have lower lactate values at submaximal exercise intensities than those with low aerobic capacities.

Measurement of lactate in blood can be performed on either whole blood or plasma. Plasma values will be about one-third higher than whole-blood values, although the relationship between plasma and blood lactate is variable from horse to horse. If samples are not to be analyzed immediately, it may be best for the blood to be collected into tubes containing fluoride/oxalate as an

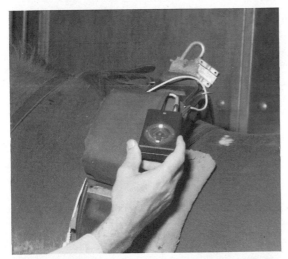

Figure 12-6. *The electrodes for recording the electrocardiogram by telemetry are maintained in position by the use of foam rubber over the electrodes, held in position by a girth which holds the telemetry transmitter.*

anticoagulant (gray top Vacutainer tubes[*]) so that glycolysis is inhibited and lactate values do not continue to increase after collection. However, we have found that provided the blood samples are kept refrigerated and the samples are analyzed within 48 hours of collection, sodium or lithium heparin is a suitable anticoagulant. Collection of blood samples during exercise is simplified by the use of a 14-gauge catheter and extension tubing so that blood samples can be withdrawn at the conclusion of each exercise step. Because little information is provided at the lower treadmill speeds, we collect samples only at 6, 8, and 10 m/s. Alternatively, a single sample collected immediately after the 10-m/s exercise step can be used. While there are a number of possible measurement methods, we use a rapid automated lactate analyzer.[†] This type of machine is simple to use and provides a reliable and cost-effective method for lactate measurement in clinical practice.

For comparison of blood or plasma lactate values between horses or in the same horse during training, the treadmill speed at a plasma lactate of 4 mmol/liter (V_{LA4}) generally has been used.[21] Overall, the higher the V_{LA4}, the fitter is the horse and the greater is the exercise capacity. Plasma values for V_{LA4} in normal, fit thoroughbred horses that are 3 years of age and over range from 8.0 to 9.5 m/s. Normal plasma lactate values in thoroughbred horses are shown in Figure 12–8. Another useful reference point that we have found is the blood or plasma lactate value at the conclusion of the 10-m/s exercise step of the incremental test described previously. The best, fit athletic horses usually will have plasma lactate concentrations less than 5.0 mmol/liter. This finding relates to most competitive equine activities, with the exception of sprinting. Over sprint distances (400 to 800 m), a high glycolytic capacity is advantageous but may not be detectable with an incremental exercise test. Horses with high anaerobic capacities have the highest peak plasma lactate values after a maximal exercise test.[34] Therefore, peak lactate may be a more useful predictor of sprint performance.

ARTERIAL BLOOD GAS ANALYSIS DURING EXERCISE

At exercise intensities above 65 percent $\dot{V}_{O_2max}$, athletic horses become hypoxemic,[35,36] with arterial blood gas tensions, at sea level, falling from mean values of around 100 mmHg at rest to 70 mmHg at or above intensities equivalent to $\dot{V}_{O_2max}$. While this is generally true, the extent of the hypoxemia appears to be much less in some individuals than in others. In horses with low $\dot{V}_{O_2max}$ values, there may be very little decrease in arterial oxygen tensions.[37]

Venous blood, while appropriate for assessing acid-base status, is inappropriate for evaluation of gas exchange during exercise. Arterial blood can be collected

[*]Becton Dickinson, Rutherford, N.J. 07070.
[†]YSI 23L or 2300L, Yellow Springs Instruments, Yellow Springs, Ohio, 45387.

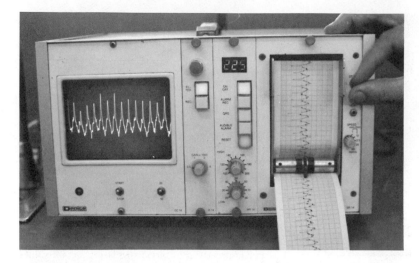

Figure 12-7. Display of the electro-cardiogram receiver recorded by telemetry during maximal exercise.

during exercise by catheterization of the transverse facial artery near the lateral canthus of the eye. Horses tolerate this procedure well after desensitization of the skin over the site with 0.2 ml of 2% lidocaine (Fig. 12–9). The volume of local anesthetic used should not be greater than 0.2 ml because the local anesthetic may diffuse and block the facial nerve. Catheterization is performed with an 18-gauge, 32-mm (1.25-in) catheter, using palpation to direct the catheter (Fig. 12–10). Once blood starts to drip from the catheter, it is advanced up the artery for 3 to 4 mm prior to withdrawal of the stylet by 5 mm. With the stylet in place to maintain rigidity, the catheter is advanced up to its hub (Fig. 12–11). The catheter is then connected to minimum-volume extension tubing previously filled with heparinized saline (4 IU heparin per milliliter of 0.9% saline) and secured in position using rapid setting glue (Fig. 12–12). Because blood temperature influences blood gas and pH results,[38,39] a central

venous thermistor also must be placed to determine blood temperature during exercise. This allows correction of the values determined at 37°C in the blood gas machine to the blood temperature, which during maximal exercise may reach 42°C.

Arterial blood gas analysis during exercise may be indicated in horses with poor performance suspected to be due to respiratory disorders. Often, we find it useful to undertake arterial blood gas determination during exercise in horses that have abnormalities on bronchoalveolar lavage cytology or where there is a suspicion of an upper respiratory tract abnormality that could interfere with gas exchange. Blood gas results during exercise in normal racehorses, a horse with mild idiopathic laryngeal hemiplegia, and a horse with severe exercise-induced pulmonary hemorrhage are shown in Figures 12–13 and 12–14.

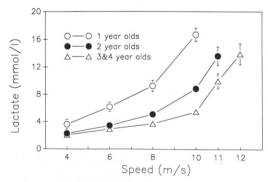

Figure 12-8. Normal plasma lactate values in yearling (○), 2-year-old (●), and 3-year-old (△) thoroughbred horses. The 2- and 3-year-old horses were in racing condition, but the yearlings were untrained. Values were obtained with the treadmill set at a 10 percent slope. (From Rose and colleagues. Aust Vet J 1990; 67:345.)

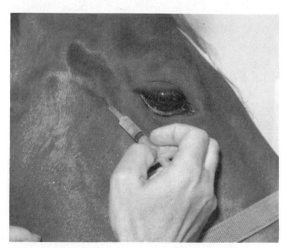

Figure 12-9. Transverse facial artery catheterization. To catheterize the transverse facial artery 0.2 ml of 2% lidocaine is injected intradermally over the artery.

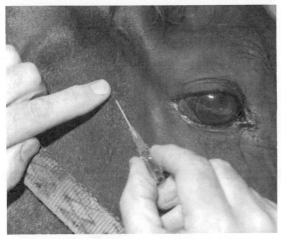

Figure 12-10. Transverse facial artery catheterization. *The catheter (18-gauge, 32-mm) is inserted through the bleb of local anesthetic after palpating the transverse facial artery.*

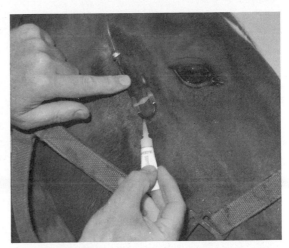

Figure 12-12. Transverse facial artery catheterization. *After advancing the catheter, it is connected to minimum-volume extension tubing previously filled with heparinized saline and secured in position using rapid setting glue.*

ENDOSCOPIC EXAMINATION OF THE UPPER RESPIRATORY TRACT DURING EXERCISE

Treadmill endoscopy also may be a useful diagnostic aid in horses in which partial upper respiratory tract obstructions are suspected.[40] We find treadmill endoscopy to be useful in assessing the significance of some cases of laryngeal asynchrony or assymmetry, as well as evaluation of cases where soft palate dislocation is suspected. Videoendoscopes are now available that provide excellent images of the upper airway during exercise. However, these machines are very expensive, and adequate images can be obtained by connecting a video camera to a normal fiberoptic endoscope. If there is no

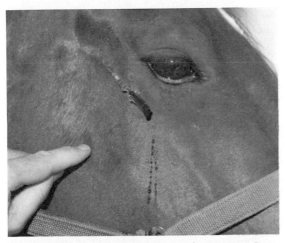

Figure 12-11. Transverse facial artery catheterization. *Once the blood starts to drip from the catheter, it is advanced up the artery for 3 to 4 mm, prior to withdrawal of the stylet by 5 mm. With the stylet in place to maintain rigidity, the catheter is advanced up to its hub.*

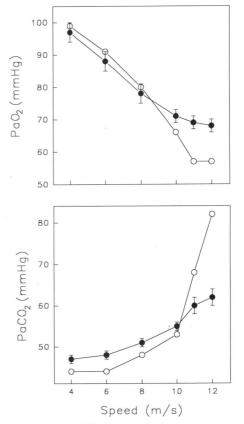

Figure 12-13. Arterial blood gas results during exercise in *normal racehorses (●) and a horse with idiopathic laryngeal hemiplegia (○).*

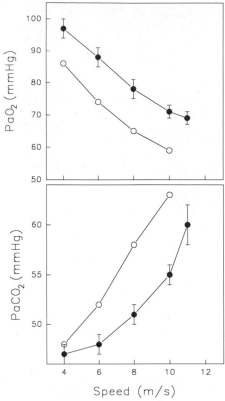

Figure 12-14. Arterial blood gas results during exercise in normal racehorses (●) and a horse with severe exercise-induced pulmonary hemorrhage (○).

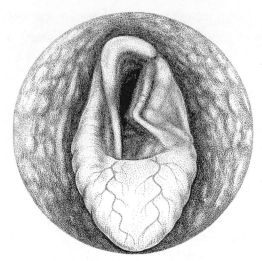

Figure 12-15. Left laryngeal dysfunction with intrusion of the left arytenoid cartilage into the airway. Drawing from the endoscopic view of the larynx during galloping exercise on a treadmill.

clear explanation for reduced athletic capacity, upper airway endoscopy during treadmill exercise sometimes provides the answer. We have seen a few horses that apparently have normal abductor and adductor laryngeal function at rest but during exercise, left laryngeal dysfunction is apparent, with intrusion of the left arytenoid cartilage into the airway (Fig. 12–15).

EXERCISING HEMATOCRIT AND TOTAL RED CELL VOLUME

Because the total volume of red cells is a major determinant of oxygen-carrying capacity in horses, measurement of red cell volume (CV) can give some index of exercise capacity.[32] Additionally, Persson[41] has reported an overtraining syndrome in standardbred trotters in which red cell hypervolemia resulted in decreased exercise capacity. The technique of red cell volume measurement is simple and reliable and utilizes Evans blue (T 1824) dye to determine plasma volume following mobilization of the splenic erythrocyte pool either by epinephrine injection or near-maximal exercise.[3] Details of the technique are given in Chapter 5. Simple measurement of postexercise hematocrit (PCV) will not be reliable as an indicator of total CV because of plasma vol-

ume variations. However, postexercise PCV will provide a rough guide to total circulating red cells.

Normal values for CV in thoroughbred horses in training have ranged from 80 to 102 ml/kg. While definitive normal ranges are not yet established, high CV values have not been found in standardbred or thoroughbred horses presented to our clinic for poor racing performance. The clinical usefulness of CV measurements to assist in evaluation of poor performance as well as performance prediction awaits further research.

OXYGEN UPTAKE

The measurement of $\dot{V}_{O_2}$ is critical in the assessment of athletic performance. Not only are measurements of submaximal $\dot{V}_{O_2}$ important in calculating the energy cost of exercise, but maximal oxygen uptake ($\dot{V}_{O_2max}$), a key indicator of exercise capacity, can be measured. Measurement of $\dot{V}_{O_2}$ is best performed using a gas-collection mask without valves via an open-flow method because masks with valves will impair respiration.[42] The open-flow method for $\dot{V}_{O_2}$ measurement uses a loose-fitting mask or a mask with holes around its perimeter so that there is no restriction to respiration. A large vacuum motor is used to suck air through the mask at flow rates between 6000 and 10,000 liters/min, and a differential pressure transducer is used to ensure that the flow rate across a Venturi device remains constant during exercise. It has been established that gas flow rates in excess of 6000 liters/min are adequate to prevent rebreathing of expired gas.[43] Samples of gas are collected, and after dehumidification, the oxygen and carbon dioxide concentrations are determined using appropriate analyzers. From measurement of the flow, gas temperature, O_2, and CO_2, the $\dot{V}_{O_2}$ and carbon dioxide production ($\dot{V}_{CO_2}$) can be measured reliably. A schematic drawing of the open-

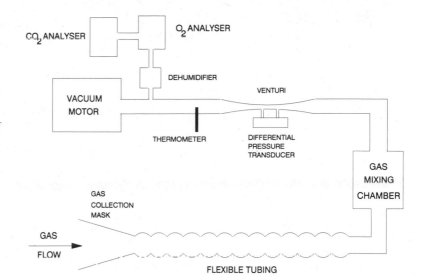

Figure 12-16. *A schematic drawing of the open-flow gas-collection system for measuremnt of $\dot{V}_{O_2}$ and $\dot{V}_{CO_2}$ in exercising horses.*

flow gas-collection system for measurement of $\dot{V}_{O_2}$ and $\dot{V}_{CO_2}$ is shown in Figure 12–16. Measurement of total gas flow can be carried out simply and reliably using a nitrogen dilution technique.[44] The coefficient of variation for $\dot{V}_{O_2}$ and $\dot{V}_{CO_2}$ determinations is in the range of 3 to 5 percent.

$\dot{V}_{CO_2}$ increases linearly as the intensity of exercise increases in a similar fashion to $\dot{V}_{O_2}$. At higher exercise intensities, $\dot{V}_{CO_2}$ increases more rapidly than $\dot{V}_{O_2}$, resulting in an increase in the respiratory exchange ratio R. At intensities approaching $\dot{V}_{O_2max}$, values for R exceed 1.0, and at $\dot{V}_{O_2max}$, R values are usually around 1.2 to 1.3 because of buffering of lactate by bicarbonate as lactate moves from exercising muscle into the blood.

Determination of $\dot{V}_{O_2max}$ has been a key measurement in assessment of exercise capacity of human athletes since the 1950s.[45] The $\dot{V}_{O_2}$ increases linearly with

increasing treadmill speed, and $\dot{V}_{O_2max}$ can be identified where there is a plateau in $\dot{V}_{O_2}$ despite an increase in speed (Fig. 12–17). In most horses, a plateau in $\dot{V}_{O_2}$ occurs despite an increase in speed (Fig. 12–17), but in some, no such plateau may be found, but rather an asymptote.[46] Where no plateau can be identified, we take the $\dot{V}_{O_2max}$ as the maximum $\dot{V}_{O_2}$ recorded in an incremental exercise test in which the horse exercises to fatigue. Seeherman and Morris[46] refer to this as the $\dot{V}_{O_2}$ peak. Noakes[47] reports that $\dot{V}_{O_2max}$ is regarded by the majority of human athletes as the "best predictor of athletic potential." Until the last few years, $\dot{V}_{O_2max}$ has been a difficult measurement to undertake in athletic horses because of difficulties in designing suitable respiratory gas-collection masks. Additionally, access to treadmills is required that enable horses to exercise at an intensity high enough for a plateau in $\dot{V}_{O_2}$ to be defined. Gas-collection masks with valves impose too much resistance to respiration, are poorly tolerated by horses, are usually quite heavy, and cause a greater degree of hypoxemia and hypercapnia than would normally be present during high-intensity exercise.[42] Exercise on a treadmill inclined at a slope of 10 percent (6 degrees) using the open-flow gas-collection system allows $\dot{V}_{O_2}$, $\dot{V}_{CO_2}$, and $\dot{V}_{O_2max}$ to be determined reliably without impeding respiration.[18,43,48] A number of studies have shown that the thoroughbred horse has $\dot{V}_{O_2max}$ values that are higher than those of many other mammalian species when expressed on a mass-specific basis. The major factor responsible for the high $\dot{V}_{O_2max}$ in athletic horses is their high oxygen-carrying capacity, which arises from a large arteriovenous oxygen content difference and a high stroke volume. Given that the HR_{max} and arteriovenous oxygen content difference do not increase with training,[31] a high value for $\dot{V}_{O_2max}$ probably represents a high maximal stroke volume. Because of the rapid kinetics of $\dot{V}_{O_2}$,[25,49] a high $\dot{V}_{O_2max}$ would seem likely to be advantageous for most athletic horses. Harkins and coworkers[19] found a

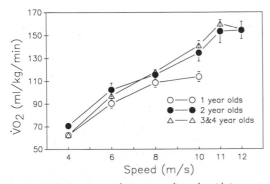

Figure 12-17. *Oxygen uptake increases linearly with increasing treadmill speed, and $\dot{V}_{O_2max}$ can be identified as the plateau in $\dot{V}_{O_2}$ despite an increase in speed. Values for $\dot{V}_{O_2}$ are shown in yearling (○), 2-year-old (●), and 3-year-old (△) thoroughbred racehorses. (From Rose and colleagues. Aust Vet J 1990; 67:345.)*

positive correlation between $\dot{V}_{O_2max}$ and running speed on an 800-m track for distances over 1200 m. While the best athletic horses are likely to have high $\dot{V}_{O_2max}$ values, it is unlikely that $\dot{V}_{O_2max}$ by itself will be a useful predictor of performance. Noakes[47] has pointed out that while $\dot{V}_{O_2max}$ is a reasonable predictor of performance in human athletes when one is evaluating subjects of different abilities, $\dot{V}_{O_2max}$ is less useful in predicting performance of a homogeneous group of athletes.

MAXIMAL OXYGEN PULSE

Oxygen pulse is $\dot{V}_{O_2}/HR$ and is expressed as milliliters per kilogram per beat. Because the arteriovenous oxygen content difference is similar for most athletic horses exercising at $\dot{V}_{O_2max}$, oxygen pulse at $\dot{V}_{O_2max}$ provides an indication of the maximal stroke volume. Values in good-quality horses that we have assessed range from 0.66 to 0.76 ml/kg per beat. Conversely, horses with cardiac problems which result in low cardiac outputs usually have values in the range 0.50 to 0.56 ml/kg per beat. The latter values also will be found in normal horses with low $\dot{V}_{O_2max}$ values. We found that maximal oxygen pulse correlated well with treadmill total run time ($r = 0.67$).[50]

STRIDE LENGTH

It has long been believed that champion horses have better stride characteristics than average horses.[51] The stride length can be measured on the track using high-speed cinematography, or simply on the treadmill by knowing the treadmill speed and counting the stride frequency. In studies at the University of Sydney Equine Performance Laboratory, we have found high correlations ($r > 0.7$) between maximal stride length and treadmill run time in the standardized treadmill exercise test described previously.

PEAK RUNNING SPEED AND TOTAL RUN TIME

Noakes[47] noted that in human athletes, a predictor of performance in middle- and long-distance athletes was the peak treadmill running speed during an incremental exercise test. Noakes considered peak running speed to be more useful than $\dot{V}_{O_2max}$ as a predictor of performance. We take the total run time as that time when the horse can no longer keep pace with the treadmill and therefore moves onto the back-restraining bar. Depending on the type and duration of exercise test, such a value may indicate either endurance or short-distance exercise capacity. In racehorses tested at the University of Sydney Equine Performance Laboratory using the incremental test protocol described, the poorest-quality horses were barely able to maintain a speed of 10 m/s for 60 s, in contrast to several high-quality race winners that were able to continue until they had completed 60 s at 13 m/s. However, this type of test does leave the horse quite fatigued and may be less acceptable to owners and trainers than a more limited test. Despite this,

we have used this type of test in more than 200 athletic horses and have found no detrimental effects.

Conclusions

Clinical exercise testing provides a way of assessing exercise capacity in an objective way, with important physiologic measurements able to be undertaken under conditions of peak metabolic demand. Such testing is an important advance to our traditional assessments of the athletic horse with reduced performance, as well as providing a method for evaluation of performance potential. While track testing is readily undertaken, the limited range of measurements possible, together with difficulties in standardizing exercise conditions, makes treadmill exercise testing the technique of choice for assessment of performance.

Poor performance often is multifactorial, with the respiratory and musculoskeletal systems being most commonly involved.[52] A careful workup of horses presented for poor performance is indicated (see Chap. 13), and in some cases, there may be a clear role for clinical exercise testing. The role of exercise testing in young horses to attempt to determine performance potential is still to be determined. However, it seems likely that exercise testing of horses prior to training has the potential to discriminate among animals of poor, moderate, and superior metabolic capacity. Simple exercise tests also enable trainers to objectively assess the effect of training on improving fitness. This type of testing, with blood or plasma lactate samples collected in response to a standardized test, has considerable potential for both track and treadmill testing.

References

1. Jones NL, Campbell EJM: Conduct of stage 2, 3, and 4 exercise tests. *In*: Clinical Exercise Testing. Philadelphia, WB Saunders Co, 1982, p 142.
2. Wasserman K, Hansen JE, Sue DY, et al: Principles of Exercise Testing and Interpretation. Philadelphia, Lea & Febiger, 1987.
3. Persson S: On blood volume and working capacity in horses. Acta Vet Scand Suppl 1967; 19:1.
4. Maier-Bock H, Ehrlein HJ: Heart rate during a defined exercise test in horses with heart and lung disease. Equine Vet J 1978; 10:235.
5. Littlejohn A, Bowles F, Aschenborn G: Cardiorespiratory adaptations to exercise in riding horses with chronic lung disease. *In* Snow DH, Persson SGB, Rose RJ (eds): Equine Exercise Physiology. Cambridge: Granta Editions, 1983, p 33.
6. Thornton JR: Exercise testing. *In* Rose RJ (ed): The Veterinary Clinics of North America: Equine Practice—Exercise Physiology. Philadelphia, WB Saunders Co, 1985, p 573.
7. Erickson HH, Lundin CS, Erickson BK, et al: Indices of performance in the racing quarter horse. *In* Persson SGB, Lindholm A, Jeffcott LB (eds): Equine Exercise Physiology 3. Davis, Calif, ICEEP Publications, 1991, p 41.
8. Hörnicke H, Meixner R, Pollman U: Respiration in exercising horses. *In* Snow DH, Rose RJ (eds): *Equine Exercise Physiology*. Cambridge: Granta Editions, 1983, p 7.
9. Hörnicke H, Weber M, Schweiker W: Pulmonary ventilation in thoroughbred horses at maximum performance. *In* Gillespie JR, Robinson NE (eds): Equine Exercise Physiology 2. Davis, Calif, ICEEP Publications, 1987, p 216.
10. Bayly WM, Grant BD, Breeze RG, et al: The effects of maximal exercise on acid-base balance and arterial blood gas tension in

thoroughbred horses. *In* Snow DH, Persson SGB, Rose RJ (eds): Equine Exercise Physiology. Cambridge: Granta Editions, 1983, p 400.

11. Littlejohn A, Kruger JM: Technique for arterial and mixed venous blood sampling in working saddle horses. Br Vet J 1976; 132:172.

12. Rose RJ, Purdue RA, Hensley W: Plasma biochemistry alterations in horses during an endurance ride. Equine Vet J 1977; 9:122.

13. Rose RJ: An evaluation of heart rate and respiratory rate recovery for assessment of fitness during endurance rides. *In* Snow DH, Persson SGB, Rose RJ (eds): Equine Exercise Physiology. Cambridge: Granta Editions, 1983, p 505.

14. Marsland WP: Heart rate response to submaximal exercise in the standardbred horse. J Appl Physiol 1968; 24:98.

15. Persson SGB, Forssberg P: Exercise tolerance in standardbred trotters with T-wave abnormalities in the electrocardiogram. *In* Gillespie JR, Robinson NE (eds): Equine Exercise Physiology 2. Davis, Calif, ICEEP Publications, 1987, p 772.

16. Persson SGB, Kallings P, Ingvast-Larsson C: Relationships between arterial oxygen tensions and cardiocirculatory function during submaximal exercise in the horse. *In* Gillespie JR, Robinson NE (eds): Equine Exercise Physiology 2. Davis, Calif, ICEEP Publications, 1987, p 161.

17. Marlin DJ, Harris RC, Harman JC, et al: Influence of post-exercise activity on rates of muscle and blood lactate disappearance in the thoroughbred horse. *In* Gillespie JR, Robinson NE (eds): Equine Exercise Physiology 2. Davis, Calif, ICEEP Publications, 1987, p 321.

18. Seeherman HM, Morris EA: Methodology and repeatability of a standardized treadmill exercise test for clinical evaluation of fitness in horses. Equine Vet J Suppl 1990; 9:20.

19. Harkins JD, Beadle RE, Kamerling SG: The correlation of running ability and physiological variables in thoroughbred racehorses. Equine Vet J 1993; 25:53.

20. Rose RJ, Hendrickson DK, Knight PK: Clinical exercise testing in the normal thoroughbred racehorse. Aust Vet J 1990;67:345.

21. Persson SGB: Evaluation of exercise tolerance and fitness in the performance horse. *In* Snow DH, Persson SGB, Rose RJ (eds): Equine Exercise Physiology. Cambridge, Granta Editions, 1983, p 441.

22. Persson SGB, Essén-Gustavsson B, Lindholm A, et al: Cardiorespiratory and metabolic effects of training of standardbred yearlings. *In* Snow DH, Persson SGB, Rose RJ (eds): Equine Exercise Physiology. Cambridge: Granta Editions, 1983, p 458.

23. Thornton J, Essén-Gustavsson B, Lindholm A, et al: Effect of training and detraining on oxygen uptake, cardiac output, blood gas tensions, pH and lactate concentrations during and after exercise in the horse. *In* Snow DH, Persson SGB, Rose RJ (eds): Equine Exercise Physiology. Cambridge: Granta Editions, 1983, p 470.

24. Evans DL, Rose RJ: Determination and repeatability of maximum oxygen uptake and other cardiorespiratory measurements in the exercising horse. Equine Vet J 1988; 20:94.

25. Rose RJ, Hodgson DR, Bayly WM, et al: Kinetics of $\dot{V}_{O_2}$ and $\dot{V}_{CO_2}$ in the horse and comparison of five methods for measurement of maximum oxygen uptake. Equine Vet J Suppl 1990; 9:39.

26. Rose RJ: Exercise and performance testing in the racehorse: Problems, limitations, and potential. *In* Proceedings of the 36th Annual Convention of the American Association of Equine Practitioners, 1990, p 491.

27. Medbø JI, Mohn A-C, Tabata I, et al: Anaerobic capacity determined by maximal accumulated O_2 deficit. J Appl Physiol 1988; 64:50.

28. Evans DL, Rose RJ: Method of investigation of the accuracy of four digitally-displayed heart rate meters suitable for use in the exercising horse. Equine Vet J 1986; 18:129.

29. Physick-Sheard PW, Harman JC, Snow DH, et al: Evaluation of factors influencing the performance of four equine heart rate meters. *In* Gillespie JR, Robinson NE (eds): Equine Exercise Physiology 2. Davis, Calif, ICEEP Publications, 1987, p 102.

30. Evans DL, Rose RJ: Cardiovascular and respiratory responses in thoroughbred horses during treadmill exercise. J Exp Biol 1988; 134:397.

31. Evans DL, Rose RJ: Cardiovascular and respiratory responses to submaximal exercise training in the thoroughbred horse. Pflugers Archiv 1988; 411:316.

32. Persson SGB, Ullberg LE: Blood volume in relation to exercise tolerance in trotters. J S Afr Vet Ass 1975; 45:293.

33. Rose RJ, Evans DL: Cardiovascular and respiratory function in the athletic horse. *In* Gillespie JR, Robinson NE (eds): Equine Exercise Physiology 2. Davis, Calif, ICEEP Publications, 1987, p 1.

34. Eaton MD, Rose RJ, Evans DL, Hodgson DR: The assessment of anaerobic capacity of thoroughbred horses using maximal accumulated oxygen deficit. Aust Equine Vet 1992; 10:86.

35. Bayly WM, Grant BD, Breeze RG, et al: The effects of maximal exercise on acid-base balance and arterial blood gas tension in thoroughbred horses. *In* Snow DH, Persson SGB, Rose RJ (eds): Equine Exercise Physiology. Cambridge: Granta Editions, 1983, p 400.

36. Bayly WM, Schulz DE, Hodgson DR, et al: Ventilatory response to exercise in horses with exercise-induced hypoxemia. *In* Gillespie JR, Robinson NE (eds): Equine Exercise Physiology 2. Davis, Calif, ICEEP Publications, 1987, p 172.

37. Evans DL, Silverman, Hodgson DR, et al: Gait and respiration in standardbred horses during pacing and galloping. Res Vet Sci (in press).

38. Fedde MR: Blood gas analyses on equine blood: Required correction factors. Equine Vet J 1991; 23:410.

39. Pan LG, Forster HV, Kaminsky RP: Arterial vs rectal temperature in ponies: Rest, exercise, CO_2 inhalation and thermal stresses. J Appl Physiol 1986; 61:1577.

40. Morris EA, Seeherman HJ: Evaluation of upper respiratory tract function during strenuous exercise in racehorses. J Am Vet Med Assos 1990; 196:431.

41. Persson SGB: Blood volume, state of training and working capacity of racehorses. Equine Vet J 1968, 1:52.

42. Evans DL, Rose RJ: Effect of a respiratory gas collection mask on some measurements of cardiovascular and respiratory function in horses exercising on a treadmill. Res Vet Sci 1988; 44:220.

43. Bayly WM, Schulz DA, Hodgson DR, et al: Ventilatory responses of the horse to exercise: effect of gas collection systems. J Appl Physiol 1987; 63:1210.

44. Fedak MA, Rome L, Seeherman HJ: One-step N_2-dilution technique for calibrating open-circuit $\dot{V}_{O_2}$ measuring systems. J Appl Physiol 1981; 51:772.

45. Taylor HL, Buskirk E, Henschel A: Maximal oxygen intake as an objective measure of cardio-respiratory performance. J Appl Physiol 1955; 8:73.

46. Seeherman HJ, Morris EA: Application of a standardised treadmill exercise test for evaluation of fitness in 10 thoroughbred racehorses. Equine Vet J Suppl 1991; 9:26.

47. Noakes TD: Implications of exercise testing for prediction of athletic performance: A contemporary perspective. Med Sci Sports Exerc 1988; 40:319.

48. Rose RJ, Hodgson DR, Kelso TB, et al: Maximum O_2 uptake, O_2 debt and deficit, and muscle metabolites in thoroughbred horses. J Appl Physiol 1988; 64:781.

49. Evans DL, Rose RJ: Dynamics of cardiorespiratory function in standardbred horses during different intensities of constant-load exercise. J Comp Physiol [B] 1988; 157:791.

50. King CM, Evans DL, Rose RJ: Physiological response of normal and lame horses during an incremental treadmill exercise test. (In preparation).

51. Pratt GW Jr: Remarks on Gait Analysis. *In* Snow DH, Persson SGB, Rose RJ (eds): Equine Exercise Physiology. Cambridge: Granta Editions, 1983, p 245.

52. Morris EA, Seeherman HJ: Clinical evaluation of poor performance in the racehorse: The results of 275 evaluations. Equine Vet J 1991; 23:169.

13

Investigation of Poor Performance

R. J. ROSE AND D. R. HODGSON

Athletic horses with poor performance have long been a challenge for owners, trainers, and veterinarians. One of the most important decisions is whether the horse has suffered a reduction in performance or simply has a lack of ability. Of those horses presented with a clear history of reduced performance, a high percentage will have few or no abnormal findings on examination. Other cases may show abnormalities either on clinical examination or on one of the diagnostic tests used, but it may be difficult to prove that these abnormalities are contributing to the poor performance. In many cases, the vet-erinarian may resort to a battery of hematology and plasma or serum biochemical measurements in an attempt to find some explanation for the problem. However, many horses show one or more measurements outside the "normal range" without any detrimental effects on athletic capacity. These facts, together with a horse presented free of overt clinical disease, may make it exceedingly difficult to arrive at a definitive diagnosis for the cause of poor performance.

In this chapter we will outline our approach to the investigation of cases presented for poor performance to

---

Table 13-1. University of Sydney Equine Performance Laboratory Poor Performance History Sheet

Horse Name:	Breed:
Date:	Age:
Clinic No.:	Sex:
OWNER:	PHONE:
TRAINER:	PHONE:

Presenting complaint:
1. Is the horse lame or uneven?
2. Is the horse showing signs of respiratory distress?
3. Is the horse doing any of the following?
   a. "Blowing" excessively after a race or slow to recover.
   b. Not running straight, running out or "hanging".
   c. Not jumping out or starting well, lacking in early speed.
   d. Tires early, "fades in its run".
   e. Inappetant after a race.

Racing and training details:
1. What distances does the horse race over?
2. How many starts this preparation?
3. For what placings?
4. How long has the horse been in training?
5. What is the average spacing between races?
6. Details of training programme:
   a. How often does the horse do pace work per week?
   b. What distance and at what pace?
   c. What other exercise does the horse do?
7. Details of earlier preparations, race starts, and placings:

8. Has the horse raced well/better this preparation?
9. When did the horse last rest, for how long, and for what reason?
10. Does the horse become overly excited or difficult to manage on race Day?

Medical history:
1. Detail recent or previous illness or injury:

2. Does the horse make an abnormal respiratory noise during exercise?
3. Does the horse cough either at rest or during exercise?
4. Has the horse ever bled from the nostrils or shown evidence of blood on "scoping"?
5. Does the horse show signs of muscle soreness after fast exercise?
6. What veterinary attention has the horse received recently?
7. Is the horse on any medication at present? If so, what?

Other:
1. Attending veterinarian:
2. Has the horse been on a treadmill before?
3. Does the horse exercise in any special gear or harness?
4. Is the horse on any special diet or supplements?
5. How fit is the horse in the opinion of the trainer?
6. What is the trainer's assessment of the horse's ability?

Comments:

the University of Sydney Equine Performance Laboratory. We adopt a standard protocol for the examination of horses presented for poor performance. In many cases, we are able to establish a likely cause, but there are a number of horses in which, despite a number of sophisticated tests, a clear diagnosis cannot be established. It is important to remember that there is often more than one cause, and multiple body systems may be involved in horses with reduced athletic capacity.[1] Therefore, the examination should not stop when an abnormality is found. The type of investigation undertaken will depend on the type of equipment and facilities available. However, the basic evaluation of any athletic horse with poor performance centers around obtaining a precise history and performing a detailed clinical examination using appropriate diagnostic aids and finally specialized techniques such as treadmill endoscopy, clinical exercise testing, and nuclear scintigraphy.

History

The history is vital in establishing the duration and severity of reduced performance. It is important to determine whether the horse has had chronic and progressive reduction in performance or an acute and unexpected decrease in exercise capacity. In the case of racehorses, careful questioning of the trainer may reveal that rather than a reduction in performance, the horse has never really shown good exercise capacity. Because racehorses seldom gallop over race distances in their track work, trainers can be given a false sense of the horse's ability by track gallops over 400 or 600 m (2 to 3 furlongs). The cause of poor performance is more likely to be determined in cases with acute reduction in performance rather than horses that have chronic and/or progressive poor exercise capacity. In racehorses presented for poor performance at the University of Sydney Equine Performance Laboratory, we use the following standard history sheet, which we find is helpful in obtaining important history details (Table 13–1). Some important questions include

- Has the decrease in exercise capacity been sudden or gradual?
- Is there respiratory distress after exercise?
- Is there any respiratory noise during exercise, and if so, at what speed does this occur?
- Is the problem continuous or intermittent?
- Is the horse's track work/training work adequate but the horse does not reproduce the form in competition?
- Is there any indication of lameness or change in gait?
- Are there any signs of ill health (weight loss, change in demeanor, coughing, etc.)?
- Are there any changes in the horse's appetite?
- Has the horse had any recent drug therapy?

These questions are by no means all-inclusive, but they help to focus on the important body systems likely to be involved. The standard history form is helpful in

ensuring that no important areas are overlooked. Once the history has been obtained, there will be some indication of the directions for further investigation. An indication of chronicity of a problem, relationship to ill health, involvement of the upper respiratory tract, or musculoskeletal problems should be evident.

Clinical Examination

A detailed clinical examination is the cornerstone of all investigations of poor performance. Too often this is the vital step that either is not performed or only a cursory examination is carried out because it is easier and quicker to take a blood sample or use an endoscope. The following key aspects of the clinical examination are related to body systems likely to affect athletic capacity.

RESPIRATORY SYSTEM

The nostrils should be checked for signs of nasal discharge, and airflow can be determined grossly at rest. It is usual to percuss over the frontal and maxillary sinuses to determine whether there is dullness or evidence of pain. This is important if the horse has any signs or history of nasal discharge. When percussing over the sinuses, it is useful to place a thumb in the interdental space to slightly open the mouth, since the sound is magnified.

One of the key aspects of a physical examination in performance horses is palpation of the larynx. Because of the high incidence of idiopathic laryngeal hemiplegia (ILH) in thoroughbred horses, digital palpation of the dorsal cricoarytenoid muscle should be undertaken in all athletic horses with reduced performance. Where there is ILH, palpation will reveal a loss of muscle mass of the left dorsal cricoarytenoid muscle resulting in increased prominence of the muscular process of the left arytenoid cartilage. Palpation of the larynx is done standing on the left side of the horse and facing toward the front of the animal. The larynx is palpated on the left and right sides using the index finger inserted under the tendon of the sternocephalicus muscle, palpating dorsally until the prominence of the muscular process of the arytenoid cartilage is felt. A more notable muscular process on the left side of the larynx indicates atrophy of the left dorsal cricoarytenoid muscle and thus the likelihood of ILH. During this palpation, it is important to note whether there is enlargement of the retropharyngeal or intermandibular lymph nodes. Following palpation of the muscular process, the cricotracheal membrane can be palpated to determine whether the cough reflex may be elicited more easily than normal.

The character of the respiration should be observed as well as the respiratory frequency to determine whether the rate is elevated or whether inspiratory or expiratory phases are prolonged. This observation provides a guide to the presence of lower airway disease. Using a stethoscope, the trachea should be auscultated as well as the lung fields on both left and right sides of the thorax to detect any abnormal sounds. Any suspicious noises ("gurgles" or "wheezes") can be accentuated further by increasing the respiratory rate and tidal volume. This is most easily done by having the horse rebreathe from a plastic bag placed over the nostrils. The bag is usually left in position for 1 to 2 minutes, and key areas of the lung fields are auscultated with a stethoscope. If there is any possibility that fluid is present in the thorax, percussion of both sides of the chest should be carried out so that dull areas can be detected.

CARDIOVASCULAR SYSTEM

Cardiovascular abnormalities are responsible for many cases of poor performance in athletic horses. In young horses, congenital abnormalities such as ventricular septal defects should be high on the list of differential diagnoses. Older horses have a number of acquired cardiovascular diseases, varying from conduction disturbances to alterations in valve function. The important components of the cardiovascular examination hinge on examination of mucous membrane color and capillary refill time, examination of the peripheral pulses (both arterial and venous), and auscultation of the heart. Very few horses with poor performance will have abnormalities of pulse quality or changes in mucous membrane color or capillary refill time. However, abnormalities of pulse rhythm may be an indication of a potential problem. It is important to note that second-degree atrioventricular block and sinoatrial block are common findings in all performance horses, and therefore, a regular missing beat is of little clinical significance when examining the pulse or heart rhythm.

When auscultating the heart, it is essential to examine routinely both the left and right sides. Too often clinicians become used to examining only the left chest and fail to auscultate over the right chest wall, thus failing to detect a number of heart murmurs. Normally, three to four heart sounds can be heard with the fourth, first and second heart sounds being most obvious. The fourth heart sound is also called the *atrial sound* because it is associated with atrial contraction at the end of diastole. The first heart sound occurs shortly after this fourth sound, and some clinicians mistakenly diagnose a split first heart sound rather than the two distinct sounds associated with atrial contraction (S_4) and atrioventricular valve closure (S_1). It is important to auscultate the heart over a wide area of the lower left and right chest walls and to listen for at least 2 to 3 minutes. Some dysrhythmias may require several minutes to evaluate, particularly when the rhythm disturbance is very irregular.

The major cardiac murmurs may be auscultated over a wide area of the chest, but some murmurs which are pathologic may be quite localized. Lower-grade systolic murmurs localized to the anterior aspect of the left chest wall are common in athletic horses and do not necessarily indicate any pathologic problem. Most commonly, these innocent murmurs (ejection murmurs) are heard well forward on the left chest wall. To assess the significance of a murmur on performance, treadmill exercise testing may be useful to examine heart rate responses as well as measurements of maximal oxygen

pulse ($\dot{V}_{O_2}$/HR), which provide an indirect method for assessment of stroke volume (see Chap. 12).

Atrial fibrillation is a common cause of dramatically reduced athletic performance and appears to be found more commonly in standardbred trotters and pacers than in other performance horses. If there is no overt cardiac disease, such cases respond well to cardioversion using quinidine sulfate administered via a nasogastric tube at a dose rate of 20 mg/kg given every 4 hours for a total of four to seven doses. There are several reports of successful racing performance in horses following the treatment of atrial fibrillation with quinidine sulfate.[2,3]

MUSCULOSKELETAL SYSTEM

A surprising number of horses presented because of poor performance are lame at the time of presentation, and this may not be recognized by the trainer or owner. While it is not possible to diagnose a musculoskeletal problem as the main contributing factor to poor performance, resolution of such problems will often result in improvement in exercise capacity. However, it is important to realize that a number of successful horses often will have low-grade lameness problems that do not appear to affect their athletic capacity. Because of the high incidence of lameness in horses with poor performance, it is important to do a careful and detailed examination of the musculoskeletal system.

Examination Procedure

The examination should commence with careful observation of the horse at rest, looking for any signs of asymmetry (muscle atrophy) or swelling around joints or tendons. After noting any areas that may require a more detailed examination, the gait of the horse is then assessed. The horse should then be walked, turned, and backed so that ataxia can be detected. Cervical spinal cord disease, which is common in young, rapidly growing horses, can result in poor performance. If there are signs of neurologic dysfunction, a complete neurologic examination can be performed.[4]

The horse is then trotted on a firm, hard surface, and any gait abnormalities are noted. Most horses presented for poor performance do not have severe lameness, and in the majority of cases, it is grade 1 or 2.[5] Following the examination at the trot, we undertake a series of flexion tests involving both the front limbs and hindlimbs. The first flexion test performed is pastern and fetlock flexion with the carpus extended and firm pressure applied to the toe. The leg is held in this position for 1 minute, and the horse is trotted off, with note being made of worsening of the lameness. Following this, carpal flexion is performed without any flexion of the pastern or fetlock, and the flexion is again applied for 1 minute, after which the horse is trotted off and any exacerbation of lameness noted. The same test is applied to the opposite front limb, after which the hindlimb flexion tests are performed. We undertake a flexion test of the hind fetlocks with as little flexion of the hock as possible, followed by a traditional spavin test, where the hock and stifle are held in flexion for 2 minutes and the horse trotted off. With all tests, one or two abnormal steps following flexion cannot be regarded as abnormal, but lameness, if apparent or worsened following flexion, should be regarded as significant.

The next part of the examination concentrates on the back. Back disorders are a common cause of poor performance.[6] In many horses with back problems, poor performance may be the only presenting sign, although changes in temperament, head shaking, and signs of pain when being ridden are also relatively frequent presenting signs. Examination of the back should concentrate initially on any changes in back contour, which is best done by the observer standing on a box or some similar object so that asymmetry of the back can be detected from behind the horse. Firm palpation along the longissimus dorsi muscles is helpful in localizing any muscular pain. Many horses with back pain will be reluctant to ventroflex or dorsiflex their backs when pressure is applied over the thoracolumbar or caudal sacral regions. This can indicate a back disorder, as can hypersensitivity in one region of the back. The thoracolumbar regions are the most common sites for lesions in pleasure horses, while sacroiliac pain, manifested by extreme hypersensitivity when applying pressure over the tuber sacrale, is a common site for back problems in standardbred pacers.

After these phases of the initial examination, a more detailed examination can be carried out to evaluate any areas of the limbs that have shown potential problems on the initial examination. Standard examination techniques are performed commencing at the hoof and working proximally to localize any painful areas. If more definitive localization is required, the use of nerve blocks and intraarticular anesthesia may be required.[7] A number of conditions can give rise to poor performance, and some of the major problems that we have found in horses presented to our clinic will be discussed.

Pedal Osteitis. This disorder is found commonly in racehorses that are shod so that the sole bears more weight than it should, and the condition can be found in horses working on hard, jarring surfaces. Most horses have the problem bilaterally in the forelimbs, with the main clinical signs being a reluctance to stretch out so that in some cases the horses look like they are stepping on hot bricks. Pain is present when the feet are examined with hoof testers. Most horses will respond to nonsteroidal anti-inflammatory drugs combined with corrective shoeing to remove some of the pressure on the sole.

Navicular Disease. Navicular disease is a common problem afflicting older horses (usually greater than 6 years of age) and is particularly common in larger horses such as warmbloods and quarter horses. It causes a chronic, progressive bilateral forelimb lameness, although in most horses one forelimb is affected more than the other. Most horses with navicular disease will show worsening of the lameness after a pastern and fetlock flexion test, although usually there is no pain on flexion itself. There

are a variety of treatment options from corrective shoeing using egg-bar shoes through treatment with isoxsuprine hydrochloride and in some cases palmar digital neurectomy.

Dorsal Metacarpal Disease ("Bucked Shins"). Bucked shins is the single most important cause of lameness and poor performance in 2-year-old racehorses. A combination of bone immaturity and inadequate training preparation results in an inflammatory reaction in the midregion of the dorsal metacarpus. The problem usually affects both forelimbs, and the horse shows a reluctance to stretch out during training and racing exercise. If horses are maintained in training, there is usually notable reduction in performance. The condition is best treated by short rest periods and administration of anti-inflammatory drugs when the acute problem is evident, followed by careful and progressive increases in training duration and intensity.

Plantar Fetlock Chips. Plantar fetlock chips occur in the hind fetlock joints and are probably more common than is realized. In the last few years, we have found a number of poorly performing standardbred pacers in which chip fractures on the plantar aspect of the proximal phalanx have been the only significant finding on examination. Many of these horses had little or no lameness at presentation, with some showing a grade 1 lameness after fetlock flexion of the appropriate hindlimb. Following arthroscopic surgery to remove the fractured pieces, a high percentage of these horses returned to their previous racing ability.

Bone Spavin. A number of horses with back disorders will have primary hock problems, particularly bone spavin. Most horses respond positively to the spavin test, and in many cases, lameness will be evident. However, because many hindlimb lamenesses may be difficult for owners or trainers to detect, they may be unaware of the hindlimb problem when the horse is presented. Treatment options include intraarticular steroids and fusion of the affected joint, which can be achieved chemically by using monoiodoacetate injections or by surgical arthrodesis.

Rhabdomyolysis ("Tying Up"). Rhabdomyolyis, or "tying up," afflicts all types of athletic horses but appears to be more common in fillies and mares than in stallions and geldings. In some horses, there may be few clinical signs apart from poor performance, and the condition may only become evident on serum or plasma biochemical tests where elevations in muscle-derived enzymes are found. In horses performing prolonged exercise, the condition is usually acute and severe, but in racehorses, it tends to be a recurrent, low-grade problem. Because electrolyte deficiencies have been incriminated in the etiology of the condition,[8] determination of fractional excretions of electrolytes may be useful so that electrolyte supplements can be added to the diet. In chronic, severe cases, treatment with phenytoin has been used successfully.[9]

Obviously, there are a wide range of other musculoskeletal problems that can contribute to poor performance. Fetlock and carpal joint disease and tendon and ligament injuries are all common in athletic horses (see Chap. 15). However, in most of these cases, the condition may manifest itself more clearly than some of the injuries discussed in the preceding list. The key in all poor performance cases is a careful and detailed examination.

Diagnostic Aids

HEMATOLOGY AND PLASMA OR SERUM BIOCHEMISTRY

The significance of a range of abnormalities occurring in the hemogram or plasma or serum biochemistry of athletic horses is discussed in detail in Chapter 5. Hematologic and plasma or serum biochemical findings are critical to any evaluation of poor performance. However, too often significance is placed on mild changes in the neutrophil/lymphocyte ratio, red cell indices, and plasma protein and minor electrolyte alterations. Our experience in horses that have normal clinical findings on examination is that a single sample of blood for hematology and biochemistry will fall within the normal ranges for the breed. Therefore, it is often helpful if previous routine hemograms and biochemical measurements have been performed, because values for an individual horse will be in a much narrower range than values for the breed. There are a number of changes that may be of significance when evaluating poor performance.

Alterations in the Leucocyte Count and Distribution. Some horses with subclinical infections will show only small increases in leukocyte count together with an increase in neutrophils. Others in the early stages of viral disease may show both a leukopenia and a neutropenia. It is important to note that the neutrophil/lymphocyte ratio fluctuates markedly during the course of the day, and therefore, care is needed in interpretation of results.

Plasma Fibrinogen Levels. Fibrinogen is elevated in any inflammatory process, and in chronic problems, values in excess of 3 g/liter (0.3 g/dl) are abnormal and may indicate a focus of inflammation or infection. This is a measurement we have found valuable in a number of horses presented for poor performance. While it is not common to find elevated fibrinogen values, a small percentage of horses with poor performance suffer from chronic low-grade infection, and in these cases, the fibrinogen values provide the most valuable clue to the problem.

Plasma or Serum Enzyme Values. A number of cases of rhabdomyolysis will not be evident from clinical examination alone. Therefore, any horse with reduced performance should have measurements of plasma creatine kinase (CK) and aspartate amino transferase (AST) performed.[10] It also may be useful to determine CK concentrations before and 1 to 2 hours after a treadmill exercise test. Horses that have more than a twofold increase in CK values may have a muscle problem.

Some clinicians attach great significance to changes in plasma or serum electrolyte concentrations. However, most horses free of clinical disease regulate the plasma or serum concentrations of these electrolytes so that abnormalities are seldom found. It is important to note that the electrolyte values in serum or plasma do not reflect total-body concentrations and that substantial changes in various other measurements occur during the course of the day. Great care should be taken, therefore, before the poor performance is attributed to an electrolyte abnormality.

UPPER RESPIRATORY TRACT ENDOSCOPY

Upper respiratory tract endoscopy should always be a routine part of evaluation with a poor performance case. In many upper airway problems there will be a history of an abnormal respiratory noise during exercise or coughing. However, in some cases, no respiratory noise may be noted. Soft palate displacement may present in some horses as a sudden and severe decrease in the horse's performance, with no abnormalities detectable in the resting examination.

The most commonly observed problems associated with poor performance are idiopathic laryngeal hemiplegia, epiglottic entrapment, and soft palate displacement. Some abnormalities do not show up in the horse at rest, with some cases of soft palate displacement and laryngeal hemiplegia becoming evident only during fast exercise. In such cases, upper respiratory tract endoscopy during treadmill exercise is useful. In examining a number of horses with histories consistent with soft palate displacement, we have found that displacement is impossible to create during routine treadmill exercise evaluation. In these cases, we use long reins and a bit to achieve poll flexion, and in some cases the soft palate displacement can be produced. It is also important to remember that some abnormalities may be of no clinical significance. For example, we have seen some horses with entrapment of the epiglottis in which the arterial blood gases during exercise have been unaffected.

BRONCHOALVEOLAR LAVAGE

Bronchoalveolar lavage (BAL) is a valuable technique for evaluating the poor performance horse because of the high incidence of viral respiratory tract disease in athletic horses. The technique is carried out in the standing horse using a special catheter (BAL catheter, Bivona Corporation, Gary, Ind.) passed via the ventral nasal meatus into the trachea and from there distally to wedge in a bronchus. In most cases, the catheter wedges in a bronchus supplying the dorsocaudal lung fields, and a cuff on the distal tip of the catheter can be inflated to seal that particular lung section off. We routinely use between 65 and 100 ml of sterile saline, lavaged into the lung segment and reaspirated. The bronchoalveolar la-

Table 13-2. Bronchoalveolar Lavage Findings (Mean ± SD) in 62 Normal Thoroughbred Racehorses in Training

Measurement	1-Year-Olds	2-Year-Olds	3-Year-Olds	4-Year-Olds and Older
Volume retrieved (ml)	38 ± 5	41 ± 4	40 ± 7	40 ± 5
Nucleated cells (/μl)	547 ± 221	721 ± 536	835 ± 609	1187 ± 639
Macrophages (%)	54 ± 5	59 ± 9	64 ± 9	57 ± 11
Hemosiderophages (% of macrophages)	2 ± 2	13 ± 18	19 ± 19	43 ± 28
Neutrophils (%)	12 ± 8	9 ± 7	7 ± 5	10 ± 6
Lymphocytes (%)	34 ± 7	32 ± 10	29 ± 9	31 ± 11
Eosinophils (%)	0.5 ± 3.1	0.2 ± 0.8	0.1 ± 0.1	1.9 ± 6.5
Epithelial cells (%)	0.1 ± 0.1	0.4 ± 0.8	0.6 ± 1.2	0.3 ± 0.5
Erythrocytes (% total cells)	0.1 ± 0.2	11 ± 20	10 ± 12	16 ± 24
Number of horses	10	20	18	14

Note: In all cases, 65 ml of saline was infused for the sample collection.
From McKane SA et al: Aust Vet J 1993; 70–401.

vage findings from 62 normal thoroughbred horses in race training are presented in Table 13–2. We have found that 100 percent of horses that are racing or ready to race will have hemosiderophages in the bronchoalveolar lavage fluid, indicating exercise-induced pulmonary hemorrhage. It is difficult in these cases to correlate presence of hemosiderophages with any adverse effects on performance. Undoubtedly, there are horses with exercise-induced pulmonary hemorrhage in which the athletic capacity is affected, but it is difficult to determine this from the BAL findings unless a blood-contaminated sample is obtained. Of more significance is the presence of large numbers of neutrophils in the BAL sample, and we regard horses with more than 15 percent neutrophils in the BAL fluid as being abnormal. Further evaluation of the significance of the BAL abnormalities can be undertaken by performing arterial blood gas analysis during exercise (see Chap. 12).

ELECTROCARDIOGRAPHY

We perform an electrocardiogram on all horses presented for poor performance. Electrocardiography is most useful for determining the cause of dysrhythmias and diagnosing conduction abnormalities. Common dysrhythmias, where there is regular dropping of beats, include second-degree atrioventricular block and sinoatrial block. Second-degree atrioventricular block is characterized by the presence of a P wave followed by no QRS complex or T wave. In some cases, this may appear intermittently on the trace, while other beats may be dropped regularly every four or five normal heartbeats. In contrast, sinoatrial block is characterized by no impulse generation, and therefore, the R-R interval is double normal as the block occurs. Both these dysrhythmias do not cause performance problems and appear to be the result of high vagal tone in the normal horse at rest, because the dysrhythmia disappears at higher heart rates when the horse exercises.

The most serious dysrhythmia, with effects on performance, is atrial fibrillation, which can be suspected

from auscultation and confirmed by electrocardiography by characteristic f, or flutter, waves between irregularly spaced QRS complexes. Conduction abnormalities that cannot be detected by auscultation include intraatrial block, where the P-wave duration is prolonged greater than 0.17 s in lead 2, and intraventricular block, where the QRS complex duration is prolonged greater than 0.16 s. In racehorses, these abnormalities appear to have a serious affect on performance, and in most cases, recovery does not occur.

Abnormalities of the T wave with typical positive and peak T waves in chest leads on the electrocardiogram are considered by many veterinarians to indicate an abnormality. Some studies[11,12] found a higher incidence of T-wave abnormalities in poorly performing horses than in a normal group. However, Evans[13] reported that in English racehorses, T-wave abnormalities appeared to be more likely to be related to training stage because horses at a more advanced stage of training had more of these "abnormalities." Furthermore, using Timeform rating as an index of performance, horses with T-wave abnormalities did not have a significantly lower level of performance. More recently, in testing carried out at the Equine Performance Laboratory at the University of Sydney, T-wave abnormalities were not found to result in abnormalities in horses tested on a high-speed treadmill.[14] Thus considerable care should be taken before ascribing the performance problem to T-wave abnormalities.

TREADMILL VIDEO GAIT ANALYSIS

Treadmill gait analysis to assess subtle gait alterations[15] that could be the cause of poor performance can be done with commercial video equipment, although more sophisticated equipment will allow greater precision. This assessment is performed with the treadmill set on the flat, and the symmetry of motion is evaluated. Some of the major aspects of gait analysis are described in Chapter 3, and further details can be found in the article by Seeherman and others.

TREADMILL EXERCISE TESTING

We find that exercise testing using a high-speed treadmill is helpful in many difficult cases to determine the cause of the poor performance. Not only is exercise testing useful for the diagnosis of problems which would otherwise be hard to detect, but also such testing can be helpful in evaluation of the significance of findings such as heart murmurs and abnormal BAL results, where the clinical significance of the findings may be questionable. Full details of exercise testing measurements are given in Chapter 12.

NUCLEAR SCINTIGRAPHY

A number of lameness disorders that may contribute to poor performance in athletic horses can be diagnosed using scintigraphy. In the past, a high-cost gamma camera was necessary for this evaluation, but more recently, the availability of a hand-held scintigraphy probe has put scintigraphy into the realm of the specialist equine practitioner. Details and indications for nuclear scintigraphy are given in Chapter 14C.

Conclusions

Determining the reasons for poor performance in athletic horses is often difficult. In some cases, few abnormalities may be found on a detailed clinical examination, or the problems found may not be contributing to the performance problem. In most cases, it is essential to undertake a careful examination that involves the judicious use of various diagnostic aids to help in narrowing the possible causes of poor performance or to enable a positive diagnosis. While more sophisticated techniques such as treadmill exercise testing, video gait analysis, and nuclear scintigraphy are helpful, the cause of poor performance can be determined in many cases by the combination of a detailed clinical examination together with standard diagnostic tests.

References

1. Seeherman HJ, Morris EA: Application of a standardised treadmill exercise test for evaluation of fitness in 10 thoroughbred racehorses. Equine Vet J Suppl 1991; 9:26.
2. Rose RJ, Davis PE: Treatment of atrial fibrillation in three racehorses. Equine Vet J 1977; 9:68.
3. Deem DA, Fregin GF: Atrial fibrillation in horses: A review of 106 clinical cases, with consideration of prevalence, clinical signs, and prognosis. J Am Vet Med Ass 1982; 180:261.
4. Mayhew IG: Large Animal Neurology: A Handbook for Veterinary Clinicians. Philadelphia, Lea & Febiger, 1989.
5. Stashak TS: Lameness. In TS Stashak (ed): Adam's Lameness in Horses. Philadelphia, Lea & Febiger, 1987, p 551.
6. Jeffcott LB: The examination of a horse with a potential back problem. In Proceedings of the 31st Convention of the American Association of Equine Practitioners, 1985, p 353.
7. Stashak TS: Diagnosis of Lameness. In Stashak TS (ed): Adam's Lameness in Horses. Philadelphia, Lea & Febiger, 1987.
8. Harris PA, Snow DH: Role of electrolyte imbalances in the pathophysiology of the equine rhabdomyolysis syndrome. In Perrson SGB, Lindholm A, Jeffcott LB (ed): Equine Exercise Physiology 3. Davis, Calif, ICEEP Publications, 1991, p 432.
9. Beech J: Equine muscle disorders. Proc Am Coll Vet Intern Med 1992; 10:397.
10. Valberg S, Haggendal J, Lindholm A: Blood chemistry and skeletal muscle metabolic responses to exercise in horses with recurrent exertional rhabdomyolysis. Equine Vet J 1993; 25:17.
11. Rose RJ, Davis PE: The use of electrocardiography in the diagnosis of poor racing performance in the horse. Aust Vet J 1978; 54:51.
12. Stewart JH, Rose RJ, Davis PE, et al: A comparison of electrocardiographic findings in racehorses presented either for routine examination or poor racing performance. In Snow DH, Persson SBG, Rose RJ (eds): Equine Exercise Physiology. Cambridge, Granta Editions, 1983, p 135.
13. Evans DL: T-waves in the equine electrocardiogram: Effects of training and implications for race performance. In Persson SGB, Lindholm A, Jeffcott LB (eds): Equine Exercise Physiology 3. Davis, Calif, ICEEP Publications, 1991, p 475.
14. King C, Rose RJ, Evans DL: The effects of electrocardiographic abnormalities and heart murmurs on exercise capacity in racehorses. (In preparation.)
15. Seeherman HJ, Morris E, O'Callaghan MW: Comprehensive clinical evaluation of performance. In Auer JA (ed): Equine Surgery. Philadelphia, WB Saunders Co, 1992; p 1106.
16. McKane SA, Canfield PJ, Rose RJ: Equine bronchoalveolar lavage cytology: Survey of thoroughbred racehorses in training. Aust Vet J 1993; 70:401.

Diagnostic Imaging in the Athletic Horse: Radiology

R. K. W. SMITH AND P. M. WEBBON

Over the last 60 years, radiographs have played an increasingly important role in equine veterinary diagnosis. Use of radiographs has increased diagnostic acuity, has enabled better monitoring of the progress of lesions, and has led to improved understanding of the nature of many diseases. Radiographs have become so widely used that horse owners may ascribe to a radiographic examination a level of diagnostic certainty denied to the other aspects of a routine clinical examination. The veterinary profession sometimes contributes to this misconception.

In its simplest form, a radiographic examination allows determination of position, number, shape, size, density, margination, and, to a limited extent, function of those structures which are radiographically visible. Like photographs, radiographs are two-dimensional and show the appearance of the subject only at the time that the exposure was made.

Repeatedly, horses are examined that remind us that it is often difficult to reconcile radiographic changes with clinical signs (Figs. 14A–1 and 14A–2) and that radiography is only part of an examination. Radiographs rarely, if ever, should be viewed alone without an appreciation of the whole clinical picture.

This section deals with the radiology of conditions that are important either because they are the result of equestrian activities or because they are likely to affect a horse's athletic performance. The section is divided to describe conformational and developmental abnormalities which may prejudice an animal's performance and those conditions which are the result of trauma, either acute or repetitive, to which athletes of any species are constantly exposed.

Conformation and Its Contribution to Athletic Injury

FOOT BALANCE

The debate continues on the contribution that conformation makes to the development of lameness in horses.

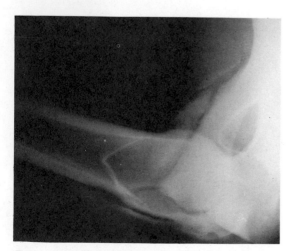

Figure 14A-1. *Flexed craniomedial-caudolateral oblique view of the elbow joint of an 8-year-old gelding kicked on the lateral aspect of its elbow joint 12 months previously. Despite the nonunion fracture, the horse was clinically sound and in work.*

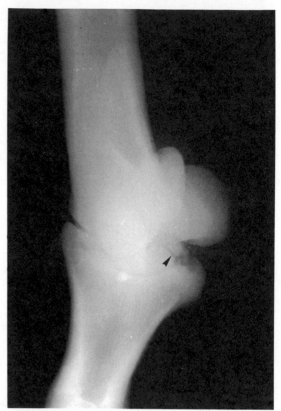

Figure 14A-2. *Dorsomedial-proximoplantarolaterodistal oblique projection of the hindlimb of a 12-year-old gelding. This osteochondral lesion (arrow) was an incidental finding.*

In the past, claims of the importance of conformation have probably been exaggerated, since many animals with poor conformation are able to compete satisfactorily. However, any departure from the ideal conformation will tend to exert specific stresses on the appendicular skeleton of the horse, the effect of which will depend on the severity of the conformational abnormality, the degree of exercise, and the innate ability of the animal to remodel its bone to neutralize such stresses. The effectiveness of bone remodeling is influenced by the age at which exercise commences and the intensity of the training schedule. Hence horses can compensate for conformational abnormalities if they are not exercised until they have reached skeletal maturity and the training method allows their bones time to remodel. This is thought to be particularly true for conformational abnormalities of the foot with respect to the pathogenesis of navicular disease.[1]

At present, the mainstay of navicular disease treatment is centered on the correction of foot balance. The parameters of ideal foot conformation are laid out in Table 14A–1 and in Figure 14A–3. Any departure from this ideal is considered detrimental to the biomechanical function of the foot, resulting in abnormal force vectors which trigger remodeling changes within the foot (especially the navicular bone) as well as soft-tissue stresses that may or may not cause lameness. While much can

Table 14A-1. Normal Foot Conformation Determined Radiographically

Lateromedial radiograph	Dorsopalmar radiograph
Dorsal wall of hoof should be 45 to 50 degrees in the forefoot and 50 to 55 degrees in the hindfoot	The height of each wall should be equal (although the medial wall should be more vertical) *provided that* there is no angular limb deformity above the foot
Walls of the heel should be parallel to the dorsal wall	
Height of heels should be approximately one-third the dorsal wall height	The thickness of the sole should be equal mediolaterally (apart from cases of angular limb deformity)
Solar surface of the distal phalanx should be angled down by 5 to 10 degrees	
A perpendicular from the center of rotation of the distal interphalangeal joint should bisect the weight-bearing surface of the foot	
Normal range of dorsal hoof wall thickness is 14.5 to 21.5mm (unpublished data)	
The solar surface of the hoof should be concave and adequately thick	

Note: Foot-pastern axis, which is also an important factor in distal limb conformation and foot balance, cannot usually be assessed radiographically because of the necessity to raise the foot on a block to obtain lateromedial radiographs of the foot

be gained from an external examination of the foot, radiographic assessment is vital before and during a course of corrective farriery, which aims to return the foot to its ideal conformation (Fig. 14A–4). This may be very difficult to achieve in those horses, often thoroughbreds, with long-toe, low-heel conformations, although the early detection and correction of poor foot conformation should help to prevent future problems.

ANGULAR LIMB DEFORMITY AND CARPAL DISEASE

Recently, emphasis has been placed on carpal conformation and its contribution to increasing the risk of carpal disease.[2] While deformities can be assessed clinically, further information can be obtained from radiographs. In the frontal plane, partial flexion of the carpus ("bucked knees") is not thought to be associated with any pathology. In contrast, overextension of the carpus ("back at the knee") predisposes the carpus to carpal disease.

In the sagittal plane, it is important to know what is normal. A certain degree of external rotation and carpal valgus is considered normal in the foal. As the foal grows, the chest widens and the forelimbs rotate inward and straighten.

Radiographic assessment involves the use of a correctly positioned dorsopalmar view. Lines are drawn along the diaphysis of the radius and metacarpus, parallel to the axis of the bone. It is therefore important to include a substantial amount of the radius and metacarpus in the radiograph, and a large 30 × 24 cm plate usually is required. These lines will meet at the center of deformity, and the angle between the two is the *angle of deformity*. The intersection of the lines will indicate the center of deformity and the origin of the deformity (e.g., carpal bone laxity, epiphyseal wedging) only if there is a single cause of the deformity. However, it is uncommon to find a single origin, in which cases the center of

Figure 14A-3. Diagram to illustrate ideal radiographic foot conformation.

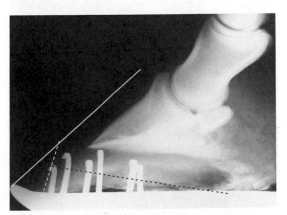

Figure 14A-4. Lateromedial projection of a grossly imbalanced foot. Radiography is useful in formulating a plan for corrective farriery. The egg bar shoe with a rolled toe indicates a previous attempt at corrective farriery. The radiograph shows that the toe of the foot is overgrown and the solar surface of P3 is deviated proximally. The solid line denotes the dorsal hoof wall. The broken lines indicate the extent of the hoof to be removed.

angulation is a summation of the different sites. It is also important to assess the morphology of the epiphyses, the carpal bones, and the heads of the third and fourth metacarpi[3] (Fig. 14A–5). Wedging and hypoplasia of these structures can be responsible for the deformity. Alterations within the physis can indicate "osteochondrosis" or type V or VI Salter-Harris injuries (see below). "Stressed" radiographs will reveal carpal laxity as the cause if the joint spaces are uneven.

Varus deformity is rare and usually precludes successful performance. Pronounced valgus can predispose the horse to chip fractures of the distal lateral radius. However, a certain degree of valgus is protective for carpal disease due to repetitive trauma because it reduces the loading of the medial aspect of the joint.

Axial deformities can be of two types: lateral offset or rotational. Lateral offset is usually centered in the radiocarpal joint and increases the loading down the medial aspect of the carpus. It therefore predisposes to injuries of the middle carpal joint. The presence of carpal valgus in this deformity will be protective and therefore should not be corrected. Similarly, combined varus deformity will exacerbate the effect of the deformity. Ro-

tational deformity has little effect on carpal disease, and a certain degree of external rotation is normal. However, it is often confused with sagittal plane deformities and will complicate the production of an accurate dorsopalmar radiograph for assessment of the sagittal plane deformity.

Developmental Conditions

OSTEOCHONDROSIS

Osteochondrosis is a term applied to a group of conditions recognized in domestic species which share, as a common feature failure of normal endochondral ossification. The condition was first described in detail in animals in 1970 (see, for example, refs. 4 to 6), with recognition and description of the cystic lesions preceding those of the dissecting flaps. The impression of most clinicians is that osteochondrosis lesions are being found with increasing frequency, although this may be due in part to the classification of a greater variety of lesions into the osteochondrosis complex.

In horses, a number of joints may be affected at a variety of sites (Table 14A–2). Osteochondrosis lesions develop when there is failure of differentiation of proliferating cartilage cells in the physis or articular cartilage. Since the cartilage matrix is neither calcified or vascularized, a thickened plug of nonradiopaque cartilage is retained. Necrosis of the basal layer of the retained cartilage precedes further development of the lesion, which is also governed by the site of the retained cartilage.[7]

Peripheral articular cartilage lesions may be "dissected" from the subchondral bone along the fissure line in the necrotic basal layer, resulting in the condition now usually known as *osteochondrosis dissecans* (OCD). Frequently, the separate flap or fragments become calcified and are then visible radiographically.

Alternatively, central lesions in the articular cartilage may collapse and fold in on themselves, leading, ultimately, to a subchondral cyst-like lesion. While these lesions are usually considered to be part of the osteochondrosis complex, there is a possibility that some cystic lesions may be secondary to traumatic fissures in the articular cartilage and others may be secondary to degenerative joint disease.

In most instances, standard radiographic technique and a reasonable level of radiologic competence will allow a diagnosis of the presence of a cystic or dissecting lesion. However, there are occasions when special projections may need to be used (Table 14A–3). Recognition of the lesion should not be too troublesome, but an accurate prediction of its clinical significance may prove more difficult (Table 14A–4). This may be difficult radiographically because it is uncommon for the size of the lesion to be correlated accurately with the severity of the clinical signs.

In general, OCD in high-motion joints results in synovial effusion and variable lameness. OCD lesions in low-motion joints may produce more insidious lameness and degenerative joint disease (DJD), although the only

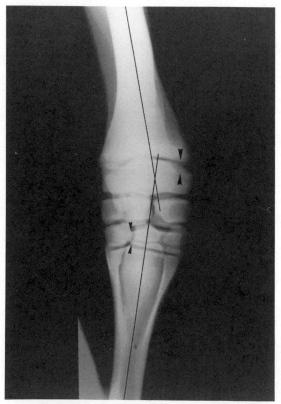

Figure 14A-5. *Dorsopalmar view of the carpus of a 1-month-old foal with a 16-degree valgus deformity of its carpus. There are wedging of the third carpal bone (short arrows) and reactive changes in the medial physis (long arrow). The intersection of the radial and metacarpal axial lines indicates the effective point of the angulation.*

Table 14A-2. Sites of Osteochondrosis and Osteochondrosis-like Lesions

| Joint | Sites of Lesions | |
	Osteochondrosis dissecans	Cystic lesions
Shoulder	Caudal humeral head Glenoid cavity	Glenoid cavity
Elbow	Anconeal process	Lateral humeral condyle Medial proximal radial head
Carpus	Cranial distal radius Distolateral ulnar carpal bone	Carpal bones Distal radius

Fetlock	Dorsal sagittal ridge distal metacarpus/tarsus
	Palmar/plantar distal metacarpus/tarsus (see traumatic
	   osteochondrosis)
	Plantar (palmar) eminences axially and peripherally
	Dorsomedial and dorsolateral proximal proximal
	   phalanx
		Distal third metacarpus/tarsus
		Proximal sesamoid bones
		Proximal, proximal phalanx

Proximal interphalangeal	Dorsoproximal middle phalanx	Distal proximal phalanx Proximal middle phalanx
Distal interphalangeal	Dorsoproximal distal phalanx (extensor process)	Distal phalanx
Hip	Femoral head Acetabulum	
Stifle	Lateral trochlear ridge Medial trochlear ridge Patella	Medial femoral condyle Proximal tibia
Hock	Cranial intermediate ridge of the distal tibia Lateral trochlea ridge of the talus Medial trochlea ridge of the talus Medial (and lateral) malleolus of the tibia	Small tarsal bones, may lead to DJD in young horses, "juvenile spavin"

Note: For proposed pathological classification, see Pool RR: Difficulties in definition of equine osteochondrosis; differentiation of developmental and acquired lesions. Equine Vet J 1993; Suppl 16:5

joints in which DJD develops rapidly and consistently secondary to OCD are the shoulder and proximal interphalangeal joints.[8] Subchondral cystic lesions tend to be responsible for intermittent lameness with insidious onset and little synovial effusion. Older horses occasionally present with a sudden onset of severe lameness which can be related to a cystic lesion, usually involving the distal femur.[8] Scintigraphy of these cases reveals an active lesion (compared with "typical" cystic lesions) presumably due to trauma to the subchondral bone plate overlying the cyst.

In general, it is agreed that where a lesion can be related to lameness, surgical intervention is indicated. Table 14A–4 indicates the frequency with which various lesions may be expected to cause lameness and the likely response to conservative management with rest, nonste-

Table 14A-3. The Radiographic Projections Required to Demonstrate Osteochondrosis

Joint	Projections required
Shoulder	ML of extended joint
Elbow	LM of extended joint CrCa of weight-bearing joint
Carpus	LM and DPa of weight-bearing joint DL-PaM and DM-PaL obliques Obliques determined by carpal bone involved
Fetlock	LM and DPa of weight-bearing joint DL-PaM and DM-PaL obliques D30^{0}Pr-PaDi oblique for cystic lesions of the distal third metacarpal bone Flexed LM for lesions on the dorsal sagittal ridge of the distal third metacarpal bone. D45^{0}L45^{0}Pr-PaMDi and D45^{0}M45^{0}Pr-PaLDi obliques for axial and peripheral plantaroproximal lesions on the proximal phalanx
Proximal interphalangeal	LM and D45°Pr-PaDi oblique of weight-bearing joint
Distal interphalangeal	LM and D60^{0}Pr-PaDi oblique of weight-bearing joint
Hip	VD with animal standing or in dorsal recumbency
Stifle	Ca15^{0}Pr-CrDi and Ca30°L-CrM obliques of weight-bearing joint and flexed LM
Hock	LM, DPl, DL PlM, and DM-PlL obliques of weight-bearing joint

Table 14A-4. The Possible Significance of Osteochondrosis Lesions

| Joint | Possible clinical significance | |
	OCD lesion	Cystic lesion
Shoulder	Humeral head and glenoid cavity Variable degree of lameness; often severe	Glenoid cavity Cysts close to the joint margin often associated with lameness. Appear to move away from the joint with time; lameness may improve
Elbow	Anconeal process*	Lateral humeral condyle and proximal radius*
Carpus	Cranial distal radius and distolateral ulnar carpal bone*	Second and ulnar carpal bones Usually insignificant Radial carpal bone Usually significant Others Variable
Metacarpopha langeal	Sagittal ridge Lameness variable. Young thoroughbreds. May affect all four limbs. Distal metacarpus (metatarsus) Often multiple, associated with marked lameness, rapidly lead to DJD. Dorsal and palmaro/plantaro-proximal phalanx Must differentiate from chip fractures. Often seen in ridden horses with poor performance rather than overt lameness. May become insignificant with time	Distal metacarpus/metatarsus and proximal phalanx Yearlings and 2 year olds. Lameness unrelated to size of lesion, more to degree of synovial effusion and size of communication with joint
Interphalangeal joints	*	Variable significance. May be associated with DJD
Hip	*	
Stifle	Lateral and medial trochlea ridges and patella Mild lameness associated with work	Distal femur and proximal tibia Onset of lameness usually later than in horses with stifle OCD. Prognosis improved if cyst small, central rather than intercondylar, and animal less than 3 years old when presented.
Hock	Distal intermediate ridge, medial and lateral malleolus and trochlea ridges Mild lameness associated with work	Tarsal bones Often associated with DJD

*Rarely seen.

roidal anti-inflammatory agents, controlled exercise, and chondroprotective medication.

Radiology of Osteochondrosis Lesions
Subchondral Cystic Lesions. Cystic lesions may be solitary or multiple. Their size is variable, and their contents have soft-tissue density. Some are surrounded by a zone of sclerosis. No matter which theory of etiology is accepted, there should be at some stage a communication between the joint and the cystic cavity. This may or may not be visible radiographically. If a cystic lesion is followed over a period of time, it may move away from the joint, lose its visible communication with the joint, or fill with bone-density material. Alternatively, the cyst may remain unchanged over time.

In the stifle joint, the most common site for cysts, two groups of lesions have been recognized.[9] In group A, the cysts are discrete, well defined, and in the center of the medial femoral condyle (Fig. 14A–6). They all communicate with the joint, either directly or via a visible neck. The majority are 1 to 2 cm in diameter and show little tendency to regress or fill in. In the smaller group (B), the cysts may be numerous and poorly defined and are found adjacent to the intercondyloid fossa of the distal femur or in the proximal tibia. They are more likely than those in group A to have a peripheral zone of sclerosis and to have no visible communication with the joint. The sites of other cystic lesions have been reviewed by McIlwraith[10] and are described in Tables 14A–2 and 14A–4.

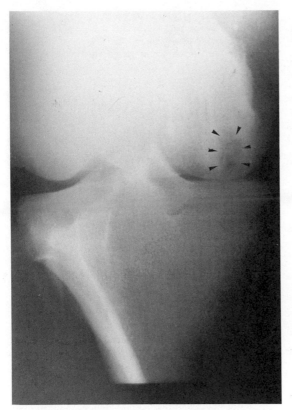

Figure 14A- 6. Caudoproximal-craniodistal projection of the stifle of a 5-year-old mare. There is a single subchondral cystic lesion in the medial femoral condyle (arrows).

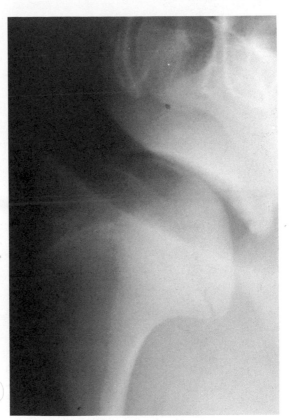

Figure 14A-7. Osteochondrosis dissecans. Lateromedial view of the shoulder joint of a 5-month-old warmblood foal. The caudal margin of the scapula is flattened with sclerosis and roughening of the subchondral bone. The humeral head is flattened. Superimposition of the affected region on the trachea aids recognition of the lesions.

Metaphyseal Osteochondrosis. The persistence of metaphyseal cartilage plugs is found in several species, including the horse, and may be associated with no clinical signs. If the failure of growth plate differentiation and calcification leads to metaphyseal microfractures (more likely in heavy, rapidly growing individuals), a series of events is initiated which leads to the condition often, but erroneously, known as *physitis.* This affects most commonly the distal radius. The metaphyseal microfractures lead to pain and stimulate metaphyseal periosteal new bone reduction, which can be seen both clinically and radiographically.

Osteochondrosis Dissecans. The appearance of these lesions varies from joint to joint but in each joint is usually characteristic. The primary lesion is a subchondral defect which may be associated with ossified or calcified, single or multiple, bodies which more or less follow the outline of the normal subchondral bone architecture. Typical examples are shown in Figures 14A–7 through 14A–9. Single, smooth fragments may be observed separated from the underlying bone by a discrete line of cleavage, or the subchondral bone defect may have a ragged appearance with disruption of the associated osseous fragments. There are, additionally, rather similar

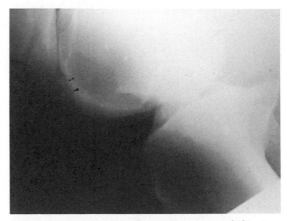

Figure 14A-8. Osteochondrosis dissecans. Lateromedial projection of the stifle of a 4-year-old thoroughbred cross gelding. There are two discrete fragments (arrows) in a defect in the subchondral bone of the lateral femoral trochlear ridge. (See Fig. 14B-31 in the Ultrasound section for corresponding ultrasonographs.)

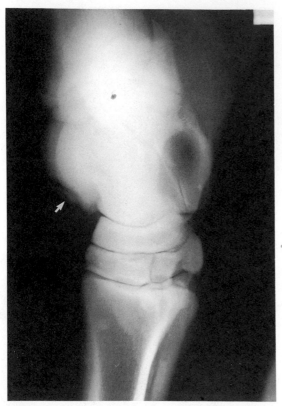

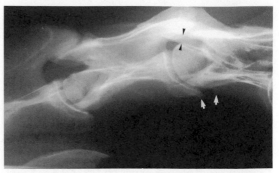

Figure 14A-10. *Lateral view of the second (C2), third (C3), and fourth (C4) cervical vertebrae of a 3-year-old thoroughbred colt. There is dorsal displacement of the cranial edge of C4 with lytic remodeling of the ventral extremity of the caudal endplate of C3 with a "kissing" lesion on the ventral body of C4 (large arrows) and narrowing of the neural canal at the C3–C4 articulation (small arrows).*

Figure 14A-9. *Osteochondrosis dissecans. Dorsomedial-plantarolateral view of the hock of an 18-month-old thoroughbred gelding. An ossified fragment can be identified on the lateral trochlear ridge of the tibial tarsal bone (arrow).*

lesions seen on the dorsoproximal margins of all three phalanges and palmaroproximally on the proximal phalanx which share some of the radiologic features of osteochondrosis.

CERVICAL VERTEBRAL MALFORMATION

Minor malformations of one or more cervical vertebrae may be responsible for few, if any, clinical signs. If the malformation leads to a degree of stenosis of the neural canal, with impingement on the spinal cord either intermittently or constantly, the animal will become ataxic or "wobble." The malformations develop during growth, but the clinical signs may be apparent only when the animal is mature. Thoroughbreds are most frequently affected.

Two main syndromes are described.[11] In the first, usually recognized in young animals, there is apparent instability or abnormal movement between adjacent vertebral bodies, typically C3–4 to C5–6 (Fig. 14A–10). Flexed and extended cervical radiographs should be taken, most easily under general anesthetic, to investigate the full range of vertebral body movement. Dorsoventral enlargement of the vertebral endplates may exacerbate the neural canal stenosis. There may be con-

current malformation of the articular facets, possibly manifestations of osteochondrosis, which may or may not be visible on plain radiographs. Shortening of the vertebral arches contributes to dorsal subluxation of the vertebral body of an affected vertebra. Reference values for the normal ranges of measurements of the dorsoventral diameter of the cervical vertebrae have been published.[12]

Static stenosis of the neural canal is found in older horses, predominantly between 1 and 4 years of age. The lesions are located in the caudal cervical vertebrae and involve the articular facets and, to a lesser extent, the dorsal laminae. Degenerative joint disease of the intervertebral articulations is demonstrable as periarticular, osteophytic proliferation with irregular opacity.

As in other species, an important component of the neural canal stenosis is due to soft tissue, particularly hypertrophy of the ligamentum flavum and joint capsules. This will not be seen on plain films, so a full evaluation of the degree and site of stenosis requires a myelogram. Myelography should only be performed when there is a clear clinical indication—the most obvious is to confirm the site of cord compression before embarking on decompressive surgery.

Most reports describe the use of metrizamide as the contrast agent,[11] but this agent has been associated with adverse reactions in addition to the possible worsening of clinical signs due to general anesthesia and vertebral manipulation.[13] The contrast agent of choice is one of the nonionic isotonic solutions, either iopamidol[14] or iohexol,[15] both of which produce a diagnostic contrast column and relatively few side effects. Whichever agent is used, care should be taken to avoid rostral flow of the agent during subarachnoid injection via the cisterna magna. This is achieved by elevating the horse's head and by using a spinal needle with the bevel directed caudally and then injecting the agent at no more than 5 ml/min. The average horse will require 30 to 40 ml of the agent for a cervical myelogram using an iodine concentration of between 300 and 370 mg/ml.

Narrowing of the contrast column ventrally on a flexed lateral projection may be normal, and both the dorsal and ventral columns must be narrowed to demonstrate cord compression. It is possible to imagine, for example, compression to occur from dorsally on the right to ventrally on the left, which would not be seen on a lateral myelogram. Fortunately, this seems to occur only rarely, and most compressive lesions can be seen using a lateral projection.

Conditions Resulting from Trauma

ACUTE TRAUMA

It is neither the purpose nor the intention of this subsection to describe and illustrate every fracture or dislocation that has ever been seen in the horse. Rather, the aim is to describe the various types of injuries that can be recognized.

Fractures Involving Growth Plates

Many horses are introduced to work before they have reached skeletal maturity, so their cartilaginous growth plates are susceptible to injury. A comprehensive list of all growth plate closure times can be found in a standard text.[16]

The Salter-Harris classification has been modified to classify physeal injuries in horses.[17] (Fig. 14A–11). The incidence and management of physeal fractures have been reviewed extensively.[18,19] All fractures occurred in horses less than 2 years of age, and the most common was type II. Injury to pressure physes generally occurred at earlier ages than those injuries involving traction physes. The most common sites were the proximal femoral physis (pressure physis) and the proximal ulnar physis (traction physis).

Accurate identification of the fracture type is important, since the prognosis tends to worsen as the fracture type number increases. After radiographic growth plate closure, there is still a line of weakness along the site of the growth plate scar. For example, although the supraglenoid tuberosity fuses with the scapula by 12 months, fractures along the fusion line may be seen in horses up to 2 years of age,[20] and indeed, it remains a predilection site for fractures in older horses.[21] These fractures are often distracted by the pull of the bicipital tendon, and oblique caudocranial projections are sometimes necessary for their demonstration.

Appendicular Fractures in the Mature Animal

Appendicular fractures can be broadly divided into three categories: those having diaphyseal and/or metaphyseal components (e.g., long bone fractures), those having only epiphyseal components (osteochondral fractures), and avulsion fractures. Osteochondral fractures can be further divided into chip fractures (involving just the periarticular margin), slab fractures (involving two articular surfaces), and fractures involving bones with no diaphysis or metaphysis (pelvis, scapula, sesamoid, patella, and third phalanx fractures).

Type I - Complete epiphyseal separation

Type II - Epiphyseal separation with metaphyseal fragment

Type III - Epiphyseal fragment

Type IV - Combined epiphyseal and metaphyseal fragment

Type V - Uniaxial physeal injury

Type VI - Uniaxial bridging of physis with bone

Figure 14A-11. *A diagram illustrating the modified Salter-Harris classification of growth plate injuries.*

Long bone fractures tend to occur at predictable sites (Table 14A–5). They may be caused by direct external trauma, spontaneously as a result of a single mechanical stress, or secondary to stress fractures. Multiple views may be necessary to identify accurately the course of a fracture and the extent to which it may involve a joint (Fig. 14A–12).

Fatigue, or stress, fractures are described later as a consequence of repetitive trauma. The frequency with which they precede complete fractures is questionable but appears to depend on the bone involved. Prefracture damage is rarely identified in cases with distal limb fractures, tending to suggest a single traumatic incident as the most important etiologic factor (Riggs, personal communication), while fractures of proximal long bones (especially the tibia, humerus, and femur) have been shown to be commonly associated with earlier incomplete fractures.[22] However, some consider that all apparently spontaneous complete fractures in horses are pre-

Table 14A-5. Common Sites of Long Bone Fractures in Adult Horses

Long bone*	Common fracture site
Humerus	Middiaphysis, spiral or oblique Lateral epicondyle
Radius	Oblique or transverse middiaphyseal ± comminution Lateral tuberosity of distal radius
Ulna	Transverse fracture of olecrannon
Femur	Middiaphyseal ± comminution
Tibia	Oblique or spiral diaphyseal ± comminution Tibial crest avulsion
Metcarpus	Lateral condylar fracture: incomplete or exiting lateral cortex Medial condylar fracture: incomplete or tending to spiral
Proximal phalanx	Sagittal: incomplete or extending to distal articular margin, lateral or medial cortices
Middle phalanx	Often comminuted

*For the purposes of this chapter, a long bone is considered to be a bone possessing an epiphysis, metaphysis, and diaphysis.

ceded by incomplete fracture, and some cases of distal limb fracture have been seen with radiographic evidence of previous incomplete fracture at the site of catastrophic fracture.

The etiopathogenesis of osteochondral fractures has two components: direct trauma and previous bone remodeling changes, similar to the etiopathogenesis of stress/fatigue fractures (e.g., carpal slab fractures). The relative importance of each of these components depends on the joint affected. Direct trauma can result from an external blow or excessive or altered joint movement. Hence dorsolateral or dorsomedial osteochondral fractures of the proximal phalanx can result from overextension of the metacarpophalangeal joint[23,24] (Fig. 14A–13). Similarly, the fragmentation of the distal aspect of the patella which may follow medial patellar ligament desmotomy[25] is thought to arise from altered tracking of the patella within the intertrochlear groove and the impingement of the distal patella on to the lateral trochlear ridge.

Chip fractures can involve a normal articular margin but are invariably the result of a more chronic process. They can result from fracture of a remodeled artic-

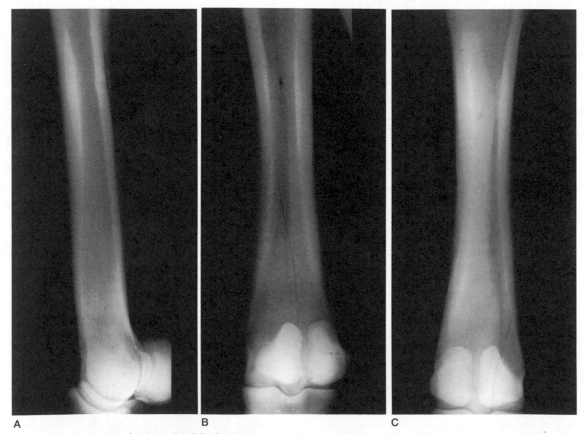

A   B   C

Figure 14A-12. A series of radiographs of the distal metacarpus of a 4-year-old thoroughbred gelding. The full extent of the fracture lines extending proximally and into the metacarpophalangeal joint can only be appreciated by examining all the projections.

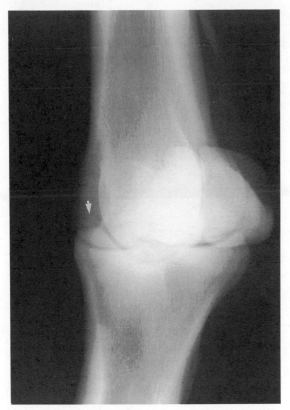

Figure 14A-13. *Dorsomedial-palmarolateral oblique projection of the metacarpophalangeal joint of a 10-year-old thoroughbred-cross mare. A discrete fracture fragment is separated from the dorsolateral articular margin of the proximal phalanx (arrow).*

ular rim or from fracture of periarticular osteophytes concurrent with degenerative joint disease.[26] Thus carpal chip fractures invariably originate from an earlier remodeling change with superimposed direct trauma. Conformational abnormalities will increase the relative contribution of the direct trauma component in the etiopathogenesis of these fractures.

Osteochondral fractures occur in two basic conformations.[24] They can involve the nonarticular portion of the cartilage and the fibrous attachments of the joint capsule and, as a result, are usually minimally displaced. In the second conformation, they involve the articular cartilage and have minimal or no attachments to the fibrous joint capsule. These are therefore commonly displaced and on occasion may become free within the joint. Knowledge of the etiopathogenesis of these fractures helps in the diagnosis of chip fractures and in assessing their significance.

Chip fractures need to be distinguished from so-called secondary centers of ossification and osteochondrosis. Histologically, osteochondrosis and traumatic chip fractures cannot be distinguished,[27,28] so it is not surprising that radiologic differentiation is also very difficult. Osteochondrosis tends to occur at predictable sites, often, but not always, different from the usual site of fractures (compare Tables 14A-2 and 14A-6). The identification of a fracture bed helps to identify a chip fracture, but this is not always present. Often the differentiation relies on the clinical signs and history, as, for example with palmar/plantar ostochondral fragments associated with the metacarpo/metatarsophalangeal joints (Table 14A-7). There is confusion in the literature over their likely etiopathogenesis.[27,29-33]

Fractures of the pelvis, scapula, distal phalanx, patella, and sesamoid bones do not readily fit into the preceding categorization. Pelvic fractures can be imaged radiographically with powerful x-ray generators. The examination can be performed with the horse anesthetized and in dorsal recumbency with a large cassette in a cassette tunnel beneath the hindquarters. However, the dangers of anesthetizing patients with pelvic fractures prompted the development of a technique to radiograph the pelvis with the animal standing.[34] The x-ray beam is directed upward toward a cassette placed above the hindquarters. Good pictures can be achieved with this method (Fig. 14A-14), but careful attention has to be paid to protection of the personnel involved. Alternative diagnostic techniques for the diagnosis of pelvic fractures may be more appropriate, in particular rectal examination, gamma scintigraphy (see Chapter 14C), and ultrasonography (see Chapter 14B).

The prognosis for pelvic fractures is difficult to assess radiographically,[35] although extensive involvement

Table 14A-6. Sites of Common Osteochondral Fractures

Distal interphalangeal joint
  Extensor process
Distal border of the navicular bone
Proximal interphalangeal joint
  Dorsoproximal P2
Metacarpo/metatarsophalangeal (fetlock) joint
  Dorsomedial and dorsolateral proximal P1
  Palmaroproximal P1
  Proximal sesamoid bone fractures
Carpus
  Middle carpal joint
    Distal radial carpal bone
    Distal intermediate carpal bone
    Proximal third carpal bone
  Antebrachiocarpal joint
    Proximal intermediate carpal bone
    Proximal radial carpal bone
    Dorsolateral distal radius
    Dorsomedial distal radius
    Proximal ulnar carpal bone
Shoulder
  Supraglenoid tubercle
Tarsus
  Lateral malleolar fracture
  Tarsal bone fracture (slab)
Stifle
  Distal fragmentation of the patella
  Medial patellar fracture

Table 14A-7. Palmar Osteochondral Fragments of the Metacarpophalangeal Joint

Type	Site	Suggested etiopathogenesis	ʼ Clinical signs
Type 1	Fragments off palmaroproximal P1, either side of the sagittal ridge	Believed to be osteochondrosis[29,30] or avulsion fractures[31]	Mild lameness only at high speed
Type 2	Fragments off the palmar processes of P1	Believed to be osteochondrosis[29,30] or ununited proximopalmar tuberosity[32]	Mild lameness only at high speed
Type 3	Avulsion fractures from the base of the proximal sesamoid bones	Avulsion fractures of the distal sesamoidean ligaments[29,30]	Moderate to severe lameness
Type 4	Ossification within the distal sesamoidean ligaments	Not an osteochondral fragment; do not communicate with joint[29]	No lameness.
Type 5	Fractures of the palmar processes of P1	Traumatic or avulsion fractures[33]	Mild to severe lameness

Based on Foerner JJ, McIlwraith CW: Othopedic surgery in the racehorse. Vet Clin North Am Equine Pract 1990; 6:147.

of the acetabular rim would suggest a poor prognosis for return to athletic function.

Dyson[21] has described the distribution of scapula fractures. In young animals, the cranial part of the glenoid cavity develops from two separate centers of ossification. These two centers unite radiographically by 9 months of age, are fused to the remainder of the scapula by 12 months, and should not be confused with fractures.[21] Fractures of the scapula body and spine are rare

Figure 14A-14. Standing ventrocranial-dorsocaudal projection of the right caudal hemipelvis of a 4-year-old Welsh Cob cross. The ischial fracture caudal to the acetabulum is easily seen.

and present a diagnostic challenge radiographically. Tangential views can be used to demonstrate the fracture, but it may be more easily and reliably detected by scintigraphy or ultrasonography.

Distal phalanx fractures have been divided into six types based on their position and conformation[36] (Table 14A–8). Type VI marginal fractures are commonly associated with laminitis, type V with solar injury, type IV with overextension of the distal interphalangeal joint, and types I to III with direct trauma. Types I and II can sometimes be difficult to identify with the standard lateromedial and dorsoproximal-palmarodistal oblique ("upright pedal") projections. Identification can be improved by using 45-degree oblique projections, angled distally by 45 degrees, of each wing or, alternatively, repeating the examination after 14 days when resorption will have occurred around the fracture line (Fig. 14A–15).

Navicular bone fractures are rare and are usually parasagittal (Fig. 14A–16). Frog shadows should not be confused with navicular bone fractures (Fig. 14A–17). If there is any doubt, the foot should be repacked and a further radiograph obtained and/or a flexor cortex view (palmaroproximal-palmarodistal oblique) taken. Margin fractures of the navicular bone involving the proximal or distal borders can be traumatic in origin but are more likely to be related to remodeling changes within the navicular bone in navicular disease.

Patella fractures may be the result of external trauma, often hitting a jump, in addition to abnormal mobility. Recognition of medial fractures requires a "skyline" projection of the patella.

Table 14A-8. Types of Distal Phalanx Fracture

Type	Conformation
I	Nonarticular wing fracture
II	Articular wing or parasagittal fracture
III	Sagittal fracture
IV	Extensor process fracture
V	Comminuted fracture
VI	Solar margin fractures (associated with laminitis)

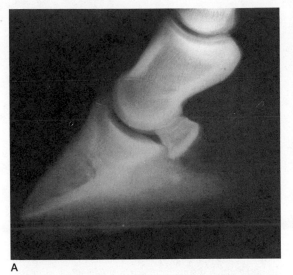
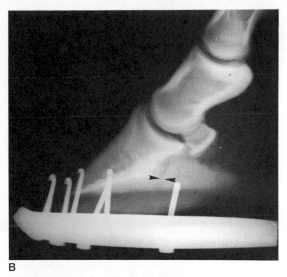

A
B

Figure 14A-15. *Lateromedial projections of the distal phalanges of the left foreleg of a 6-year-old quarter horse gelding. The first radiograph (left) was taken 24 hours after the horse was seen to be lame. No fracture was visible. A second radiograph was taken 14 days later (right), by which time an intra-articular wing fracture of the distal phalanx was visible (arrows).*

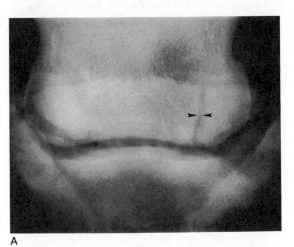
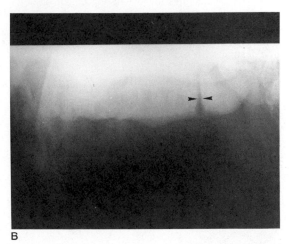

A
B

Figure 14A-16. *Dorsoproximal-palmarodistal (left) and palmaroproximal-palmarodistal (right) views of the navicular bone of a 15-year-old hunter mare with a parasagittal fracture (arrows).*

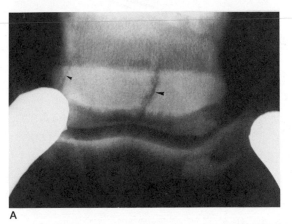
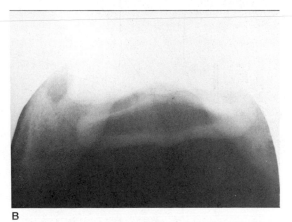

A
B

Figure 14A-17. *Dorsoproximal-palmarodistal (left) and palmaroproximal-palmarodistal (right) views of a navicular bone with packing artifacts mimicking a parasagittal fracture (large arrow) and a wing fracture (small arrow) on one projection. No fracture was visible on any other projection.*

279

Table 14A-9. Proximal Sesamoid Bone Fractures

Type	Conformation
Apical	Involving less than a third of the proximal portion of the sesamoid bone
Midbody	Involving more than a third but less than two-thirds of the sesamoid bone
Basilar	Involving less than a third of the distal portion of the sesamoid bone
Abaxial	Involving the abaxial surface of the proximal sesamoid bone and not usually articular; often associated with suspensory ligament or palmar/platar annular ligament avulsion
Axial/sagittal	Involving the axial portion of the sesamoid bone and often articular; often associated with metacarpal/metatarsal condylar fractures
Foal	Often midbody with distraction; possibly fractures through the cartilage precursor

Avulsion fractures involve an attachment of either a tendon or ligament. Proximal sesamoid bone fractures can be included into this group because most are related to pull of the suspensory ligament or the distal sesamoidean ligaments and are therefore commonly distracted. They have been categorized into a number of types[37-39] (Table 14A–9) and have been related to the stage of training of the animal.[40]

In the early stages of training, soft-tissue injuries predominate, i.e., suspensory ligament strains, while in the later stage of training, proximal sesamoid bone fractures are more common because bone adapts less quickly than soft tissues. Some proximal sesamoid bone fractures are associated with other pathology,[26] commonly suspensory ligament desmitis or lesions on the palmar aspect of the distal metacarpus,[41] while axial sesamoid fractures are often associated with palmar/plantar metacarpal/metatarsal condylar fractures.[38] Oblique projections have been described to examine the basal, apical, and abaxial regions of the sesamoid bones[42,43] (Fig. 14A–18).

A ruptured peroneus tertius commonly has avulsion fragments at its origin on the distal femur. Similarly, cruciate ligament injuries in the horse can be confirmed radiographically by the presence of avulsed fragments at the insertion of either the cranial or caudal cruciate ligaments (Fig. 14A–19). Fracture of the intercondylar eminence of the tibia was thought to be an avulsion fracture, since it was occasionally observed in conjunction with cranial cruciate ligament ruptures. However, the cruciate ligaments do not insert on this eminence, and its fracture is more likely to be related to instability of the stifle which results from a cruciate ligament rupture.

Axial Fractures
Cervical fractures are usually the consequence of a "nose-dive" fall and may or may not be associated with neurologic abnormalities. Any fracture involving the neural canal or resulting in instability of the cervical spine will provoke neurologic signs. Fracture of other areas of the cervical vertebrae will generate neck pain in the acute stage, but with time, dramatic radiographic signs may develop with no clinical abnormalities. A radiographic examination of the spine in cases where neurologic signs result from trauma should include the proximal thoracic vertebrae, since damage to these can be responsible for signs similar to those of cervical vertebral fractures.

Skull fractures are commonly depressed (Fig. 14A–20). Their recognition can present a radiographic challenge, and for safety as well as radiographic quality, it is

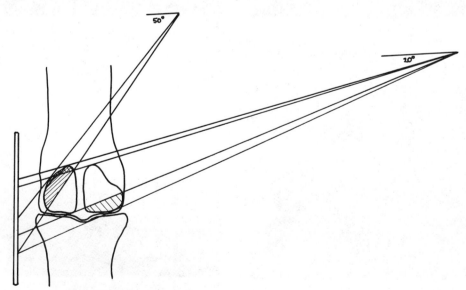

Figure 14A-18. Oblique projections to examine the basal, apical (20 degrees), and abaxial (50 degrees) regions of the sesamoid bones.

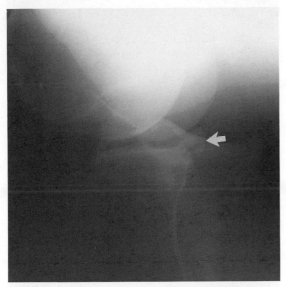

Figure 14A-19. *Lateromedial projection of the stifle of a 9-year-old hunter gelding with a triangular avulsion fracture at the site of the insertion of the caudal cruciate ligament* (arrow).

often preferable to perform a detailed radiographic examination with the horse under general anesthesia. If the paranasal sinuses are involved, hemorrhage within the sinus may be recognized as a fluid line or generalized opacity, depending on the position of the horse.

Vestibular signs following a fall are often associated with fracture of the petrous temporal bone. Radiologic diagnosis of this fracture is difficult, but on a good lateral projection, a fracture can be seen as an interruption to the line of bone below the calvarium.

Mandibular fractures can involve both rami, so oblique radiographs of both rami should be included in any radiographic examination. If the investigation is per-

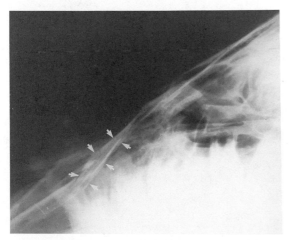

Figure 14A-20. *Lateral view of the maxillary region of 9-year-old Irish draught cross mare with a depressed fracture* (arrows).

formed under general anesthesia, intraoral nonscreened film can be cut to size to fit in the mouth to take a ventrodorsal view of the rostral part of both mandibles and the symphysis.

Luxations/Subluxations

Luxations are easily recognized but fortunately are rare. Subluxations can be more subtle to detect. In both instances, the full extent of the instability and, by inference, the damage to the supporting soft tissues sometimes can only be demonstrated by the use of "stressed" radiographs (Fig. 14A–21). A mild injury to collateral ligaments will result in an uneven joint space, although this should not be confused with the mild uniaxial widening of a normal joint space when stressed uniaxially or narrowing due to uniaxial cartilage loss (Fig. 14A–22). Injury to the supporting structures of a joint can be accompanied by small avulsion fractures (see above). Injuries to the components of the stay apparatus of the distal limb can result in characteristic subluxations. Thus injury to the suspensory ligament and distal sesamoidean ligaments, can result in dorsal subluxation of the proximal interphalangeal joint (Fig. 14A–23). Subluxation of the proximal interphalangeal joint also has been described in young animals associated with flexure deformity of the distal interphalangeal joint.[44] Injury to the deep digital flexor tendon can result in subluxation of the distal interphalangeal joint (Fig. 14A–24).

PROBLEMS SECONDARY TO ACUTE TRAUMA

Infection

Radiographic signs characteristic of infection can be seen in both soft tissues and bone. There is usually considerable soft-tissue swelling, especially with infection of the extremities. If there is an accompanying skin wound, this can sometimes be identified radiographically. Radiolucencies within the soft tissues indicate the presence of gas, either of bacterial origin or most commonly from aspiration of air through the open wound. Careful inspection of such lucencies is important, since radiolucent foreign bodies, e.g., wood (Fig. 14A–25), can occasionally be demonstrated as linear gas shadows.

When a bone is infected, it is important to try to differentiate between osteitis and osteomyelitis. Osteitis is a superficial infection of the cortex. The clinical signs usually are mild, with limited lameness. In contrast, osteomyelitis also involves the medullary cavity and commonly results in moderate to severe lameness. The radiographic findings suggestive of bony infection are mixed lysis and sclerosis (Fig. 14A–26). The pattern of the changes will depend on the organism involved, the age of the animal, the duration of the infection, and the presence of foreign bodies or surgical implants. The changes usually develop rapidly when compared with other bony pathology and may be dramatic. In chronic infections, the sequestration of necrotic bone fragments is a common finding. The sequestrum almost invariably lies within a less radiopaque involucrum, which, in the horse, usually is shallow (Fig. 14A–27).

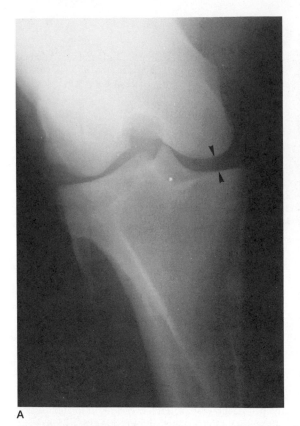 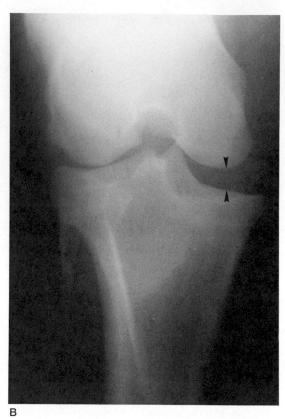

A   B

Figure 14A-21. *Caudoproximal-craniodistal projections of the stifle of an 8-year-old pony mare. The medial joint space (arrows) is equivocally enlarged in an unstressed non-weight-bearing study (left), but a stressed radiograph (right) confirmed severe ligamentous disruption. An autopsy revealed rupture of the medial collateral and both cruciate ligaments and a medial meniscal tear.*

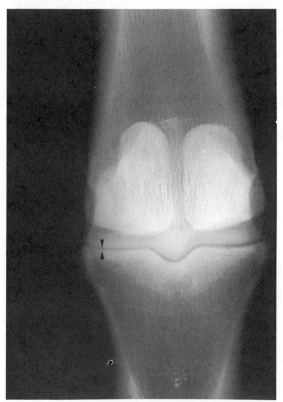

Figure 14A-22. *Dorsopalmar view of the metacarpophalangeal joint of a 14-year-old New Forest pony mare with chronic lameness. There is uniaxial cartilage loss seen as narrowing of the lateral joint space in a weight-bearing study.*

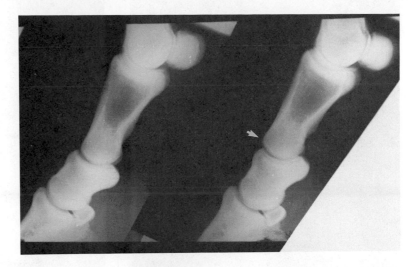

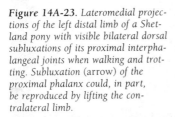

Figure 14A-23. Lateromedial projections of the left distal limb of a Shetland pony with visible bilateral dorsal subluxations of its proximal interphalangeal joints when walking and trotting. Subluxation (arrow) of the proximal phalanx could, in part, be reproduced by lifting the contralateral limb.

One unusual manifestation of infection which has recently been described[45] is osteomyelitis of the axial surface of the proximal sesamoid bones. The etiopathogenesis of this condition is still unclear. There is often no wound, both limbs may be involved, and the most likely explanation is hematogenous infection. Lysis with surrounding sclerosis can be identified in the dorsopalmar/plantar radiograph (Fig. 14A-28). Both limbs should always be radiographed.

The limits of infected wounds, fistulous tracts, and sinuses can be determined by using positive contrast medium or, alternatively, ultrasonography (see Chap. 14B). To ascertain the approximate direction of the tract, a blunt-ended metal probe can be inserted *gently* into its opening, but overenthusiastic use of the probe can cause

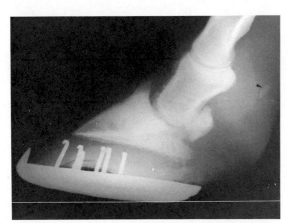

Figure 14A-24. Lateromedial projection of the distal limb of a 15-year-old horse with a history of chronic lameness alleviated by a palmar digital neurectomy. There are advanced chronic accretions of bone on the dorsal surface of the middle phalanx and marked degenerative disease of the distal interphalangeal joint and dystrophic calcification at the site of the neurectomy (arrows). The deep digital flexor tendon has ruptured, leading to a secondary subluxation of the distal interphalangeal joint. The white line indicates the block on which the horse was standing.

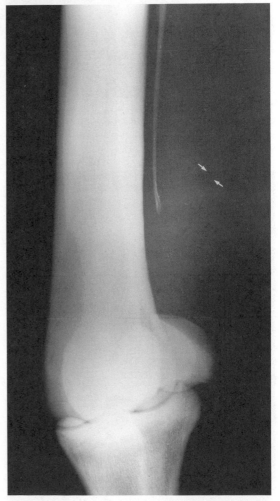

Figure 14A-25. Oblique view of the distal metacarpal region of a horse with a recurrent discharging sinus. Linear gas shadows (arrows) are faintly visible in the soft tissues, characteristic of a wooden foreign body.

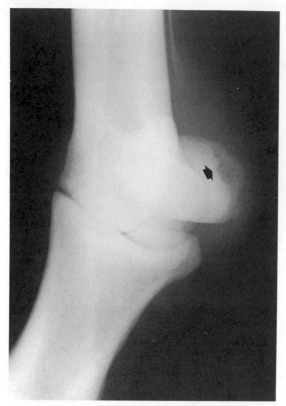

Figure 14A-26. *Osteomyelitis in a proximal sesamoid bone. The destructive focus (arrows) is accompanied by new bone adjacent distal to the lesion. The absence of a sclerotic margin to the lesion suggests that it is active and progressive.*

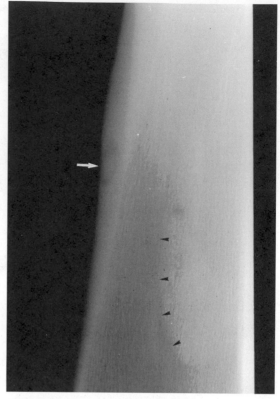

Figure 14A-27. *Chronic radial osteomyelitis with a small sequestrum (large arrows). Sequestra are necrotic bone fragments. They usually are denser than the surrounding hyperemic bone, with well-defined margins and no evidence of periosteal reactivity. Also visible is an incomplete fracture (small arrows).*

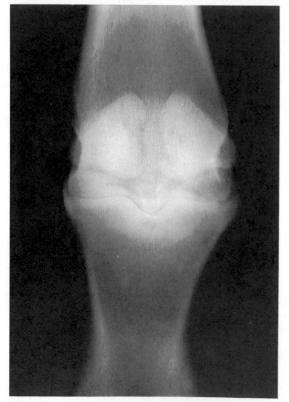

Figure 14A-28. *Dorsoplantar projection of the right hind metacarpophalangeal joint of an 8-year-old thoroughbred mare. The axial border of both proximal sesamoid bones is eroded and poorly defined. These changes are typical of axial border osteomyelitis. In this case there was concurrent infection of the metacarpophalangeal joint, manifested radiographically on this projection as narrowing of the joint space.*

further damage and penetrate as yet unviolated synovial cavities. For a better assessment of the extent of the tract, a water-soluble contrast medium can be introduced into it using a dog urinary catheter.[46] Adequate sealing of the catheter at the skin is essential to ensure complete opacification of the tract. In cases where synovial sepsis is suspected, it is often more helpful to introduce the contrast medium directly into the synovial cavity first to determine whether it is intact. Figure 14A–29 illustrates a suggested protocol for the investigation of a penetrating wound to the foot which provides a good example of a contrast study.

Disuse Osteopenia

Prolonged reduced weight bearing, because of either severe lameness or immobilization within a cast, results in the loss of mineral from bone. Radiographically, this is manifested as a mottled appearance to the distal limb bones with obvious shell-like cortical margins. Changes are usually first noted in the proximal sesamoid bones, where small punched-out lytic regions can be identified (Fig. 14A–30). As the osteopenia progresses, these bones become generally radiolucent and have been described as "ghost sesamoids."[47]

Soft-Tissue Abnormalities

Acute or insidious (chronic) damage to ligamentous structures, including fibrous joint capsules, can result in avulsion fractures and osseous accretions at the ligament-bone junction. These, strictly, are termed *enthesiophytes,* since their pathogenesis is different from that of osteophytes, which represent secondary ossification of a remodeled cartilage rim. Enthesiophytes are commonly seen adjacent to joints exhibiting signs of degenerative joint disease, formed as a result of capsular strain and/or joint instability. Another common site is within the insertional region of the suspensory ligament branches onto the proximal sesamoid bones. Their precise identification often requires oblique projections to highlight the abaxial surfaces of the proximal sesamoid bones.[42] The condition, termed *sesamoiditis,* was thought originally to be characterized by lytic processes, so-called vascular channels, within the proximal sesamoid bones as a result of hyperemia (Fig. 14A–31). Poulos[48] demonstrated that these changes actually represented an overall increase in bone. Enthesiophytes are generated around the vascular channels in response to suspensory ligament damage, thus making them more prominent and giving the characteristic radiographic appearance. If

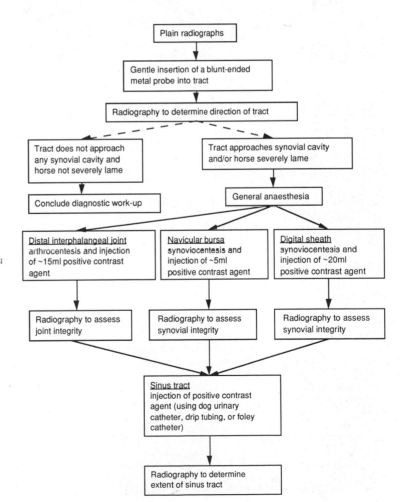

Figure 14A-29. A suggested protocol for the investigation, with contrast media, of a penetrating wound to the foot.

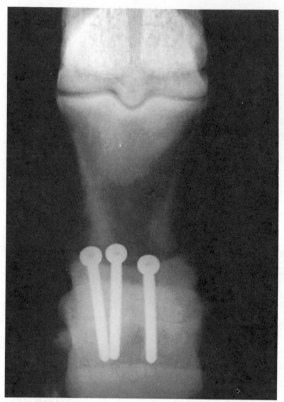

Figure 14A-30. *The right hindlimb of this 16-year-old mare was immobilized in a cast for 6 weeks after arthrodesis of the proximal interphalangeal joint. Disuse osteopenia is most easily seen in the proximal sesamoid bones as numerous, punctate, foci of reduced radiopacity.*

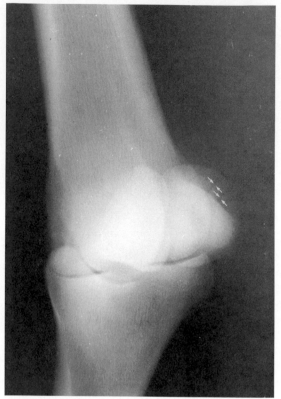

Figure 14A-31. *Linear vascular channels in the proximal sesamoid bones (arrows) are accentuated by enthesiophytes around the channels rather than by demineralization of the channels themselves.*

such changes are identified, ultrasonographic examination of the suspensory ligament is recommended.

Some soft-tissue injuries occur concurrently with bone injuries, such as the association between suspensory ligament injuries and small metacarpal/metatarsal bone fractures (Fig. 14A–32). The mechanism of the association is unclear. The fractures may be avulsions caused by the second or fourth interosseous muscles or may result from vibration forces in the suspensory ligament.

Other soft tissue lesions, such as chronic proliferative synovitis of the metacarpophalangeal (fetlock) joint, may be seen as erosions of adjacent bone. The hypertrophic synovium can be demonstrated using positive contrast or air arthrography or ultrasonography.

Metastatic calcification can occur within soft tissues in response to the local injection of corticosteroids, especially the depot preparations. This is common particularly if corticosteroids have been injected into a tendon or ligament and also can be identified in the synovial membrane of synovial cavities injected with corticosteroids, (Fig. 14A–33). Calcification within tendons or ligaments can occur secondary to injury without steroid injection (Fig. 14A–34).

Chronic or repetitive trauma is thought to be capable of triggering soft-tissue calcification, the mechanism that is thought to be responsible for the formation of "calcinosis circumscripta" masses on the lateral aspect of the stifle, over the tibial crest. These lesions have a particular pattern of calcification characterized by "whorls" of radiodensities (Fig. 14A–35).

REPETITIVE TRAUMA

Fatigue (Stress) Fractures

Fatigue fractures occur in athletes of all species. They are the result of repeated loading during training and racing and occur at specific sites related to the biomechanics of the applied forces. The exact mechanism of fatigue fractures in horses has not been determined, but Riggs and Evans[49] propose that undetected microdamage will lead first to osteon resorption and then to deposition of secondary osteons. There is concurrent periosteal and endosteal production of new bone which adds little to the mechanical stability of the bone. Osteon resorption and secondary osteon development take 2 to 3 months, and full mineralization of the secondary osteon requires a further 4 to 5 months. A correctly designed training

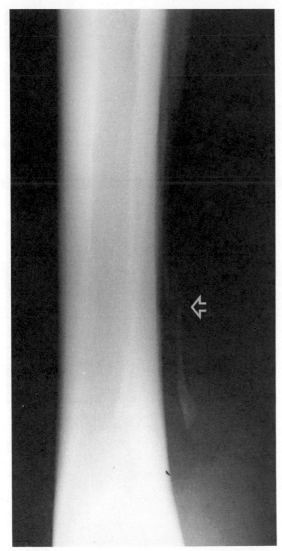

Figure 14A-32. *Fractures of the distal segment of the second or fourth metacarpal/metatarsal bones (arrow) may be associated with injuries to the suspensory ligament (third interosseous muscle).*

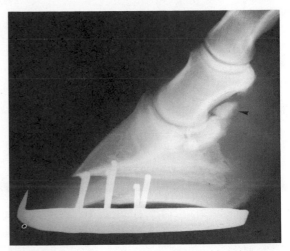

Figure 14A-33. *Lateromedial projection of the foot of a 13-year-old gelding. The discrete radiopacity proximal to the navicular bone (arrows) is metastatic calcification in the navicular bursa and was assumed to result from the repeated intrabursal injection of long-acting corticosteroid.*

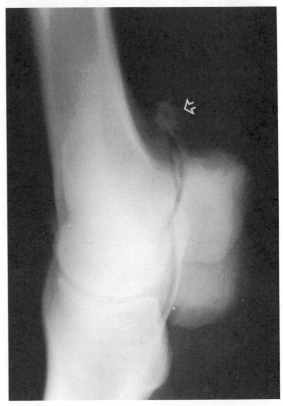

Figure 14A-34. *Lateroproximal-mediodistal projection of the metacarpophalangeal joint of a 9-year-old thoroughbred cross gelding. Previous damage to the suspensory apparatus resulted in an abaxial avulsion fracture of the medial proximal sesamoid bone and calcification of the damaged suspensory ligament (interosseous muscle) branch (arrow).*

schedule should proceed at a rate that allows remodeling to keep pace with loading (see Chap. 14C). Strenuous training and racing during this period may lead to stress fractures, which may themselves precede catastrophic long bone fractures in some individuals or may present as cortical fractures that will heal satisfactorily with rest or appropriate surgical intervention. Not all cortical fractures are fatigue fractures, because it is possible that they may result from a single traumatic episode, but once they have occurred, they too may lead to major long bone fractures if they are ignored.

In their early stages, stress fractures may not be apparent radiographically. Their recognition may be made easier if radiography is repeated after 2 to 3 weeks, if

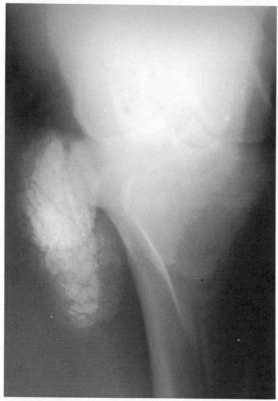

Figure 14A-35. *Calcinosis circumscripta. Characteristic calcified lesions over the lateral tibia.*

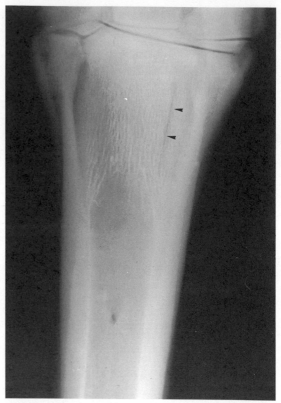

Figure 14A- 36. *Dorsopalmar view of the proximal metacarpus of a 5-year-old warmblood mare showing a linear longitudinal fracture of the palmar metacarpal cortex (arrows).*

high-detail imaging systems are used, and if special projections are employed. Scintigraphy is particularly useful in the diagnosis of stress fractures and should be used whenever the clinical signs indicate the possibility of a fracture but there is no clinical or radiographic evidence of the lesion.[50,51]

The most common manifestation of stress or fatigue fractures is the "bucked shin" complex in 2- to 4-year-old racehorses. Horses may exhibit no radiographic signs, with the lesions thought to be the result of a mismatch between the exercise regime and the remodeling within the metacarpus. If exercise continues, dorsal cortical fractures can appear. These are usually situated on the dorsolateral aspect of the metacarpus at the junction between the middle and distal thirds[29,38,52] and can be accompanied by a periosteal reaction. The fracture line is usually oblique through the dorsal cortex but can occasionally exit the surface of the cortex, giving a saucer fracture.

Unicortical fractures are seen in other locations. Palmar cortical fractures of the proximal metacarpus/metatarsus are thought to represent fatigue or stress fractures,[53,54] although in some cases there may be a relationship with desmitis of the origin of the suspensory ligament (proximal suspensory disease).[53,55] The fractures can be either longitudinal or transverse (Fig. 14A–36). Recently, unicortical fractures of the dorsoproximal

metatarsus have been seen (Pilsworth, personal communication), but these may represent avulsion-like injuries by the peroneus tertius.

Carpal Fractures
Carpal fractures provide a good example of the way in which repetitive stress may lead to changes that modify a bone's biomechanical function and, ultimately, to fracture. The normal carpus relies on a mediolateral dissipation of concussive forces through lateral and medial movement of the individual carpal bones and energy absorption by the carpal soft tissues.[56] However, the medial aspect of the carpus is inadequately protected, so forces are concentrated on the radial and third carpal bones, which are, therefore, most susceptible to damage by either chronic stress accumulation or acute overloading.

Adaptation of the carpus to prevent such injury depends on responses within both the soft tissues and the bone. Early in training, the soft tissues are most susceptible to injury, and inflammation of the intercarpal ligaments and the fibrous joint capsule results in a condition inappropriately termed *carpitis*. Radiographically, this is evident as enthesiophytosis on the dorsal surface of the carpal bones (Fig. 14A–37). These changes are a reflection of the increased stresses on the carpus and are not necessarily related to overt lameness. If action is

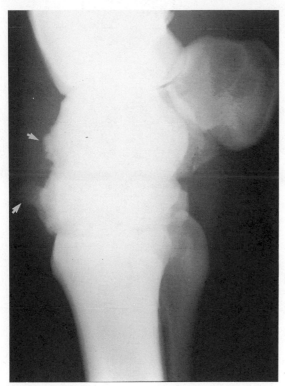

Figure 14A-37. Prominent enthesiophytes on the dorsal surface of both proximal and distal rows of carpal bones (arrows).

taken to reduce the loading of the carpus, the enthesiophytes will remodel.

The soft tissues adapt more quickly than the bone, and continued loading of the carpus produces changes within the carpal bones, some of which can be identified radiographically. The earliest alteration is a change in the contour of the dorsodistal radial carpal bone produced as a result of softening of the dorsal border of the bone. Radiographically, there is a change in contour and a loss of density on the dorsodistal aspect. As a result, forces are concentrated further on the third carpal bone, and similar changes appear in the third carpal bone as a loss in radiodensity in the skyline view. As the remodeling progresses, new bone can be seen as sclerosis of the third carpal bone in the skyline view, and in a dorsolateral-palmaromedial oblique projection, the proximal and distal subchondral bone plates of the radial carpal bone become joined.

If the carpal bones are subjected to unphysiologic loading or the remodeling process cannot keep pace with the cyclical loading provided by training and racing, there is a "material failure," and fracture occurs. Because of the structure of the carpus, these fractures tend to occur at predictable sites. If the loading has produced a large remodeling response, fracture can occur through the whole of the carpal bone, namely a slab fracture involving two articular surfaces. If fracture occurs at a less advanced stage of remodeling, it usually involves one or more articular rims.

The distribution of fractures varies between continents and breeds,[57] with a higher incidence of radial carpal bone fractures occurring in the United Kingdom than in the United States. A full set of views is necessary not only to identify the extent of the remodeling process but also to recognize multiple fragments. The contralateral limb also should be radiographed, since a high proportion of cases are found to be bilateral.

If the remodeling process is able to accommodate the loading and prevent fracture, degenerative joint disease can still ensue as a result of subchondral sclerosis, poor shock absorption, and cartilage damage. Hence radiographic signs of degenerative joint disease can be present without obvious signs of a fracture. Acute overloading also can be responsible for carpal bone fracture. Again, because of the construction of the carpus, these fractures have predictable sites (see Table 14A–6). Such fractures often have no remodeling changes within the affected bones. Figure 14A 38 summarizes the etiopathogenesis of carpal bone fractures with the resulting radiographic characteristics of carpal disease.

"Traumatic Osteochondrosis" of the Distal Metacarpus/Metatarsus

Although this condition has been described as part of the osteochondrosis complex, it is, in fact, a consequence of repetitive trauma to the distal metacarpus/metatarsus which causes sclerotic remodeling and subsequent ischemic necrosis. The 125-degree dorsodistal-palmaro/plantaroproximal projection[58,59] is ideal for detecting these lesions.

Spinous Process Impingement

The detection of impinging dorsal spinous processes radiographically presents a diagnostic challenge, since not all such findings are significant. Changes vary from the mildest form where the spines are positioned close to one another to evidence of active bone turnover with areas of sclerosis and lysis within the abutting spinous processes (Fig. 14A–39). The presence of the latter implies a significant lesion. Further confirmation can be supplied using gamma scintigraphy or by obtaining a clinical response to the introduction of local anesthetic into the appropriate interspinous space(s).

Degenerative Joint Disease

The pathophysiology of degenerative joint disease (DJD) is complex. Radiographically, affected joints can be divided into those which show no radiographic changes (and therefore carry a reasonable prognosis), those which show the characteristic radiographic changes of established DJD (Fig. 14A–40), and those which have signs of a primary lesion, e.g., an intraarticular fracture, with or without the radiographic signs of DJD.

Joints that undergo clinically obvious sudden-onset, acute changes with no radiographic signs other than joint capsule distension are the high-motion joints, particularly the carpus and metacarpo(tarso)phalangeal joints. Low-motion joints, notably the intertarsal and proximal interphalangeal joints, demonstrate a more in-

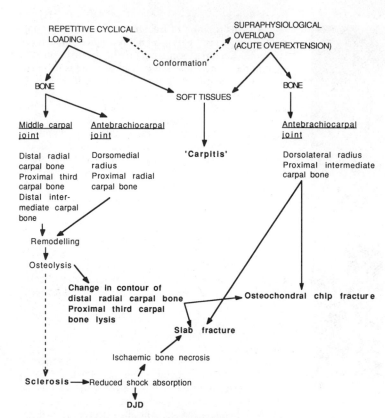

Figure 14A-38. *A summary of the etio-pathogenesis of carpal bone fractures and the radiographic characteristics of carpal bone disease. (Based on Bramlage, Schneider, and Gabel, 1988.[56])*

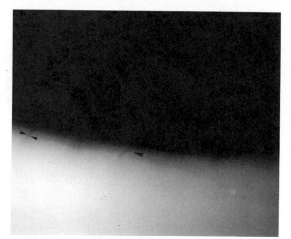

Figure 14A-39. *Lateral radiograph of the spinous processes of a 9-year-old pony mare. Spinous processes, which are unusually closely apposed (small arrow) or in contact with secondary changes of cavitation and remodeling (large arrow), may be seen in horses with no signs of back pain. Radiographs with markers allow the accurate infiltration of local anaesthetic to assess the significance of the lesions.*

sidious onset of lameness usually associated with radiographic changes.

The radiographic signs of DJD are usually listed (based on the radiographic changes in human patients) as narrowing of the joint space in weight-bearing studies (due to articular cartilage depletion), marginal osteophytes, subchondral sclerosis, and/or cysts. In horses, frequently the only sign to be seen is marginal osteophytes/enthesiophytes in high-motion joints. Narrowing of the joint space is rare, except in very advanced cases, and it is unusual to see subchondral changes.

In low-motion joints, the radiographic changes are more characteristic of DJD in humans (Figs. 14A–41 and 14A–42). In spavin, changes are seen most frequently on a dorsolateral-plantaromedial oblique projection, but in some cases they are better seen on a lateral or dorsomedial-plantarolateral oblique view. All the changes listed above are significant. However, common incidental findings in horses which are not lame are dorsal and dorsomedial enthesiophytes at the attachments of the dorsal ligament of the tarsus which may be mistaken for marginal osteophytes. We see very few cases with florid, verrucose proliferations of bone around the intertarsal or tarsometatarsal joints and therefore few joints in which ankylosis appears to be a likely consequence in the foreseeable future. In contrast, we see a number of horses in which bilateral distal intertarsal joint fusion has occurred, although the owner has been aware of no lameness.

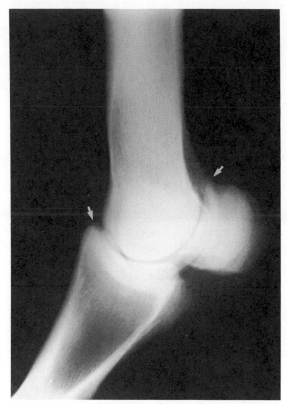

Figure 14A-40. *Lateromedial projection of a metacarpophalangeal joint showing established degenerative changes. Well-developed osteophytes on the proximal articular margins of the proximal sesamoid bones and the dorsoproximal border of the proximal phalanx (arrows).*

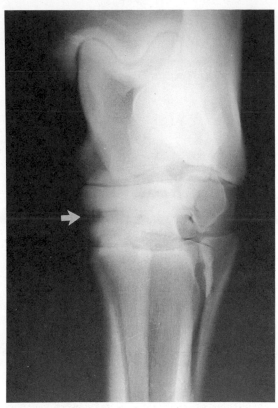

Figure 14A-41. *Dorsolateral-plantaromedial oblique view of the hock of a 9-year-old thoroughbred cross. Degenerative joint disease of the distal intertarsal joint and tarsometatarsal joints (spavin) is seen, predominantly, as subchondral bone lysis (arrow) and narrowing of the joint space.*

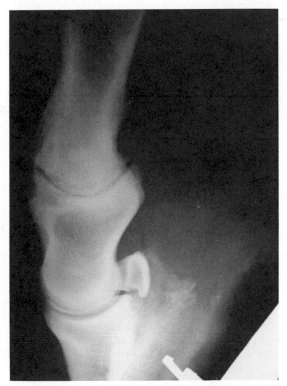

Figure 14A-42. *Degenerative joint disease of the proximal interphalangeal joint. Cartilage depletion is seen as a narrowed joint space, and there is extensive periarticular bone remodeling.*

The same low-motion joint changes can be seen in the navicular bone in navicular disease. This, and other pathophysiologic similarities, has led to the suggestion that navicular disease is another manifestation of DJD.[1]

CHRONIC FOOT LAMENESS

Navicular Disease

Few subjects have caused more confusion than navicular disease. The name itself is inadequate and is as meaningless as would be *humerus disease* or *mandible disease.* The substitution of *syndrome* for *disease* is an attempt to indicate the diversity of the pathologic changes that may culminate in the same clinical presentation. Neither *navicular disease* nor *navicular syndrome* tells us anything about the pathophysiology or etiology of the condition, and since the former has, until recently, stood the test of time, it should be used until the nature of the entity is more clearly defined and a more logical system of nomenclature is suggested.

Navicular disease, or chronic lameness associated with pain and pathologic changes in the navicular bone (almost invariably affecting one or both forelimbs but occasionally seen in a hindlimb), was first recognized and described on clinicopathologic grounds long before x-rays and their diagnostic potential were discovered. Although some of the earliest published radiographs were of animals, it was several years before radiography was used in veterinary diagnosis to investigate more than fractures and obvious bone lesions. A notable but infrequently acknowledged development in veterinary radiology was made by veterinary officers in the Royal Army Veterinary Corps. In 1935, Oxspring,[60] developing the original work of his colleagues, published his description of the radiography, radiology, and pathology of navicular disease. He described three of the four standard views still used for navicular radiography, and his descriptions of both the gross pathology and radiographic changes which may be encountered in the navicular bone remain unchallenged.

It was, however, as a result of his work that the idea developed that navicular disease could be diagnosed solely or definitively by radiography, and he contended that he could diagnose the incipient condition before clinical signs were established. This idea persisted for many years and is still a view held by many horse owners and some veterinary surgeons. Nevertheless, it is now generally accepted that navicular disease is a clinical entity capable of definition in clinical terms only. Once the diagnosis has been made, radiography allows an examination of the contours and radiopacity of the navicular bone. It also rules out other conditions that may, depending on the stringency of the clinical examination, mimic navicular disease clinically.

A full radiographic examination of the navicular bone requires three views: a lateromedial projection centered on the navicular bone, a dorsoproximal-palmarodistal (upright pedal or high coronary) oblique view, and a palmaroproximal-palmarodistal ("skyline") oblique view (Figs. 14A–43 and 14A–44). None of the radiographic changes described in Table 14A–10 are pathognomonic for navicular disease,[61–63] and none has been unequivocally related to the prognosis after treatment, although Wright[64] has recorded an association between flexor cortex defects, proximal border enthesiophytes, mineralization of the deep digital flexor tendon, medullary trabecular disruption and medullary sclerosis, and the response to navicular suspensory desmotomy.[64]

Pedal Osteitis

Frequently, a radiographic examination of a lame horse's feet reveals changes in the distal phalanx. These take the form of new bone on the solar and mural surfaces, remodeling of the dorsosolar junction, generalized osteopenia, and localized bone resorption around the vascu-

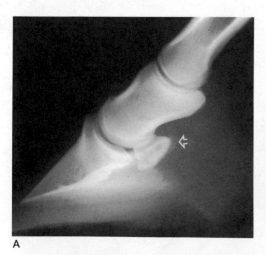 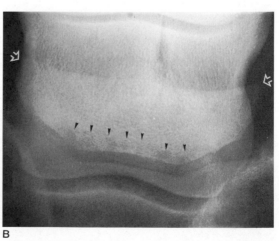

A   B

Figure 14A-43. *Dorsoproximal-palmarodistal* (left) *and lateromedial* (right) *views of a foot showing enthesious bone at the insertion of the suspensory ligaments of the navicular bone* (open arrows). *There are seven globular synovial fossae on the ventral border of the navicular bone* (closed arrows).

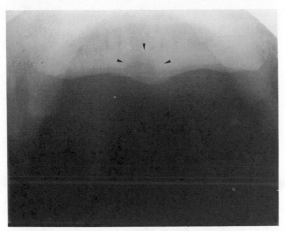

Figure 14A-44. *Palmaroproximal-palmarodistal view of a navicular bone showing an erosive lesion in the flexor cortex (arrows).*

lar channels. The changes may occur in any combination and indeed may be seen to some extent in some apparently normal horses,[65] but remodeling of the dorsosolar junction is usually associated with chronic laminitis (Fig. 14A–45), and new bone on the margin of the solar surface may be seen in poorly balanced feet. Chronic inflammatory changes in the distal phalanx, therefore, are usually secondary to another condition. While they may be described as pedal osteitis, this is not a useful concept because it does not encourage the clinician to look for and correct the primary problem. In those rare cases where no primary cause of the radiographic changes can be discovered and the clinical signs are consistent with distal phalangeal pain, a diagnosis of idiopathic pedal osteitis is justified.

Type 6 distal phalangeal fractures (see Table 14A–8) in the acute stage will undoubtedly cause inflammation the distal phalanx, but they should not be thought of as pedal osteitis, as some authors recommend.

Table 14A-10. The Changes That May be Seen on Radiographs of the Navicular Bone and Their Possible Significance

Radiologic sign	Possible significance
Lateromedial projection	
New bone along the proximal border	Present in 5 percent of horses with no signs of lameness; more important if unilateral; may not be associated with pain
Distal elongation of the flexor surface	Present in 35 percent of horses with no signs of lameness
Osteoporosis of the flexor subchondral bone	Clinically significant in all horses of 6 years old or more
Thinning of the flexor cortex	May be insignificant in older horses in light work
Osteosclerosis of the medullary cavity	Frequently present in lame horses with navicular disease but seen in about 1.5 percent of horses with no clinical signs
Loss of corticomedullary definition	May result from flexor cortex osteoporosis medullary sclerosis
Calcification of the impar ligament	Present in about 2 percent of horses with no signs of lameness; more frequently seen in horses with navicular disease
Calcification of the soft tissues adjacent to the navicular bone	May represent long standing deep flexor tendon degeneration or metastatic calcification following corticosteroid injection
Fragment on distal border	May be found in normal animals; may be bilateral
Variations in trabecular pattern	Trabeculation variable in animals with no signs of lameness
Dorsoproximal-palmarodistal oblique projection	
Change in shape, including suspensory ligament enthesiophytes	The shape of navicular bones from horses with no signs of lameness is very variable; in 10 percent of horses with no signs of lameness the left and right navicular bones were asymmetrical
Central loss of radiopacity	One of the signs of navicular disease first described; usually associated with lameness but not pathognomonic for the disease
Number, shape, and position of synovial fossae	In general, poorly correlated with clinical signs
Palmaroproximal-palmarodistal projection	
Roughening/calcification of the flexor cortex	Seen in up to 2 percent of horses with no signs of lameness; usually associated with lameness
Defects in the flexor cortex	Seen in less than 1 percent of horses with no sign of lameness; usually significant
Indistinct corticomedullary border	Seen in 17 percent of horses with no sign of lameness; influenced by angle of incident beam relative to the navicular bone

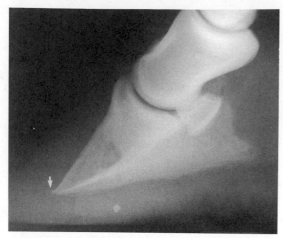

Figure 14A-45. *Remodeling of the dorsal solar margin of the distal phalanx (arrow) is usually secondary to chronic laminitis and rotation of the distal phalanx.*

Distal Interphalangeal Arthropathy

Pain emanating from the distal interphalangeal joint is common, yet few references are made to its possible causes.[66] Acute cases of synovitis may present similarly to subsolar infection. There are no radiographic changes in the acute phase, and subtle evidence of chronic degenerative joint disease may take several months to appear. Other cases present as chronic lamenesses, almost indistinguishable clinically from navicular disease. The contribution of the distal interphalangeal joint and the navicular bone and bursa to the pain causing lameness in horses with navicular disease has not been established, but it is clear that both are involved to a greater or lesser extent. In those cases where intraarticular an-

esthesia confirms the involvement of the distal interphalangeal joint, there may or may not be radiographic evidence of degenerative joint disease.[67] The changes are usually subtle and appear as small osteophytes on the dorsoproximal edge of the distal phalanx, on the dorsodistal edge of the middle phalanx, and on the proximal articular border of the navicular bone adjacent to the middle phalanx (Fig. 14A-46). The most profound radiographic changes involving the distal interphalangeal joint are secondary to fracture of the extensor process of the distal phalanx.

Conclusion

Evaluation of limb injuries in athletic horses requires both clinical and radiologic skills. Some radiographic lesions are of little clinical significance, while others may have profound implications for athletic performance. These comments have particular significance when applied to the area of prepurchase examination in performance horses, where "screening" radiographs of the distal limbs are often requested by the potential purchaser.

Radiographs often are used by clinicians to determine the prognosis for various treatment strategies, and yet there are few prospective studies to allow such evaluations to be made accurately. However, while ultrasound and scintigraphy have become used more widely in recent years for the diagnosis and prognosis of musculoskeletal injuries, radiography is still the cornerstone.

References

1. Pool RR, Meagher DM, Stover SM: Pathophysiology of navicular disease. Vet Clin North Am 1989; 5:109.
2. Bramlage LR: Conformation and carpal disease (abstract). In Proceedings of the 31st British Equine Veterinary Association Congress, 1992.
3. Bertone AL, Park RD, Turner AS: Periosteal transection and stripping for treatment of angular limb deformities in foals: Radiographic observations. J Am Vet Med Assoc 1985; 187:153.
4. Olsson SE, Reiland S: The nature of osteochondrosis in animals. Acta Radiol Suppl 1978; 358:153.
5. Birkeland R, Haakenstad LH: Intracapsular bony fragments of the distal tibia of the horse. J Am Vet Med Assoc 1986; 152:1526.
6. De Moor A, Verschooten F, Desmet P, et al: Osteochondritis dissecans of the tibiotarsal joint in the horse. Equine Vet J 1972; 4:139.
7. Stromberg B: A review of the salient features of osteochondrosis in the horse. Equine Vet J 1979; 11:211.
8. Watkins JP: Osteochondrosis. In Auer JA (ed): Equine Surgery. Philadelphia, WB Saunders Co, 1992, p 971.
9. Jeffcott LB, Kold SE: Clinical and radiological aspects of stifle bone cysts in the horse. Equine Vet J 1982; 14:40.
10. McIlwraith CW: Subchondral cystic lesions in the horse: The indications, methods, and results of surgery. Equine Vet Ed 1990; 2:75.
11. Nixon AJ: The Wobbler syndrome. In Stashak ES (ed): Adams's Lameness in Horses. Philadelphia, Lea & Febiger, 1987, p 772.
12. Mayhew IG, Whitlock RH, de Lahunta A: Spinal cord disease in the horse; Electromyographic and radiographic studies. Cornell Vet 1978; 68:suppl. 6:44.
13. Coyne CP, Cox J: Neurological examination. In Robinson NE (ed): Current Therapy in Equine Medicine. Philadelphia, WB Saunders Co, 1992, p 521.
14. May SA, Wyn-Jones G, Church S, et al: Iopamidol myelography in the horse. Equine Vet J 1986; 18:199.
15. Burbidge HM, Kannegieter N, Dickson LR, Goulden BE, Badcoe L: Iohexol myelography in the horse. Equine Vet J 1989; 21:347.

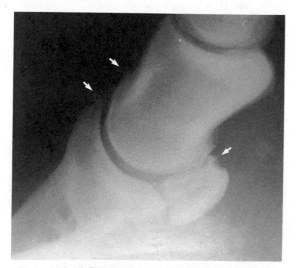

Figure 14A-46. *Degenerative joint disease of the distal interphalangeal joint. Osteophytes may be seen on the proximal articular border of the navicular bone and dorsally on the distal middle phalanx and proximal distal phalanx.*

16. Butler JA, Colles CM, Dyson SJ, et al: Clinical Radiology of the Horse. London, Blackwell Scientific Publications, 1993.

17. Watkins JP, Auer JA: Physeal injuries. Comp Cont Ed Pract Vet 1984; 6:S226.

18. Embertson RM, Bramlage LR, Herring DS, et al: Physeal fractures in the horse: I. Classification and incidence. Vet Surg 1986; 15:223.

19. Embertson RM, Bramlage LR, Gabel AA: Physeal fractures in the horse: II. Management and outcome. Vet Surg 1986; 15:230.

20. Leitch M: A review of treatment of tuber scapulae fractures in the horse. J Equine Med Surg 1977; 1:234.

21. Dyson SJ: Sixteen fractures of the shoulder region in the horse. Equine Vet J 1985; 17:104.

22. Stover S, Johnson BJ, Daft BM, et al: An association between complete and incomplete stress fractures of the humerus in racehorses. Equine Vet J 1992; 24:260.

23. Copelan RW, Bramlage LR: Surgery of the fetlock joint. Vet Clin North Am Large Anim Pract 1983; 5:221.

24. McIlwraith CW: Diseases of joints, tendons, ligaments, and related structures. In Stashak ES (ed): Adam's Lameness in Horses. Philadelphia, Lea & Febiger, 1987, p 339.

25. McIlwraith CW: Fragmentation of the distal aspect of the patella. Equine Vet J 1990; 22:157.

26. Pool RR, Meagher DM: Pathologic findings and pathogenesis of racetrack injuries. Vet Clin North Am Equine Pract 1990; 6:1.

27. Pool RR: Difficulties in definition of equine osteochondrosis; differentiation of developmental and acquired lesions. Equine Vet J 1993; suppl. 16:5.

28. Jeffcott LB: Osteochondrosis in the horse: Searching for the key to pathogenesis. Equine Vet J 1991; 23:331.

29. Foerner JJ, McIlwraith CW: Orthopedic surgery in the racehorse. Vet Clin North Am Equine Pract 1990; 6:147.

30. Foerner JJ, Barclay WP, Phillips TN, et al: Osteochondral fragments of the palmar/plantar aspect of the fetlock joint. In Proceedings of the American Association of Equine Practitioners, 1987, p 739.

31. Pettersson H, Ryden G: Avulsion fractures of the caudoproximal extremity of the first phalanx. Equine Vet J 1982; 14:333.

32. Grøndahl AM: Incidence and development of ununited proximoplantar tuberosity of the proximal phalanx in standardbred trotters. Vet Radiol Ultrasound 1992; 33:18.

33. Bukowiecki CF, Bramlage LR, Gabel AA: Palmar/plantar process fractures of the proximal phalanx in 15 horses. Vet Surg 1986; 15:383.

34. May SA, Patterson LJ, Peacock PJ, et al: Radiographic technique for the pelvis in the standing horse. Equine Vet J 1991; 23:312.

35. Rutowski JA, Richardson DW: A retrospective study of 100 pelvic fractures in horses. Equine Vet J 1989; 21:256.

36. Honnas CM, O'Brien TR, Linford RL: Distal phalanx fractures in horses: A survey of 274 horses with radiographic assessment of healing in 36 horses. Vet Radiol 1988; 29:98.

37. Schneider RK: Incidence and location of fractures of the proximal sesamoids and proximal extremity of the first phalanx. In Proceedings, Annual Convention of the American Association of Equine Practitioners 1979, p 25.

38. Barclay WP, Foerner JJ, Phillips TN: Axial sesamoid injuries associated with lateral condylar fractures in the horse. J Am Vet Med Assoc 1985; 186:278.

39. Ellis DR: Fractures of the proximal sesamoid bones in thoroughbred foals. Equine Vet J 1979; 11:48.

40. Bramlage LR, Bukowiecki CW, Gabel AA: The effect of training on the suspensory apparatus of the horse. In Proceedings, Annual Convention of the American Association of Equine Practitioners 1990, p 245.

41. Ferraro GL: Lameness diagnosis and treatment in the thoroughbred racehorse. Vet Clin North Am Equine Pract 1990; 6:63.

42. Palmer SE: Radiography of the abaxial surface of the proximal sesamoid bones of the horse. J Am Vet Med Assoc 1982; 181:264.

43. Dik KJ: Special radiographic projections for the equine proximal sesamoid bones and the caudoproximal extremity of the first phalanx. Equine Vet J 1985; 17:244.

44. Shiroma JT, Engel HN, Wagner PC, et al: Dorsal subluxation of the proximal interphalangeal joint of the pelvic limb in three horses. J Am Vet Med Assoc 1989; 195:777.

45. Wisner ER, O'Brien TR, Pool RR, et al: Osteomyelitis of the axial border of the proximal sesamoid bone in seven horses. Equine Vet J 1991; 23:383.

46. Lamb CR: Contrast radiography of equine joints, tendon sheaths, and draining tracts. Vet Clin North Am Equine Pract 1991; 7:211.

47. Wyn-Jones G: Equine Lameness. Oxford, Blackwell Scientific Publications, 1988.

48. Poulos PW: Radiographic and histologic assessment of proximal sesamoid bone changes in young and working horses. In Proceedings, Annual Convention of the American Association of Equine Practitioners 1988, p 347.

49. Riggs CM, Evans GP: The microstructural basis of the mechanical properties of equine bone. Equine Vet Ed 1990; 2:197.

50. Webbon PM: Scintigraphic detection of equine fractures. In Proceedings of the 26th British Equine Veterinary Association Congress, 1987.

51. Pilsworth R, Webbon PM: The use of radionuclide bone scanning in the diagnosis of tibial "stress" fractures in the horse: a review of five cases. Equine Vet J 1988; (suppl 6):60.

52. Richardson DW: Dorsal cortical fractures of the equine metacarpus. Comp Cont Ed 1984; 6:S248.

53. Dyson SJ: Some observations on lameness associated with pain in the proximal metacarpal region. Equine Vet J 1988; (suppl 6):43.

54. Wright IM, Platt D, Houlton JEF, et al: Management of intracortical fractures of the palmaroproximal third metacarpal bone in a horse by surgical forage. Equine Vet J 1990; 22:142.

55. Dyson S: Proximal suspensory desmitis: Clinical, ultrasonographic and radiographic features. Equine Vet J 1991; 23:25.

56. Bramlage LR, Schneider RK, Gabel AA: A clinical perspective on lameness originating in the carpus. Equine Vet J 1988; (suppl 6):12.

57. McIlwraith CW, Yovich JV, Martin GS: Arthroscopic surgery for the treatment of osteochondral chip fractures in the equine carpus. J Am Vet Med Assoc 1987; 191:531.

58. Hornof WJ, O'Brien TR: Radiographic evaluation of the palmar aspect of the equine metacarpal condyles: A new projection. Vet Radiol 1980; 21:161.

59. Pilsworth RC, Hopes R, Greet TRC: A flexed dorsopalmar projection of the equine fetlock in demonstrating lesions of the distal third metacarpus. Vet Rec 1988; 122:323.

60. Oxspring GE: The radiology of navicular disease, with observations on its pathology. Vet Rec 1935; 15:1433.

61. Turner TA: Diagnosis and treatment of navicular syndrome in horses. Vet Clin North Am Equine Pract 1989; 5:131.

62. Verschooten F: The importance of the lateromedial view for the radiographic diagnosis of navicular disease. Vet Ann 1990; 30:172.

63. Kaser-Hotz B, Ueltschi G: Radiographic appearance of the navicular bone in sound horses. Vet Radiol Ultrasound 1992; 33:9.

64. Wright IM: A study of 118 cases of navicular disease: treatment by navicular suspensory desmotomy. Equine Vet J 1993; 25:501.

65. Rendano VT, Grant B: The equine third phalanx: Its radiographic appearance. J Am Vet Radiol Soc 1978; 19:125.

66. McIlwraith CW, Goodman NL: Conditions of the interphalangeal joints. Vet Clin North Am Equine Pract 1989; 5:161.

67. Dyson SJ: Lameness due to pain associated with the distal interphalangeal joint: 45 cases. Equine Vet J 1992; 23:128.

Diagnostic Imaging in the Athletic Horse: Musculoskeletal Ultrasonography

R. K. W. SMITH AND P. M. WEBBON

Glossary of Terminology

Ultrasound terminology is sometimes used rather loosely and, therefore, inaccurately. The following guidelines are suggested for descriptive terminology:

- *Echogenicity:* the ability of a tissue to produce reflections (echoes)
- *Anechogenic:* producing no echoes; black, or anechoic, on the screen
- *Hyperechogenic:* producing high-intensity echoes; bright, or hyperechoic, on the screen
- *Hypoechogenic:* producing low-intensity echoes; dark, or hypoechoic, on the screen
- *Isoechogenic:* producing similar-intensity echoes to another area
- *Normoechogenic:* producing the expected intensity of echoes for the tissue
- *Ultrasonograph:* image produced by the ultrasound scanner.

The terms *echolucent* and *sonolucent* are incorrect, since *lucent* refers to the transmission of electromagnetic radiation and not to the reflection of a physical wave such as sound. They should therefore not be used.

Applications of Ultrasonography in the Athletic Horse

Ultrasonography was first used routinely in horses to examine the urogenital tract in mares. It soon became clear that similar equipment could be used to examine the soft tissues in the distal limbs.[1] While this application is now commonplace, it is becoming clear that there are other applications in the proximal limb, in examining bones and joints, in investigating wounds, and in detecting radiolucent foreign bodies. This section reviews the common uses of diagnostic ultrasound and illustrates some of its less frequent applications.

Diagnostic Ultrasound Physics and Equipment

A detailed description of ultrasound physics and the equipment available is beyond the scope of this text. Those who are interested should refer to the references.[2-7] Ultrasound frequencies are above 20 kHz, the upper limit of normal human hearing. Diagnostic ultrasound frequencies usually are between 2.25 to 10 MHz, and for musculoskeletal ultrasonography, the most commonly used frequency is 7.5 MHz. Ultrasound is generated by the piezoelectric effect when a pulsed voltage is applied to the crystal (sector probe) or crystals (linear array) in the scan head. Tissue interfaces reflect the sound waves to an extent dependent on the difference in the acoustic impedance between the adjacent tissues. Thus, at soft-tissue/air and soft-tissue/bone boundaries, over 90 percent of the sound is reflected, effectively acting as a barrier to deeper imaging.

The ultrasound echoes deform the crystal(s) in the scan head in the intervals between the generating pulses, and the resulting voltage is processed to produce the ultrasound image.

The equipment used to produce the illustrations for this section was a Concept 2000 (Dynamic Imaging, Livingston, Scotland) with a 7.5-MHz linear array head and, when appropriate, a nonechogenic stand-off pad (Sonokit TM, Sonogel Vertriebs GMBH, Idstein, Germany).

Common Artifacts

The ease with which artifacts can be generated necessitates a critical appraisal of all ultrasound images before any diagnostic conclusions are reached. The ultrasound machine and the scan head which are used impose restrictions on the axial resolution (dependent on the pulse length and frequency of the transducer), lateral resolution, and section thickness (dependent on the crystal size and focusing). If the scan head is not positioned at 90 degrees to the structure to be examined, it may appear to have a hypoechogenic center.[5,8,9]

The gain controls should be standardized as far as possible and should only be altered if the picture is too dark or too light. It is common to find the gain controls set too high,[2,5,10] which will obscure tissue detail.

Poor contact between the scan head and the skin will obstruct the return of echoes. The consequence will be either a poor-quality picture or dark, anechoic bands in the image.[5] Too much pressure exerted on the limb not only may cause the horse to fidget but also will distort the normal anatomy and may prevent the identification of peritendinous edema.[5]

Air, other gases, or metallic foreign bodies, either in the tissues or between the scan head and the limb, will result in a *reverberation artifact,* a series of concentric, echoic rings. Refraction causes the beam to be bent as the sound travels across a boundary between two areas with different acoustic impedance; positioning errors will be produced as a result. If sound returns to the probe in a different way from its transmission due to multiple reflections, the reflector will be misplaced on the screen. For instance, a second reflection from a highly reflective surface can produce a mirror image of the more superficial soft tissues deep to the reflective surface.

Shadowing is caused either by a highly reflective boundary, e.g., bone, or occurs at the edge of a reflective curved surface when the beam is tangential to it, so-called edge refraction or shadowing. This is particularly evident on transverse scans of the suspensory ligament branches when the edges of the flexor tendons produce a shadow through each branch.

Enhancement occurs deep to an area of low attenuation, usually fluid, providing it is at least 2 to 3 cm in diameter, making the deeper structures seem more echogenic. With the use of sector scanners, the central area of the beam generates more echoes than the periphery. This is known as *focal enhancement.*

The presence of either shadowing or enhancement can be used to the operator's benefit to help recognize calcification or fluid.

Tissue Characteristics

Ultrasound images are generated as a result of echoes within a heterogeneous tissue (nonspecular reflection) or at the interface between two tissues (specular reflection). The pattern of echoes is often not characteristic, so ultrasound cannot be used reliably to identify individual tissues. However, as a basic principle, "cystic," or nonechoic, areas represent uniform structures, and "solid," or echoic, areas represent nonuniform structures. Homogeneous fluids are anechogenic, often with acoustic enhancement in the deeper tissues. Blood varies between hypoechogenic and hyperechogenic depending on the degree to which it is clotted.[11] Normal blood vessels are hypoechogenic. The appearance of pus depends on its consistency, but it will have a variable number of internal echoes and reverberation artifacts if gas is present.

Skeletal muscle is heterogeneous with hyperechogenic fascial planes interspersed between the relatively hypoechogenic muscle fibers, producing a herringbone pattern. Fat is relatively hyperechogenic, while tendons and ligaments have a dotted internal architecture when the probe lies at right angles to the structure and a striated pattern when the probe is parallel. Bone is highly reflective and produces acoustic shadowing deep to it, while gas will produce shadowing and reverberation artifacts unless suspended in small bubbles, which generate bright, speckled reflections. Foreign bodies are usually strongly hyperechogenic, producing either acoustic shadowing or a reverberation artifact, the so-called comet tail.

Preparation and General Technique

The procedure is painless, but nervous horses may need to be sedated or restrained with a twitch. To obtain good contact between the probe and the skin, the hair is removed with fine-bladed electric clippers. Surgical scrub solution is used to clean the area thoroughly, and then surgical alcohol is applied to help dissolve wax and greases on the skin. Finally, the region is wiped dry.

High-viscosity contact gel is applied liberally to the skin and probe and, if used, to the stand-off. Generally, in the metacarpal and metatarsal region, a stand-off is used for investigating tendon and ligament injuries, but examination of the suspensory ligament and accessory ligament of the deep digital flexor tendon should also be carried out without one. Other areas of the musculoskeletal system are usually scanned without the stand-off unless very superficial structures are to be investigated or the contours of the area are such that a linear probe has poor contact. Whenever possible, structures should be examined in at least two planes.

Tendons and Ligaments

PALMAR/PLANTAR ASPECT OF THE METACARPAL/ METATARSAL AND PHALANGEAL REGIONS

The procedure adopted for examination must be methodical (Table 14B–1 and Figs. 14B–1 and 14B–2). Any

Table 14B-1. Protocol for Routine Examination of the Metacarpal, Metatarsal, and Phalangeal Regions

Metacarpal region	Seven transverse scans Three longitudinal scans
Plantar tarsal and metatarsal region	Nine transverse scans Four longitudinal scans
Phalangeal region	Three transverse scans (two more distal levels can be scanned with a sector probe)[18] One longitudinal scan

system must allow comparative views to be taken between limbs and for follow-up examination. Methods currently in use rely either on transverse scans at equidistant arbitrary points (seven in the metacarpal region, nine for the plantar tarsus and metatarsus, three to five for the phalanges)[4,12–17] or record the distance of the probe below the accessory carpal bone.[7,18] The horse should be standing squarely with its weight evenly distributed; otherwise, its tendons can vary in size and shape.

If resolution of the outline of the structures is difficult, slight tilting of the probe will highlight the borders of tendons and ligaments, although this also will generate artifacts within the tissue. Always scan both forelimbs or hindlimbs, both for comparison and to detect bilateral injuries.

The skin is represented by an echoic line. The subcutaneous tissues are usually less echogenic than the skin and 1 to 2 mm thick in the average horse. In horses with a lot of "feather," the thickness of the skin and subcutaneous tissues can increase substantially (up to 2 cm). This may impair the image obtained of the tendons and ligaments.

The superficial digital flexor tendon (SDFT) is closely associated with the deep digital flexor tendon (DDFT) throughout most of its length. From its musculotendinous junction it courses within the carpal sheath through the carpal canal. Proximally, in the metacarpal/metatarsal region, it is ovoid and separated from the DDFT by a diagonal line running in a palmarolateral to dorsomedial direction. Distally, it is crescentic. At the level of the proximal sesamoid bones, the SDFT encircles the DDFT. The dorsal part of the encircling ring can be seen as a clearly defined, thin, echoic line. Distal to the metacarpo/metatarsophalangeal (fetlock) joint, it divides into two branches which can be adequately examined only if the probe is moved around the limb laterally and medially. In transverse ultrasonographs a normal SDFT appears as a fine array of dots enclosed in a echogenic paratenon. In longitudinal images, the tendon is seen as a series of striations.

In the hindlimb, the SDFT lies lateral to the DDFT throughout most of the metatarsal region, only reaching the midline in the distal third of the metatarsus. It has a smaller cross-sectional area than the corresponding forelimb tendon. Proximally, in the forelimb, the DDFT lies with the SDFT within the carpal canal. It is oval on transverse views, and its internal architecture is similar to the SDFT, although generally more echogenic.

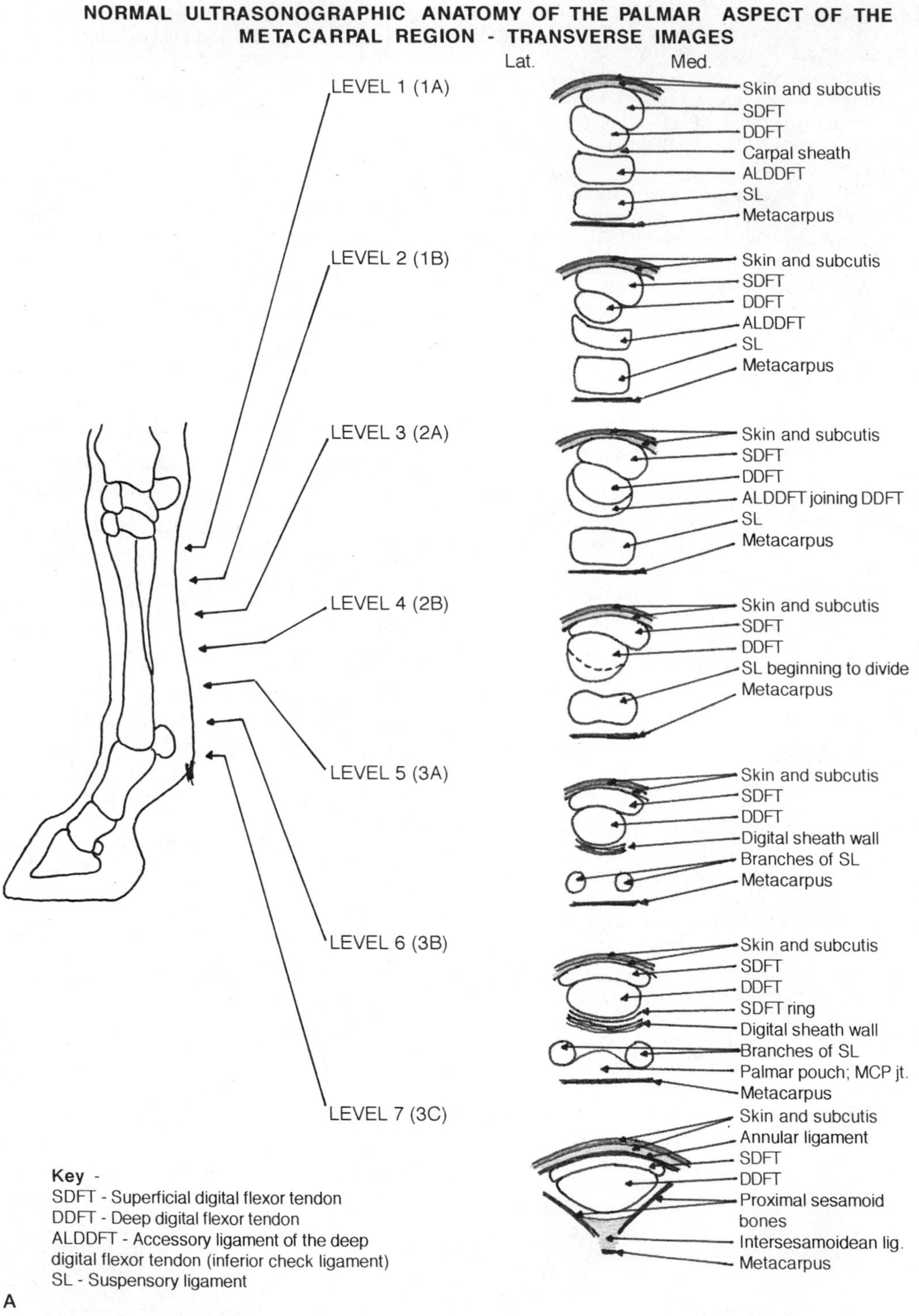

NORMAL ULTRASONOGRAPHIC ANATOMY OF THE PALMAR ASPECT OF THE METACARPAL REGION - TRANSVERSE IMAGES

LEVEL 1 (1A)

Lat.   Med.

Skin and subcutis
SDFT
DDFT
Carpal sheath
ALDDFT
SL
Metacarpus

LEVEL 2 (1B)

Skin and subcutis
SDFT
DDFT
ALDDFT
SL
Metacarpus

LEVEL 3 (2A)

Skin and subcutis
SDFT
DDFT
ALDDFT joining DDFT
SL
Metacarpus

LEVEL 4 (2B)

Skin and subcutis
SDFT
DDFT
SL beginning to divide
Metacarpus

LEVEL 5 (3A)

Skin and subcutis
SDFT
DDFT
Digital sheath wall
Branches of SL
Metacarpus

LEVEL 6 (3B)

Skin and subcutis
SDFT
DDFT
SDFT ring
Digital sheath wall
Branches of SL
Palmar pouch; MCP jt.
Metacarpus

LEVEL 7 (3C)

Skin and subcutis
Annular ligament
SDFT
DDFT
Proximal sesamoid bones
Intersesamoidean lig.
Metacarpus

Key -
SDFT - Superficial digital flexor tendon
DDFT - Deep digital flexor tendon
ALDDFT - Accessory ligament of the deep digital flexor tendon (inferior check ligament)
SL - Suspensory ligament

A

Figure 14B-1. Diagrams showing the normal ultrasonographic anatomy of the palmar aspect of the metacarpal region: (A) transverse,

NORMAL ULTRASONOGRAPHIC ANATOMY OF THE PALMAR ASPECT OF THE METACARPAL REGION - LONGITUDINAL IMAGES

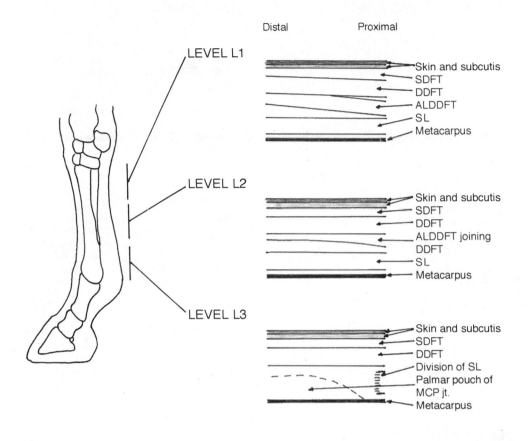

Key-
SDFT - Superficial digital flexor tendon
DDFT - Deep digital flexor tendon
ALDDFT - Accessory ligament of the deep digital flexor tendon (Inferior check ligament)
SL - Suspensory ligament
MCP jt. - Metacarpophalangeal joint

B

Figure 14B-1. Continued (B) longitudinal.

In the proximal hindlimb, the DDFT is medial to the plantar ligament and plantaromedial to the suspensory ligament. All these structures are similar in size at this level. In the proximal metatarsal region, the plantar ligament is no longer present, and the DDFT assumes a more central position. There is a small medial head of the DDFT which is poorly visible and which joins the DDFT medially in the proximal metatarsal region.

The third interosseous muscle is more commonly referred to as the *suspensory ligament* (SL). The amount of muscle in the SL is variable and not related to age, but it is responsible for the heterogeneous appearance of the SL compared with that of the SDFT and DDFT. It divides into two branches in its distal third to insert on the proximal sesamoid bones. These branches can be imaged both from the palmar/plantar aspect so that a comparison of their size can be made and also from the medial and lateral aspects, when they appear as teardrop-shaped, echoic bodies.

The straight distal sesamoidean ligament is the most echogenic of the soft-tissue structures on the palmar/plantar aspect of the phalanges. It is triangular in section proximally, becoming oval distally. The oblique distal sesamoidean ligaments are also identifiable in the

NORMAL ULTRASONOGRAPHIC ANATOMY OF THE PALMAR/PLANTAR ASPECT OF THE PHALANGES.

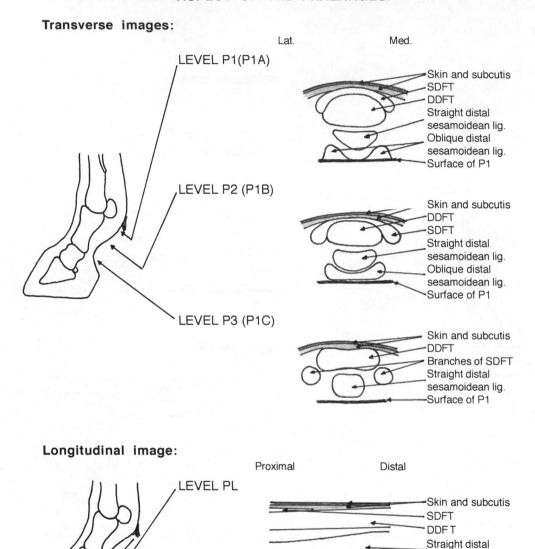

Transverse images:

Lat.   Med.

LEVEL P1(P1A)

Skin and subcutis
SDFT
DDFT
Straight distal
sesamoidean lig.
Oblique distal
sesamoidean lig.
Surface of P1

LEVEL P2 (P1B)

Skin and subcutis
DDFT
SDFT
Straight distal
sesamoidean lig.
Oblique distal
sesamoidean lig.
Surface of P1

LEVEL P3 (P1C)

Skin and subcutis
DDFT
Branches of SDFT
Straight distal
sesamoidean lig.
Surface of P1

Longitudinal image:

Proximal   Distal

LEVEL PL

Skin and subcutis
SDFT
DDFT
Straight distal
sesamoidean lig.
Oblique distal
sesamoidean lig.
Surface of P1

Key -
SDFT - Superficial digital flexor tendon
DDFT - Deep digital flexor tendon
P1 - First phalanx

Figure 14B-2. Diagram showing the normal ultrasonographic anatomy of the palmar/plantar aspect of the phalangeal region.

proximal phalangeal region medial and lateral to the straight distal sesamoidean ligament. An adequate examination requires rotation of the scan head medially and laterally through 45 degrees. The cruciate and short distal sesamoidean ligaments are not visible ultrasonographically.

The accessory ligament of the DDFT or inferior check ligament (CL) joins the DDFT in the midmetacarpal region, but its fibers remain distinguishable both macroscopically and ultrasonographically more distally. It is often, but not always, the most echogenic of the palmar soft-tissue structures. In the hindlimb the structure is very small, but it can be larger in draught horses and, very occasionally, other breeds.

The palmar/plantar annular ligament (AL) blends medially and laterally with the collateral sesamoidean ligaments and maintains the flexor tendons in the sesamoidean groove. It can be demonstrated ultrasonographically in a normal horse as a thin (1 to 2 mm) echogenic band immediately adjacent to the surface of the SDFT at the level of the proximal sesamoid bones.

A synovial attachment between the SDFT and the AL is not an adhesion but one of the routes by which blood reaches the SDFT as it encircles the DDFT. The proximal and distal digital annular ligaments are only clearly visible, superficial to the SDFT and DDFT, when they are enlarged.

The digital sheath encompasses both the SDFT and the DDFT from the level of the distal third of the metacarpus to a region proximal to the navicular bursa and palmar pouch of the distal interphalangeal joint. In addition to the very short mesotenon attaching the AL to the SDFT, there is a longer distal vinculum at the level of the proximal interphalangeal joint (to the DDFT). The distal vinculum is only occasionally identifiable, usually with distension of the sheath, which provides negative contrast. There is a normal synovial reflection joining the DDFT laterally and medially in the proximal sheath which should not be mistaken for an adhesion. The thickness of the sheath capsule can be assessed palmar to the SL branches where it is identifiable as an echoic band dorsal to the DDFT.

The carpal sheath may be seen ultrasonographically between the DDFT and the CL in the proximal metacarpal region. The tarsal sheath extends from proximal to the medial malleolus to the proximal quarter of the metatarsus. It can be seen ultrasonographically between the SL and the DDFT on the plantar aspect of the proximal metatarsus, medially over the tarsus, and deep to the gastrocnemius tendon proximal to the point of the hock.

The plantar ligament of the tarsus originates from the plantar surface of the os calcis and inserts on the proximal fourth tarsal bone and proximal fourth metatarsal bone. It is visible ultrasonographically on the lateral aspect of the os calcis. For further descriptions of technique and ultrasound anatomy, readers are referred to the references.[4,7–9,13,14,16,18,20,21]

Attempts have been made to relate soft-tissue ultrasonographic changes to their histopathologic appearance. The proposed correlation, based on experimental evidence[22,23] is that the initial injury results in fiber disruption, hemorrhage, and fibrin accumulation, which is largely anechogenic. Granulation tissue then forms, which is hypoechogenic. The peritendinous edema which often accompanies acute injuries disappears early in the convalescence. As healing progresses hypoechogenic immature fibrous tissue is produced, which subsequently remodels and "matures." This is seen as a steady increase in echogenicity to approach that of normal tendon,[24] although densely packed fibrous tissue is hyperechogenic.

Therefore, chronic injuries tend to have a mottled appearance. The experimental work has been confirmed in some clinical cases.[25–29] In one study,[25] however, only minor alteration to the echogenicity of the lesion was observed until the fibrous tissue matured. These observations are true in general, but individual tissues may exhibit different patterns of change and heal at different rates.

Superficial Digital Flexor Tendon Abnormalities

Most acute tendon injuries can be seen either as generalized, normoechogenic, or hypoechogenic enlargement, as core or eccentric lesions, or as ruptures. Occasionally, no ultrasonographic changes are visible when an acute injury is suspected from the history or clinical examination. In these cases, rescan the limbs after 1 to 2 weeks, since changes can develop at a later date, especially if the limb was scanned for the first time very soon after the injury.

In early or subclinical injuries, often the only finding is tendon enlargement. It is essential to compare both limbs, bearing in mind that the lesion may be bilateral. Enlargement over 20 percent should be regarded as clinically significant (Table 14B–2).

Most commonly, SDFT injuries are seen as core lesions (Fig. 14B–3). A hypoechoic (occasionally anechoic) lesion of variable size is visible in the center of the tendon, usually most obviously in the midmetacar-

Table 14B-2. Ultrasonographic Cross-Sectional Areas of the Digital Flexor Tendons of 15 Thoroughbred Horses

Level*	Area of SDFT in mm² to the nearest 10 mm²			Area of DDFT in mm² to the nearest 10 mm²		
	Mean	Upper limit†	Lower limit†	Mean	Upper limit†	Lower limit†
1	140	160	110	130	160	100
2	130	160	100	100	120	80
3	120	150	100	180	230	140
4	130	160	90	170	210	140
5	130	160	90	170	210	120
6	140	180	100	170	210	130
7	150	180	120	210	260	170

*For explanation of level, see Figures 14B–1 and 14B–2.
†1.96 standard deviations above/below the mean, which includes 95.0 percent of the population.

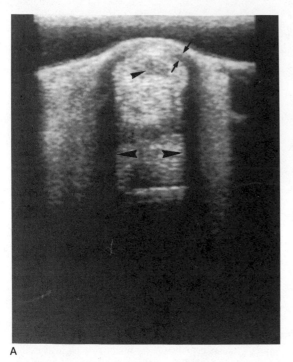

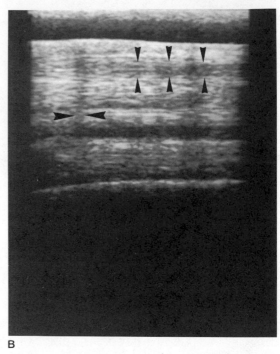

A   B

Figure 14B-3. *Superficial digital flexor tendonitis. (A) A central hypoechoic "core lesion" (medium arrow) in the midmetacarpal region (level 4). Note the hypoechoic ring of edema (small arrows) surrounding the tendon which increases its definition. Edge refraction is responsible for the incomplete appearance of both suspensory branches as they divide (large arrows). (B) Longitudinal ultrasonograph of the midmetacarpal region (level L2). There is a linear hypoechoic region within the tendon (small arrows), and the two flexor tendons can be distinguished. Note the striated pattern of the normal tendon as demonstrated by the DDFT and the poor contact artifacts causing hypoechoic lines (large arrows).*

pal region. If the injury is more proximal or at or below the metacarpophalangeal joint, this is often secondary to a previous injury in the midmetacarpal region. The tendon is usually enlarged, frequently to a greater extent than can be explained by the core lesion, probably because of intratendinous edema or peripheral damage. Although a core lesion can appear completely anechoic, it is unlikely that it will be completely devoid of intact tendon fibrils. As the hemorrhage resolves, these fibrils become identifiable (Genovese, personal communication).

Less commonly, the lesion will be eccentric when it can be dorsally, palmarly (Fig. 14B–4), medially, or laterally situated. The dorsal lesions are said to be more painful, possibly because of the restricted space between the tendons for the lesion to expand. This type of injury is an uncommon manifestation in the thoroughbred. However, in the standardbred, medial or lateral lesions are the most common (Genovese, personal communication).

A generalized hypoechoic appearance of the tendon may represent an acute injury or a tendon that is healing, from which the core lesion has already disappeared. If the injury is recent, however, this appearance is thought to represent extensive fiber disruption, hemorrhage, and intratendinous edema.[30] Rupture of the SDFT is manifest by an almost totally anechogenic region sur-

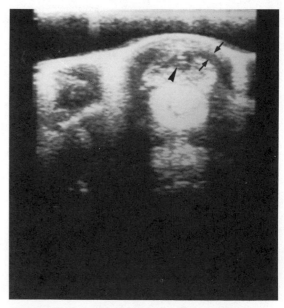

Figure 14B-4. *A palmar border hypoechoic lesion (large arrow) in the SDFT in the proximal midmetacarpal region (level 3). The surface of the tendon appears disrupted. There is substantial hypoechogenic edema surrounding the tendon (small arrows).*

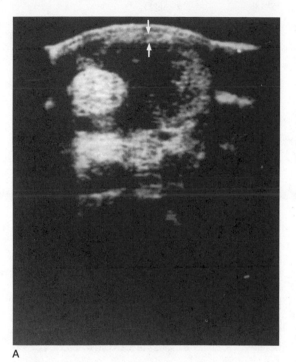
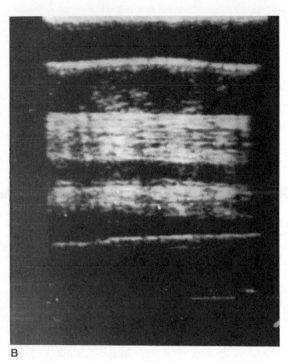

Figure 14B-5. Superficial digital flexor tendon (SDFT) rupture. (A) Transverse ultrasonograph in the midmetacarpal region (level 3) of a horse with almost complete rupture of the SDFT. Note that there is still some echogenic material at the periphery of the tendon (arrows), and in these cases, the paratenon usually remains intact. The gross swelling of the tendon has displaced the deep digital flexor tendon (DDFT) laterally. (B) Longitudinal ultrasonograph in the midmetacarpal region (level L2) of the same case as (A). There is almost complete loss of the echogenicity in the region of the SDFT.

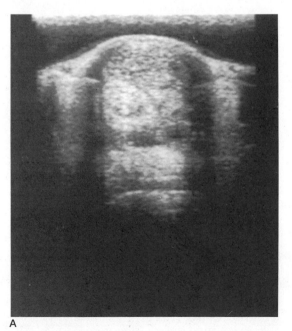
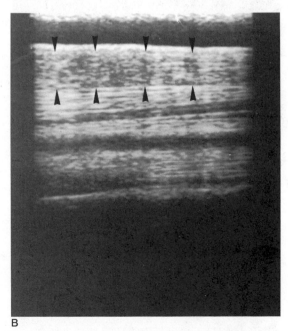

Figure 14B-6. Chronic tendonitis. (A) Transverse ultrasonograph in the midmetacarpal region (level 3) of a case of chronic tendonitis. Note the enlargement, the hypoechogenicity and mottled appearance to the internal architecture of the tendon, and the displacement of the deep digital flexor tendon (DDFT) laterally. (B) Longitudinal ultrasonograph in the midmetacarpal region (level L2) of the same horse as in (A). The superficial digital flexor tendon (SDFT) is hypoechogenic (arrows) and lacks a good striated pattern. The prognosis for this horse to return to full work would be poor based on these findings.

rounded by a thin echogenic line, the paratenon (Fig. 14B–5). Evidence of damage also will be apparent proximal and distal to the rupture.

The ultrasound characteristics of chronic tendon injuries are subtle. The tendon is often still enlarged, but its echogenicity varies from hypoechogenic through normoechogenic to hyperechogenic if the initial injury was severe and substantial fibrosis has occurred. The intratendinous pattern usually is more coarse (Fig. 14B–6). Rarely, dystrophic calcification occurs, usually a result of the intratendinous injection of corticosteroids, and this leads to acoustic shadowing (Fig. 14B–7).

Superficial digital flexor tendon lesions have been typed 1 to 4[4,12,31] in order to allow comparison between sequential scans and to assign them a degree of severity. Type 1 is marginally hypoechoic, while Type 4 is anechoic. By combining the size of the lesion and its degree of hypoechogenicity, a severity rating can be adduced for the lesion.[32]

Local trauma can cause either localized peritendinous edema with no evidence of intratendinous damage (Fig. 14B–8) or localized hypoechogenic/anechogenic lesions on the palmar or plantar surface of the tendon (Fig. 14B–9). Sepsis is usually seen as an anechogenic lesion, often with a communicating tract to the periphery of the tendon. Aspiration of the lesion will yield a sample containing large numbers of degenerate neutrophils and possibly bacteria. These lesions change rapidly

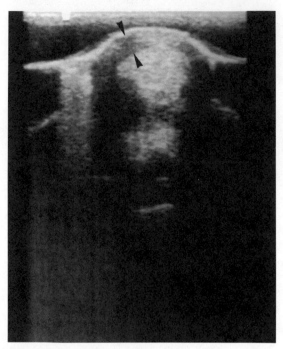

Figure 14B-8. *Subcutaneous edema with no tendon damage, presumed to be due to local trauma to the palmar aspect of the limb in the midmetacarpal region (level 4). Note the good definition of the palmar border of the superficial digital flexor tendon (SDFT) in particular and the hypoechoic region palmar to the tendon which represents the edema (arrows).*

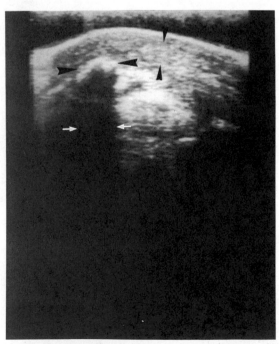

Figure 14B-7. *Transverse ultrasonograph in the distal metacarpal region (level 6) of a case with calcification (large arrows) within the superficial digital flexor tendon (SDFT). This is causing a shadow (white arrows) to be cast over the deep digital flexor tendon (DDFT). Note also the extensive fibrosis (small arrows) in the subcutaneous tissues.*

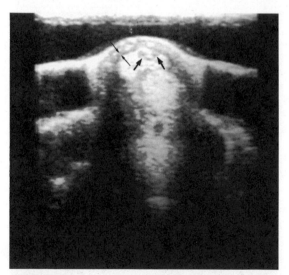

Figure 14B-9. *Transverse ultrasonograph of the proximal metatarsal region (level 4). There is a small, localized, hypoechoic lesion (large arrows) on the plantar aspect of the superficial digital flexor tendon (SDFT). Note the usual position of the SDFT in the proximal hindlimb, lateral to the deep digital flexor tendon (DDFT), and the ring of hypoechogenic edema (small arrows) surrounding the tendon. This lesion had not been identified 2 weeks earlier, so the ultrasonographic examination was repeated because the peritendinous edema had not resolved as expected.*

in time (increasing or decreasing) compared with the slow resolution of a core lesion.

Abnormalities of the Accessory Ligament of the Deep Digital Flexor Tendon

The damaged ligament is hypoechogenic, either diffusely or focally (Fig. 14B–10). It is usually enlarged and may extend and adhere to the margins of the SDFT. There may be a concurrent SDFT injury.[33]

Suspensory Ligament Abnormalities

Three syndromes are encountered. In the proximal metacarpal/metatarsal syndrome, or "high suspensory disease," the abnormal ultrasonographic appearance of the SL overlaps with its normal appearance. In normal horses, the presence of hypoechogenic foci in the proximal SL is common (Fig. 14B–11), and therefore, their significance must be determined by the clinical findings (swelling, pain on palpation) and the effects of diagnostic local anesthesia. Those considered to be true lesions will vary in time, so repeat examinations are useful to confirm their significance. Other clinically significant changes that have been described include enlargement of the SL in the dorsopalmar direction (Fig. 14B–12), poor definition to its margins (especially dorsally), single or multiple poorly defined areas of focal hypoechogenicity, or diffuse hypoechogenicity.[34] Avulsion fractures, enthesiophytosis, or palmar/plantar cortical bone changes at the origin of the SL, which are readily detectable ra-

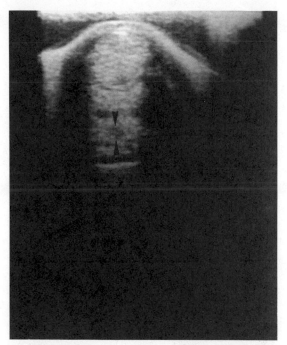

Figure 14B-11. Transverse ultrasonograph of the proximal metacarpal region (level 1) of a normal horse demonstrating an insignificant central hypoechoic region (arrows) within the suspensory ligament (SL).

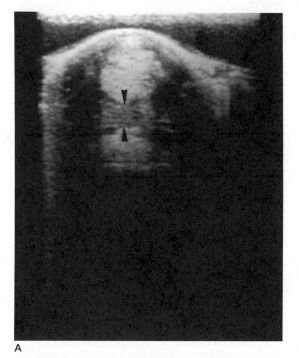

A

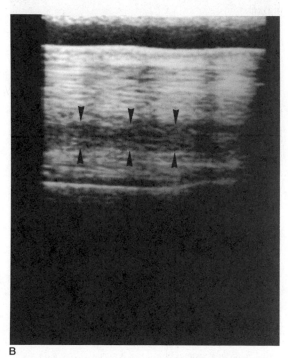

B

Figure 14B-10. Desmitis of the ALDDFT. (A) Transverse ultrasonograph in the proximal metacarpal region (level 1). Note the hypoechogenicity of the ALDDFT (arrows), which usually is the most echogenic structure in this region in a normal horse. (B) Longitudinal ultrasonograph in the proximal metacarpal region (level L1) of the same horse as in (A). The ALDDFT is hypoechogenic (arrows). Note also the loss of the normal "space" between the suspensory ligament (SL) and the ALDDFT because of the latter's enlargement.

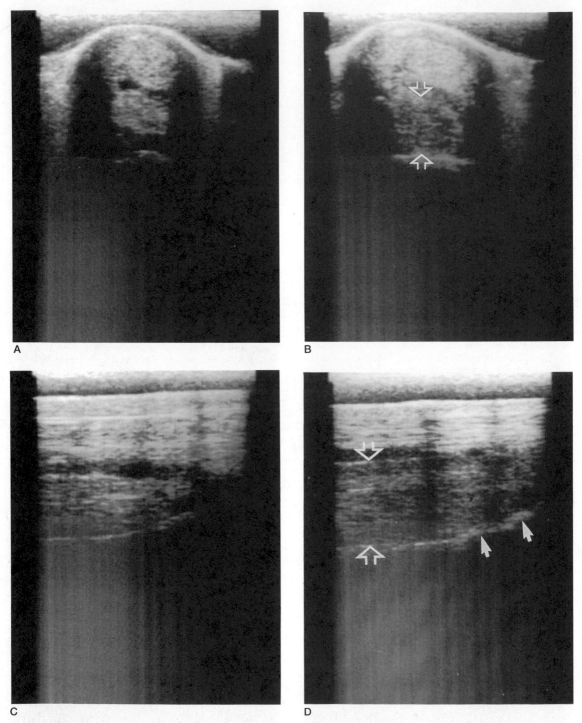

Figure 14B-12. Proximal suspensory ligament (SL) desmitis. (A) Normal proximal metatarsal region (level 3)—transverse ultrason-ograph. (B) Transverse ultrasonograph of the same level but the contralateral limb to that in (A). Note the hypoechogenicity and enlargement of the proximal SL (arrows). This horse had been lame on this limb for 6 months prior to this examination. Swelling was palpable in the proximal metatarsal region. (C) Normal proximal metatarsal region (level L2)—longitudinal ultrasonograph. (D) Lon-gitudinal ultrasonograph of the contralateral proximal metatarsal region (level L2). There is considerable hypoechogenic enlargement in the dorsoplantar direction (open arrows). There is also some evidence of enthesiophytosis at the origin of the suspensory ligament, demonstrated by greater irregularity of the plantar surface of the metatarsus (closed arrows).

diographically, also may be seen during an ultrasonographic examination.

Injuries to the body of the SL usually result in generalized hypoechogenicity with a heterogeneous pattern and enlargement (Fig. 14B–13). If one or both of the branches are involved, the most common SL injury, a core lesion, or more generalized involvement of the branch is seen ultrasonographically (Fig. 14B–14). It is useful to examine the branches from the medial or lateral aspect as well as from the palmar aspect because of the edge refraction shadowing that commonly obscures the branches in transverse images. The injury can extend proximally into the body of the SL. Body and branch SL injuries can be associated with splint bone fractures or periostitis, sesamoiditis, distal sesamoidean ligament pathology, and fetlock joint changes, so radiography is mandatory in these cases.

Some horses will have bilaterally hypoechogenic and enlarged SL branches without clinical signs (Fig. 14B–15). This may represent previous or insidious trauma or degenerative changes. The increasing incidence of SL body and branch injury with age suggests a degenerative component to the condition. In our experience, approximately one-third of cases have bilateral changes ultrasonographically, so both limbs should be examined at the initial presentation and subsequently.

In standardbreds, the SL is injured more commonly in the hindlimb, while in thoroughbreds, the forelimbs are most commonly affected. Furthermore, in standardbreds, the hindlimb SL is the palmar/plantar soft-tissue structure most commonly injured in comparison with thoroughbreds, which more often injure the forelimb SDFT.[35]

Healing of SL injuries often results in considerable fibrosis between the branch and the skin (Fig. 14B–16). Not all cases will show ultrasonographic evidence of healing. Lesions may remain unchanged over many months, although, clinically, the horse may be unaltered, improved, or sound. Such cases may be returned to work, but with a guarded prognosis.

Annular Ligament Syndrome

A suggested scheme for the etiopathogenesis of the annular ligament syndrome (ALS) is depicted in Figure 14B–17. Four causes of thickening of the palmar/plantar aspect of the fetlock joint, which may be differentiated with ultrasound,[36] have been described: primary AL thickening to over 2 mm (Fig. 14B–18), distension and thickening of the digital sheath without AL enlargement, SDFT/DDFT injury with secondary AL enlargement (Fig. 14B–19), and subcutaneous fibrosis. Primary ALS will have no ultrasonographic evidence of damage to the

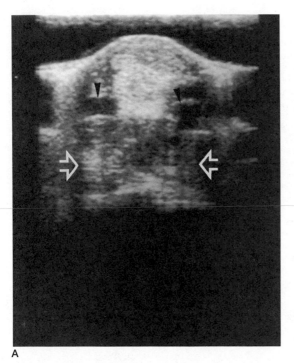

A

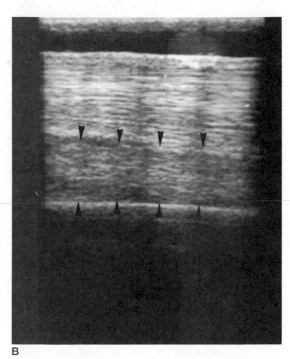

B

Figure 14B-13. *Desmitis of the body of the suspensory ligament (SL). (A) Transverse ultrasonograph of the midmetacarpal region (level 4). There is disruption of the normal internal architecture of the SL, with enlargement and hypoechogenicity (open arrows). Note also the distended vasculature on either side of the deep digital flexor tendon (DDFT) and superficial to the damaged SL (arrows). (B) Longitudinal ultrasonograph in the midmetacarpal region (level L2) demonstrating enlargement and hypoechogenicity of the body of the SL (arrows). Note the loss of the normal "space" between the ALDDFT and SL.*

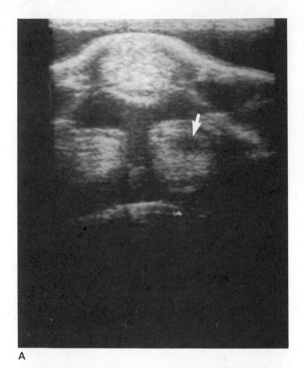

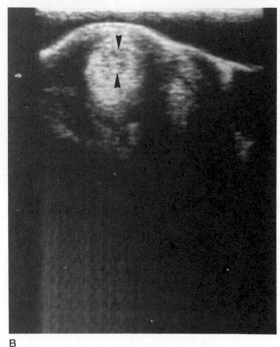

A

B

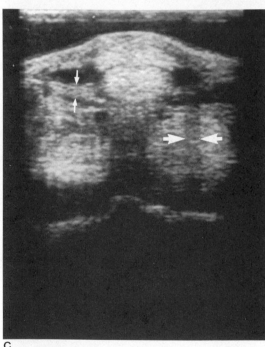

C

Figure 14B-14. *Suspensory ligament (SL) branch desmitis. (A) Transverse ultrasonograph of the distal metacarpal region (level 5) from a horse with SL branch desmitis. There is enlargement of both branches, with greater enlargement and a central hypoechoic region within the medial branch (arrow). (B) Ultrasonograph from a horse suffering from lateral suspensory branch desmitis. The image is obtained by placing the probe in a transverse fashion across the lateral aspect of the limb directly over the lateral SL branch. The branch is well delineated and reveals a hypoechoic region close to the abaxial surface of the branch (arrows). (C) Transverse ultrasonograph of the distal metatarsal region (level 7) of a horse showing generalized enlargement of the medial and to some extent the lateral SL branch. An edge refraction shadow can be seen from the medial side of the superficial digital flexor tendon (SDFT) extending through the medial SL branch (large arrows). This artifact is responsible for the poor imaging of the SL branches from the palmar aspect of the limb in most cases. Here, the gross enlargement of the SL branches has limited the compromise of the image by the edge refraction. Concurrent digital sheath distension provides negative contrast to allow easy identification of the synovial plica (small arrows) attaching to the lateral side of the deep digital flexor tendon (DDFT), which is a normal finding (see Fig. 14B–21).*

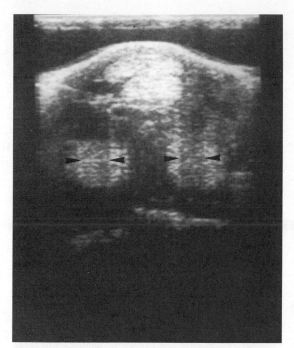

Figure 14B-15. *Transverse ultrasonograph of the distal metatarsal region (level 6) of the contralateral limb to that shown in Figure 14B–14C. Although the horse was not lame on this limb, there is biaxial enlargement (compare with Fig. 14B–20) and hypoechogenicity of the two suspensory ligament (SL) branches. This horse subsequently presented with an acute injury to the medial SL branch of this limb. Note the edge refraction shadowing through both branches (arrows).*

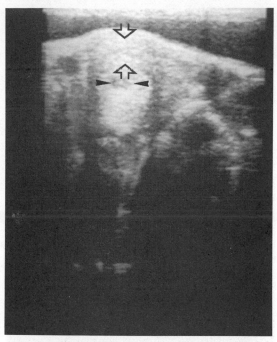

Figure 14B-16. *Lateral transverse ultrasonograph from a horse suffering from lateral suspensory ligament (SL) desmitis. Although a hypoechoic lesion still exists with the branch (closed arrows), there is considerable periligamentous fibrosis (open arrows).*

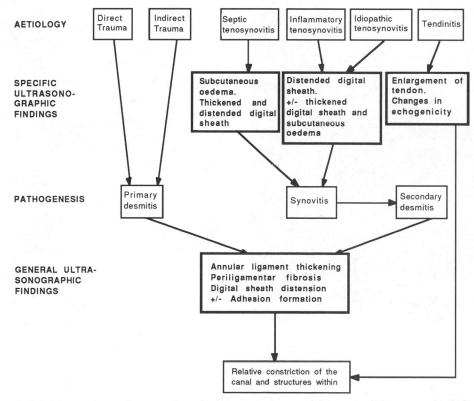

Figure 14B-17. *Suggested etiopathogenesis of annular ligament syndrome and the associated ultrasonographic findings.*

311

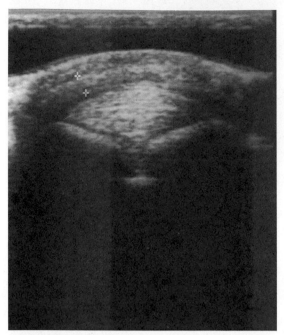

Figure 14B-18. *Transverse ultrasonograph over the palmar aspect of the metacarpophalangeal joint (level 7) of a horse with primary annular ligament syndrome. There is enlargement of the annular ligament (between crosses) to about 4 mm.*

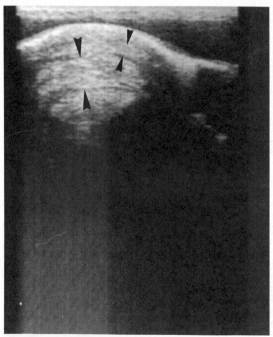

Figure 14B-19. *Transverse ultrasonograph over the palmar aspect of the metacarpophalangeal joint (level 7) of a horse with secondary annular ligament syndrome. There is enlargement of the annular ligament (small arrows) secondary to a superficial digital flexor tendon (SDFT) injury (large arrows) in the region of the metacarpophalangeal joint.*

flexor tendons, but occasionally, in the early stages of the condition, there may be signs of desmitis of the annular ligament (hypoechogenicity and regions of anechogenicity). There is digital sheath synovial effusion, and less commonly, echogenic adhesions are formed (Fig. 14B–20). The normal lateral synovial reflection in the proximal digital sheath (Fig. 14B–21) should not be mistaken for an adhesion.

Intersesamoidean Ligament Sepsis
Osteomyelitis of the axial border of the proximal sesamoid bones has been described.[37] In such cases, it is possible to demonstrate localized areas of hypoechogenicity, representing sepsis, within the intersesamoidean ligament (Fig. 14B–22).

Conditions of the Phalangeal Region
If any of the supporting structures on the palmar/plantar aspect of the phalanges are damaged, extensive subcutaneous fibrosis often develops as the injury heals. There may be concomitant bony damage, e.g., osteochondral chip fractures of the palmar/plantar aspect of the fetlock joint, so radiography also should be employed in these

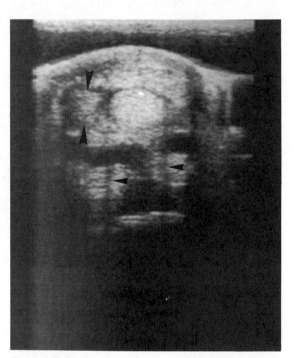

Figure 14B-20. *Transverse ultrasonograph in the distal meta-carpal region (level 5) of a horse which sustained a local injury in the region of the annular ligament. The horse developed annular ligament syndrome, and during surgical release, an ulcer was found on the surface of the superficial digital flexor tendon (SDFT) beneath the annular ligament. The horse was treated postoperatively with intrasynovial hyaluronic acid and became sound. Six months later, it suddenly became lame. Repeat ultrasonography reveals adhesions (large arrows) within the digital sheath. Note again the edge refraction shadowing extending through both suspensory ligament (SL) branches (small arrows).*

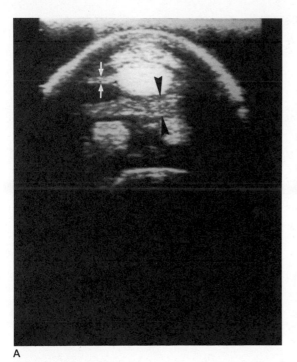

A

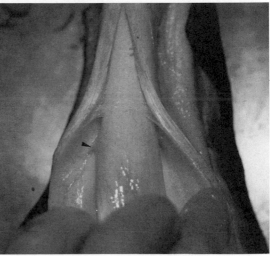

B

Figure 14B-21. (A) *Transverse ultrasonograph of the distal metacarpal region (level 5) from a horse suffering from annular ligament syndrome. The normal lateral synovial plica (white arrows) joining the sheath wall to the deep digital flexor tendon (DDFT) is easily visible because of the negative contrast provided by the digital sheath effusion. There is thickening of the digital sheath wall dorsally (black arrows) and slight thickening of the plica, indicating an inflammatory tenosynovitis. The plicae should not be confused with adhesions—none were found during an open annular ligament desmotomy. (B) Dissection of the proximal digital sheath region in a cadaver limb demonstrating the biaxial plicae joining the DDFT. The lateral plica (arrow) is more substantial and usually extends further distally than the medial plica, and the more marked lateral distension of the proximal sheath means that the plica is more often identified laterally [see (A)].*

cases. Injury to the SDFT in the region of the metacarpophalangeal joint usually includes the SDFT branches and often occurs secondarily to injury to the midmetacarpal region of the SDFT. The SDFT branches are enlarged and are best imaged with 45-degree oblique views medially and laterally, which can be compared with the contralateral limb (Fig. 14B–23). Enlargement and hypoechogenicity of either or both of the middle and straight (Fig. 14B–24) distal sesamoidean ligaments can be identified ultrasonographically. The same 45-degree oblique views are useful to examine the middle distal sesamoidean ligaments. Healing of these injuries is unpredictable both clinically and ultrasonographically, and it is common to find them unchanged after many months of convalescence. The DDFT is rarely injured proximal to the fetlock joint, but it may be injured at the level of the fetlock joint and in the region of the phalanges, when, characteristically, it is enlarged and disrupted by hypoechogenic fissures (Fig. 14B–25). It is rare to record marked ultrasonographic changes in cases of navicular disease, but this probably reflects our inability to scan successfully more distally than the proximal interphalangeal joint with a linear probe.

Sepsis of the DDFT, which may be accompanied by digital sheath sepsis, is occasionally found following

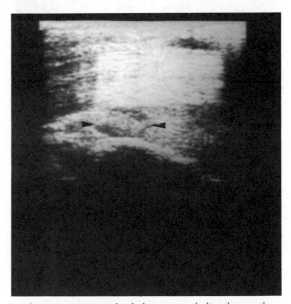

Figure 14B-22. *Longitudinal ultrasonograph directly over the intersesamoidean ligament of the metacarpophalangeal joint. An hypoechoic region within the ligament can be identified (arrows) which was subsequently confirmed to be an abscess on postmortem examination (photograph A. Kent).*

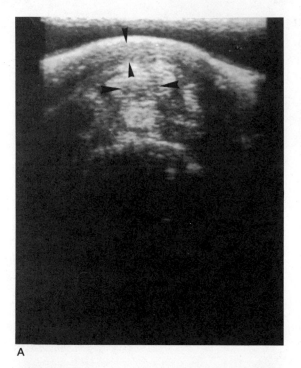

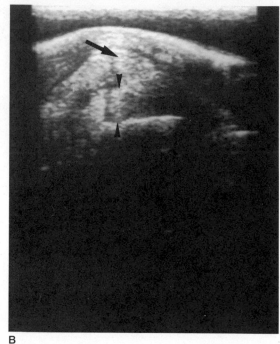

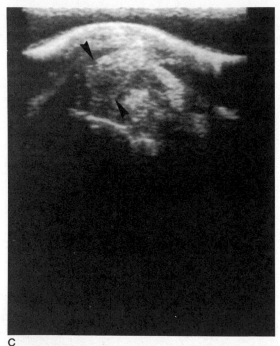

Figure 14B-23. *Tendonitis of the superficial digital flexor tendon (SDFT) branches. (A) Transverse ultrasonograph of the midphalangeal region (level P2) in a horse with tendonitis of the branches of the SDFT. The branches are poorly identifiable. There is considerable subcutaneous fibrosis (small arrows) which follows an injury to any of the soft tissues of the palmar aspect of the phalanges. Note the central hypoechoic region (large arrows) in the deep digital flexor tendon (DDFT), which is artifactual because of the angulation of the probe. (B) A 45-degree oblique transverse ultrasonograph at the same level as (A). Both the medial oblique distal sesamoidean ligament (small arrows) and the medial SDFT branch can be identified (large arrow). The latter is enlarged and heterogeneous. (C) A 45-degree oblique transverse ultrasonograph of the lateral aspect. The lateral SDFT branch is enlarged (arrows) and contains a more hypoechoic region.*

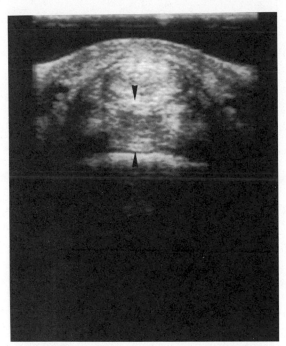

Figure 14B-24. Transverse ultrasonograph of the midphalangeal region (level P2) in a horse with desmitis of the distal sesamoidean ligaments. There is enlargement of the straight distal sesamoidean ligaments, which are also hypoechogenic (arrows). Note the nonspecific subcutaneous fibrosis.

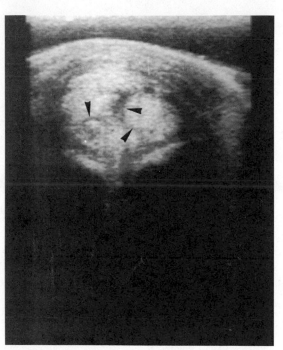

Figure 14B-25. Transverse ultrasonograph over the palmar aspect of the metacarpophalangeal joint (level 7) of a horse with a deep flexor tendon (DDFT) injury. There is enlargement of the DDFT, which contains hypoechoic fissures (arrows) and subcutaneous fibrosis.

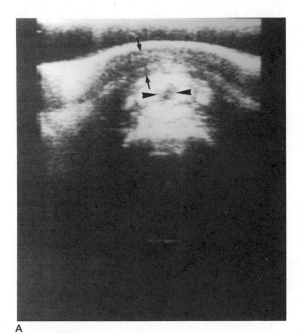

A

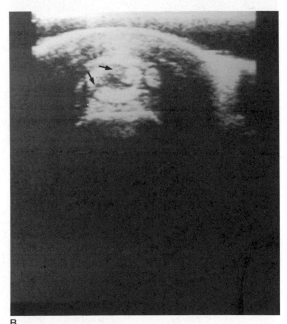

B

Figure 14B-26. Septic deep digital flexor tendonitis (DDFT) in the phalangeal region. (A) Transverse ultrasonograph of the midphalangeal region (level P2) in a pony with a septic DDFT lesion. There is an irregular hypoechoic region (large arrows) within the tendon, but the tendon is not greatly enlarged, unlike a traumatic tendonitis. There is substantial subcutaneous edema, which is hypoechogenic (small arrows). (B) Transverse ultrasonograph at the same level as (A) 7 days later. There is considerable enlargement of the hypoechoic lesion with tracts extending to the periphery of the tendon (arrows).

penetrating wounds in the region of the phalanges (Fig. 14B–26).

OTHER TENDONS

Bicipital Tendon and Bursa

The bicipital tendon and its bursa can be investigated easily using a 7.5-MHz linear probe without a stand-off. If the area is swollen, contact is made more easily. The bicipital tendon is imaged at the point of the shoulder and, more distally, cranial to the deltoid tuberosity. It is bilobed, and the bursa can be identified as a thin anechoic line deep to it. Bicipital bursal distension (Fig. 14B–27) is readily diagnosed by an increased amount of fluid within the bursa. In bursal sepsis, the effusion is often floccular. Bicipital tendon disease is rare in our experience but is manifest as a large and heterogeneous tendon with or without (Fig. 14B–28) bursal distension.[38,39]

Common Calcaneal Tendon and Deep Digital Flexor Tendon Proximal to the Tarsus

The common calcaneal tendon consists of two major tendons, the gastrocnemius and the SDFT. The common calcaneal tendon also includes the tarsal tendons of the biceps femoris, gracilis, soleus, semimembranosus, and semitendinosus muscles which unite to form a complex tendinous insertion into the os calcis.

With the probe transversely across the tendons, just proximally to the point of the hock, the SDFT is seen as

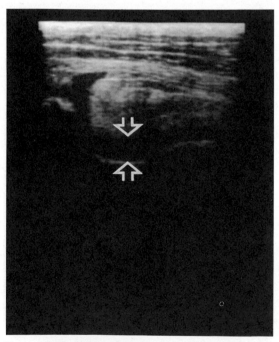

Figure 14B-27. Transverse ultrasonograph of the lateral aspect of the bicipital tendon and bursa at the level of the humeral tubercles of a horse that had sustained a small chip fracture of one of the tubercles. The bicipital tendon is not grossly enlarged, but there is increased fluid within the bicipital bursa (arrows).

a thin strip of tissue. Deep to it is the gastrocnemius tendon, which is almost circular. As the probe is advanced proximally, the SDFT becomes more circular. It is similar in size to the gastrocnemius tendon, to which it lies medially. The tendons become undiscernible further proximally at their musculotendinous junctions, where the characteristic herringbone pattern of muscle is identified. Care must be taken when examining both the common calcaneal tendon and the DDFT not to mistake normal muscle at the proximal extremity of the tendons for a hypoechoic lesion.

Ultrasonographic abnormalities of the gastrocnemius tendon include enlargement, poorly defined borders, and various hypoechogenic areas within the tendon.[40] Abnormalities in the other components of the common calcaneal tendon also have been described.[41] Effusion in the calcaneal bursa can be identified as an anechogenic separation between the SDFT and the common calcaneal tendon (Fig. 14B–29). Abnormalities of the SDFT are often related to its position, because the tendon is usually displaced laterally when it is avulsed from the point of the hock (Fig. 14B–30).

Proximal to the os calcis, the DDFT can be identified deep to the common calcaneal tendon; a 5-MHz scan head may be required. If the scan head is moved distally and medially, the DDFT within the tarsal sheath can be imaged more easily, especially if there is effusion within the sheath. At the same time, the surface of the sustentaculum tali can be identified with the DDFT superficial to it. In cases with tarsal sheath effusion (thoroughpin), an ultrasound examination will differentiate between those with DDFT damage, those with changes affecting the sustentaculum tali, and those which are primary synovitides with or without adhesions.

Extensor Tendons on the Dorsal Aspect of the Carpus

The extensor carpi radialis and common and lateral digital extensor tendons can be readily identified in that order moving from the midline laterally with a transversely positioned probe. Their sheaths can be examined for effusion and adhesions. Intrasynovial rupture of the common digital extensor tendon is a relatively common occurrence in neonatal foals. The two ends of the tendon can be identified within the negative contrast provided by the distended sheath on the dorsolateral aspect of the carpus.

Peroneus Tertius

This is easily identified on the craniolateral aspect of the crus as an elliptical hyperechogenic structure between the muscle bellies of the long digital extensor and the tibialis cranialis. Subcutaneous rupture of the peroneus tertius makes it look thinner. Healing is by fibrosis, although recovery seems to depend primarily on the hypertrophy of the surrounding muscles.[42]

BENEFITS OF ULTRASONOGRAPHIC EXAMINATION OF TENDON AND LIGAMENT INJURIES

Palpation of a swollen limb is extremely important in the diagnosis of tendon and ligament disease but can be very

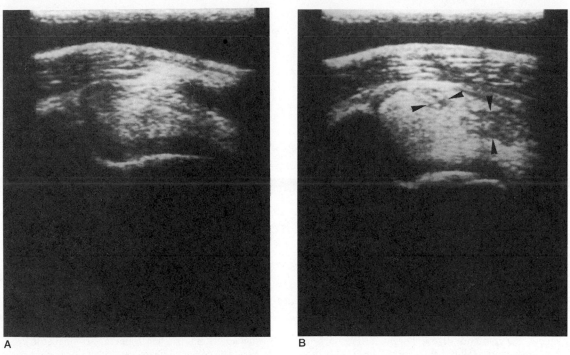

A B

Figure 14B-28. Transverse ultrasonographs of the lateral aspect of the bicipital tendon. (A) Normal bicipital tendon and bursa at the level of the humeral tubercles. (B) Bicipital tendonitis. Note the enlargement and areas of hypoechoicity within the tendon (arrows).

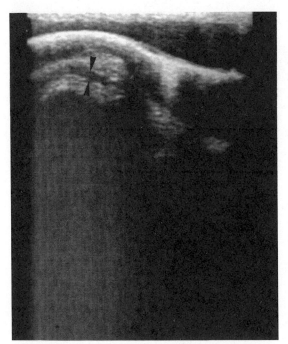

Figure 14B-29. Transverse ultrasonograph at the level of the point of the hock of a horse with septic calcaneal bursitis. An anechoic region (arrows) can be seen separating the superficial digital flexor tendon (SDFT) and the common calcaneal tendon, indicating the presence of fluid within the bursa.

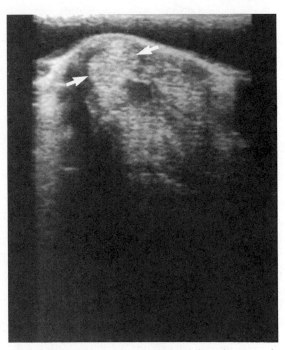

Figure 14B-30. Transverse ultrasonograph from the proximal metatarsal region (level 2) of a horse with lateral luxation of the superficial digital flexor tendon (SDFT) from the point of the hock. Note the lateral displacement (arrows) of the SDFT.

misleading. Ultrasonography allows identification or confirmation of the structure involved and facilitates an assessment of the severity of the damage. When only mild swelling of the limb has been noticed clinically, ultrasonography may reveal subtle signs, especially increases in the cross-sectional area of the tendon with no alteration in its internal architecture, which are harbingers of more severe injury. Recognition of these changes should help to avert an acute, overt tendon injury, which will result in a prolonged convalescence culminating in a healed tendon that has inferior strength to the original. Alternatively, a similar swelling may prove to be due to peritendinous edema with no tendon involvement and a good prognosis for a rapid return to work.

It is possible that ultrasonographic monitoring has made the most important contribution to the successful outcome of tendon injuries in recent years. Ultrasound examination performed at 2- to 3-month intervals allows a judgment to be made of when the horse can return to graded gentle and then strenuous work. Before the horse is returned to full exercise, the healed tendon ideally should show homogeneous longitudinal and transverse patterns with no hypoechogenic regions and no adhesions. It has been shown that a tendon ultrasonograph does not return to normal until healing is completed.[25] A persistently hypoechogenic lesion does not indicate that no healing has occurred, because hemorrhage and granulation tissue may have organized, yet little or no difference may be seen ultrasonographically. The tendon must, however, be considered to be inferior functionally.

Nevertheless, some horses, particularly standardbreds rather than thoroughbreds, are able to compete even though ultrasonographic lesions remain. These cases should be followed ultrasonographically very carefully (preferably after each race/competition) to determine if the tendon is deteriorating and so hopefully to prevent a catastrophic failure. Not every case will return to normoechogenicity. The quality of healing varies between animals and is dependent on a number of factors, including the structure damaged, the severity of the injury, the age of the horse, the breed, and the purpose for which the animal is used. In racehorses, SDFT injuries appear to heal less well ultrasonographically than those in other horses. Some aspects of the rehabilitation of horses with tendon injuries are covered in Chapter 16.

Joints

Joint effusions are usually anechogenic. Synovial thickening, villous proliferation, and adhesions also can be demonstrated.[43] Collateral ligaments can be hard to identify ultrasonographically because they tend to be less discrete than tendons. Damage to them is best identified by the accompanying hemorrhage, which is hypoechogenic. Menisci are echogenic with a fine homogeneous internal architecture. Meniscal tears can be imaged provided that they involve the part of the meniscus that can be seen ultrasonographically.

The articular cartilage is very thin in the distal joints of the limb. It can be identified as a thin, anechoic line superficial to the bright, subchondral bone, but because it is so thin, the detection of minor erosions is difficult. The more proximal joints, especially the stifle, have thicker cartilage, which is easily examined using a 7.5-MHz probe. Articular erosions and osteochondral defects, e.g., osteochondrosis and the opening to intraarticular cysts, can be identified, especially in the stifle, provided that the probe can be positioned over the defect. The thickness of the cartilage varies with both individual and age, so the contralateral limb must be examined for comparison.[43] If fractures involve a joint surface that is amenable to ultrasound examination, ultrasound is very useful in conjunction with radiography, to examine the articular portion of the fracture, to assess joint comminution and cartilage damage, and to locate accurately its position.

STIFLE

The ultrasonographic appearance of the stifle region has been described.[44] The identifiable structures include the three patellar ligaments, the collateral ligaments, the articular cartilage on the trochlear ridges, and the medial and lateral menisci. The middle patellar ligament is the easiest of the three patellar ligaments to identify. The medial and lateral patellar ligaments are smaller in cross section. The collateral ligaments are elliptical and poorly defined on the most medial and lateral margins of the joint. The articular cartilage of the trochlear ridges in

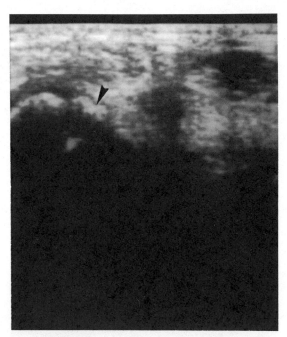

Figure 14B-31. *Transverse ultrasonograph of the trochlear ridges of the femoropatellar joint of a horse with osteochondrosis of the lateral trochlear ridges. An ossified fragment* (arrow) *can be identified on the axial surface of the lateral trochlear ridge with a defect beneath it visible between the fragment and the normal subchondral bone.*

adult horses is usually 1 to 2 mm in thickness. In cases of osteochondrosis, areas of thickened cartilage with or without bone fragmentation can be identified in both transverse and longitudinal scans of the trochlear ridges (Fig. 14B–31). The entrance to medial condylar cysts cannot be imaged ultrasonographically unless they are situated very close to the medial edge of the condyle.

The menisci can be identified with the probe held longitudinally caudally to the medial or lateral patellar ligament or between the middle patellar ligament and the medial or lateral patellar ligament. They are triangular in this view. The cruciate ligaments cannot be imaged unless the stifle is maintained in severe flexion,[44,45] when they are hypoechogenic within a relatively hyperechogenic fat pad.

TARSUS

The trochlear ridges are easily examined, although they are very superficial, and a stand-off pad is useful. Thinning of the articular cartilage is difficult to assess with certainty (Fig. 14B–32). In contrast, thickening of the articular cartilage, secondary ossification of cartilage flaps, and/or fragmentation of the subchondral bone (as in osteochondrosis) can be readily identified. The lateral trochlear ridge of the talus can be assessed easily for such lesions, while the distal intermediate ridge of the tibia, another common site of osteochondrosis in the tarsus, is less easily imaged because of the difficulty in placing the probe directly above the lesion. Large defects are visible, but smaller fragments close to the trochlear ridges may be missed. The collateral ligaments are identifiable, and the long and short collateral ligaments can be individually imaged (Fig. 14B–33).

ELBOW

The medial and lateral collateral ligaments can be identified ultrasonographically[45] because they lie superficially on the limb. They are best seen in a longitudinal view.

FETLOCK JOINT

The dorsal aspect of this joint can be scanned easily in the standing horse with the limb flexed. The sagittal ridge of the distal metacarpus/metatarsus can be identified, but the articular cartilage is very thin (<1 mm), so its accurate examination is very difficult. Effusion can be imaged both dorsally and laterally and medially in the palmar/plantar pouches. An ultrasonographic examination permits an assessment of the thickness of the synovial membrane and any echogenic material within the joint. Soft-tissue masses attached to the joint capsule dorsally also can be visualized, for example, in villonodular synovitis.[46,47]

On the dorsal aspect of the joint, many horses have a bursa related to the common and lateral digital extensor tendons which, if septic, can mimic clinically a joint infection. Ultrasonographically, the infected bursa can be seen as a separate, distended structure (Fig. 14B–34).

Muscle

Skeletal muscle consists of relatively hypoechogenic muscle fibers separated by hyperechogenic fibroadipose septa. This gives a characteristic herringbone pattern.[48–50] Initially, hematomas can be very difficult to identify, since fresh hemorrhage is echogenic, and all that may be seen is a loss of the normal herringbone pattern. As the hemorrhage begins to organize, the hematoma becomes hypoechogenic. It may contain small, bright echoes, which are thought to represent fibrin clots. It is consequently very difficult to distinguish a hematoma from an abscess. However, an ultrasound-guided aspiration of the cavity will usually provide positive differentiation.[51]

An abscess may be anechogenic (Fig. 14B–35) with acoustic enhancement deep to it. The amount of internal echoes will depend on the consistency of the pus, thick pus being more echogenic. A chronic abscess will often have a hyperechogenic capsule.

Ultrasonography has been suggested for confirmation of the diagnosis of fibrotic myopathy.[45] Fibrosis will be hyperechogenic, and calcification casts acoustic shadows. Musculoskeletal tumors are encountered infrequently in the horse, but sarcomas and rhabdomyosarcomas have been described and their ultrasonographic appearance recorded.[50,52,53]

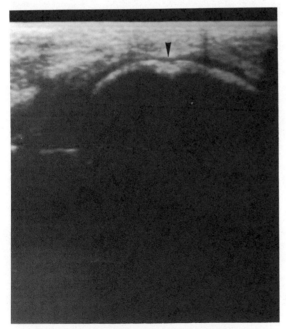

Figure 14B-32. Longitudinal ultrasonograph of the lateral trochlear ridge of the talus of a horse that had sustained a wound over the lateral aspect of the tarsocrural joint. A defect can be seen in the trochlear ridge (arrow) with thinning of the overlying cartilage (compare with the cartilage either side of the defect).

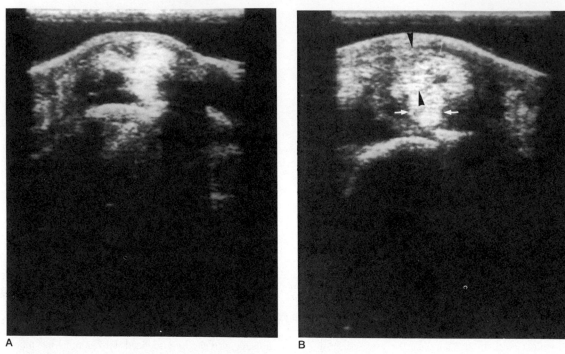

Figure 14B-33. *Transverse ultrasonographs of the medial collateral ligaments of the tarsocrural joints in (A) a normal limb and (B) the contralateral limb with desmitis of the medial collateral ligaments. Note the enlargement of both the short (white arrows) and long (black arrows) medial collateral ligaments.*

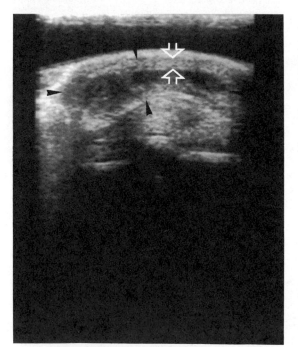

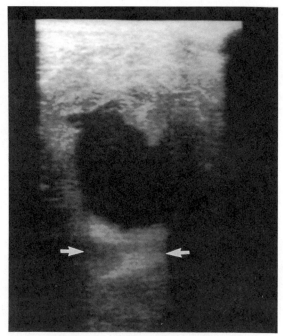

Figure 14B-34. *Transverse ultrasonograph over the dorsal aspect of the metacarpophalangeal joint in a horse with septic bursitis of the dorsal subcutaneous bursa. An anechoic region (black arrows) is surrounded by a capsule (white arrows). The dorsal sagittal ridge of the distal metacarpus can be identified, and the bursa is superficial to the joint and the extensor tendon.*

Figure 14B-35. *Transverse ultrasonograph of the medial aspect of the thigh in a horse with a muscle abscess. There is an irregularly shaped anechoic region with acoustic enhancement deep to it (arrows). A clearly defined abscess capsule is identifiable.*

Blood Vessels

Blood vessels are generally circumscribed and anechogenic. They are easily identified in the region of the metacarpus while scanning for tendon and/or ligament injuries. If there is thrombosis within a vessel, the thrombus appears hyperechogenic, as in cases of aorto-iliac thrombosis.[54–56]

Bone

Ultrasonography has long been considered of most value in examining soft tissues. However, it is used increasingly in assessing the surface of bone, where, in combination with other imaging techniques, especially radiography, it allows a more complete picture of bony problems to be assessed.[48,57] Because of the acoustic shadowing caused by bone, the area of interest should be examined in as many planes as possible.

FRACTURES

Fractures can be identified in areas not readily amenable to radiography, such as the ribs and pelvis.[58] In the latter, diagnosis using ultrasonography may avoid risking further damage by anesthetizing the animal, although standing pelvic radiographs are feasible (see Chap. 14A). The degree of fragmentation and any associated soft-tissue damage, an important component in successful fracture repair, can be examined ultrasonographically.

Ultrasonographs can identify and locate small fragments precisely, especially those which are intraarticular, which may have been missed radiographically. This is especially true of regions where appropriate tangential views cannot be taken, for example, to determine the axial or abaxial position of a lesion on the trochlear ridge of the stifle or tarsus (Fig. 14B–36) or in the proximal limb where swelling has reduced the quality of the radiographs because of increased scatter and poor contrast (Fig. 14B–37). By manipulating the probe, the ultrasonographer can build up a three-dimensional image of the injured area. Nondisplaced or incomplete fractures can be identified ultrasonographically, although with difficulty, as a thin echogenic line visible deep to the subchondral bone.

The progress of fracture healing also can be assessed. Initially, the unmineralized callus can be identified between the two ends of bone. As healing progresses, mineralized callus is identified casting an acoustic shadow (Fig. 14B–38). Immature callus is seen ultrasonographically before it is visible radiographically as mineralized, mature callus.[59]

INFECTION

In chronic osteomyelitis, a characteristically anechogenic or hypoechogenic involucrum with one or more central, highly reflective sequestra is easily identified[45,60] (Fig. 14B–39). In some cases (Fig. 14B–40), no involucrum develops, and the infected area of bone is roughened with an anechogenic fluid collection and several bone fragments.[49,61]

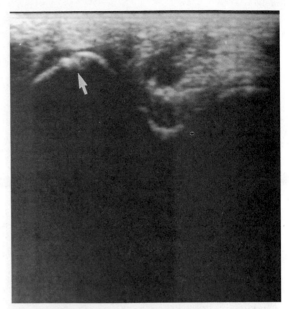

Figure 14B-36. *Transverse ultrasonograph of the trochlear ridges of the talus of a horse with an injury to the dorsolateral aspect of the tarsocrural joint (see also Fig. 14B–32). A defect is seen abaxially on the lateral trochlear ridge (arrow).*

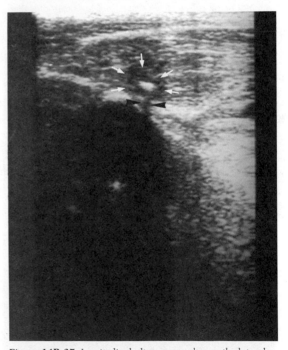

Figure 14B-37. *Longitudinal ultrasonograph over the lateral aspect of the proximal humerus of a horse with a penetrating wound over the deltoid tuberosity. A bony fragment, causing shadowing deep to it (black arrows), is visible off the distal extremity of the deltoid tuberosity. It is surrounded by an anechoic area suggestive of fluid (white arrows). Because of the small size of the fragment and the swelling of the proximal limb, this fragment was only identified radiographically after the swelling of the limb had decreased.*

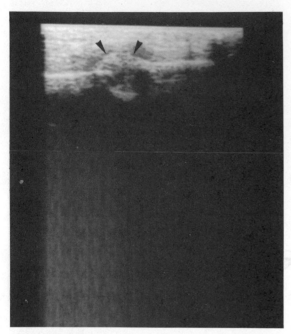

Figure 14B-38. Longitudinal ultrasonograph over a lateral splint bone that had a fracture of 2 weeks' duration. The developing callus is identifiable between the two bone ends (arrows) with insufficient calcification to cause complete acoustic shadowing.

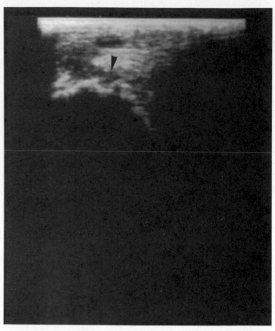

Figure 14B-40. Transverse ultrasonograph of the craniomedial surface of the radius of a horse with a discharging wound. There is an irregular contour to the bone with an anechoic region (arrow) superficial to it, strongly suggestive of osteitis (osteomyelitis).

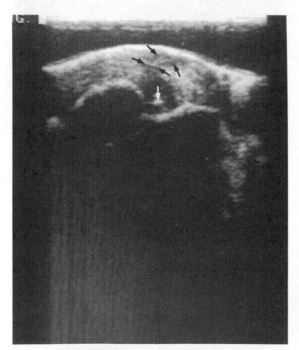

Figure 14B-39. Transverse ultrasonograph over the medial malleolus of the tibia of a horse with a healed wound. A small sequestrum (white arrow) can be seen within an involucrum and surrounded by anechogenic fluid. Note the hypoechogenic healing tract (black arrows) overlying the involucrum curving to the right (caudally) toward the skin.

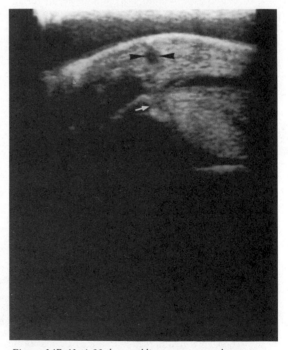

Figure 14B-41. A 30-degree oblique transverse ultrasonograph over the palmarolateral aspect of the metacarpophalangeal joint of a horse with a wound over the lateral proximal sesamoid bone. A tract between the skin and distended digital sheath contains pockets of anechogenic fluid (black arrows). A defect, probably due to infection, in the axial surface of the lateral proximal sesamoid bone also can be identified (white arrow). These findings were confirmed at surgery.

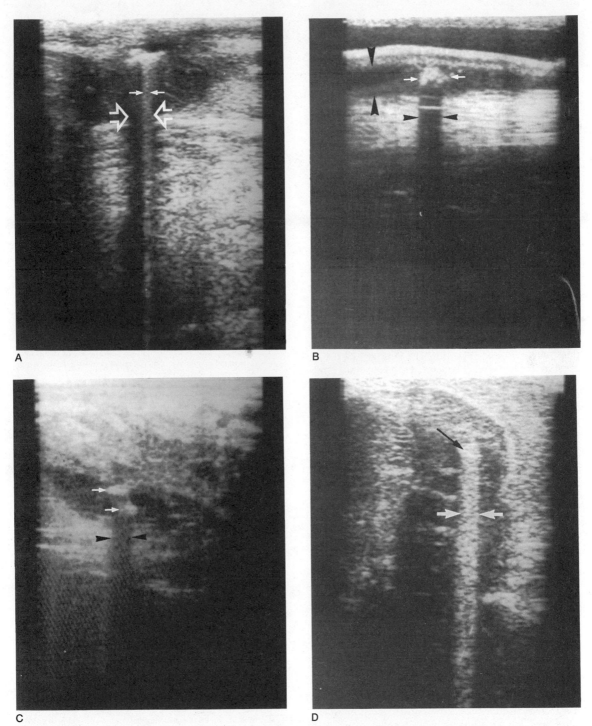

Figure 14B-42. (A) The appearance of air on an ultrasonograph, here within a shoulder wound. There is acoustic shadowing (large arrows) combined with a "comet-tail" (reverberation) artifact (small arrows). (B) Longitudinal ultrasonograph of the distal metacarpal region (level L3) of a horse with a wooden foreign body lodged within the superficial digital flexor tendon (SDFT) just proximal to the digital sheath. The foreign body is highly reflective (white arrows), with a hyperechoic surface reflection and a deep acoustic shadow (small arrows). Note the anechoic region superficial to the tendons which was an abscess cavity (large arrows). (C) A suture foreign body within an abscess in the inguinal region of a horse that had been castrated 7 years earlier. The loops of suture material (white arrows) cast an acoustic shadow (black arrows). (D) A metallic foreign body (a bullet) lodged in the caudal thigh muscles of a pony (black arrow) which has caused a "comet-tail" artifact deep to it instead of an acoustic shadow (white arrows). The foreign body did not appear to affect the animal, and the absence of fluid surrounding it suggests that it is quiescent.

IMMATURE BONE

The periosteum in a foal is considerably thicker than in the adult and is demonstrable as a thick, hypoechoic line superficial to the surface of the bone. In very young foals, regions of the skeleton are unmineralized, and their cartilaginous precursors can be imaged ultrasonographically but not radiographically.[49] Physes are identified ultrasonographically as thin, echoic lines separating the bright echoes from the subchondral bone. The appearance is very similar to that of a fracture but should not be confused with one in a young animal.

Wounds

Much can be gained from an ultrasonographic examination of wounds. The degree of soft-tissue damage and the components of the swelling around the wound can be determined, and foreign bodies (acoustic shadowing), fibrosis (hyperechogenic), edema (hypoechogenic), or fluid, such as an abscess or seroma (anechogenic), can all be recognized. Associated injuries to tendons and ligaments can be identified, and the extent of the penetration can be assessed (Fig. 14B–41). Damage to articular cartilage can occasionally be seen, especially in the proximal limb joints. Synovial thickening and effusion in cases of synovial sepsis also will be evident. Fracture fragments and sequestra can be identified easily and located precisely together with other bony changes such as the formation of callus and periosteal new bone. It is essential to avoid the misdiagnosis of a bone fragment or foreign body when there is air or gas present in the wound. The appearance can be very similar, although air or gas tends to give multiple shadows with "comet-tail" artifacts. Foreign bodies are mostly highly reflective, and using ultrasound, foreign bodies that are not visible radiographically, e.g., plastics, wood, and sutures (Fig. 14B–42), can be reliably demonstrated.[11,45,60,62,63] The exact size and depth of the foreign body can be measured using the electronic callipers, allowing removal through a small incision, if appropriate.

Imaging in just one plane will show the surface of the foreign body but not the structures below because of the acoustic shadowing. It is therefore imperative to examine rigorously the area in multiple planes so that the structure in which it is embedded can be identified.

Conclusion

The range of structures imaged by diagnostic ultrasound has increased dramatically over the past 3 to 4 years. Ultrasound examination has now become an essential component of the diagnostic protocol in evaluation of athletic horses with musculoskeletal problems. The major problem for the ultrasonographer is the discrimination of normal structures from clinically significant ultrasonographic findings. The use of ultrasonography to follow up various soft-tissue lesions will permit more accurate assessment of prognosis. In the future it is likely that more sophisticated ultrasound equipment will permit better-quality images to be obtained and should enhance the value of diagnostic ultrasound.

References

1. Rantanen NW: The use of diagnostic ultrasound in limb disorders of the horse: A preliminary report. J Equine Vet Sci 1982; 2:62.
2. Bentley H, Dyson S: Practical ultrasound physics: How to make optimal use of your machine. Equine Vet Ed 1991; 3:227.
3. Dyson S: Selecting a machine for diagnostic ultrasound examinations in horses. Equine Vet Ed 1991; 3:161.
4. Genovese RL, Rantanen NW, Hauser ML, et al: Diagnostic ultrasonography of equine limbs. Vet Clin North Am Equine Pract 1986; 2:145.
5. Neuwirth LA, Selcer BA, Mahaffey MB: Equine tendon ultrasonography: Common artifacts. Equine Vet Ed 1991; 3:149.
6. Rantanen NW: Principles of ultrasound use in the horse. *In* Proceedings of the Annual Convention of the American Association of Equine Practitioners, 1985, p 685.
7. Steyn PF, McIlwraith CW, Rawcliff N: The ultrasonographic examination of the palmar metacarpal tendons and ligaments of the equine digit: A review. Equine Pract 1991; 13:24.
8. Colby J: Artifacts and image quality in ultrasound. J Equine Vet Sci 1985; 5:295.
9. Rantanen NW: Ultrasonographic examination of equine tendons and ligaments. J Equine Vet Sci 1989; 10:163.
10. Dyson S: The use of ultrasonography for the assessment of tendon damage. Equine Vet Ed 1989; 1:42.
11. Wilson DJ: Ultrasonic imaging of soft tissues. Clin Radiol 1989; 40:341.
12. Genovese RL, Rantanen NW, Simpson BS: The use of ultrasonography in the diagnosis and management of injuries to the equine limb. Comp Cont Ed 1987; 9:945.
13. Hauser ML: Ultrasonographic appearance and correlative anatomy of the soft tissues of the distal extremities in the horse. Vet Clin North Am Equine Pract 1986; 2:127.
14. Hauser ML, Rantanen NW, Genovese RL: Ultrasound anatomy and scanning technique of the distal extremities in the horse. *In* Proceedings of the Annual Convention of the American Association of Equine Practitioners, 1985, p 693.
15. McClellan PD: A proposal for the standardization in sonographic imaging: I. Metacarpus and metatarsus. J Equine Vet Sci 1986; 6:327.
16. McClellan PD, Colby J: Ultrasonic structure of the pastern. J Equine Vet Sci 1986; 6:99.
17. Redding WR: Ultrasonographic imaging of the structures of the digital flexor tendon sheath. Comp Cont Ed Eur Edition 1991; 13:E752.
18. Dyson S: Ultrasonographic examination of the metacarpal and metatarsal regions in the horse. Equine Vet Ed 1992;4:139.
19. Hauser ML, Rantanen NW, Modransky PD: Ultrasound examination of the distal interphalangeal joint, navicular bursa, navicular bone and deep digital tendon. J Equine Vet Sci 1982; 2:95.
20. Pharr JW, Nyland TG: Sonography of the equine palmar metacarpal soft tissues. Vet Radiol 1984; 25:265.
21. Rantanen NW: Ultrasound standoff techniques. J Equine Vet Sci 1989; 10:17.
22. Henry GA, Patton CS, Goble DO: Ultrasonographic evaluation of iatrogenic injuries of the equine accessory (carpal check) ligament and superficial digital flexor tendon. Vet Radiol 1986; 27:132.
23. Spurlock GH, Spurlock SL, Parker GA: Ultrasonographic, gross, and histologic evaluation of a tendinitis disease model in the horse. Vet Radiol 1989; 30:184.
24. Reef VB, Martin BB, Elser A: Types of tendon and ligament injuries detected with diagnostic ultrasound: description and followup. *In* Proceedings of the Annual Convention of the American Association of Equine Practitioners, 1988, p 245.
25. Crass JR, Genovese RL, Render JA, et al: Magnetic resonance, ultrasound, and histopathologic correlation of acute and healing tendon injuries. Vet Radiol Ultrasound 1992; 33:206.
26. Denoix JM, Mailot M, Levy I: Etude anatomo-pathologique des lesions associees aux image echographiques anormales des tendons et ligaments chez le cheval. Rec Med Vet 1990; 166:45.
27. Marr CM, McMillan I, Boyd JS, et al: Ultrasonographic and histopathological findings in equine superficial digital flexor tendon injury. Equine Vet J 1993; 25:23.
28. Nicoll RG, Wood AKW, Rothwell TLW: Ultrasonographical and

pathological studies of equine superficial digital flexor tendons; initial observations including tissue characterisation by analysis of image grey scale in a thoroughbred gelding. Equine Vet J 1992; 24:318.

29. Reef VB, Martin BB, Stebbins K: Comparison of ultrasonographic, gross, and histologic appearance of tendon injuries in performance horses (abstract). *In* Proceedings of the Annual Convention of the American Association of Equine Practitioners, 1989, p 279.

30. Steyn PF, McIlwraith CW, Rawcliff N: The use of ultrasonographic examination in conditions affecting the palmar metacarpal soft tissues of the equine limb. Equine Pract 1991; 13:8.

31. Genovese RL, Rantanen NW, Hauser ML, et al: Clinical application of diagnostic ultrasound to the equine limb. *In* Proceedings of the Annual Convention of the American Association of Equine Practitioners, 1985, p 701.

32. Genovese RL, Rantanen NW, Simpson BS, et al: Clinical experience with quantitative analysis of superficial digital flexor tendon injuries in thoroughbred and standardbred racehorses. Vet Clin North Am Equine Pract 1990, 6.129.

33. Dyson S: Desmitis of the accessory ligament of the deep digital flexor tendon: 27 cases (1986–1990). Equine Vet J 1991; 23:438.

34. Dyson S: Proximal suspensory desmitis: Clinical, ultrasonographic and radiographic features. Equine Vet J 1991; 23:25.

35. McIlwraith CW: Diseases of joints, tendons, ligaments and related structures. *In* Stashak ES (ed): Adam's Lameness in Horses. Philadelphia, Lea & Febiger, 1987, p 339.

36. Dik KJ, van den Belt AJM, Keg PR: Ultrasonographic evaluation of fetlock annular ligament constriction in the horse. Equine Vet J 1991; 23:285.

37. Wisner ER, O'Brien TR, Pool RR, et al: Osteomyelitis of the axial border of the proximal sesamoid bone in seven horses. Equine Vet J 1991; 23:383.

38. Adams SB, Blevins WE: Shoulder lameness in horses, part I. Comp Cont Ed 1989; 11:64.

39. Bone A, Papageorges M, Grant BD: Ultrasonographic evaluation and surgical treatment of humeral osteitis and bicipital tenosynovitis in a horse. J Am Vet Med Assoc 1992; 201:305.

40. Dyson SJ, Kidd L: Five cases of gastrocnemius tendinitis in the horse. Equine Vet J 1992; 24:351.

41. Proudman CJ: Common calcaneal tendinitis in a horse. Equine Vet Ed 1992; 4:277.

42. Dik KJ: Ultrasonography of the equine peroneus tertius muscle (abstract). Vet Radiol Ultrasound 1992; 33:126.

43. Gibbon WW: Ultrasound in the diagnosis of joint disease. RAD Magazine 1991; 17:17.

44. Penninck DG, Nyland TG, O'Brien TR, et al: Ultrasonography of the equine stifle. Vet Radiol 1990; 31:293.

45. Dik KJ: Ultrasonography in the diagnosis of equine lameness. Vet Ann 1990; 30:162.

46. Modransky PD, Rantanen NW, Hauser ML, et al: Diagnostic ultrasound examination of the dorsal aspects of the equine metacarpophalangeal joint. J Equine Vet Sci 1983; 3:56.

47. Steyn PF, Schmitz D, Watkins J, et al: The sonographic diagnosis of chronic proliferative synovitis in the metacarpophalangeal joints of a horse. Vet Radiol 1989; 30:125.

48. Coral A: Musculoskeletal ultrasound: Extending its use. RAD Magazine 1992; 18:10.

49. Kaplan PA, Matamoros A, Anderson JC: Sonography of the musculoskeletal system. Am J Radiol 1990; 155:237.

50. Wilson DJ: Diagnostic ultrasound in the musculoskeletal system. Curr Orthop 1988; 2:41.

51. Baxter GM, Humphries GB: Percutaneous drainage of an abscess in the lateral region of a horse. J Am Vet Med Assoc 1991; 198:660.

52. Clegg PD, Coumbe A: Alveolar rhabdomyosarcoma: An unusual cause of lameness in a pony. Equine Vet J 1993, 25, 547.

53. Danton CAS, Peacock PJ, May SA, et al: Anaplastic sarcoma in the caudal thigh of a horse. Vet Rec 1992; 131:188.

54. Edwards GB, Allen WE: Aorto-iliac thrombosis in two horses: clinical course of the disease and the use of real-time ultrasonography to confirm the diagnosis. Equine Vet J 1988; 20:384.

55. Reef VB, Roby KA, Richardson DW, et al: Use of ultrasonography for the detection of aortic-iliac thrombosis in horses. J Am Vet Med Assoc 1987; 190:286.

56. Tithof PK, Rebhun WC Dietze AE: Ultrasonographic diagnosis of aorto-iliac thrombosis. Cornell Vet 1985; 75:540.

57. Steiner GM, Sprigg A: The value of ultrasound in the assessment of bone. Br J Radiol 1992; 65:589.

58. Reef VB: Diagnosis of pelvic fractures in horses using ultrasonography (abstract). Vet Radiol Ultrasound 1992; 33:121.

59. Derbyshire NDJ, Simpson AHRW: A role for ultrasound in limb lengthening. Br J Radiol 1992; 65:576.

60. Cartee RE, Rumph PF: Ultrasonographic detection of fistulous tracts and foreign objects in muscles of horses. J Am Vet Med Assoc 1984; 184:1127.

61. Reef VB: Ultrasonographic findings in horses with osteomyelitis (abstract). Vet Radiol Ultrasound 1992; 33:119.

62. Modransky PD, Welker B, Moon M: Subcutaneous foreign body in a horse resembling fistulous withers. Vet Radiol 1989; 30:282.

63. Shah ZR, Crass JR, Oravec DC, et al: Ultrasonographic detection of foreign bodies in soft tissues using turkey muscle as a model. Vet Radiol Ultrasound 1992; 33:94.

Diagnostic Imaging in the Athletic Horse: Scintigraphy

M. C. SCHRAMME AND P. M. WEBBON

Technique and General Principles

RADIOPHARMACEUTICALS

Radioisotope scanning relies on the ability of tissues to sequester chemical compounds called *radiopharmaceuticals*. A radiopharmaceutical (RP) consists of a tissue tracer coupled with a *radionuclide,* which is an isotope attempting to reach a stable condition by emitting radiation. Technetium-99m (^{99m}Tc) is the radionuclide most commonly used for scintigraphy because of its 6-hour half-life and its 140-keV primary photon energy. Tissue-specific tracers are stable chemicals that are localized by organs or tissues. By using different tissue tracers, a variety of organs or diseases can be investigated, but in performance horses, the musculoskeletal system and the lungs are most frequently examined.

RADIOPHARMACEUTICALS FOR MUSCULOSKELETAL SCINTIGRAPHY

Diphosphonates, e.g., methyldiphosphonate (MDP), are the most commonly used tracers in skeletal imaging. They adsorb onto the exposed surface of hydroxyapatite crystals in areas of active bone resorption or formation. Technetium-99m MDP also has been used effectively for the selective localization of areas of muscle damage (myocardium, skeletal muscles).[1] The mechanism by which the RP is deposited in the damaged muscle is not clear, but the soft-tissue localization of MDP is often associated with high calcium levels either locally or systemically.[2] Both the increased deposition of calcium in the injured cells and the increased concentration of amorphous calcium-macromolecular complexes in damaged muscles may therefore be responsible for the observed accumulation of MDP. Another suggestion is that release of colloidal calcium phosphate from the mitochondria of damaged muscle cells allows formation of hydroxyapatite crystals in the extracellular fluid.[3]

Radionuclides also can be used independently of a tissue tracer in regional perfusion studies. Following the injection of xenon-133 (an inert and relatively insoluble gas with a half-life of 5.3 days and an energy emission of 81 keV) into a tissue, its clearance rate may be used as an indication of the blood flow in that area. Clearance from the gluteal muscles and the coronary band has been used to measure muscular perfusion in cases of rhabdomyolysis and digital blood flow in cases of laminitis, respectively.[4]

RADIOPHARMACEUTICALS FOR PULMONARY SCINTIGRAPHY

Scintigraphy of the lungs in horses can be used to study perfusion, ventilation, or the two combined. A lung perfusion scan is obtained after the intravenous injection of ^{99m}Tc tagged to macroaggregated albumin (MAA) particles. When the particles pass through the pulmonary arteries, they become trapped in the alveolar vascular bed. Imaging immediately after injection reflects the blood flow distribution in the lung.

Lung ventilation imaging, using an inhaled radioactive gas or aerosol, practically is more difficult and much less commonly performed. The aerosol of choice in equine ventilation studies is ^{99m}Tc DTPA. Aerosol droplet size is critical to ensure aerosol delivery to the alveoli and terminal bronchioles, where droplet deposition occurs by inertia impaction or sedimentation. The breathing system and mask must be constructed safely to avoid any radioactive contamination of the imaging room. Ventilation scans are acquired immediately after a 4-minute nebulization period.

DETECTION OF DISTRIBUTION/CONCENTRATION OF RADIOPHARMACEUTICALS

Gamma ray emission is detected with a sodium iodide crystal. Each gamma ray absorbed by the crystal generates a light flash that is converted into an electrical impulse by a photomultiplier tube. A gamma camera contains a single, large sodium iodide crystal and a number of photomultiplier tubes. The position of a light flash generated in the crystal can be determined by the response of a specific tube. A typical image (scintigraph) of the RP distribution and concentration of an area is composed of approximately 100,000 to 200,000 counts and requires an acquisition time of 30 to 60 seconds.

Simple, inexpensive, hand-held systems are also available. A manual scintillation, or point-counting, detector consists of a much smaller sodium iodide crystal, a single photomultiplier tube, both shielded in lead casing, and a ratemeter (Fig. 14C–1). This point-counting system numerically displays the amount of radioactivity measured per second at a particular site. The spatial resolution of this technique has been estimated as 1 to 2 cm,[5,6] and by placing the probe over a number of predetermined anatomic sites, the clinician can map out the RP distribution as a scintigram.

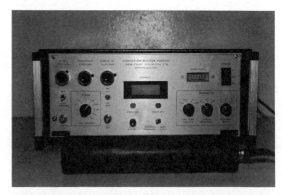

Figure 14C-1. *A manual scintillation (point counting) detector consisting of a sodium iodide crystal and a single photomultiplier tube, both shielded in lead casing, and a ratemeter.*

INTERPRETATION OF RESULTS

Computer Links

All data from a gamma camera for computer analysis is acquired in a matrix. The usual image matrix sizes, measured in picture elements (pixels) along each side of the matrix, are 64 × 64 and 128 × 128. Depending on the computer used, each pixel is composed of 8 or 16 bits. The matrix size determines the image resolution, so a 32 × 32 matrix has relatively few pixels and an image on a 256 × 256 acquisition matrix is much more detailed.

The examiner can define regions of interest (ROI) on a scintigraph, in which the total activity and the activity per pixel will be displayed. Clinical interpretation of the counts generated by the manual scintillation counter, which is used almost entirely for bone scanning, relies on two parameters for each measured point in a limb. The first is an expression of activity at each point in relation to the count of a reference point (usually the atlas), and the second is the activity relative to the corresponding point in the contralateral limb. A software program has been developed to provide a visual presentation that facilitates the clinical interpretation of these counts (Equiscint, Oakfield Instruments, Ltd., Oxford, U.K.). Histograms are used to present the collected counts in the two different ways. One graph shows the absolute values of each point in both limbs as bars on either side of the ordinate axis. This allows for quick recognition of the scale of the measured activity in each point, as well as left/right differences (Fig. 14C–2). Under normal conditions, this bar graph should be symmetrical for each pair of limbs. A second histogram expresses the differences between the limbs, with a bar for each measured point (Figs 14C–3). Only differences greater than 10 percent are shown. The bars allow for immediate identification of activity peaks, or "hot spots."

CONSTRUCTION OF A GAMMA CAMERA FACILITY FOR LARGE ANIMALS

Some basic requirements are needed for a large animal nuclear medicine facility. Because of the danger of damage to the gamma camera crystal, the room temperature should be thermostatically controlled. Animal restraint can be provided by open-sided stocks, which must be adjustable to allow camera access to all parts of the body. To keep the animal stationary during a scan, it may need to be sedated. Alternatively, the procedure can be performed under general anesthesia, provided induction and recovery facilities are available in the nuclear medicine unit. Lead shielding of at least 1 mm thickness should be available to eliminate radiation emanating from other limbs within the field of view of the camera.

The room should have solid walls, which will be reasonable barriers for the emitted radiation, and have a

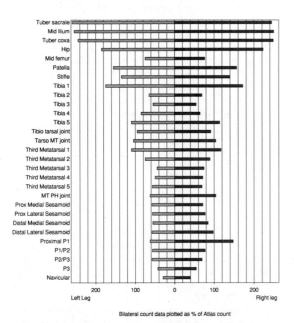

Figure 14C-2. *Point-count values expressed as a percentage of the axis count from both hindlimbs displayed as bars on either side of the ordinate axis. The bar graph should be symmetrical for each pair of limbs of a normal horse. In this case there is a peak of activity over the proximal part of P1 caused by a sagittal fracture.*

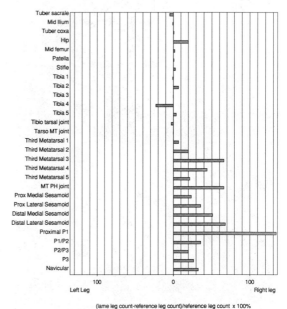

Figure 14C-3. *The same point-count values as in Fig. 14C-2 displayed to show the differences between contralateral limbs with a bar for each measured point. Only differences greater than 10 percent are shown. The bars allow immediate identification of the activity peak or "hot spot" centered on proximal P1.*

floor which is easily cleaned if the horse passes radio-active urine in the examination area.

However, in order to obtain maximal benefits from the system, the most important feature is the mounting of the heavy camera head to an appropriate support. The criteria for such a support system are low cost, high safety, and a wide range of movement of the camera head. It is essential that the camera can be used on all parts of the body of the restrained, stationary patient. This applies in particular to the less accessible areas of the pelvis, the thoracolumbar region, and the distal limbs.

A number of different support systems are presently in use at veterinary hospitals in Europe and North America. Most gamma cameras are still mounted on a gantry or a vertical fixed stand intended primarily for use with human patients (Fig. 14C–4). This arrangement requires that the patient is sufficiently cooperative to be presented to the camera in whatever position is necessary. This is unsatisfactory for equine patients, most of which, even when sedated, are suspicious of the camera and reluctant to approach it too closely.

To present the camera to the patient, rather than vice versa, the camera support must be mobile. This has been achieved by mounting the camera head on a yoke,

which allows rotational movement, on a mobile fork lift/trolley,[7] on a hydraulic knuckleboom crane,[8] or suspending it from multidirectional ceiling tracks.

Practical difficulties are also encountered when attempting to view a horse's distal limb because the camera cannot be lowered sufficiently to provide diagnostic images of the foot. To avoid this, the design of the restraining stocks can be modified to include a floor pit into which the camera can be lowered for solar views or an elevated floor to facilitate centering of the field of view on the foot. Alternatively, the foot can be elevated manually on a block or, for solar views, held directly on top of a piece of plexiglas covering the face of the camera, although it is not always easy to keep the limb stationary in these positions.

RADIATION SAFETY

The use and storage of radioactive materials and the disposal of radioactive waste are generally subject to control by the appropriate authority. Rules should be drawn up locally to ensure staff safety, but the following general comments apply to the use of ^{99m}Tc-MDP for bone scintigraphy.

The exposure rate at the skin surface of a horse at the time of its scintigraphic examination is typically 10 to 50 µSv/h depending on the dose administered. In most instances, this is reduced, at 0.5 m from the horse, to below the threshold of 7.5 µSv/h laid down by the Ionizing Radiation Regulations, in the United Kingdom, for the classification of radiation workers.

All personnel should wear whole-body and, if required, extremity radiation dosemeters. Disposable gloves should be worn when handling the radionuclide, and a syringe shield should be used when the horse is injected. Because as much as 50 percent of the injected activity is excreted renally, the animal's stable should be labeled to control access, and the soiled bedding must not be handled until the day after injection. Routine radiation surveys of both horse and stable[9] have shown that it is acceptable to remove the bedding, continue the lameness examination, or discharge the horse from the hospital on the day after the scan.

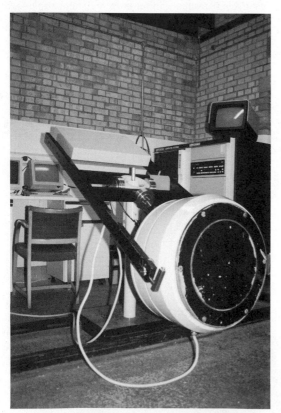

Figure 14C-4. A gamma camera mounted on a fixed stand intended primarily for use with human patients. It is difficult to position a conscious horse sufficiently close to the camera to ensure the best possible resolution.

Scintigraphy in Musculoskeletal Disease

Bone has traditionally been imaged radiographically, which reveals established structural changes that may have taken a long time to develop. Radiographs, therefore, depict structure via radiation absorption. Scintigraphs, on the other hand, depict the functional or pathophysiologic status of bone via radionuclide distribution.

An objective assessment of skeletal activity can be obtained with the definition of three regions of interest: ROI1 over the highest activity concentration, ROI2 in soft tissues, and ROI3 over a consistent area of normal bone turnover. Quotient 1 (ROI1/ROI2) is an indication of the quality of the bone labeling. A high Q1 value reflects low soft-tissue activity with a good bone/soft-tissue ratio. A low Q1 value is due to high soft-tissue activity or low bone activity. Quotient 2 (ROI1/ROI3) measures the local concentration of radioactivity in the area of highest radiation on the scan.[10]

A 10 percent isocontour ROI also can be used as a standardized area for each image. The activity within each ROI can be divided by the 10 percent isocontour ROI to compensate for any variation in overall activity within the limb.

How large the measured difference in radiation must be to indicate the presence of bone pathology remains somewhat empirical and depends on the area of interest, but generally, an activity increase or decrease of at least 25 percent is needed to indicate the presence of skeletal pathology. This relatively high threshold reflects the *recruiting phenomenon* of the skeletal capillary system. In normal bone, only 75 percent of the osteons link up with the osseous blood supply. The resting osteons can become activated by autonomic stimulation and increase the radionuclide uptake by the bone.[11]

DISTRIBUTION OF ^{99m}Tc-MDP

Following systemic administration, the ^{99m}Tc-MDP is distributed between the circulation, the extracellular fluid (ECF), and bone tissue. This distribution of the RP is characterized by three phases. During phase 1 the RP is still predominantly present in the large blood vessels as a nuclear angiogram. During phase 2, the RP is distributed throughout the capillary beds and ECF. This soft-tissue phase persists for 10 to 20 minutes (soft-tissue image). Finally, during phase 3, the RP is predominantly present in bone, while the activity in the blood and soft tissue significantly decreases (Fig. 14C–5). A delay of 3 hours after injection is required for renal excretion of the soft-tissue RP. Approximately 40 to 50 percent of the total activity is excreted, and the remainder adsorbs onto bone, where it remains and decays. Bone scans are performed in the third phase of distribution.

FACTORS INFLUENCING BONE TRACER UPTAKE

The dose rate at which the RP is administered by intravenous injection ranges from 2 MBq/kg for manual scintillation detection to 8 MBq/kg for gamma camera detection. Several factors influence uptake of the RP, involving its delivery to, deposition in, or elimination from the target tissue (bone) or the background.

The delivery of the RP depends on the regional blood flow, the permeability of the capillary bed, and the local ECF volume. At subnormal and normal rates of blood flow to bone, the RP uptake by the skeleton is proportional to the blood flow, but at higher rates of blood flow, the uptake is proportional to the available hydroxyapatite crystal surface.

The deposition of the RP in bone is determined by the available bone crystal surface, the volume of bone per unit of area, and the trabecular/cortical bone ratio Trabecular bone adsorbs more RP than cortical bone, so there is higher activity over the epiphyses compared with the diaphysis of a normal long bone.

The RP is eliminated by urinary excretion. Decreased urinary excretion due to hypovolemia or reduced cardiac output will result in diffuse RP retention in the soft tissues. A similarly poor bone/soft-tissue ratio can occur with increased ECF volume.

There are a number of nonskeletal artifacts that can result in a confusing distribution of the RP and reduce the diagnostic value of the scan. These include skin contamination with radioactive urine, a false "hot spot" at the injection site, and recent intramuscular injections, particularly with irritating agents. However, from the clinician's point of view, the most important factors that may interfere with a bone scan are alterations in the peripheral circulation in the limbs, regional anesthesia, urinary accumulation of the RP, and secondary or induced skeletal changes.

Peripheral Circulation

Anything that hinders normal distal limb blood flow can decrease the skeletal uptake of the RP. Low ambient temperatures cause peripheral vasoconstriction, sometimes unilaterally, while decreased peripheral perfusion is present in 10 to 20 percent of normal horses (especially older animals) distal to the carpus/tarsus. Consequently, these animals have poor RP uptake in their distal limbs. Some clinicians routinely advise bandaging or administration of vasodilating drugs prior to scanning to eliminate the problems arising from poor peripheral circulation.[11] However, tight bandaging can impair normal blood flow, and venous pooling proximal to a limb bandage may increase activity in that region.

Regional Anesthesia

If gamma scintigraphy is used following perineural or intraarticular anesthesia, false "hot spots" can result[12,13] (Fig. 14-C–5). This has prompted a number of studies of the effect of commonly performed regional anesthetic techniques on both soft-tissue and bone phase scintigraphy in the horse.[14–16] These studies are summarized in Table 14C–1.

Some studies[15,16] showed a significant increase in gamma emission on soft-tissue phase images at the sites of recent palmar digital and palmar/palmar metacarpal nerve blocks and intraarticular anesthesia of the carpus. None of the studies[14–16] demonstrated any significant effects on bone phase scintigraphs. Because this was not in agreement with our own clinical findings, we performed a small study on four healthy horses with no history or sign of lameness that were scanned with a point counter prior to regional anesthesia. A palmar/palmar metacarpal (low four-point) nerve block was performed (4 × 3 ml) in the left forelimb and a plantar (abaxial sesamoid) nerve block was performed in the left hindlimb (2 × 4 ml) with 2% prilocaine hydrochloride, while the contralateral limbs served as controls. The horses were then scanned from 0 to 10 days after the nerve blocks.

Figures 14C–6 and 14C–7 show the difference in gamma ray emission between the injected and control limbs. Three of the four horses showed increased activity in the injected front limbs from the day of injection

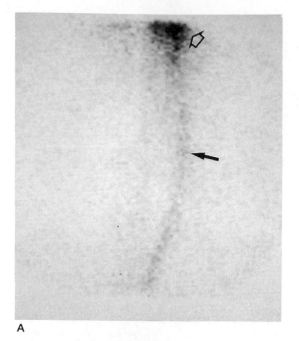

A

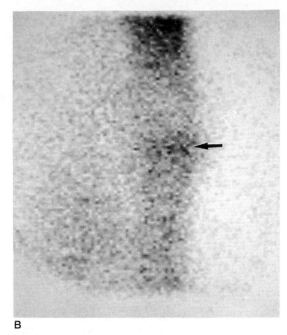

B

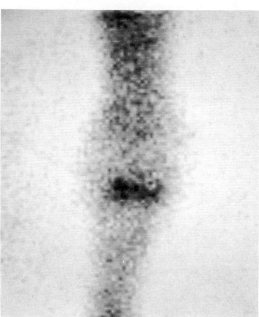

C

Figure 14C-5. A "three-phase" dorsopalmar examination of the right carpus of a 9-year-old thoroughbred with a chip fracture of the third carpal bone. During phase 1 (A: 220 s after the IV administration of 3.5 GBq of ^{99m}Tc-MDP), the RP is still predominantly present in the large blood vessels (arrow), but there is intense uptake at the sites of a median and ulnar nerve block performed 4 days previously (open arrow). During phase 2 (B: 10 min after injection), the RP is distributed throughout the capillary beds and ECF, and there is marginally increased uptake in the third carpal bone (arrow). Finally, during phase 3 (C: 3 h after injection), the RP has accumulated in the third carpal bone, while the activity in the soft tissue has significantly decreased.

for 3 days. From day 4 onward, no differences between the injected and the control limbs were found. In the hindlimbs, there was no significant increase in gamma ray emission in any of the injected limbs.

Unlike the previous studies, our findings confirmed, at least partly, our clinical observation that nerve blocks can create false-positive "hot spots" on bone phase images for a period of at least 3 days after injec-tion. We therefore postpone scintigraphy for a minimum of 3 days after regional or intraarticular anesthesia.

Urinary Excretion
Up to 50 percent of the intravenous RP dose is eliminated via the urinary tract. The activity in the bladder causes a considerable rise in gamma ray emission in the caudal spine and pelvic area that will mask changes in

Table 14C-1. Summary of the Effects on RP Uptake of Regional Anesthetic Studies

Nerve block	Anesthetic solution	Time after injection	Soft-tissue phase increase	Bone phase increase
PDNB	Lidocaine 2%	0–17 days	Mild/3 days	None[15]
	Mepivacaine 2%	2 days	—	None[13]
ASNB	Lidocaine 2%	0–17 days	Mild/1 day	None[15]
	Mepivacaine 2%	4 & 24 hours	—	None[14]
	Bupivacaine 2%	4 & 24 hours	—	None[14]
Low palmar	Lidocaine 2%	0–17 days	Strong/7 days	None[15]
High palmar	Lidocaine 2%	0–17 days	Strong/17 days	None[15]
Ulnar	Mepivacaine 2%	1 & 2 days	—	Strong/mild[13]
Fetlock joint	Lidocaine 2%	0–14 days	Mild/8 days	None[16]
Intercarpal joint	Mepivacaine 2%	4 & 24 hours	—	None[14]
	Bupivacaine 2%	4 & 24 hours	—	None[14]
Radiocarpal joint	Lidocaine 2%	0–14 days	Strong/14 days	None[16]
Tarsocrural joint	Lidocaine 2%	0–14 days	Mild/8 days	None[16]
Tarsometatarsal joint	Lidocaine 2%	0–14 days	None	None[16]

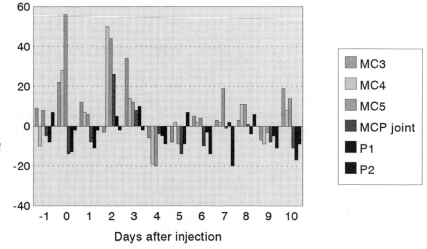

Figure 14C-6. *The mean percentage difference in* ^{99m}*Tc-MDP uptake between left (palmar/palmar metacarpal nerve block on day 0) and right (control) forelimbs of four horses in the distal metacarpus (MC3, 4, 5), metacarpophalangeal joint (MCP), and proximal (P1) and middle (P2) phalanges.*

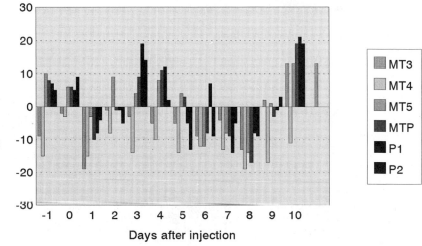

Figure 14C-7. *The mean percentage difference in* ^{99m}*Tc-MDP uptake between left (abaxial sesamoid nerve block on day 0) and right (control) hindlimbs of four horses in the distal metatarsus (MT3, 4, 5), metatarsophalangeal joint (MTP), and proximal (P1) and middle (P2) phalanges.*

bone activity in these areas. To investigate the effect of furosemide-induced diuresis, six healthy horses were scanned using the point-counting method at 13 predetermined arbitrary points along the spine and sacrococcygeal area (Fig. 14C–8) before and after furosemide-induced urination 3 hours after administration of the RP (Fig. 14C–9).

As soon as urination occurred, a fall of up to 400 percent in radioactivity was registered in the lumbar and pelvic area of all six horses. Regular rescanning over the next 3 hours indicated that refilling of the bladder did not result in a renewed increase in measured radiation because the RP had been eliminated from the soft tissues and circulation at this stage. The only remaining RP was that linked to bone.

We concluded that the bladder should be emptied at least once prior to obtaining bone phase scintigraphs/scintigrams of the lumbosacral spine and pelvis. Alternatively, scanning can be delayed until adequate spontaneous urination has occurred. This may take up to 5 hours from the time of injection of the RP.

Secondary or Induced Skeletal Responses
It is possible to recognize a number of consistent, but confusing, patterns of radionuclide distribution that interfere with the diagnostic quality of bone phase scintigraphs/scintigrams. Distal to a site of bone pathology, radionuclide activity can be significantly decreased; non-weight-bearing lameness can lead to this pattern of RP distribution in a matter of days. In chronic lameness, a generalized increase in radionuclide activity can be registered throughout the entire lame leg. This distribution pattern can hinder the recognition of "hot spots," reflecting a true site of pathology (Fig. 14C–10). Chronic lameness also can lead to a pattern of generalized activity increase at all sites of the sound, possibly overloaded limb.

A specifically confusing pattern of RP distribution occasionally arises in horses with chronic heel pain and a positive response to palmar digital nerve anesthesia. In these horses, bone phase scintigrams may identify the dorsal aspect of the fetlock joint as the site of highest gamma ray emission. Exactly what causes these aberrant

distributions of the RP remains unclear, but it is probable that they reflect altered levels of bone metabolism in response to changes in stress patterns or blood flow distribution. Steckel[9] formulated a set of useful guidelines for the interpretation of bone scans in horses (Table 14C–2).

INDICATIONS FOR SCINTIGRAPHY IN MUSCULOSKELETAL DISEASE

A comprehensive list of indications for the use of bone scintigraphy in lameness diagnosis is shown in Table 14C–3. A bone scan can be performed either as a screening procedure for the first identification of a lesion or lesions or as a specific imaging technique focused on a known site of abnormality (Fig. 14C–11).

Our experience with both the gamma camera and the manual scintillation counter has enabled us to redefine the animals suitable for manual scintillation probe scanning[18] (Table 14C–4). This profile fits perfectly the young thoroughbred in training, which has the additional advantage of a highly active bone metabolism. It is therefore not surprising to find that the accessibility and versatility of the manual scintillation counter have made it a well-established diagnostic tool in racehorse practice in the United Kingdom.

"Normal" Racehorse Scan
Because the main target group for the detection of exercise-induced orthopedic injury is composed of 2- and 3-year-old racehorses in training, we embarked on a study to investigate the normal scintigraphic appearance of the 2-year-old skeleton and its response to training. The aim of the study was to determine whether sequential scintigraphy could demonstrate adaptation of the immature equine skeleton to training stress. We suspected that training would disrupt the normal scintigraphic symmetry between contralateral limbs until the horse had adapted to the level of exercise, at which stage symmetry would be restored. Further, it seemed possible that, in some horses, failure to restore skeletal symmetry might presage overt lameness.

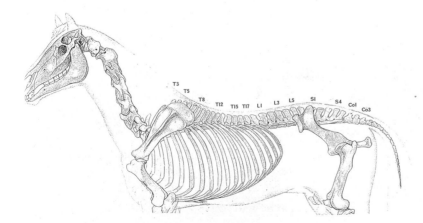

Figure 14C-8. *To investigate the effect of furosemide-induced diuresis, six healthy horses were scanned using the point-counting method at 13 predetermined arbitrary points along the spine and sacrococcygeal area before and after furosemide-induced urination.*

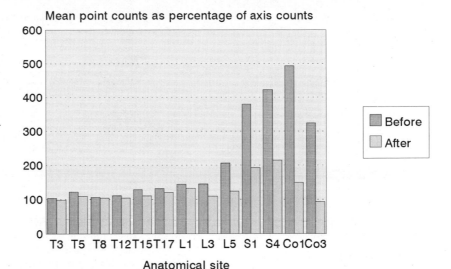

Mean point counts as percentage of axis counts

Figure 14C-9. Three hours after administration of the RP. Immediately after urination, a fall of up to 350 percent in radioactivity was registered in the lumbar and pelvic area.

Five thoroughbreds that remained free of orthopedic disease were followed throughout their first training/racing season. Every 4 weeks each horse was injected with 0.5 GBq of ^{99m}Tc-MDP and scanned 3 hours later with a manual scintillation counter by positioning the probe over specific, arbitrary, anatomic sites.

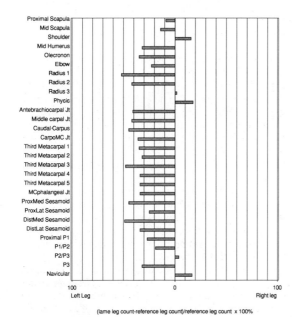

Figure 14C-10. Point counts from an 11-year-old thoroughbred intermittently lame on the left forelimb over 2 years. There is generalized ^{99m}Tc-MDP uptake throughout the lame limb without a focal increase in activity which might indicate the site of lameness.

Each horse was scanned twice, and the readings were standardized relative to the atlas for each horse.

To assess the reproducibility of the technique, the differences between the two measurements of the same points on the same day were analyzed. In the distal limb, the maximal variation between two consecutive readings of the same point was 10 percent of the mean measured value. For the proximal radius and the proximal and distal tibia, the variation was greater (Fig. 14C–12). This was probably due to the proximity of highly active growth plates, which made slightly inaccurate positioning of the probe more significant.

Symmetry between contralateral limbs was assessed by comparing the mean readings at corresponding points. At some points, differences amounted to over 20 percent (Fig. 14C–13). Additionally, for each point, the measurements were graphically displayed as a function of time. A regression curve was fitted to the points, and the regression coefficient was calculated to reflect the upward or downward trend of radionuclide uptake at a given anatomic point throughout the 28-week trial period (Fig. 14C–14).

When comparing variation within the limbs (reproducibility) with variation between limbs (symmetry),

Table 14C-2. Guidelines for Bone Phase Scintigraph Interpretation

Young animals produce "hotter" scintigraphs than adults.

Epiphyses and physes of long bones are normal "hot" areas in young horses.

Major joints retain more RP than the rest of the skeleton in all age groups.

Dehydration results in poor RP uptake in the skeleton.

Regional derangement in sympathetic innervation may cause an unexpected increase of RP uptake in certain bones.

After Steckel RR: The role of scintigraphy in lameness evaluation. Vet Clin North Am Equine Pract 1991; 7:207, with permission.

Table 14C-3. Criteria for Bone Scintigraphy

Whole-body screening
  Poor performance, stiffness, and subtle lameness unsuitable for
    the use of local anesthesia
  Obvious lameness that fails to respond to routine local anesthesia
    (especially proximal limb, torso, and pelvis).
  Multiple sites of lameness
  Suspected acute bone lesions prior to their radiographic
    appearance (especially occult, incomplete, and stress
    fractures in young racehorse)
Focused scintigraph
  Positive regional anesthesia, negative radiography
  Assessment of known radiographic lesion
  Monitoring bone healing (fractures, osteostixis)
  Specific soft-tissue scan (bursitis, villonodular synovitis,
    tendinitis, desmitis, rhabdomyolysis) or differentiation of
    bone versus soft-tissue inflammation in mixed injuries
  Presumptive diagnosis of thoracolumbar or sacroiliac pain
Unsuitable for scintigraphy
  Purely lytic lesions, not accompanied by inflammatory remodeling
  Myelomas, etc.
  Many osteochondrosis dissecans lesions
  Many subchondral cystic lesions

After O'Callaghan MW: The integration of radiography and alternative imaging methods in the diagnosis of equine orthopedic disease. Vet Clin North Am Equine Pract 1991; 7:339, with permission.

Table 14C-4. Criteria for Use of the Manual Point Counter

Ideal case
  Lameness acute in onset
  Lameness at least moderately severe
  No obvious clinical signs to guide radiography
  No recent regional anesthesia
  Within 2 to 5 days of lameness
Least suitable case
  Chronic low-grade lameness
  Chronic degenerative conditions (navicular syndrome, spavin)
  Developmental lesions (OCD and some subchondral cystic
    lesions)

proximal to the carpus, both graphs mirror each other. Distal to the carpus, the mean difference between limbs exceeds the normal variation of the reading (Fig. 14C–15).

These findings partially supported our hypothesis in that the symmetry between distal contralateral limbs was disturbed. However, the asymmetry seen in the lower limbs of each of these 2-year-olds individually reflected a considerable amount of variation, and in only one of the five sampled horses could a trend from disturbed to restored symmetry between the distal forelimbs be observed (Fig. 14C–16).

In other centers, the use of scintigraphic whole-body screening in the investigation of poor performance in young racehorses, particularly standardbreds, has shown that a large number of these horses have multiple sites of abnormally intense uptake, indicating abnormal bone turnover.[9,17,19] This syndrome of *stress-induced bone sclerosis* was identified as a specific cause of lameness in young horses in training, paralleling a well-described syndrome in young human athletes,[3] where early detection allowed modification of training regimens to facilitate more gradual bone adaptation. Similarly, 2 or 3 months of rest and/or controlled exercise appears to be a successful approach to this syndrome in the horse.

Nuclear Imaging of Stress and Incomplete Cortical Fractures

Fatigue/stress damage is the progressive loss of strength of a material under cyclic loading. The initial consequence of fatigue is the accumulation of microdamage in the area subjected to the cyclic stress.

Bone responds to this microdamage by initiating its remodeling processes. These consist of the initial resorption of cortical bone and the production of endosteal and/or periosteal callus. The very process of repair, which can take as long as 8 months, may predispose the bone to failure at normal loads until the resorbed bone is replaced by secondary osteons. It is therefore clear that early recognition of these injuries is necessary before further deterioration of the bone matrix occurs, leading to stress fracture.

Radiography does not always reveal the presence of stress or incomplete cortical fractures. The subtle alterations in trabecular detail may be easily overlooked, and bone lysis is not visible until 30 percent of the bone has been demineralized. Usually, there is a gap of several weeks before bone pathology results in radiographic changes. Moreover, the character of many of these lesions often precludes their identification on standard radiographic views, and specialized views may be necessary following a positive scintigraph (Fig. 14C–17).

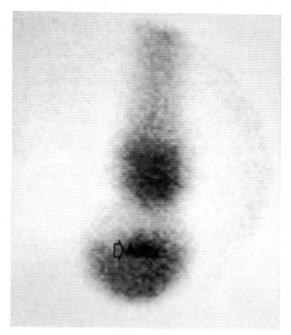

Figure 14C-11. *An 8-year-old event horse with pain localized to the navicular bone region. Radiographs suggested an avulsion fracture from the distal border of the navicular bone, and a bone-phase scintigraph showed marked uptake of the ^{99m}Tc-MDP by the navicular bone (arrow).*

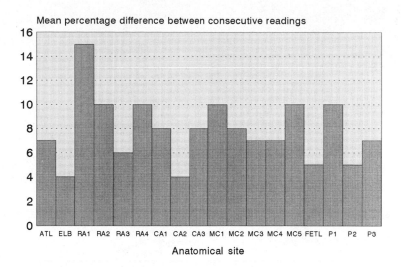

Mean percentage difference between consecutive readings

Figure 14C-12. A 2-year-old thorough-bred study. In the distal limb, the mean variation between two consecutive readings of the same point was 10 percent or less. For the proximal radius (and the proximal and distal tibia), the variation was greater.

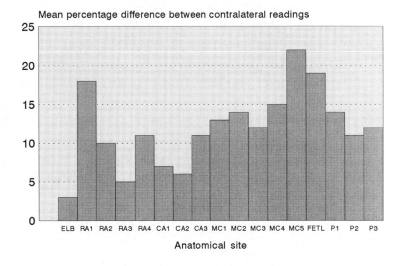

Mean percentage difference between contralateral readings

Figure 14C-13. A 2-year-old thorough-bred study. Symmetry between ^{99m}Tc-MDP uptake in contralateral limbs was assessed by comparing the mean readings at corresponding points.

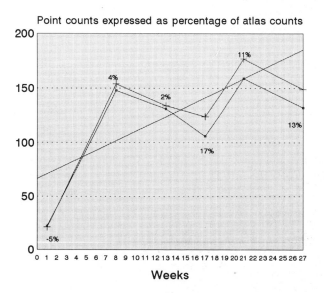
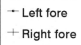

Point counts expressed as percentage of atlas counts

Figure 14C-14. A 2-year-old thoroughbred Tb study. For each point, the activity in contralateral limbs was graphically shown as a function of time with the percentage difference between points displayed. A regression curve was fitted to the points, and the regression coefficient was calculated to reflect the trend of ^{99m}Tc-MDP uptake at a given anatomic point throughout the trial period.

337

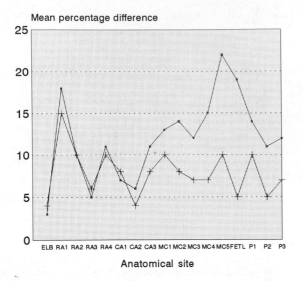

Figure 14C-15. *A 2-year-old thoroughbred study. The reproducibility and symmetry of the point counts from the group of horses was similar proximal to the carpus, suggesting that variation between contralateral limbs may be due to the error in reproducibility. Distal to the carpus the asymmetry exceeded the reproducibility, implying that the group demonstrated true asymmetry, due to variations in bone metabolism or limb perfusion, in their distal forelimbs.*

It is in the recognition of this stress-induced damage at specific sites (Table 14C–5) that scintigraphy is most useful in racehorse practice. Without scintigraphy, many of these lesions can be missed and go on to become fractures.

Nuclear Imaging of the Vertebral Column and Pelvis

All equine practitioners are regularly presented with vague complaints about a horse's back and pelvis. The first, and often biggest, problem in the investigation of these cases is to decide whether or not the horse is genuinely and primarily suffering from back/pelvic pain. A clinical examination may be inconclusive, and radiography is difficult due to the large overlying soft-tissue masses. Scintigraphy can yield valuable additional information (Fig. 14C–18).

The most commonly diagnosed spinal lesion is that of *overriding dorsal spinous processes*. Our experience has supported previous observations that there is a very

strong correlation between increased RP uptake in the dorsal spinous processes and radiologic evidence of bone remodeling at the contact points.[9,20] Manual radiation detection is performed at 20 arbitrary points along the midline of the horse's back. The results are displayed as a bar-graph representation of absolute counts, expressed as a percentage of the atlas count. The technique allows only comparison with adjacent sites and does not allow spatial resolution between different skeletal structures, but regions of increased RP uptake may be detected. Contrary to previous reports, there is an increasing realization that injuries to the equine pelvis resulting from routine athletic activity are quite common. Pilsworth[6] describes several cases where a pelvic fracture was preceded by intermittent hindlimb lameness, which may have been a sign of stress damage to the pelvis. Nuclear bone scanning can detect this stress damage before a catastrophic fracture occurs. The examination can be performed with a gamma camera (Fig. 14C–18) or a man-

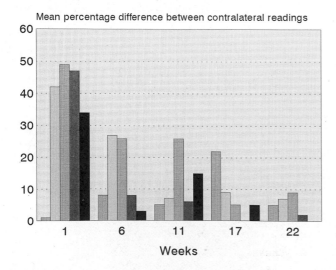

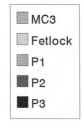

Figure 14C-16. *A 2-year-old thoroughbred study. In only one of the five sampled horses, could a trend from disturbed to restored symmetry between the distal forelimbs be observed.*

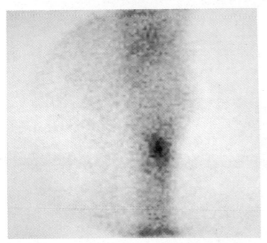

Figure 14C-17. *Focal increased* [99mTc-MDP] *bone-phase uptake seen in a dorsopalmar view of a palmar cortical stress fracture of the proximal metacarpus of a 4-year-old thoroughbred. Radiographs of the corresponding site showed only equivocal changes.*

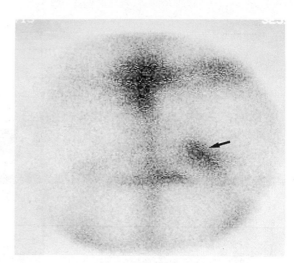

Figure 14C-18. *Dorsoventral bone-phase projection of a pony with a dislocated right hip and acetabular rim fracture of 2 weeks' duration (arrow).*

ual scintillation probe, when the detector is positioned over 110 points symmetrically arranged over the horse's hind quarters. With the aid of a computer program (Equiscint, Oakfield Instruments, Ltd., Oxford, U.K.), a three-dimensional graph of gamma ray emission across the quarters is constructed to represent the RP uptake by the pelvis and sacrum (Fig. 14C–19).

Caution is necessary when significant unilateral muscle wastage is present over the hind quarters. Because the tissue half-thickness for [99mTc] gamma rays is 4 cm (4 cm of muscle effectively halves the amount of gamma radiation measured), muscle atrophy can result in important artifacts.[6]

Sprain or subluxation of the sacroiliac joint is an-

Table 14C-5. Common Sites of Abnormal Bone Turnover in the Athletic Horse

Bone/joint	Location	Condition
Distal phalanx	Medial quarter	"Pedal osteitis"[17]
Navicular bone		Navicular disease[23]
Proximal phalanx	Sagittal groove	"Split pastern"[24,25]
	Dorsal cortex	Stress-induced bone remodeling[17,26]
Proximal sesamoid bones		Stress-induced bone remodeling[17,19]
Metacarpus	Distal condyles	Stress-induced bone remodeling[9,17,19,27]
	Dorsal cortex	Stress-induced bone remodeling/fracture[9,28]
	Proximal palmar cortex	Incomplete cortical fracture/enthesopathy[10,29,30]
	Proximal dorsomedial cortex	Incomplete cortical fracture/enthesopathy[31]
Metatarsus	Distal condyles	Stress-induced bone remodeling[9]
	Dorsal cortex	Stress-induced bone remodeling[9]
	Proximal plantar cortex	Incomplete cortical fracture/enthesopathy[9,10]
	Proximal dorsal cortex	Incomplete cortical fracture[32]
Carpus	Medial facet of third carpal bone	Stress-induced bone sclerosis[9,19]
Tarsus	Central/third tarsal bone	Stress-induced bone sclerosis/incomplete fracture[33]
	Lateral collateral ligament	Enthesopathy/enthesitis[34]
Radius	Middiaphysis	Stress fracture[35]
Tibia	Proximal lateral cortex	Stress fracture[36]
	Diaphysis	Stress fracture[35,37]
	Distal caudolateral cortex	Stress fracture[35]
Humerus	Proximal caudolateral cortex	Stress fracture[35]
	Distal craniomedial cortex	Stress fracture[35]
Stifle	Insertion of anterior cruciate ligament	Enthesopathy[9,17]
	Patella	Stress-induced bone remodeling[17]
	Tibial crest	Enthesopathy[17]
Pelvis	Ilium	Stress/spontaneous fracture[32]

Cranial

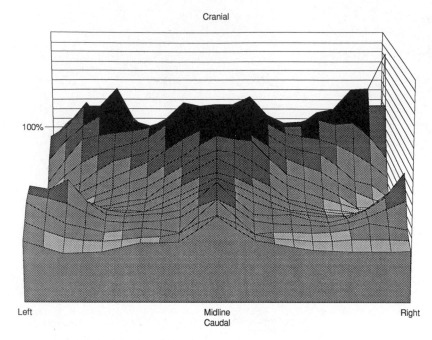

100%—

Left   Midline   Right
                                        Caudal

Figure 14C-19. Computer-generated three-dimensional pelvic image based on a grid of 110 point counts symmetrically arranged over the horse's hindquarters.

other tentative diagnosis in performance horses with vague hindlimb lameness. Clinically, a distinction can be made between acute luxations, with external asymmetry of the pelvis, and chronic subluxation, with few clinical signs except for gluteal atrophy leading to a "hunter's bump." Scintigraphic imaging and scintillation counting of the pelvis appear to confirm the presence of two separate entities. Acute luxation generally results in increased radionuclide uptake over the "sunken" side of the pelvis, whereas chronic subluxation can cause increased gamma ray emission along the midline over the sacrum. In either event, bone scanning has been reported to be extremely accurate in confirming suspected cases.[9]

Nuclear Imaging of Skeletal Muscle Damage
Bone-seeking RPs have been shown to localize in damaged skeletal and myocardial muscle.[3] The mechanism for this localization is still poorly understood, but it has a direct application in the horse for the identification of damaged muscles and quantification of the degree of damage in the rhabdomyolysis syndrome. Scintigraphs are obtained during the bone phase of RP distribution on the day following strenuous exercise. Increased RP uptake has been correlated with histologic evidence of myofiber degeneration, necrosis, and regeneration consistent with a diagnosis of rhabdomyolysis.[1] Uptake of the RP appears to correlate more closely with these histologic changes than with increases in plasma CK levels.

Scintigraphic imaging following the injection of ^{99m}Tc pertechnetate does not result in increased gamma radiation over the affected muscle sites, suggesting that there is no increase in blood flow to the damaged muscles in the acute phase of rhabdomyolysis.

Regional perfusion in the gluteal muscles of horses with the rhabdomyolysis syndrome also has been investigated by assessing the clearance of locally injected xenon-133.[4] The washout of xenon-133 from a tissue is proportional to its blood flow and related to the absolute blood flow by the diffusion coefficient for the tissue. Preliminary results from horses with recurrent rhabdomyolysis suggest that the onset of clinical signs is preceded by a reduction in perfusion of the affected muscle. In such horses, vasodilators such as isoxuprine may maintain perfusion and inhibit rhabdomyolysis.

Scintigraphy in Respiratory Disease

There are several reports of the use of scintigraphy in the study of equine respiratory diseases, particularly exercise-induced pulmonary hemorrhage (EIPH) and chronic obstructive pulmonary disease (COPD). Much of the work has been done by O'Callaghan and colleagues, to whose original work reference should be made for a more complete description of the techniques and their application.[21]

On ^{99m}Tc-MAA scans, deficits in lung perfusion are shown as "cold spots" (localized absence of gamma ray emission). Patterns of reduction of capillary perfusion may be related to specific diseases. COPD (small airway disease) results in patchy lung perfusion images. Focal lung perfusion deficits are caused by lung abscesses, but EIPH is associated with a perfusion deficit in the dorsocaudal angle of both lungs. Pneumonia can produce a varied pattern but tends to cause more perfusion deficits in the dependent areas of the lung.[22]

EIPH show a mild reduction
the dorsocaudal lung field.
haracteristic concentration
ger airways as well as a
periphery.[21]

computer program, the ventilation
ages can be overlaid for analysis of re-
ation-perfusion matching.[21] In COPD, per-
deficits generally match the ventilation deficits.
In EIPH, however, the perfusion deficit is unmatched,
which results in higher ventilation/perfusion ratios.

Conclusions

While gamma cameras will continue to be outside the range of equipment available to veterinarians in most equine practices, the portable machines described in this chapter are cost-effective and will allow the use of scintigraphy in many practices that deal with acute injuries in athletic horses. However, one of the problems with the use of scintigraphy is that the technique is sometimes employed in cases where it is not necessary rather than a detailed clinical examination being undertaken. Judicious use of scintigraphy for evaluation of musculoskeletal disorders involves a careful clinical and radiographic examination prior to scintigraphy.

References

1. Morris E, Seeherman HJ, O'Callaghan MW, et al: Scintigraphic identification of skeletal muscle damage in horses 24 hours after strenuous exercise. Equine Vet J 1991; 23:347.
2. Palmer AM, Watt I, Dieppe PA: Soft tissue localization of ^{99m}Tc-hydroxymethylene diphosphonate due to interaction with calcium. Clin Radiol 1992; 45:326.
3. Matin P: Basic principles of nuclear medicine techniques for detection and evaluation of trauma and sports medicine injuries. Semin Nucl Med 1988; 18:90.
4. Webbon PM: Unpublished data, 1988.
5. Attenburrow DP, Bowring CS, Vennart W: Radioisotope bone scanning in horses. Equine Vet J 1984; 16:121.
6. Pilsworth RC: Can a pelvic fracture be detected by probe scintigraphy? Vet Rec 1992; 131:123.
7. Attenburrow DP, Portergill MJ, Vennart W: Development of an equine nuclear medicine facility for gamma camera imaging. Equine Vet J 1989; 21:86.
8. Riddols LJ, Willoughby RA, Dobson H: A method of mounting a gamma detector and yoke assembly for equine nuclear imaging. Vet Radiol 1991; 32:78.
9. Steckel RR: The role of scintigraphy in lameness evaluation. Vet Clin North Am Equine Pract 1991; 7:207.
10. Ueltschi G: Zur Diagnose von Interosseuslesionen an der Ursprungstelle. Pferdeheilk 1989; 5:65.
11. Ueltschi G: Die Skelettszintigraphie beim Pferd 1. Teil: Einfahrung. Pferdeheilk 1989; 3:99.
12. Schramme MC: Unpublished data, 1991.
13. Allhands RV, Twardock AR, Boero MJ: Uptake of ^{99m}Tc-MDP in muscle associated with a peripheral nerve block. Vet Radiol 1987; 28:181.
14. Gaughan EM, Wallace RJ, Kallfelz FA: Local anesthetics and nuclear medical bone images of the equine forelimb. Vet Surg 1990; 19:131.
15. Trout DR, Hornof WJ, Liskey CC, Fisher PE: The effects of regional perineural anaesthesia on soft tissue and bone phase scintigraphy in the horse. Vet Radiol 1991; 32:140.
16. Trout DR, Hornof WJ, Fisher PE: The effects of intraarticular esthesia on soft tissue and bone phase scintigraphy in the ho. Vet Radiol 1991; 32:140.
17. O'Callaghan MW: The integration of radiography and alternativ imaging methods in the diagnosis of equine orthopedic disease Vet Clin North Am Equine Pract 1991; 7:339.
18. Webbon PM: Bone scintigraphy: indications and limitations. *In* Proceedings of the 27th Annual Congress of the British Equine Veterinary Association, 1987, p 34.
19. Seeherman HJ, Morris E, O'Callaghan MW: The use of sports medicine techniques in evaluating the problem athlete. Vet Clin North Am Equine Pract 1990; 6:239.
20. Ueltschi G: Roentgenologische und szintigrafische Untersuchungen an der Brust- und Lendenwirbelsaule des Pferdes. *In* Proceedings of the 7th Tagung uber Pferdekrankheiten—Equitana Essen, 1987.
21. O'Callaghan MW: Nuclear imaging techniques for equine respiratory disease. Vet Clin North Am Equine Pract 1991; 7:417.
22. Twardock AR, Allhands RV, Boero MJ, et al: Nuclear scintigraphy of the equine skeletal and pulmonary systems: Overview of the technique, its capabilities and limitations. *In* Proceedings of the American Association of Equine Practitioners, 1986, p 495.
23. Trout DR, Hornof WJ, O'Brien TR: Soft tissue and bone phase scintigraphy for diagnosis of navicular disease in horses. J Am Vet Med Assoc 1991; 198:73.
24. Markel MD, Richardson DW: Non comminuted fractures of the proximal phalanx in 69 horses. J Am Vet Med Assoc 1985; 86:573.
25. Ellis DR, Simpson DJ, Greenwood RES, Crowhurst JS: Observations and management of fractures of the proximal phalanx in young thoroughbreds. Equine Vet J 1987; 19:43.
26. Metcalf MR, Forrest LJ, Sellett LC: Scintigraphic pattern of ^{99m}Tc-MDP uptake in exercise induced proximal phalangeal trauma in horses. Vet Radiol 1990; 31:17.
27. Koblik PD, Hornof WJ, Seeherman HJ: Scintigraphic appearance of stress induced trauma of the dorsal cortex of the third metacarpal bone in racing thoroughbred horses: 121 cases (1978–1986). J Am Vet Med Assoc 1988; 192:90.
28. Kent Lloyd CK, Koblik PD, Ragle C, et al: Incomplete palmar fracture of the proximal extremity of the third metacarpal bone in horses: Ten cases (1981–1986). J Am Vet Med Assoc 1988; 192:798.
29. Wright IM, Platt D, Houlton JEF, Webbon PM: Management of intracortical fractures of the palmaroproximal third metacarpal bone in a horse by surgical forage. Equine Vet J 1990; 22:142.
30. Scott Pleasant R, Baker GJ, Muhlbauer MC, et al: Stress reactions and stress fractures of the proximal palmar aspect of the third metacarpal bone in horses: 58 cases (1980–1990). J Am Vet Med Assoc 1992; 201:1918.
31. Ross MW, Martin BB: Dorsomedial articular fracture of the proximal aspect of the third metacarpal bone in standardbred racehorses: Seven cases (1978–1990). J Am Vet Med Assoc 1992; 201:332.
32. Pilsworth RC: Incomplete fracture of the dorsal aspect of the proximal cortex of the third metatarsal bone as a cause of hind-limb lameness in the racing thoroughbred: A review of three cases. Equine Vet J 1992; 24:147.
33. Stover SM, Hornof WJ, Richardson GL, Meagher DM: Bone scintigraphy as an aid in the diagnosis of occult distal tarsal bone trauma in three horses. J Am Vet Med Assoc 1986; 188:624.
34. Boero MJ, Kneller SK, Baker GJ, et al: Clinical, radiographic, and scintigraphic findings associated with enthesitis of the lateral collateral ligaments of the tarsocrural joint in standardbred racehorses. Equine Vet J 1988; (suppl 6):53.
35. Mackey VS, Trout DR, Meagher DM, Hornof WJ: Stress fractures of the humerus, radius and tibia in horses: Clinical features and radiographic and/or scintigraphic appearance. Vet Radiol 1987; 28:26.
36. Pilsworth RC, Webbon PM: The use of radionuclide bone scanning in the diagnosis of tibial "stress" fractures in the horse: A review of five cases. Equine Vet J 1988; (suppl 6):60.
37. Johnson PJ, Allhands RV, Baker GJ, et al: Incomplete linear tibial fractures in two horses. J Am Vet Med Assoc 1988; 192:522.

15

Lameness: Approaches to Therapy and Rehabilitation

V. C. SPEIRS

There are several textbooks that deal with diseases that cause lameness in horses, and these should be read in order to obtain an appreciation of all aspects of lameness evaluation and treatment. This chapter covers the therapeutic options and prognosis for some of the problems that cause lameness in athletic horses and for which there is a chance of a return to athletic activity. The catastrophic conditions resulting in complete and immediate removal from athletic activity are not considered. Since appropriate management of many of the problems affecting athletic horses requires knowledge of the etiology and pathogenesis of lameness, this information is provided where necessary. A knowledge of anatomy appropriate to the body systems involved is assumed, as too are the details of the sporting activity peculiar to each type of athletic endeavor.

Definition of Lameness

Lameness can be defined as an abnormality of gait resulting from pain, loss of normal neuromuscular control, or mechanical factors restricting normal movement. Consequently, lameness can be the result of injury to or malfunction of any body component involved in locomotion. To provide a basis for discussing lameness and to focus attention at the organ level, the flowchart in Figure 15–1 has been devised.

Objectives for Management of Lameness in Athletic Horses

Because major injuries usually carry a prognosis that effectively precludes return to athletic activity, manage-

ment of injuries to athletic horses is directed mainly toward treating relatively minor lesions and controlling inflammation and degeneration while attempting to maximize activity and avoid excessive loss of time. Although injuries usually can be classified as acute or chronic, management in both categories is usually undertaken with the same questions in mind:

- What immediate treatment is required?
- Can the horse continue with training or competition while treatment is administered?
- If a period of rest is required, how long should it be, and when can training and competition be resumed?
- What is the prognosis?

To provide answers to these questions and to maximize performance, a thorough understanding is required of the nature of injury and repair, as well as knowledge of the specific conditions causing lameness.

Physical Therapy

The objective of physical therapy is to increase tissue repair by utilizing the properties of heat, cold, light, ultrasound, and electricity to stimulate normal physiologic processes. This form of managing musculoskeletal injuries has been used extensively in humans, and although some modalities have been used to treat horses, very little scientific data exist that are directly applicable to horses. While there are many forms of physical therapy, only those which have been shown to be of benefit will be mentioned here.

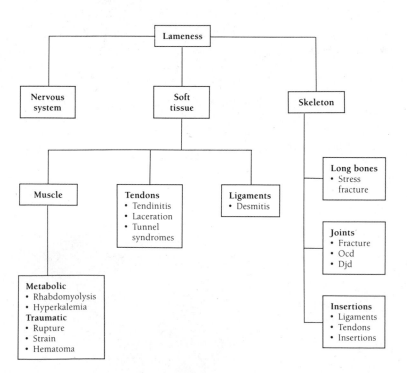

Figure 15-1. Flow diagram illustrating some problems experienced by athletic horses according to body system.

COLD

The application to tissue of a cold medium results in removal of heat from the tissue and stimulates vasoconstriction, reduces blood flow and metabolism, and causes some analgesia.[1,2] These responses are useful in minimizing edema and hematoma formation during the first 48 hours after an injury. The beneficial effects are obtained without freezing the tissues and by application times of approximately 30 minutes carried out three to four times daily. Prolonged use or use of lower temperatures has no value and may be injurious. The effectiveness of cryotherapy is shown by a study in horses where application of a gel wrap cooled to 4°C to the metacarpal region for 30 minutes resulted in a 6°C difference between treated and untreated limbs immediately after removal of the wrap, the dorsal metacarpus being the slowest region to rewarm with a difference of 4°C after 4 hours.[3] There are a number of ways to utilize cryotherapy.

Hose Pipe. This is a simple but time-consuming and relatively ineffective method (Fig. 15–2).

Tub, Whirlpool, or Turbulator Boot. These are less consuming in terms of manpower but are also relatively inefficient unless crushed ice is added to the water.

Ice Cup. A Styrofoam cup containing ice, prepared by placing the water-filled cup in a freezer, is an effective way to apply cryotherapy to a localized region (Fig. 15–3). It is done by peeling away some of the rim of the cup and then massaging the affected region by hand, using the cup as insulation for the hand.[4]

Gel Wrap. Commercially available gel wraps can be cooled in the refrigerator and then applied in a self-retaining nylon covering. The equine Orthoform hot/cold therapy boot (Hufmeister Co., Inc., Orthoform Division Equine Therapeutic Products, 145 Bridge St., Suite D, P.O. Box 1347, Arroyo Grande, Calif. 93421) fitted with a Polar Pack (Midlands Chemical Co., Inc., Omaha, Neb.), consisting of a sodium acetate gel, is an example of such a device which can be cooled in the refrigerator and used repeatedly (Fig. 15–4). As demonstrated above, this is an effective cooling technique.

Crushed Ice and Water in a Plastic Bag. This is an effective, cheap, and convenient way of applying cold, since it easy to apply and conforms to surface contours (Fig. 15–5).

HEAT

The application of heat causes an elevation in tissue temperature, which subsequently produces vasodilation and

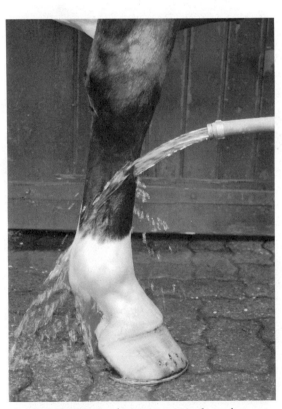

Figure 15-2. Cryotherapy using water from a hose.

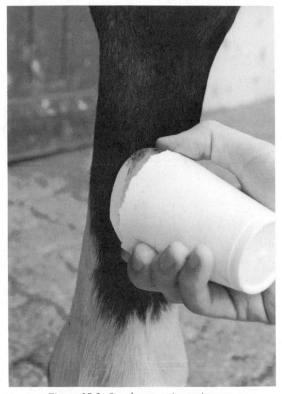

Figure 15-3. Cryotherapy using an ice cup.

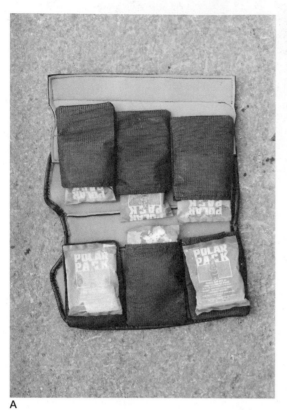
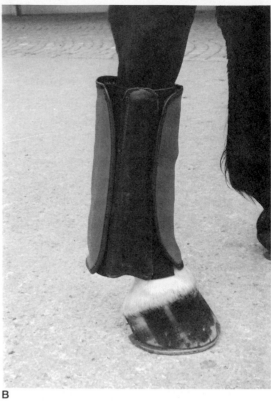

A   B

Figure 15-4. *Cryotherapy using a frozen gel pack (Polar Pack, Midlands Chemical Co., Inc., Omaha, Neb.). (A) Frozen gel packs inserted into a boot applicator. (B) Boot applicator positioned on the right metacarpus.*

increased metabolism.[1,5] This response is harmful in the early stages of injury, when there is potential for edema and hematoma, but after approximately 48 hours, this danger is passed and heat can be used to stimulate healing.

Heat can be applied superficially as radiant (infrared energy) or conductive heat (hot water bottles, pads, or poultices) and deeply as conversive heat produced in tissues as a result of resistance to the passage of high-frequency electrical energy (diathermy) and sound waves (ultrasound). Conductive heat is used most commonly in the form of hot water poultices and heating pads, an example of which is the equine Orthoform hot/cold therapy boot fitted with a Safe and Warm gel pack (Safe and Warm, Inc.), which contains a metal strip that can be bent to activate the heating process (Fig. 15–6). This device is reusable, and the pad can be reactivated by boiling. When using water, a massage effect can be added by using a high-pressure pulsating jet or a turbulator, which uses a motor to create water turbulence. A study in horses showed that application of a chemical gel wrap heated to 40°C for 30 minutes increased the temperature of the metacarpal region by 5°C immediately after the wrap was removed.[3] The temperature remained 2°C higher than control after 4 hours. Some mild edema was noted in most horses. This study also found that after beginning to cool, the temperature of the treated limb temporarily increased 30 to 45 minutes af-

ter removal of the wrap, judged to be a reflex vasodilation. The authors recommended application of a bandage after removal to prevent heat loss and edema.

Production of deep heat by diathermy is not practical in horses because of the difficulty in using the equipment, whereas therapeutic ultrasound has a much greater application (see below).

MAGNETIC FIELD THERAPY

The effects of electric current on tissue healing have received considerable attention in recent years, especially for management of nonunion fractures. Invasive methods of producing an electric current involve insertion of one or two electrodes, while the noninvasive techniques utilize the ability of a magnetic field to induce an electric current in tissues exposed to the field. Although there is evidence that electrical energy influences biologic systems, there is a lack of controlled data to indicate a specific use in horses. One controlled study failed to demonstrate an increase in limb temperature with application of a flexible biomagnet.[3]

ULTRASOUND

The cellular effects of therapeutic ultrasound can be grouped into those predominantly of thermal origin and those mainly nonthermal.[6] Nonthermal effects include

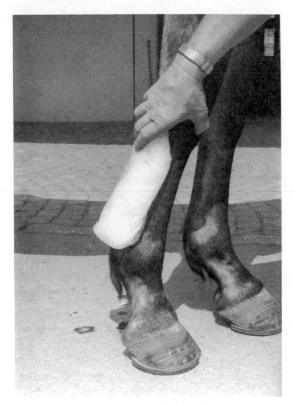

Figure 15-5. *Cryotherapy using crushed ice in a plastic bag applied to the limb.*

standing waves, acoustic streaming, microstreaming, and cavitation.[6] Thermal effects occur as a result of deep heat production through tissue vibration,[7] with subsequent improvement in tissue metabolism.[8-10] Ultrasound is reportedly useful in increasing tissue healing.[11] Although its effect on healing in horses is unknown, it is documented[3] as producing increased skin temperature for at least 4 hours after treatment with 1.0 W/cm². Ex-

cessive application has the potential to damage bone, periosteum, vascular membranes, and cells and, accordingly, should be used carefully.

Soft Tissues

GENERAL RESPONSE TO INJURY AND PRINCIPLES OF MANAGEMENT

Following injury to soft tissue, the initial inflammatory response is characterized by swelling, edema, increased temperature, and pain, with the degree of disability depending on the extent and the site of injury. Hematoma formation is often a complicating factor in muscle injuries. Later, as the inflammation subsides, pain and disability decrease, and the repair stage begins to provide gradual increase in strength. Optimal management of soft-tissue trauma is based on a thorough understanding of the processes involved, with different therapies being used at different stages.

The general principles of management are summarized in Figure 15–7. In general, during the acute phase, treatment is directed toward controlling the inflammatory response and minimizing further injury, and later, during the maturation phase, it is to apply mechanical stress in order to attain the maximum possible functional adaptation of the new tissue.

The main objectives of management and the means of attaining them are summarized as follows:

- Control inflammation
    Cryotherapy
    Anti-inflammatory agents
    Wound support
- Provide analgesia
    Wound support
    Analgesics
- Evacuate hematoma
- Prevent further injury
    Immediate reduction or cessation of exercise
    Provision of support to limbs

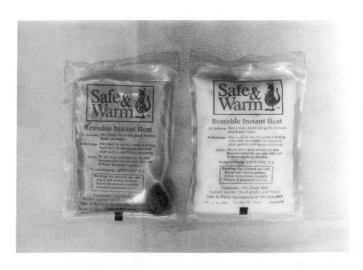

Figure 15-6. *Conductive heat therapy using a chemically activated gel pack (Safe and Warm, Safe and Warm, Inc.). The inactivated (left) and activated (right) forms of the pack are shown. The activated pack is applied using the same pouch system shown in Figure 15–4.*

Acute injury
• Prevent/minimize inflammation
   Reduce/eliminate exercise
   Provide physical support (bandage, splint, cast)
   Anti-inflammatory drugs (e.g., NSAIDs)
   Cryotherapy
• Provide analgesia
   NSAIDs
   Physical support (bandage, splint, cast)
   Cryotherapy
• Evacuate hematomata
• Prevent further injury
   Reduce/eliminate activity
   Provide physical support (bandage, splint, cast)
• Stimulate healing (after 48 hours)
   Application of heat (superficial, deep)
Chronic injury
• Gradual increase in physical activity
• Monitor progress—reduce activity if lameness returns

Figure 15-7. *Principles of management of soft-tissue injuries.*

TENDON

Specific Response to Injury

Tendon injury varies between mild strain, with little disruption of tissue, and complete rupture. In mild cases the repair process involves resorption of edema fluid and blood with restoration of a relatively normal tendon, while in more severe injuries there is formation of a dense, highly cellular granulation tissue and later fibrous tissue that contributes to a large increase in the cross-sectional area of the tendon. When there is significant disruption of tendon, the repair process originates mainly from tissues outside the tendon, so-called extrinsic repair. Intrinsic repair does occur but appears to be of limited significance, except in regions where the extrinsic process is restricted by the tendon sheath or in cases where the injury is confined to the interior of the tendon.

The significant differences between normal tendon tissue and tendon scar tissue are the presence of disordered fibrous tissue, increased cellularity, and reduced content of collagen. Type III collagen is the predominant form of collagen in scar tissue, in contrast to normal tendon, where it is type I. The fact that type III collagen has less tensile strength than type I is probably an important factor in the poor prognosis for tendinitis. It would appear, therefore, that the prognosis could be improved if existing tenocytes could be induced to produce type I collagen and if the production of type III collagen could be minimized.[12]

Tendinitis, or strain, is primarily a disease of athletic horses and is predisposed to by biomechanical stresses that occur during exercise. The precise mechanism is not known, and there is disagreement as to whether the lesion occurs suddenly when an excessive load is applied to a normal tendon[13,14] or whether continual exercise causes an accumulation of microdamage in the tendon which then predisposes it to break down when even a normal load is imposed.[14,15] Both mechanisms may apply on occasions. Sufficient load could be applied during exercise if there is a loss of footing or

abnormal muscular activity.[16] The fact that most clinical lesions occur in regions of the tendon where cross-sectional area is least has been used to support the single-event theory.[17] However, cross-sectional area has been shown to be independent of tendon strength.[18,19] Evidence to support the alternate theory, that of accumulation of microdamage, is the fact that in the sites where tendinitis is observed most commonly, many "normal" tendons contain gross and microscopic evidence of previous injury and repair.[15] The consensus probably supports the latter theory based on the accumulation of microdamage.

Tendinitis

Clinical Signs and Diagnosis. Injuries to the flexor tendons are more likely to be in a foreleg and to involve the superficial flexor tendon (SFT) than the deep flexor tendon (DFT).[14] In the SFT, the most common site for a lesion is the region between the distal aspect of the carpal sheath and the proximal region of the digital sheath.[20] In the acute phase, there is swelling, pain, increased skin temperature, and mild lameness. If the lesion involves major disruption or rupture of the tendons, the fetlock on that side will be overextended ("dropped fetlock") because of a loss of support from the tendons. The chronic phase is characterized by localized or extensive firm swelling composed of fibrous tissue. The lesion is usually painful on palpation, particularly when palpated with weight off the leg. When the lesion is sufficiently enlarged and located distally in the metacarpal or metatarsal region, there is often an associated inflammation of the digital sheath as a result of a relative constriction of the annular ligament.

Diagnosis of tendinitis traditionally has been made by detecting the presence of swelling, pain, and elevated tissue temperature, by palpation, and by visual examination. This simple examination readily allows clinical disease to be detected; however, the existence of lesions not producing clinical signs may remain unnoticed. Identification of silent lesions can be improved by measuring limb temperature thermographically or by evaluating tendon structure ultrasonographically (see Chap. 14B). The use of ultrasound has revolutionized evaluation of tendons in that it facilitates recognition of early lesions, aids in their accurate localization, and allows the progression of the disease to be monitored.

Ultrasonographic Signs. The technique of tendon ultrasonography is well described.[21] It is usual to scan in transverse and longitudinal planes, with the transverse scan being used to identify the type and extent of injury and the longitudinal scan for examining the longitudinal fiber arrangement. The limb is scanned systematically from proximal to distal, and photographs are made of abnormal findings.

In the acute phase, a significant injury with disruption of tendon fibers and localized hemorrhage is characterized by an anechoic core (core lesion), while a less severe lesion with less fiber damage and without local accumulation of blood produces a mottled appearance. As the repair process proceeds, the core lesion becomes more echogenic as granulation tissue is produced and is then replaced first by immature nonaligned fibrous tissue and later by more organized tissue. Eventually, the structure may resemble normal tendon, although the presence of peritendinous adhesions may render its borders difficult to visualize accurately. In order to allow repair to be monitored, it is necessary to locate and measure, accurately, the cross-sectional area and the longitudinal extent of the lesion.

Good correlation exists between the gross, histologic, and ultrasonographic findings in tendinitis,[22] which is the basis for an ultrasonographic grading system:

- *Type 1:* Mature fibrous tissue.
- *Types 2 and 3:* Hypoechoic lesion indicating the presence of granulation tissue and immature fibrous tissue.
- *Type 4:* Anechoic lesion indicating the presence of a fresh hematoma.

The lesion should be graded according to the preceding system,[23] as well as to its extent.[24] The extent of the lesion can be assessed by reference to the deep flexor tendon[25] or by using an index combining the preceding grading system and the cross-sectional area.[24]

Management. The management varies depending on whether the lesion is acute or chronic.

ACUTE TENDINITIS. Management should be directed toward controlling the acute signs in such a way as to maximize the chance of the horse returning to athletic activity. Current knowledge of the inferior mechanical properties of scar tissue makes it logical to minimize scar formation in the region of the injury and to maximize the functional adaptation of that which is formed. Therefore, the objectives of the immediate therapy of the acute case are as follows:

- Decrease inflammation and the associated edema and pain.
- Minimize bleeding and hematoma formation.
- Minimize the deposition of excessive scar tissue.
- Encourage, as far as possible, the restoration of normal tendon architecture.

To accommodate these objectives, management consists of the following steps:

1. *Immediate cessation of exercise.* It is important that no further trauma is superimposed on the original lesion as a result of continued training or competition. A horse should be removed immediately from hard exercise, although the extent of this is dependent on the severity of the injury. Less severe lesions may still allow exercise of reduced intensity; however, this should be at the discretion of the veterinarian and is best based on careful palpation and ultrasonography so that core lesions can be identified. In severe cases, the horse should be confined to a stall.

2. *Cryotherapy.* In the first 48 hours after injury, appropriate use of cryotherapy is a very effective way to minimize bleeding and edema. This is effectively done by wrapping the limb in a plastic bag containing crushed ice with a little water added to facilitate uniform tissue contact or with a chemical cold pack. Cryotherapy is carried out for 30 minutes at a time and is repeated several times a day until the acute phase of inflammation has been controlled.

3. *Support bandage.* Applying a firm support bandage to the lower limb helps to reduce swelling and discomfort.

4. *Nonsteroidal anti-inflammatory drugs (NSAIDs).* The careful use of NSAIDs is very useful for limiting the inflammatory reaction and the associated pain and extravasation of intravascular fluid and protein into the injured tissue. Phenylbutazone (initial dose of 4.4 mg/kg every 12 hours) is satisfactory for this purpose and has minimal effect on the repair process. The potential for toxicity should always be considered, and dose rate and duration of treatment should be changed as necessary.

5. *Corticosteroids.* Judicious use of corticosteroids in the acute phase is a very effective method of limiting inflammation; however, prolonged therapy is contraindicated because of the inhibitory effect on many aspects of wound healing. The effectiveness of the reduction in inflammation and pain often results in overuse of the leg either because the horse feels better or because the trainer is misled by the apparently successful treatment. Intratendinous injection is contraindicated because of the tendency to produce necrosis and collagenolysis,[26] as well as intratendinous calcification.[27]

6. *Provision of analgesia.* Analgesia is provided by the cryotherapy, NSAIDs, and provision of support.

7. *Immobilization.* Confinement in a stall with a support bandage provides an easy and effective way of restricting movement, but in severe cases, this may not be sufficient. In more severe injuries, a cast or a board splint can be applied to eliminate weight bearing by the tendon. The duration of immobilization is difficult to prescribe, but in view of the known beneficial effects of early controlled motion in other species, it appears desirable to begin some form of activity as soon as the acute painful phase is over, usually about 2 weeks or earlier, if possible. If a cast is applied, it should be removed after about 2 weeks in order to allow controlled activity to begin.

8. *Dimethylsulfoxide (DMSO).* DMSO is frequently used topically, but although its solvent, anti-inflammatory, and free radical–scavenging properties are well known, the benefits of its direct application in tendon repair have not yet been established.

9. *Sodium hyaluronate (NaHa).* Sodium hyaluronate has been shown to be capable of influencing tissue repair,[28] especially the higher-molecular-weight forms.[29] The precise role for this drug in tendon healing has not been established, although in a collagenase-induced tendinitis model, there is support for[30] and against[31] its use. It also has been shown to reduce peritendinous adhesions in animals.[32,33] However, although reduction of adhesions after tendon injury in humans is very important, the significance of adhesions in horses is not known. In horses, it is likely that adhesion formation in

the usual site of tendinitis between the carpal and digital sheaths is not a problem, although within the digital sheath the situation may be analogous to that for the digital flexors in humans. The drug can be administered peri- or intratendinously, which might explain some of the discrepancies between published data.

10. *Polysulfated glycosaminoglycans (PSGAGs).* This group of drugs also has been employed to treat tendinitis. However, even though they are important components of soft tissues, their precise role in tendon repair is not known. Intralesional injection is performed.[34]

11. *Ultrasound.* Therapeutic ultrasound has shown benefit in treating chemically induced tendinitis,[35] as well as after tendon-splitting surgery.[36] While its use in clinical disease is not established, benefit has been claimed in a small clinical series.[37]

12. *Surgery.* Until recently, surgery usually was not considered in the treatment of acute cases of tendinitis. However, the emphasis given to reducing, rather than stimulating, scar tissue formation has revived interest in percutaneous tendon splitting or stabbing under ultrasonic guidance as a means of evacuating intratendinous hematomas and reducing edema. This approach has shown value in a collagenase-induced tendinitis model, where it reduced tendon diameter, lesion size, and grade and improved the quality of repair tissue.[38] Its value in clinical cases has yet to be fully ascertained, although it seems likely to become part of the early intensive management of tendon injuries when a core lesion is present, as detected by use of ultrasound.

CHRONIC TENDINITIS. The management of chronic tendinitis has always been a controversial topic, and many different methods have been tried. Of the variety of surgical treatments, none has stood the test of time. Some of the objectives behind these techniques have been stimulation of the inflammatory response in order to increase deposition of fibrous tissue (thermal cautery or "firing," injection of sclerosing agents, insertion of carbon fibers), exposure of the tendon core to facilitate internal healing (open or percutaneous tendon splitting or stabbing), insertion of a tendon graft to provide a framework for the orderly production of repair tissue, and provision of a synthetic scaffolding to provide extra mechanical strength as well as a framework for new tissue. The majority of these methods have not been scientifically evaluated, and with the possible exception of percutaneous tendon stabbing or splitting,[39,40] most techniques have fallen into disuse after an initial period of enthusiasm. The most recent technique is superior check ligament (SCL) desmotomy, the beneficial effects of which have been reported in clinical[41,42] and experimental[43] investigations. This method is now under extensive worldwide clinical evaluation. The rationale for the surgery is based on the supposition that after desmotomy, a greater portion of the tensile load will be carried by the flexor muscle, which can elongate, rather than the tendon and the check ligament, which have limited ability to extend. Since the ligament will subsequently heal, albeit probably lengthened, the putative beneficial effect may result from either temporary reduction in tensile load immediately after the desmotomy,

from permanent reduction in tensile load as a result of lengthening of the ligament, or from both of these. After SCL desmotomy, a period of 60 days of stall confinement with regular hand walking during the last 6 weeks, followed by 60 days of turnout to pasture or light exercise, before gradually returning to training is recommended.

Exercise Plan. Regardless of the method used for the immediate treatment, the rehabilitation of an injured tendon requires an initial period of rest. This is then followed by a long period of controlled exercise, during which the tendon is exposed to loads gradually increasing in frequency and magnitude in order to encourage the orderly alignment of new tissue. Exactly how best to achieve this is not known, and details of management are at the discretion of the veterinarian. There is ample evidence that the repair stage of a tendon is a long one and, depending on the extent of fiber damage, may require 12 to 18 months. During this phase, ultrasonography is of considerable assistance because it reveals the extent of the injury, especially the existence of a core lesion, and thus allows an individual plan of management to be devised.

The following program is based on regular ultrasonographic examinations carried out at approximately monthly intervals:

- *An anechoic region present in the substance of the tendon:* Horse should be confined to stall with hand walking.
- *A hypoechoic region present:* As the lesion becomes more echogenic, indicative of repair, controlled exercise, consisting of periods of walking and trotting, should be instituted. Under conditions of good supervision and if the horse is docile, it may be turned out during this stage, but it is important that enough exercise is provided to ensure that the tendon experiences the tensile loading necessary to stimulate fiber alignment.
- *Tendon has normal appearance:* Exercise of greater intensity can begin. During this phase, ultrasonographic examinations are carried out after exercise to detect recurrence before a major injury occurs. Any clinical or ultrasonographic evidence of recurrence indicates that the workload should be reduced.

Prognosis. Prognosis is related to a number of different factors:

- Severe tendon disruption with rupture of many fibers greatly reduces prognosis because there is simply insufficient normal tendon remaining to withstand the mechanical loads.
- The inadequate mechanical capability of scar tissue contributes to a poor prognosis.
- Tendon repair and scar maturation are a lengthy procedure, requiring up to a year or more. This period of time is not always available to horses in activities such as racing, where the competitive life span is relatively short.

- Projected use of the horse. Horses used for racing will always have a worse prognosis than those used for less rigorous activities.

When adequate time for convalescence cannot be ensured, or when there is extensive injury, the prognosis is very poor. Because of the lack of data from prospective trials, it is very difficult to provide a reliable figure for prognosis. However, the poor prognosis for conservative and surgical management of tendinitis is well recognized, and figures on the order of 20 percent for return to athletic activity are available. The advent of ultrasonography has provided an imaging method that undoubtedly improves management of tendinitis, and new treatment methods aside, it is probably responsible for an improvement in prognosis simply by providing more reliable information about the lesion and the state of repair, thus facilitating diagnosis and management.

LESIONS OF THE SUSPENSORY (INTEROSSEOUS) LIGAMENT

Desmitis

Suspensory desmitis is primarily a problem of racehorses, especially standardbreds, where it occurs more often in the hindlimbs, in contrast to thoroughbreds, where it is seen mainly in the forelegs.[39,44] Injury to the suspensory ligament can occur in the region of its origin on the proximal palmar (plantar) aspect of the third metacarpal (tarsal) bone, its body, and its branches and at its distal attachments to the proximal sesamoid bones. The most common site is in the branches.

The histologic changes seen in suspensory ligament desmitis are similar to those seen in flexor tendinitis, which is not unexpected because it serves a similar function and has a similar structure, the major difference being its content of muscle fibers. As described for flexor tendinitis, tissue changes in the acute phase can range between minor separation of fibers with peri- and intraligamentous edema and bleeding to cases with significant fiber damage or complete rupture. In chronic lesions, the emphasis is on scar tissue deposition with enlargement of the ligament. The ligament's muscle component, more in standardbreds than thoroughbreds,[45] is thought to be involved in damping vibration under load, although whether it is significant in relation to injury is unknown.

Injury to the Body and Branches of the Ligament
Clinical Signs and Diagnosis. Clinical signs and diagnosis are similar to those for flexor tendinitis. However, the condition is frequently complicated by fracture of the distal aspect of the second or fourth metacarpal (tarsal) bones, as well as sesamoiditis, and evaluation should always include examination of these structures. Lameness and swelling are always present, but they are often not as acute as in tendinitis.

Management. The management of desmitis is similar to that for tendinitis, with splitting and stabbing being more useful in standardbreds than in thoroughbreds.[39,44]

Management consists of stall rest for 4 weeks with daily hand exercise, followed by a gradual return to harder work over the next 3 months. Ultrasonography can be used to monitor progress and modify the convalescence if necessary. Since desmitis may be complicated by lesions of the proximal sesamoid bones and the small metacarpal or metatarsal bones, management will often involve treatment of these structures.

Lameness Associated with the Origin of the Ligament
Clinical Signs and Diagnosis. Injury in the region of the origin can involve damage to the soft-tissue components or can be an avulsion fracture (see section on insertions). Signs are dominated by a moderate to acute unilateral or bilateral lameness in either forelimbs or hindlimbs that is exacerbated by exercise. Since there is little or no swelling, and because regional diagnostic anesthesia is imprecise, the lesion is often difficult to localize. Diagnosis is made by using careful palpation and appropriate regional anesthesia and imaging techniques. Lesions to the soft tissue are often visible in an ultrasonogram, fractures and chronic changes to the bone in the vicinity of the origin are visible radiographically (dorsopalmar view of proximal MC3), and both may be imaged with scintigraphy. Careful examination is necessary to differentiate lesions of the suspensory ligament from lesions of the deep flexor tendon and its accessory ligament (inferior check ligament).

Management. Absolute rest is necessary in the acute stages, after which controlled exercise in the form of hand walking can be instituted. A return to hard training should not occur before 3 months, and cases in which an avulsion fracture is present may require longer. No surgery is required.

Prognosis. The prognosis is good for a return to previous levels of competition in almost all cases.

FETLOCK TUNNEL SYNDROME (ANNULAR LIGAMENT CONSTRICTION OR DESMITIS)

Whenever there is insufficient room within the fetlock canal to accommodate the flexor tendons, their subsequent restriction may result in physical irritation, inflammation, pain, and lameness. The cause may be an enlarged tendon resulting from tendinitis, thickening and fibrosis of the annular ligament as a result of desmitis, or both of these.[46–48] The more the tendon is enlarged, the greater is the chance that its movement will be compromised. The cause of annular ligament desmitis in the absence of obvious trauma is unknown.

Clinical Signs and Diagnosis. The lesion is characterized by persistent lameness which is usually unilateral and equally distributed between forelimbs and hindlimbs. The affected tendon sheath is distended and bulges proximally and occasionally distally, where it is not confined by the annular ligament. When viewed from the lateral aspect, there is a characteristic notch on the palmar aspect of the fetlock where the distended tendon sheath narrows to enter the digital canal. Flexion usually elicits a pain response, and lameness is reduced or abolished by intrathecal anesthesia. The status of the annular ligament and the flexor tendons can be assessed ultrasonographically,[48] as well as by contrast radiography using air injected into the sheath and subcutaneously.[47] It is important to establish the status of the tendon because it can be a limiting factor for prognosis if significant tendinitis exists.

Management. In acute cases, conservative treatment in the form of anti-inflammatory therapy should be tried; however, the prognosis is not good. In cases that do not respond to therapy or which are already chronic, desmotomy of the annular ligament has been shown to be of value.[46,49] The surgical technique is well described[49] and involves sectioning the ligament longitudinally. This can be done either by using a skin incision that runs the full length of the ligament or by inserting scissors through a small incision and cutting the ligament blindly. The latter technique is simpler and less traumatic, and in cases where the tendon is not affected, it is the method of choice. However, if it is necessary to examine the tendon, e.g., to evacuate a core lesion, the former method is indicated.

Postoperative management consists of bandage support for 2 weeks until healing is complete. Anti-inflammatory therapy is indicated for a few days to minimize the synovitis. Hand walking is recommended after the first few days, and controlled riding can commence as early as 14 days if the lesion is free of pain.

Prognosis. In uncomplicated cases of desmitis with no tendon lesion, a success rate for full recovery of 64 percent (16 of 25) is reported.[47] In another series in which local trauma was incriminated in 25 percent of cases, an almost identical recovery rate of 67 percent (16 of 24) was recorded.[46]

SKELETAL MUSCLE

Specific Response to Injury

Skeletal muscle has considerable powers of regeneration at the level of the myofibril; however, the results depend on the specific injury and the treatment. Restoration of function requires regeneration of muscle tissue, including nerves and blood vessels, rather than fibrosis. Therefore, the repair process depends greatly on the extent of the injury. In athletic horses, muscle problems are most likely associated with exercise of a greater duration or intensity than that to which they are accustomed or to acute trauma. Traumatic clinical problems are most likely to be contraction injuries, lacerations, contusions, and ischemia, with contraction injuries and contusions being of most significance to athletic horses. Contusions are frequently accompanied by hematomas and are seen most often in the thigh muscles of jumping horses as a consequence of accidents. This injury probably parallels that reported in the quadriceps muscles in human athletes, where ossification of the lesion frequently occurs.[50] Although the optimal method of treating muscle

injuries is not established, it is of significance that muscle tends to regain tensile strength faster when it is mobilized as part of management.[51]

Muscle Strain Injuries

Indirect injury to muscle as a result of muscle activation or stretching is most likely to occur in the region of the highly specialized myotendinous junction. The injury varies with the severity of the trauma and can be separated into categories based on tissue trauma:

- *Delayed muscle soreness.* This type of muscle injury occurs after intense exercise and is characterized by mild discomfort beginning within a few hours of exercise and reaching a maximum after 1 to 3 days.[52] The soreness is most marked at the myotendinous junction, is reversible, and is associated with temporary weakness.[53] There is also evidence to suggest that it may be associated with release of intramuscular enzymes into the serum[54] and breakdown of collagen.[55] There is probably only a fine distinction between this entity and the more obvious muscle injury known as a strain.
- *Muscle strain (pull, tear).* Strains can be complete or incomplete and usually result from sudden stress that stretches the muscle beyond its usual limits, produces excessive tension, or results in a combination of these. Injuries tend to occur in the region of the myotendinous junction. Incomplete injuries are more common than complete ones.

Clinical Signs and Diagnosis. There is little documentation of specific muscle injuries available, although fibrotic or ossifying myopathy in the caudal thigh region is relatively common, and fibrotic myopathy of the gracilis muscle[56] and tendinitis of the calcanean tendon[57] have been reported. In the acute phase, there is usually some interference with gait, although whether this is in the form of an obvious lameness or just stiffness depends on the site and severity of the injury. Injury to certain muscles, such as the caudal thigh group, result in specific lameness that is pathognomonic for the muscle.[58] Muscle pain in the region of the loin and croup is likely to cause stiffness and toe dragging, while injury to caudal thigh muscles is more likely to result in obvious lameness with a characteristic shortened anterior phase of the stride and a rapid slapping of the hoof to the ground at the end of the stride.[59]

Identification requires recognition of the specific lameness if possible and localization of swelling and pain on firm palpation. The large muscle mass in horses makes deep palpation difficult, and great care is required to localize a painful injury. Imaging techniques such as thermography and even scintigraphy are useful in detecting changes in local temperature and tissue activity. Faradic stimulation is not commonly employed these days but is useful for detecting resentment to induced muscle contraction, which may be used to indicate pain. Occasionally, in severe injuries, a hematoma is present, and ultrasonography is useful for identification.

The dearth of information about muscle injuries in horses is probably a reflection of the fact that, in general, the prognosis is good and the course is of short duration. In the event of severe injury or injury to vital structures, the prognosis is poorer.

Management. Management of the acute case is directed toward minimizing edema and hemorrhage and restricting activity while the pain is present. This is done with cryotherapy and NSAIDs. Evacuation of a hematoma is often necessary when it is large; however, this should not be done for a few days until it is apparent that bleeding has stopped. Occasionally, such hemorrhage can be very extensive, even fatal, if a large vessel is involved, and in such cases, early drainage is contraindicated. In severe cases, surgical exploration may be attempted, but the prognosis is poor because it is so difficult to find the exact site of bleeding. After a few days, when the pain has subsided, controlled exercise should be instituted to aid in dissipation of fluid and to encourage adaptation of the new scar tissue. Muscle tissue will heal best when it is exposed to tensile loading as long as it is carefully monitored to avoid producing more trauma. Controlled activity can be provided and extended as long as there is not a return of pain and lameness.

Return to full activity is dependent on the extent of the injury but should not occur until a full range of pain-free movement is possible. Naturally, it is far more difficult to control activity in a horse than it is in a smaller animal, such as a greyhound, but efforts should be made to provide physiotherapy in the form of stretching and walking. Massage is a difficult modality to utilize in such a large animal, but vigorous manipulation may be helpful. Treatment directed toward improving blood supply by means such as ultrasound has not been evaluated in horses. Injuries to the caudal thigh muscles have a guarded prognosis because of their tendency to undergo fibrosis and ossification when muscle activity is restricted.

When a case is presented as a chronic problem, it usually indicates that there is serious gait restriction as a result of fibroplasia and perhaps pain. In these cases, the objective is to relieve the restriction by physiotherapy or by surgical means. The size of the horse means that surgical treatment is necessary, and in this instance, most experience has been with injury to the caudal thigh muscles, in particular the semitendinosis muscle. Surgical treatment, consisting of resection of the injured muscle and scar tissue,[59,60] adhesionolysis,[61] or semitendinosis tenotomy,[62] is useful, but prognosis for a return to full athletic activity is often poor. The preferred technique is the tenotomy.

INJURY OF INSERTIONS OF LIGAMENTS, TENDONS, AND JOINT CAPSULES ONTO BONES

The junction between soft tissue and bone is very complex, with transformation from soft tissue to bone occurring within a few millimeters. Injuries to this region traditionally have been detected radiologically by noting the production of new bone. However, with the advent of scintigraphy, the tissue response to injury can be seen earlier, and attention has been focused on the many other insertion sites not hitherto identified in lameness evaluation. The superficial fibers around the periphery of the junction are continuous with the periosteum, while the deeper fibers inserting into the bone pass through four distinct zones comprising tendon or ligament proper, fibrocartilage, mineralized fibrocartilage, and finally, bone. In oblique insertions, the contribution of the superficial fibers is relatively greater than that of the transitional zones. The significance of this region is its susceptibility to injury. Some insertion sites where evidence of injury is often seen are

- Joint capsule insertions
  Carpal joints
  Metacarpo(metatarso)phalangeal (fetlock) joints
  Proximal interphalangeal (pastern) joints
- Ligament and tendon insertions and origins
  Radius–radial tuberosity (biceps brachii muscle)
  Humerus–deltoid tuberosity (deltoid muscle)
  Vertebral interspinous processes
  Metacarpal (tarsal) 3 — proximal aspect of palmar surface (origin of interosseus ligament)
  Proximal sesamoid bones — attachments of interosseous ligament and all sesamoidean ligaments
  Proximal phalanx — proximolateral aspect (tendon of lateral digital extensor muscle), palmar aspect (oblique sesamoidean ligaments)
  Distal phalanx (pedal bone) — extensor process (tendon of common digital extensor muscle)
  Interosseous (suspensory) ligaments between the small metacarpal (tarsal) bones and metacarpal (tarsal) III
  Navicular bone — attachments of all ligaments

Response to Injury
Injury to insertion sites produces a painful lesion, particularly when a joint is involved. The acute injury is characterized by pain and an inflammatory response. What subsequently occurs is dependent on the extent of the injury, with minor injuries resolving with little or no residual signs and more extensive lesions associated with an osseous outgrowth in and around the insertion. In both cases, the lesions usually heal and allow a return to athletic activity. Whenever the joint capsules are involved, there is always the possibility that the lesion is part of degenerative joint disease (DJD), with the clinical syndrome and its management being dominated by the more significant involvement of the articular surface. When lesions are localized to the sites of insertion, they are also significant, causing pain and disability, but they have a much better prognosis because they will heal.

Clinical Signs and Diagnosis. The signs and diagnosis vary with the site and the extent of the lesion. Lesions in the distal limbs are relatively well described and are localized using standard diagnostic techniques. Lesions located in the proximal regions of the limbs are more difficult to localize, and it is only with the advent of scintigraphy that they have been identified.

Management. In the acute phase, the emphasis is on reduction of workload, anti-inflammatory therapy, and occasionally, provision of analgesia. In chronic cases, the most important aspect of therapy is to ensure that adequate time is given for fibroplasia and ossification to be completed.

Prognosis. In uncomplicated cases, the prognosis is good, but if there is extensive new bone formation in joint capsule insertions, the prognosis is not so favorable. Lesions involving the distal sesamoidean ligaments also carry a less favorable prognosis.

Hard Tissues

This section on hard tissues is subdivided into two subsections, long bones and joints. In these tissues, the lesions of greatest interest are the bucked shin complex involving the third metacarpal bone (MC3) and degenerative joint disease (DJD). While there is no doubt that many injuries to long bones and joints in athletic horses occur as a result of sudden, excessive loads, there is mounting evidence that the mechanisms behind the majority of lesions are related to the accumulation of tissue changes caused by the cyclic stresses associated with athletic activity. In order to better understand how these injuries arise and to treat them, one must have an idea of how these tissues respond to stress.

LONG BONES

Response to Exercise
There are certain concepts and aspects of the osseous response to exercise that are relevant to the problems experienced by athletic horses.

- *Remodeling* applies to the events associated with the removal and replacement of a small packet of bone, the cells and bone tissue involved being defined as the *basic multicellular unit* (BMU). The process is responsible for the gradual turnover of all bone tissue, and each sequence of resorption (R) and formation (F) first requires activation (A) of osteoclasts, hence the sequence ARF. *Modeling* is the term used to describe the process whereby the shape and dimensions of a bone are controlled, thus determining the dimensions of the periosteal and endosteal envelopes and therefore the volume of compact cortical bone present.
- The concept of *microdamage* and subsequent *mechanical incompetence* has been proposed as a mechanism leading to a reduction in bone quality.[63] These concepts recognize the occurrence of small foci of damage to bone which then undergo repair as a BMU, the number of foci being related to frequency of loading, magnitude of the load, and bone quality. The difference between the extent of damage and its repair is termed the *microdamage burden,*

with an increase in microdamage being equated to increased bone fragility.[63]

- Repeated use of bone reduces the strain required to produce a fracture, presumably because of accumulation of microdamage. For example, fresh, wet, normal human lamellar bone can endure at least 10^6 strain cycles at less than 2000 microstrain, 10^6 cycles at 2000 microstrain, but only 20,000 cycles if strain is 4000 microstrain.[64-66] The significance of this is that a fracture can follow application of a load that would normally not be capable of producing a fracture. Such fractures, termed *stress fractures,* occur in the dorsal aspect of the third metacarpal bone of racehorses soon after they are first introduced to training and racing,[67] as well as in other long bones at less well defined ages.[68]
- It has been suggested that for bone modeling to occur, the prevailing strain should exceed 1500 to 3000 microstrain (minimum effective strain, or MES) and that remodeling requires strain on the order of 100 to 300 microstrain[69] and is possibly inhibited by large strains.
- The speed of ultrasound and bone mineral density increases in horses exercised at high speeds.[70] This is caused by the increase in new bone and the decrease in porosity in the exercised horses, as described above. The velocity of ultrasound decreases when horses suffer from shin soreness.[71]
- The dorsal region of MC3 experiences high compressive strains during exercise.[72]
- The cortical hypertrophy is greater in thoroughbreds than in standardbreds,[73] although there is no significant difference in bone quality.[74]
- The increased cortical thickness improves the ability of the bone to tolerate the loads associated with high-speed exercise by reducing stress and local strain.
- The ability of bone to resist imposed loads is related to many factors, including geometry, collagen fiber orientation, and degree of mineralization.[75-78] Therefore, loss of strength with remodeling[79-83] and increased porosity[81] are not unexpected. Resistance to fracture is reduced approximately 10 to 35 percent by remodeling of primary bone[79,82,83] and approximately 20 percent by increased porosity.[84]

Dorsal Metacarpal Disease: ("Bucked Shin Syndrome," Shin Soreness, Shin Splints, Stress Fracture, Dorsal Metacarpal Periostitis)
This syndrome is very common in young racing thoroughbreds, quarter horses, and occasionally standardbreds soon after they begin fast training. The lesion is thought to be a response by bone to the acute stress of fast exercise, before there has been sufficient time for the necessary protective modeling to occur. The exact manner in which the lesion(s) arises and its form are not well understood. However, clinical and research data indicate that at one extreme it appears to be associated with production of new bone, which may or may not be painful, and at the other it is a stress fracture akin to similar fractures in humans. This appears to be supported by

the events occurring in the MC3 of young horses exposed to intense exercise, where there is increased bone apposition on the dorsomedial periosteal and endosteal surfaces (modeling) and decreased cortical bone remodeling.[70] In contrast, confined horses showed increased remodeling associated with increased porosity but without an increase in modeling. Although in cases of clinical disease there is often a painful lesion containing new bone, new bone is not always associated with pain either in clinical cases or in research horses exercised on a treadmill.[70] The range of the clinical condition has always been thought to be a manifestation of the extremes of the one process, namely, subperiosteal hematomas, extending to microfractures and later to periosteal callus. This may not be the case. It is possible that the new bone, which is not as mechanically robust as mature bone, can be injured and result in pain or that the denser bone in the dorsal cortex resulting from a lack of remodeling and which is more susceptible to fracture can fracture and also result in pain.

Clinical Signs and Diagnosis. The clinical syndrome has been described[85] and can be considered better if graded into different types.

Type 1 disease is found usually in horses exposed to fast exercise for the first time regardless of age, although the nature of horse racing dictates that they are usually 2-year-olds. It occurs after exercise, and horses typically exhibit an acute pain response to palpation of the dorsal metacarpal region. Radiographs at this time are usually negative, although occasionally fractures are seen.

Type 2 disease is regarded as being the chronic form of type 1 disease that has failed to heal. The lesion is characterized by a hard, painful callus on the dorsomedial aspect of the limb.

Type 3 disease is characterized by a fracture on the dorsal-dorsolateral aspect. Diagnosis of the developed disease is easy, based on palpation, radiography, and scintigraphy. The onset of the problem is preceded by a decrease in the velocity of ultrasound.[70]

Management. Type 1 lesions will generally respond to a period of rest or at least a period of reduced exercise intensity. The speed with which some of these horses recover suggests that healing is not dependent on rapid repair of microfractures but perhaps on maturation of newly forming bone tissue. Type 2 disease is managed by reducing workload and instituting a training program, although these cases are sometimes refractory. Type 3 disease usually also will heal after rest, but in chronic cases and when the owner requires the best possible chance of an early return to training, surgery is recommended. When multiple fractures are present, conservative therapy is indicated. Two surgical methods are commonly used:

- Forage—in which holes are drilled through the dorsal cortex, encouraging healing by a mechanism(s) not well understood. This is a simple method and, in the absence of controlled data, is probably the method of choice.

- Screw fixation—placement of screw(s) through one or both cortices to compress and stabilize the fracture. Removal of the screw(s) is carried out after healing has occurred and before a gradual return to training, usually beginning about 3 months after surgery.

In all cases, an adequate rest from hard exercise is necessary, and a controlled exercise program should be provided to ensure osseous adaptation to exercise. It is important that in addition to a program of sufficient duration, there is also a gradual increase in the intensity of training so that the bone is conditioned to the loads likely to be experienced during competition. Although the exact mechanism involved in the development of this syndrome is not understood, the present methods of therapy appear to be justified on the basis of current knowledge.

Prognosis. The prognosis for type 1 disease is good. For the other two it is less optimistic, and recurrence is not uncommon, probably related to the fact that convalescence often consists of paddock rest followed by a sudden return to the same stresses that produced the lesions in the first place. The importance of a controlled exercise program cannot be overemphasized. Since there is considerable movement of bone during exercise, screw removal is recommended, especially when it has been placed through both cortices. If screws are not removed, lysis frequently occurs around the head of the screw, and vague lameness is often present.

Prevention is important, and a graded exercise program is necessary as all horses enter intensive training. It is apparent that horses require submaximal exercise to produce the protective modeling, and training on a treadmill can provide the controlled exercise. It appears important for horses to run on footing that allows the foot to rotate rather than slide, as evidenced by the increased incidence of the problem on dirt tracks.

Stress Fractures in Other Sites

Stress fractures also occur in the proximal palmar cortex of MC3,[86-88] where they are seen radiographically as incomplete longitudinal lines. Diagnosis may be facilitated by scintigraphy.[86] Since this region is also the site of desmitis of the proximal suspensory ligament and avulsion fracture of its origin, care is required to ensure that the diagnosis is correct. Treatment involves withdrawal from training and competition for at least 3 months. The prognosis for a return to previous levels of performance is good. Use of surgical forage to successfully treat a refractory case is described, but such therapy usually is unnecessary.[89]

There are several reports of stress fractures in other sites in MC3 as well as in other long bones, including the humerus, radius, and tibia, and these lesions are being recognized with greater frequency as imaging techniques have improved.[68,90-93] Fractures tend to occur in younger horses and at specific locations within each bone, presumably as a result of stress concentration in bones that have not adapted to exercise-induced strains.

Because they are located in the upper limb, they are often difficult to localize even though the lameness can be quite severe. In such cases, scintigraphy followed by radiology is a very useful combination of imaging techniques for detecting and then characterizing the fracture. In the majority of cases, the fracture is visible on a radiograph once the site of the lesion is known. Although acute fractures in long bones can occur after the application of sudden excessive loads, it is important to realize that they also can occur as an extension of an undiagnosed or unsuspected stress fracture, as has been demonstrated for the humerus.[94]

Once identified, treatment consists of stall rest with hand walking for a period of approximately 3 months. Most of these fractures heal without any complication, but a real danger is that they can transform into a major fracture; hence all exercise should be under firm restraint, and transport is better avoided during the early phase of healing. Prognosis is good for a return to athletic activity.

JOINTS

Pathogenesis and Management of Traumatic Joint Disease
Articulations consist of articular cartilage supported by subchondral bone plates and trabeculae, joint capsule consisting of a tough outer fibrous and a delicate inner synovial layer, supporting ligaments, and synovial fluid. *Degenerative joint disease* (DJD), the term used to describe all forms of osteoarthritis, describes a syndrome in which there is deterioration of all or some of these components, whether or not an obvious cause is apparent.[95] The development of DJD is very complex, and the reader is referred to one of the several reviews of the pathogenesis of cartilage degradation[96] or DJD in horses.[97]

Degradation of cartilage is an important aspect of DJD, being influenced by mechanical loading and induced matrix resorption. Activity has a significant influence on joint health, and management of joint problems requires recognition of this. At one extreme, total immobilization is deleterious to cartilage, causing enhanced degradation of collagen,[98] a reduction in the concentration of glycosaminoglycans in association with thinning and softening of cartilage, and increased susceptibility to injury.[99] Therefore, in athletic horses, prolonged joint immobilization has the potential to significantly limit prognosis regardless of the primary condition. At the other extreme, excessive activity is also injurious, especially so when some cartilage damage is present already. In between these extremes is an activity level that is beneficial to and necessary for joint well-being, with such exercise contributing to cartilage remodeling through an increase in chondrocyte activity manifest as an increase in collagen and proteoglycan synthesis.

Numerous proteinases can degrade cartilage, including cathepsins, plasmin, elastase, stromelysin, collagenase, and gelatinase. The synthesis of other inactive precursors of these enzymes is influenced by various of the factors, such as cytokines, growth factors, and hormones, which are, in turn, under some control from inhibitors. There is thus a delicate balance between the synthesis and degradation of the components of cartilage, and an understanding of the mechanisms involved indicates that the general directions for prevention and management of DJD may lie with control of mechanical trauma, removal of the proteinases responsible for matrix resorption, and enhancement of agents capable of inhibiting enzyme function.

The pathologic changes characteristic of DJD are wear lines, discoloration, fibrillation, and ulceration of cartilage; sclerosis and trabecular thickening of subchondral bone; fibrosis and thickening of the capsule; lipping of joint margins due to remodeling of cartilage and subchondral bone; formation of periarticular osteophytes (enthesophytes) at capsular attachments; and chip fractures of joint margins due to fragmentation of the margin or of the new bone. Although the pathology of the problem is simplified to a certain extent by taking the overview, the fact remains that the clinician does not see all manifestations in all cases. Accordingly, a management plan should be made based on the visible lesion specifically and on an understanding of DJD generally. To assist in management, it is useful to consider the problem under the clinically recognizable entities:

- *Synovitis and capsulitis without apparent osseous or cartilaginous lesions.* This form is particularly common in the carpal and metacarpophalangeal (fetlock) joints of young racehorses and, with continued trauma, will progress to more advanced forms of the syndrome. Logically, in these cases, the management is directed toward controlling the soft-tissue pain and inflammation and preventing development of the secondary cartilaginous lesions.
- *Acute osseous lesions, such as chip or fissure fractures, not obviously associated with degenerative changes.* The importance of these lesions is that they are painful and will stimulate the development of DJD if exercise is continued. Although chip fractures will often heal without excision, a period of 3 to 6 months is required, which is in conflict with the career demands of a performance horse. Consequently, they are usually treated by arthroscopic excision in order to facilitate the fastest possible return to athletic activity, with the side benefit that the joint can be fully inspected and undiagnosed lesions identified and treated. The major significance of a linear fracture extending into the joint is the possibility of a defect in the joint surface, which also will contribute to DJD when activity is imposed. Therefore, this lesion is treated whenever possible by reconstruction of the joint surface.
- *Fractures associated with DJD.* In these cases, it is apparent that treatment probably will only be of short-term value, since the DJD will be the limiting factor in prognosis. In these cases, the clinician should not embark on surgical procedures with a cure in mind. Although general joint debridement and lavage to remove bone fragments, hypertrophied synovial membrane, some marginal osteo-

phytes, and soft degenerate cartilage, combined with symptomatic management of the DJD, are often useful in the short term, a similar response often is obtained by conservative management.

- *Degenerative joint disease with no apparent indication for surgery.* The management here must be directed toward controlling the pain and inflammation, minimizing progression of the disease, and adjusting the workload to a tolerable level.

Specific Treatment of DJD
The simple objectives are to manage soft-tissue inflammation, prevent further cartilage degradation, and remove damaged cartilage and bone. Superimposed on this ideal approach are restraints such as economic considerations, age and use of the horse, and performance schedules. The objectives are summarized in Figure 15–8.

Rest and Physiotherapy. Reduction in or cessation of exercise is the first and most obvious necessity, and the extent of rest is dependent on the severity of the injury. Total restriction of joint motion is contraindicated, and although passive continuous motion without weight bearing has been shown to be beneficial, this is impossible to produce in clinical cases. Regular controlled hand, swimming, or treadmill exercise is attainable and is recommended. The precise level of activity that is most beneficial is not known, but it should certainly not produce an exacerbation of the existing problem. The use of cryotherapy is indicated in the acute case and can sometimes allow activity to continue under close observation.

Joint Lavage. Joint lavage is an effective way to remove intraarticular fragments of bone and cartilage as well as the many mediators that contribute to DJD. This is an integral part of arthroscopic surgery, but in selected cases, it also has value as a single procedure. It can be performed under general or local anesthesia.

- Prevent further physical damage to cartilage
  Reduce or eliminate exercise
  Chondroprotective agent (PSGAG)
- Control pain
  NSAIDs
  Reduce exercise
- Eliminate production of mediators
  Reduce exercise
  Improve soft-tissue lubrication (HA)
  NSAIDs
  Cryotherapy
  Corticosteroids (?)
- Remove preformed mediators from joint by joint lavage
- Allow sufficient time for maximal cartilage healing
- Institute gradual return to training
- Monitor progress and adjust exercise and/or administer therapy as necessary

Figure 15–8. Principles of management of degenerative disease.

Sodium Hyaluronate. This drug appears to be of value for treating synovitis but is of little use when chip fractures or significant DJD is present. The beneficial effect of sodium hyaluronate is mainly related to its function as the soft-tissue boundary lubricant[100] but also to its ability to filter certain compounds from the synovial fluid and also to some anti-inflammatory properties.[101] The molecular weights of available preparations vary, and although there are theoretical reasons to use those of higher molecular weight,[102,103] the clinical significance of this is not yet clear.[104]

Polysulfated Glycosaminoglycans (PSGAGs). The pharmacologic properties of these drugs and their application to DJD have been reviewed.[105] They have demonstrated chondroprotective properties through their ability to inhibit the production or release of many destructive proteinases, the synthesis of prostaglandins and interleukins, the release of free radicals, as well as the stimulation of sodium hyaluronic synthesis and chondrocyte metabolism. The drug diffuses into articular cartilage within hours of intraarticular or intramuscular administration. It has been shown to be of value in a clinical trial[106] and chondroprotective in experimental situations in horses,[106–108] although an ability to improve healing of existing cartilage defects has not been demonstrated.[107,108] Intramuscular administration in a chemically induced carpitis model (500 mg, seven times, 4 days apart) is reported to have had beneficial effects,[109] but this was not confirmed in a similar model that included artificial cartilaginous defects.[108] Its intraarticular use is associated with an enhanced susceptibility to joint infection, but this may be controlled with careful aseptic injection techniques as well as the simultaneous use of an intraarticular antibiotic with 250 mg PSGAG.[110] At present, the drug is recommended for intraarticular use in cases where there is a high probability of cartilage damage, thus utilizing its chondroprotective properties.

Intraarticular Corticosteroids. When corticosteroids are administered intraarticularly, they exert a potent anti-inflammatory effect, although because they also have the potential to injure cartilage, there is considerable argument over their intraarticular use. The beneficial effects of a reduction in metalloproteinases contributing to proteoglycan destruction[111,112] are counterbalanced by the well-recognized suppression of chondrocyte metabolism.[113–116] Furthermore, there is evidence to indicate that a deleterious effect is more likely to result in joints with preexisting injury.[117,118] Consequently, there appears to be a role for the judicious use of intraarticular corticosteroids when synovitis and soft-tissue inflammation predominate in cases with intact cartilage and no fractures. It is important to remember that these are powerful drugs and that their effects, which result in a dramatic reduction in pain, should not be interpreted as a cure. The best drug to use and the appropriate dose rate remain to be elucidated. Commonly used drugs are betamethasone acetate, methylprednisolone acetate, and triamcinolone acetonide, with the former being favored for its rapid onset of action and the latter for its prolonged effect.[119]

Dimethylsulfoxide (DMSO). This drug has a number of properties of potential use in the treatment of DJD, including an ability to inactivate oxygen-derived free radicals, suppress prostaglandin production, and inhibit depolymerization of sodium hyaluronate by oxygen-derived free radicals.[120] It has been shown to have some effect in reducing the severity of a chemical-induced synovitis model in horses,[121] although its value in clinical cases is not established.

Some Problems of Specific Joints

Carpus. The carpus is an important site of injury in racehorses, especially thoroughbreds and quarter horses, but carpal lameness is relatively uncommon in horses that compete as show horses, pleasure horses, western and rodeo horses, hunters, and jumpers. Horses that race on dirt tracks seem to have a special predisposition. Carpal lameness is a significant cause of wastage for racehorses.[122]

CARPITIS. The load applied to the carpus during exercise is supported by the bones participating in the joint, as well as the fibrous capsule and intercarpal ligaments. As explained earlier, the soft tissues and their insertions into bone can be injured by the stress of high-speed cyclic loading and also must be adapted to such conditions by a period of training. When these tissues are injured, generalized carpal inflammation (carpitis) is produced. Carpitis, specifically synovitis, is also produced in response to early degeneration of bone and cartilage before a fracture occurs, as well as after a fracture if exercise is continued (see Osteochondral Chip Fractures, below). The characteristic signs of carpitis are pain on flexion, increased synovial effusion, soft-tissue swelling, and thickening of the joint capsule.

In cases where only soft tissues and their insertions are involved, the level of exercise must be reduced to allow healing to proceed, sometimes as little as a few weeks. Anti-inflammatory treatment with NSAIDs and other forms of therapy are useful (see below) but should not mask the disease, because a major problem can ensue if pain is controlled so effectively that hard exercise can continue. Lesions of the intracarpal ligaments are being recognized more frequently with the increased use of arthroscopy, and although it is not certain if surgical debridement is necessary, precise diagnosis is possible only during arthroscopy.[123–126]

OSTEOCHONDRAL CHIP FRACTURES. These fractures involve the dorsal border of the distal radius; the proximal and distal borders of the radial, intermediate, and ulnar carpal bones; and the proximal surface of the third carpal bone.[127,128] Although injury can result from direct trauma,[129] there is mounting evidence to show that fractures and DJD also occur after the bone structure has modified in response to repetitive exercise.[130] Although many of these fractures can heal, especially when there is minimal displacement of the fragment, the urgent need to return race horses to competition as soon as possible favors surgical removal and joint debridement.

Arthroscopic surgery enables this to be carried out relatively atraumatically, allows multiple joints to be operated on during a single period of anesthesia, and enables return to training and competition at the earliest opportunity. Surgery consists of removal of bone chips and debri, deep curettage of the cartilaginous defect into subchondral bone in order to encourage a good healing response from that region, production of a defect with vertical rather than sloping edges, and conservative smoothing and removal of new bone from the dorsal surface of the bone.

Postoperative management varies with the extent of the injury and the preference of the veterinarian. It is important that the lesion be given an opportunity to heal before any hard exercise is begun. Horses are confined to a stall for 4 weeks, the first without exercise and the last three with hand walking for 10 minutes twice daily. If a rapid return to competition is planned, swimming and water treadmill exercise may be used to maintain muscle tone and cardiovascular fitness until exercise can be commenced. The original hope that horses could return to training almost immediately after arthroscopy has not materialized, and it is now obvious that some time is required to allow healing to begin and for joint inflammation to be controlled. The time lapse between surgery and return to training varies considerably from 6 weeks to 6 months. For horses that require a longer convalescence, the best procedure after the initial stage of intense management is not known. Normally, horses would be turned out, but it is possible that some form of exercise is necessary to encourage the best possible bone repair.[131] Certainly a gradual return to training is indicated in order to prevent the immediate onset of a new sequence of trauma and injury once training is recommenced. The inability of hyaline cartilage to reconstitute itself is responsible for continuation or development of DJD in many horses after surgery. The search for methods to restore normal hyaline cartilage to regions of injury has so far been unsuccessful.

Prognosis depends first on the extent of the injury and the severity of preexisting arthritis and second on the later development of DJD. A recent evaluation of 445 racehorses showed that when lesions were graded according to severity, 71.1 percent (133 of 187) with grade 1 damage, 75 percent (108 of 144) with grade 2 damage, 53.2 percent (41 of 77) with grade 3 damage, and 54.1 percent (20 of 37) with grade 4 damage returned to racing at an equal or better level than before injury.[128] As a rule, lesions located medially carry a poorer prognosis than those located laterally, and distal lesions have a poorer prognosis than proximal ones.

THIRD CARPAL BONE DISEASE. The radial fossa, especially the dorsal third, of the third carpal bone in training and racing thoroughbreds shows cancellous bone remodeling and sclerosis.[132–134] This is a normal response to exercise and results in an increase in stiffness of the affected bone.[135] In many cases it appears to be associated with a zone of ischemia extending distally from the dorsal margin of the articular surface, which undergoes remodeling consisting initially of resorption.[136] Small regions of resorption can be tolerated, but larger ones cause collapse of overlying cartilage and produce a defect that predisposes to slab fracture. The full spectrum of third carpal fracture has been described.[137]

Regions of subchondral lucency in the dorsal aspect of the bone in standardbred horses have been described as a cause of lameness.[138] It is logical to think that this is part of the same process as just described for thoroughbreds, but the cause of the lesion is unknown.

Treatment of the lucent lesions consists of debridement under arthroscopic vision, which often reveals degenerate cartilage overlying the lucent regions. The prognosis for this problem, based on a limited series of standardbreds, showed that 89 percent (8 of 9) returned to racing, of which six performed at the same level of competition as before the surgery.

Treatment of slab fractures consists in most cases of compression screw fixation and, in a minority, removal of the slab of bone when it is very thin and will not support a screw and conservative therapy when there is no displacement of the fragment. Surgery may be via arthrotomy, arthroscopy, or a combination of both. The time between admission to hospital and first race averaged 11.5 months for standardbreds and 10.4 months for thoroughbreds.[139] The results from 61 standardbreds and 72 thoroughbreds with simple frontal plane slab fractures show that the prognosis for thoroughbreds is less favorable than for standardbreds, with 57 percent of standardbreds and 30 percent of thoroughbreds racing in the highest classification after surgery.[139] The thoroughbreds also had significantly lower earnings per start after surgery than before surgery. The data for thoroughbreds are supported by information from another series of 31 cases using claiming value as an index.[140]

Fetlock. The fetlock is subject to a number of different lesions that, although they often require individual treatment, are the result of chronic or acute overload of the joint. Although acute bending stress can damage collateral ligaments, the usual form of overload is overextension, which places the capsule and suspensory apparatus under stress and apposes the dorsal surfaces of the proximal phalanx and the distal MC3 and the dorsal surfaces of the proximal sesamoid bones and palmar surface of MC3. When this occurs acutely, injury can result, but the usual experience in athletic horses is a complex of lesions with a major presenting lesion predominating. The significance of this is that the clinician must be aware of the possible existence of other lesions, know where and how to detect them, and understand how they affect the overall prognosis.

CHRONIC PROLIFERATIVE SYNOVITIS OF THE DORSAL ASPECT OF THE CAPSULE. This lesion, often termed *villonodular synovitis,* is assumed to be caused by contact between the proximodorsal aspect of the proximal phalanx and the distal end of MC3 and consists of a range of changes including inflammation, hypertrophy, fibrosis, and ossification of the synovial pad; ulceration of adjacent articular cartilage; and resorption of adjacent bone.[141] It is characterized by low-grade, chronic, often bilateral lameness. Diagnosis usually is by clinical eval-

uation and plain and contrast radiology, although ultrasonography has been shown to be useful.[142] Mild lesions may be treated conservatively with rest and anti-inflammatory therapy. However, with more advanced lesions, the results are better if the mass is removed by sharp dissection and the cartilage and bone lesions debrided. It should be noted that this syndrome is related to overextension, and therefore, the problem probably will recur and is often part of a generalized arthropathy.

CHIP FRACTURES AND REMODELING OF THE PROXIMODORSAL MARGIN OF THE PROXIMAL PHALANX. Overextension contributes to this complex of lesions on the dorsal articular margin of the proximal phalanx. Chip fractures appear to be the result of a chronic process of stress and degeneration.[136] Diagnosis is made by radiology. Treatment is usually by excision of the fragment, formerly by arthrotomy and now usually by arthroscopy. Both arthrotomy[143] and arthroscopy result in a high chance of return to successful competition, 82.6 percent in the case of arthroscopy,[144] although deleterious effects of arthrotomy have been recorded.[145] The question of the necessity of surgical excision is important here, because many horses have such fractures as incidental findings. In racing animals, where time is such an important factor, surgery is indicated to facilitate a rapid return to training and to detect and allow treatment of other, unsuspected fetlock disease.

SUPRACONDYLAR LYSIS OF THE PALMAR CORTEX OF THE DISTAL CANNON BONE. Lysis of the palmar aspect of MC3 in the region of the palmar pouch of the joint capsule is found in athletic horses. This lesion is thought to be the result of osteoclastic activity associated with chronic synovitis.[136]

TRAUMATIC OSTEOCHONDROSIS OF THE PALMAR/PLANTAR SURFACE OF THE CONDYLE OF THE CANNON BONE. This problem is found mainly in the forelimbs of mature racehorses and is located either side of the sagittal ridge just caudal to the transverse ridge. In advanced cases it consists of ulcerative lesions of the cartilage overlying regions of subchondral bone collapse.[136] The development is possibly another manifestation of an intense local response to chronic overload through the mechanism of sclerosis and ischemia.[136]

TRANSVERSE RIDGE ARTHROSIS. This lesion, also known as *gullwing arthrosis,*[146] is similar to the lesion just described and is confined to the transverse ridge, primarily in the forelimb. It has been proposed as being caused by trauma from the base of the proximal sesamoid bones during overextension and also by stress concentration along the ridge because of the abrupt change in subchondral bone density in the region.[136]

OSTEOCHONDRITIS DISSECANS OF THE SAGITTAL RIDGE OF MC3 OR MT3. This relatively common lesion usually involves the forelimb and may consist of a defect or fragmentation in the ridge or a loose body.[147] Surgical excision and debridement are indicated when fragmentation is present, and in cases where the lesion is localized the prognosis is good. Lesions with extensive cartilage damage carry a bad prognosis.

LATERAL CONDYLAR FRACTURE OF THE CANNON BONE. These fractures may occur in the medial or lateral condyles of MT3 or MC3; however, the common location is the lateral condyle in the racing thoroughbred.[148] There is some argument as to whether they are[149] or are not[136] associated with existing lesions. The lateral fractures range from incomplete to complete, with and without displacement. When the medial condyle is involved, the fracture is usually incomplete and extends proximally a considerable distance into the diaphysis. The diagnosis is made by radiology, but special care should be given to evaluation of the joint surface in order to detect malalignment or fragmentation.[148]

Incomplete fractures can be managed conservatively by confinement to a stall, although some surgeons prefer to operate on these cases to ensure that the fracture does not propagate further and become a complete or even displaced fracture. Nondisplaced complete fractures or incomplete fractures that have the potential to become complete should be treated with compression screw fixation. Incomplete fractures that extend a long way proximally without the tendency to break out from the cortex are particularly dangerous because even after surgery they have the potential to propagate into a major fracture. These fractures are best treated conservatively.

If displacement is present, the treatment is identical, except that the articular surface should be inspected using either an arthrotomy or arthroscopy. An external cast is recommended at least for the recovery from anesthesia, but care is advised for complicated fractures or those in which the fracture extends a long way proximally because of the danger of stress concentration caused by the cast. In these cases, a full leg cast or even a Kimsey splint can be used. After surgery, stall confinement is recommended for about 6 to 8 weeks with regular hand walking, to be followed by paddock rest until 6 months after the injury.

A radiographic evaluation of healing is recommended during convalescence. Some surgeons prefer to remove the screws before training commences, but experience has shown that this is not always necessary. Therefore, the options exist to remove the screws from all horses or only when they produce lameness, a decision that is at the discretion of the clinician.

The prognosis is better for incomplete fractures than for complete fractures; for complete fractures, the prognosis is better when the fragment is not displaced. In one series of thoroughbred horses treated surgically, 31.6 percent (12 of 38) with complete displaced fractures (0 of 6 treated conservatively), 66.6 percent (4 of 6) with complete nondisplaced fractures, and 81.8 percent (9 of 11) with incomplete fractures (9 of 10 treated conservatively) continued racing.[148]

DISEASE OF THE PROXIMAL SESAMOID BONES. The proximal sesamoid bones suffer fractures and sesamoiditis and also participate in chronic fetlock arthritis.

Fractures are common in racing thoroughbreds, standardbreds and quarter horses. They can be classified as apical, abaxial (articular or nonarticular), axial, midbody, basilar, and comminuted. They occur most commonly in the forelimbs of thoroughbreds and quarter horses and in the hindlimbs of standardbreds. Occasionally, both bones in the same leg or even both bones in

both legs fracture, thereby disrupting the suspensory apparatus and constituting a disaster for athletic horses and meaning the end of any athletic career. The etiology of fractures is not well understood, but it appears that while the majority are acute, there are some that are related to preexisting disease.[136] The details of the clinical signs, diagnosis, and treatment are readily available.

The proximal sesamoid bones are vital components in the suspensory apparatus, and for acute cases, the prognosis for proximal and distal fractures is related to the extent that the suspensory ligament and the distal sesamoidean ligaments, respectively, are disrupted. For midbody fractures, the problem of achieving osseous union without subsequent resorption is the limiting factor. When the fracture is chronic, the existence of DJD has a negative effect on prognosis. Abaxial and axial fractures have a good prognosis. Of the remainder, only apical fractures involving less than 25 percent (approximately) of the bone and that are treated before the onset of DJD have a favorable prognosis. In a series of 109 standardbreds with apical fractures, 60 percent of those treated within 30 days of injury returned to racing.[150] Negative factors for prognosis were suspensory desmitis and lack of a racing career before surgery. The return to an athletic career for all fracture types, despite a variety of repair techniques, is poor.

DJD of the High-Load, Low-Motion Joints (Distal Intertarsal, Tarsometatarsal, and Proximal Interphalangeal Joints). Most horses with DJD of these joints are adults, although young animals can be affected. The striking difference between DJD in these and the high-motion joints is the presence of focal regions of resorption and new bone production in the subchondral bone which merge with similar regions in the opposing articular surface to create ankylosis. Because these joints have only a limited range of movement, the mechanism(s) involved in the development of DJD may not be identical with that seen in high-motion joints. For example, the absence of excessive high-velocity motion might indicate that soft-tissue lubrication is less important, and the concentration of loads in smaller areas might indicate that compressive load and hydrostatic lubrication are relatively more important. The association between abnormalities of conformation and DJD could be taken as support for this idea.

PROXIMAL INTERPHALANGEAL JOINT. The lesion of the proximal interphalangeal joint is one of the components of the *articular ring bone complex,* the other being that of the distal interphalangeal joint, which is not classed as a disease of the athletic horse. This lesion is most common in horses that perform at a high speed while being asked to turn, twist, and stop quickly, such as polo ponies. Poor conformation may be a contributory factor. Very early cases may respond to conservative therapy, but any significant damage to the articular surface will result in a chronic, incurable lesion. With production of new bone there is often spontaneous joint fusion, which usually results in resolution of the pain. Surgical arthrodesis may be undertaken with the same objective, there being a number of surgical methods used to stabilize the joint while fusion occurs. The prognosis for an athletic career cannot be guaranteed, but under favorable circumstances, a return to soundness in around 75 percent can be expected, with better results for hindlimbs versus forelimbs.[151,152]

TARSITIS (SPAVIN). The lesion in the tarsometatarsal, distal intertarsal, and occasionally the proximal intertarsal joints is colloquially known as *bone spavin*. It occurs in all types of horses but, interestingly, is relatively rare in thoroughbred racehorses. The diagnosis is usually made with the assistance of radiology; however, the early disease is radiologically silent, and intraarticular anesthesia is necessary to confirm the diagnosis. The contribution of cunean bursitis is controversial, but intrabursal anesthesia will allow a positive diagnosis to be made.

Cunean bursitis is best treated by anti-inflammatory therapy, reduction in workload, and elimination of improper shoeing. Because it may be associated with joint disease, the prognosis is often poor, but in uncomplicated cases, good results are possible. Cunean tenotomy or tenectomy has been a popular form of therapy but is documented as being of little value.[153]

Spavin has been the subject of many surgical treatments, but the relatively unreliable response, as well as the long convalescence, dictates that conservative therapy be considered first. In acute cases, the emphasis should be on managing the arthritis, namely, anti-inflammatory therapy and corrective shoeing.[154] In young racehorses, this is the only feasible option, because they have such a short career. In these horses it is also common to inject corticosteroids and sodium hyaluronate. In horses with chronic disease and those which have a longer career, surgical treatment is a useful option. Although a number of surgical methods are available, the only practical procedures at present involve removal of sufficient articular cartilage to facilitate growth of bone across the joint space.[155] The most reliable method and that associated with the least postoperative pain has been described.[156,157] A nonsurgical method involving chemical destruction of the cartilage is also under investigation.[158] Joint fusion may require almost a year in some cases, but 6 months is average. In one series of selected cases treated by drilling the cartilage, 85 percent (17 of 20) of horses and ponies returned to activities ranging from light saddle work to hunting and jumping.[156] This return is very high and is not normally achieved in horses engaged in more athletic pursuits, where a figure on the order of approximately 50 percent may be more realistic.

Osteochondrosis

Osteochondrosis (OCD) is a clinical entity that is of great significance for athletic horses. Although the lesions associated with the syndrome can be asymptomatic, they are often associated with lameness and DJD and, as such, require treatment. The disease is a developmental one, and evidence of its presence is often apparent in young horses that have not begun an athletic career, where it may cause joint effusion without lameness. It is seen most frequently in younger animals when they are exposed to hard exercise and the preexisting

lesions are traumatized. The sites usually involved in athletic horses are the femoropatellar joint (lateral and medial trochlear ridges of the femur, patella), tarsocrural joint (distal intermediate ridge of the tibia, lateral and medial trochlear ridges of the talus, lateral and medial malleoli of tibia), and fetlock joint (sagittal ridge of distal end of MC3, MT3, and distal MC3).

Management. When lameness is present, the usual form of treatment is to remove free osteochondral fragments and any adjacent soft and degenerate tissue. The objective is to leave healthy bone to be covered later by fibrocartilage, which will, hopefully, support athletic activity. The joint is usually examined and the fragments and debris removed by arthroscopy or arthrotomy. The advantages of arthroscopy for treatment of OCD are identical to those for treatment of fractures: minimal trauma and ease of joint exploration. As stated earlier, many lesions do not result in lameness, and in these cases, surgery is not necessary, although joints with effusions will often become painful when training is instituted. If it is not feasible to carry out surgical treatment, the same conservative management as used for treating DJD is indicated, although this line of treatment is usually palliative and the joint will ultimately degenerate under the stress of continued athletic activity.

Prognosis. In the absence of preexisting DJD or extensive involvement of the joint surface, the prognosis is surprisingly good.

- *Femoropatellar joint.* In one report (161 horses, 261 joints), 86 of 134 horses (64 percent) for which follow-up records were available returned to intended use.[159] A further 7 percent were in training, 16 percent had residual problems related to the femoropatellar joint or the reason was unclear, and 13 percent were unsuccessful for other reasons. Forty-nine of 79 (62 percent) racehorses and 37 of 55 (67 percent) nonracehorses returned to racing or their intended use, respectively. The presence of patellar lesions or loose bodies had no effect on the outcome, although when lesions were graded according to increasing severity on a scale of 1 to 3, return to intended use was 78, 63 and 54 percent, respectively.
- *Tarsocrural joint.* The results of a case series involving 318 joints in 225 horses, of which 183 were available for evaluation, indicated that subsequent functional ability and cosmetic appearance were excellent, with age, sex, limb involvement (left versus right versus bilateral), or site of lesion having no bearing on outcome.[160] The size of the intermediate ridge lesions was not significant, but the presence of cartilage degeneration decreased prognosis. Resolution of the effusion occurred in 117 of 131 (89.3 percent) joints of racehorses and in 64 of 86 (74.4 percent) joints of nonracehorses. Of the 154 racehorses, 124 were available for follow-up, of which 90 (72.6 percent) returned to racing. Of 71 nonracehorses, 59 were available for follow-up, of

which 50 (84.7 percent) performed at their expected level.

- *Distal aspect of the distal sagittal ridge of the metacarpus and metatarsus.* The osseous lesions seen in this syndrome vary from focal regions of lysis in the distal aspect of the ridge to fragmentation.[161] Lytic lesions are usually managed conservatively, and when fragmentation is present, surgical debridement is necessary. Prognosis is guarded.

SOME PROBLEMS LOCATED IN THE HOOF REGION

Navicular Disease

Although navicular disease (ND) is a common cause of lameness, it is relatively uncommon in racehorses and is seen more frequently in older horses used for a variety of different activities. The cause and pathogenesis are poorly understood, and although the pathologic, radiographic, and scintigraphic characteristics are well described, there is little agreement on their etiologic significance. Further discussion on these aspects is not relevant here, but in order to consider management, some thought should be given to the cause of pain. The lesions found in the bone and surrounding soft tissues are presumably painful, as are similar lesions in other locations. Therefore, it is not unexpected that analgesics and corrective shoeing and hoof management are of some value, albeit usually only palliative. Pain due to elevation in intraosseous blood pressure is well described in humans and should be considered as a possible cause of at least part of the pain in this syndrome now that increased intraosseous blood pressure also has been identified in ND.[162,163] The beneficial effects of rheologic drugs may be associated in some way with the altered circulation. Certain aspects have made the management of ND extremely difficult:

- The diagnosis of ND has been a matter of controversy, and the requirements for a positive diagnosis have undergone a significant evolution so that what constitutes a positive diagnosis for one radiologist or clinician may be negative for another. This means that the results of different treatment regimens are difficult to compare unless blind trials have been conducted.
- A cure is unlikely once the characteristic pathologic process has begun and extensive tissue damage is present.
- The onset of ND is insidious, and the early signs are difficult and probably impossible to detect, with the result that by the time it is diagnosed, significant tissue changes will have occurred.

Management. At this time, the management of ND is based on incomplete knowledge, but in accordance with current understanding, it should be directed toward achieving the following objectives:

- Prevent the continued degeneration in the navicular bone and adjacent soft tissues and provide conditions that allow tissue repair to proceed. This is done by reducing the loads experienced by the deep flexor tendon, navicular bursa, and flexor surface of the navicular bone by corrective shoeing and hoof trimming. Traditionally, this has been achieved by elevating the heels and shortening the toe of the hoof.[164] A number of home made and commercially available leather and synthetic pads have been used to produce elevation. To counteract the hoof contraction that is frequently present, a full pad with silicone injected between the hoof and pad is often used. An alternative approach to reducing the load has been to provide support by means of the egg-bar shoe, a round, closed shoe that extends caudally from the heels.[165] The beneficial effects of the egg-bar shoe have been demonstrated histologically[166] and in a noncontrolled clinical trial.[165]
- Improve the microcirculation in the navicular bone. The observation that ND is associated with certain pathologic changes in the vasculature[167] stimulated efforts to reduce thrombosis and to produce vascularization. This was originally attempted with warfarin[168,169] and more recently with isoxuprine hydrochloride.[170,171] Although of some benefit, the difficulty in monitoring and maintaining normal blood coagulation made the use of warfarin potentially dangerous as well as tedious. Isoxuprine hydrochloride has been shown to be of benefit in randomized, double-blind studies.[170,171] Based on these data, a dosage of 0.6 mg/kg PO every 12 hours, given 30 minutes before feeding, is recommended. The duration of treatment is 12 weeks; however, retreatment is possible if there is recurrence. Higher dosages are regarded as being of no significant benefit.[171]

Prognosis. Navicular disease is usually progressive, and current treatments are probably palliative at best, although a sustained improvement is possible if a diagnosis is made early enough, appropriate measures are taken, and the workload is modified.

Lameness Associated with the Distal Interphalangeal Joint

There are a number of well-described lesions that produce pain in and around the distal interphalangeal joint (DIP), including articular ringbone, periostitis, and fracture of the extensor process of the distal phalanx and fracture of the distal phalanx (pedal bone). These lesions are easily diagnosed, and treatment is relatively simple using recognized methods. However, a syndrome that at least in part involves this joint and which is difficult to characterize is becoming increasingly recognized.[172,173] It is manifested as a lameness that is eliminated or improved by anesthesia of the DIP. Lameness also is frequently improved or alleviated by palmar digital nerve blocks, although a palmar (abaxial sesamoid) nerve block is often necessary to eliminate the lameness. The response to anesthesia of the DIP is usually rapid and in most cases eliminates the lameness or results in substantial improvement. The lameness rarely changes to the contralateral side after successful anesthesia.

In some cases, a cause for the lameness can be identified, such as the more obvious conditions mentioned above, or discrete osteophytosis can be identified with careful radiography.[174] Navicular disease is always a consideration with these cases because of the signs and responses to local anesthesia. However, the tendency for unilateral lameness, radiologically normal navicular bones, and rapid response to intraarticular anesthesia point to another cause. The present confusion regarding which sites are anesthetized with articular and palmar digital anesthesia, communication between the DIP and the navicular bursa, and the effect of diffusion of anesthetic out of the joint add to the difficulty. It can probably be assumed that there is at least a synovitis present, although the cause of this is not known. The most likely explanations are trauma-induced injury associated with exercise, poor hoof conformation, poor farriery, or combinations of these.

Management. Treatment, after elimination of other causes, is usually with sodium hyaluronate. If the severity of the lameness warrants it, NSAIDs can be used. Chronic cases unresponsive to initial therapy may respond to intraarticular corticosteroids. Care should be taken to ensure that shoeing and hoof conformation are adequate to maintain good hoof balance.

Prognosis. The prognosis for horses with radiographic evidence of osseous change is poor,[173] and for the others, recovery is better, ranging from approximately 30 percent[173] to favorable.[172] Repeated treatment may be necessary and many horses remain lame or suffer recurrences.

Pedal Osteitis

In athletic horses persistent concussion can lead to inflammation and demineralization of the distal phalanx (P3). The characteristic osseous signs are visible radiographically as a roughened solar border of P3 anywhere between the toe and the lateral wings.[173] Care should be taken not to confuse the normal crena with demineralization, as well as to remember that the osseous changes are often present in sound horses. Diagnosis must be made on evidence of pain over the soles or heels and lameness, with radiography being used to eliminate other possibilities and to indicate the severity of osseous change. Horses may be predisposed to the problem because of thin or low soles, poor shoeing, exercise on hard or stoney ground, or combinations of these. Treatment is directed toward removing predisposing causes and providing protection for the sole. Simply providing good shoeing will often be curative, but the use of synthetic or leather pads under the shoe is often necessary. Antiinflammatory therapy is indicated for a short time in severe cases. The prognosis for this condition is always guarded because poor conformation is so frequently the primary cause.

Hoof Lesions

There are some conditions of the hoof to which the athletic horse is particularly prone. These are bruising, wall cracks, and sheared heels and can be related to conformation, poor shoeing, exercise on hard or rough surfaces, or combinations of these. In an inactive horse such lesions are of no consequence or are relatively easily controlled, whereas in athletic horses a cure often is required under situations where a period of rest cannot be utilized. Therefore, treatment must be carried out in a horse that remains in training or competition. The objectives of such therapy are to protect existing sensitive tissues and to provide stability to the hoof so as to allow continuation of athletic activity. The methods for doing this involve various combinations of hoof trimming, corrective and protective shoeing, and use of rapidly polymerizing resins to fill hoof defects.[176,177] The use of specially constructed shoes designed to reduce concussion may have an application in cases with chronic problems not readily corrected by conventional means.[178]

PROBLEMS OF THE BACK

Gait and performance abnormalities associated with back problems pose a diagnostic and therapeutic dilemma, the details of which can be found elsewhere.[179,180] As far as can be ascertained, the clinical signs appear to be associated mainly with arthrosis of intervertebral articulations, inflammation of dorsal and lateral spinous processes where adjacent processes impinge on one another, and with unspecified soft-tissue injury. Of relevance to athletic horses are the categories comprising soft-tissue injury and lesions of the thoracolumbar vertebrae, in which the three most common diagnoses are nonspecific soft-tissue injury, overriding of the dorsal spinous processes, and sacroiliac strain.[179] It is important when investigating back problems to realize that back pain is often secondary to abnormal or excessive use of back structures when a horse is forced to exercise while it has pain elsewhere, especially in a hindlimb. Consequently, care is indicated in diagnosis. Furthermore, signs of back pain are frequently obscure and localization difficult, and the mere presence of radiographic lesions or heightened scintigraphic activity does not necessarily provide a diagnosis.

Management

The management of back problems is discussed against the background of the difficulties in defining the syndrome in the first place, identifying significant clinical signs, and making an accurate diagnosis. The choices consist of correction of problems related to tack or riding habits, rest, medical therapy, physiotherapy, manipulation, natural medicines, and surgery.

Conservative Therapy. Conservative therapy is often successful. In a series of 190 horses, full recoveries were made by 57 percent regardless of treatment, with recovery rates for specific conditions being 73 percent for soft-tissue injuries, 45 percent for sacroiliac joint strain, 57 percent for overriding dorsal spinous processes, and 9 percent for spondylosis[179] The problem for the clinician is the choice of management in the individual case. When there is no specific diagnosis, or when soft-tissue injury is diagnosed, a period of reduced activity or stall confinement may be all that is required. In such cases, time, during which healing can occur, is the important factor. However, since total inactivity is detrimental to the strength of ligament, tendon, muscle, and their insertions, it is advised that, where possible, a reduced exercise schedule be maintained. Judicious use of NSAIDs is necessary in many cases. The return to hard exercise should always be done gradually. The choice of physiotherapy is probably limited to massage, faradic stimulation, and swimming, with the former being of doubtful efficacy.

The management of overriding of the dorsal spinous process is more complicated. Surgery, consisting of resection of the summits of the processes, can be successful.[181-183] However, it is difficult to know which cases to treat in this way, since there is no question that many cases will heal with conservative therapy. Injection of corticosteroids between the spinous processes is often useful in suppressing signs, but retreatment is usually necessary. Experience with resection has shown that the period of convalescence is shorter and that recurrence is less common than with conservative therapy. In view of the relatively high recovery rate with conservative therapy, it is difficult to recommend surgery in all cases, but the option and its advantages should be discussed with the owner before a decision is made. Resection certainly is indicated in cases that have not responded to other methods of treatment.

Acupuncture appears to be of value for treating back pain. In a study of 200 horses with "back pain," four different methods of stimulating acupuncture points was investigated: needle, infrared laser, injection of saline, and a combination of saline and methylprednisolone injection.[184] Horses were treated weekly, an average of eight times. All methods produced some improvement, less for the saline-steroid combination. Acupuncture deserves further investigation in a controlled trial to assess its worth. At present, its use should be discussed with the owner before a decision on treatment is made. Although it can be classed as a noninvasive treatment, the necessity for multiple treatments can be tedious.

Management of sacroiliac strain is difficult because of the chronic instability and subsequent lack of hind quarter propulsion that remain after any significant injury.[185] Simply prescribing a period of rest yields very poor results in all but the mildest cases. The only form of treatment that appears to be useful is to provide support for the joints by increasing the bulk and strength of bask and hind quarter musculature, a logical therapy in view of the type of injury. Diagnosis is not always easy because this condition can exist in a subtle form with a detrimental effect on performance, as described for standardbred trotters and pacers.[186] Some pacers respond to a change in training, with less hobbled work and more galloping exercise.

In summary, rest or reduction in exercise, administration of NSAIDs, adjustment of tack and riding habits, when necessary, and development of back musculature are recommended as a useful and relatively reliable

treatment schedule for all back cases. Resection of dorsal spinous processes should be reserved for chronic cases, it being hard to recommend surgery for all animals when conservative therapy is known to be relatively successful.

STIFLE PROBLEMS

In athletic horses, functional abnormalities and subchondral bone cysts are two conditions that commonly affect the stifle joint.

Subchondral Bone Cysts

The majority of cysts occur in the medial condyle of the femur and less often in the lateral condyle and the tibia.[187,188] The condition is usually unilateral, although bilateral lesions are present in a small percentage of cases. Lameness usually is noticed when horses are first exposed to training, although extensive lesions may cause pain earlier than this.

Management. Conservative management is reported to result in complete or almost complete recovery in approximately 60 percent of those cases where the cyst is located in the medial femoral condyle and to have a poor prognosis for cysts in other locations.[187] Intraarticular medication is useful in controlling signs but has no effect on the cyst. At present, surgical management is popular and associated with a high success rate. In view of the significant number of animals that recover spontaneously, it is reasonable to reserve surgical treatment for horses in which significant improvement has not occurred after a 3-month period of conservative management. Surgery involves curettage of the cyst cavity, forage, and removal of degenerate bone and cartilage using arthrotomy[189] or arthroscopic[190] techniques. The use of cancellous bone grafts to pack the cyst cavity after debridement also has been described.[191,192] Postoperative management consists of stall confinement for 60 days and then paddock rest for 4 months, which is extended if the horse is still lame while trotting.

Prognosis. Results for complete recovery of 83.3 percent (35 of 42) and 50.7 percent (34 of 67) have been reported after arthrotomy[189] and arthroscopy, respectively.[190] Despite what appears to be a superior prognosis with arthrotomy, the ease of arthroscopy and the lack of complications with wound healing render it the preferred method. The results of using bone grafts do not indicate any advantage over simple curettage. More information is required to explain why some horses do not recover and to determine if they would respond to alternate therapy, perhaps grafting.

Patellar Fixation and Mechanical Abnormalities of the Stifle

Patellar Fixation. This condition is a common problem in many types of horses. It ranges in severity from an acute fixation with complete inability to flex the hindlimb to momentary interference with flexing followed by exaggerated flexing ("hiking"). Some horses negate the need for flexion by circumducting the leg, thus producing one of the characteristic gait abnormalities, that of a swinging-leg lameness. The mechanism of the problem is not known, and since patellar fixation is a normal process under neuromuscular control when utilized in normal circumstances, one must assume that when present as a clinical problem there is some abnormality of the control mechanisms. This is supported by its occurrence in poorly muscled horses, in those with upright limb conformation, and in trotters and pacers required to perform at high speeds.

Management. In poorly muscled horses, management first should be directed toward developing muscle mass by slowly increasing the intensity of training or in saddle horses by exercising on soft ground. In horses that do not respond to this treatment or in those in which such management is not appropriate, a medial patellar desmotomy is commonly carried out. Injection of irritant agents around the distal patellar ligaments is also frequently used in racehorses, the rationale being to "tighten" the ligaments.

Prognosis. There is often a dramatic response to improved muscle mass, but there is frequent recurrence if muscle mass is lost or if the condition is related to conformation. Methods involving injection of irritant agents also seem to result in rapid improvement, but these too are often associated with recurrence. Patellar desmotomy offers the best chance of a permanent cure in chronic or severe cases, but since it has been reported to be associated with fragmentation of the distal patella, it should not be carried out indiscriminately.[193,194]

Mechanical Abnormality of the Stifle. Trotters and pacers often appear to suffer from a syndrome that is characterized by laxity and easy manual displacement of the patella, a gait abnormality indicative of intermittent patellar fixation and an inability to run at speed, particularly around bends. To what extent this exists as a syndrome separate from that just described as patellar fixation is not known. The common occurrence is trotters and pacers probably indicates an association with the gaits of these horses. It seems likely that when adequate muscle mass and coordination are lacking, forced exercise may result in abnormal patellar function. The result is a compensatory gait and development of pain at sites stressed, such as muscle and ligamentous attachments to the patella and gluteal and lumbar musculature. It is likely that the compensatory gait, initially utilized to avoid patellar fixation and use of the stifle, fails to stimulate the muscle hypertrophy necessary for good limb function, with the result that the problem becomes worse and training cannot advance.

In all cases it is desirable to develop muscle mass in order to improve joint function. This is usually done by reducing the high-speed workload in order to allow time for muscles to develop. Medial patellar desmotomy occasionally is carried out as a last resort, but the method is not without complications and does not always restore normal gait in these horses. The injection of irritant materials around the origins and insertions of the distal patellar ligaments and the insertion of the quadriceps muscles onto the proximal patella is a common form of therapy with recognized benefit. In addition, injection can be made more proximally into lumbar acupuncture sites. How such therapy provides benefit is not known.

Conclusions

The main objective in writing this chapter was to focus on the etiology, pathogenesis, and prognosis of the major conditions affecting athletic horses. I have avoided many of the specific aspects of diagnosis and treatment, which are well covered in other texts. The selection of conditions to be included posed the initial difficulty, and although there is no doubt as to the major problems affecting athletic horses, there will probably be readers who would have preferred a different emphasis as well as the inclusion of other topics. Although there is a considerable volume of data related to other species, especially the human athlete, the applicability of such information to horses is in many cases unknown or at least unclear. Consequently, there are much data that have not been included because their relevance to horses have not been shown or proven.

A major concern when attempting to evaluate treatments and provide data on prognosis is the lack of controlled trials. Most data are based on retrospective evaluation, which, although very useful and better than nothing, simply provides the success rate for the treatment currently in favor, and lacks the scientific rigor of a prospective trial, blind or otherwise, comparing different treatments. Appropriate evaluation is difficult to carry out because of the way in which the veterinary profession functions and interacts with clients who request the very latest in therapy. An example of this is superficial digital flexor tendonitis, which, in recent years, has been treated in many different ways, with each new technique initially being accompanied by favorable reports only to fade later from the scene.

To encourage a logical and scientific approach to therapy and evaluation, an effort has been made to focus attention on the basic manner in which lesions are produced and to provide the most reliable data based, whenever possible, on reasonable case numbers. I hope that by doing this, a more scientific approach to athletic injuries will be encouraged and that blind acceptance of the latest fads will be reduced.

References

1. Stashak TS: Methods of therapy. *In* Stashak TS (ed): Adam's Lameness in Horses. Philadelphia, Lea & Febiger, 1987, p 840.
2. Ivers T: Cryotherapy. Equine Pract 1987; 9:17.
3. Turner TA, Wolfsdorf K, Jourdenais J: Effects of heat, cold, biomagnets and ultrasound on skin circulation in the horse. *In* Proceedings of the Annual Convention of the American Association of Equine Practitioners, 1991, p 249.
4. Porter M: Equine sports therapy. Equine Vet Sci 1992; 12:193.
5. Downer AH: Conductive heat therapy. Mod Vet Pract 1979; 60:525.

6. Dyson M: Nonthermal cellular effects of ultrasound. Br J Cancer 1982; 45(suppl 5):165.
7. Downer AH: Ultrasound therapy for animals. Mod Vet Pract 1976; 57:523.
8. Lang DC: Ultrasonic treatment of musculoskeletal conditions in the horse, dog and cat. Vet Rec 1980; 106:427.
9. Stevenson JH, Pang CV, Undsay WK, et al: Functional, mechanical, and biochemical assessment of ultrasound therapy on tendon healing in the chicken toe. Plast Reconstr Surg 1986; 77:965.
10. Binder A: Is therapeutic ultrasound effective in treating soft tissue lesions? Br Med J 1985; 290:512.
11. Turner SM, Powell GS: The effect of ultrasound on the healing of repaired tendon. J Hand Surg 1989; 14B:428.
12. Williams IF, Heaton, A, McCullagh KG: Cell morphology and collagen types in equine tendon scar. Res Vet Sci 1980; 28:302.
13. McCullagh KG, Goodship AE, Silver IA: Tendon injuries and their treatment in the horse. Vet Rec 1979; 105:54.
14. Webbon PM: A postmortem study of equine digital flexor tendons. Equine Vet J 1977; 9:61.
15. Strömberg B: The normal and diseased superficial flexor tendon in racehorses: A morphological and physiological investigation. Acta Radiol 1971; (suppl 305):1–94.
16. McCullagh KG: Tendon injury in the horse. Vet Ann 1981; 21:144.
17. Webbon PM: Equine tendon stress injuries. Equine Vet J 1973; 5:58.
18. Riemersma DJ, Schamhardt HC: In vitro mechanical properties of equine tendons in relation to cross-sectional area and collagen content. Res Vet Sci 1985; 39:263.
19. Riemersma DJ, De Bruyn P: Variation in cross-sectional area and composition of equine tendons with regard to their mechanical function. Res Vet Sci 1986; 41:7.
20. Nilsson G, Björck G: Surgical treatment of chronic tendinitis in the horse. J Am Vet Med Assoc 1969; 155:920.
21. Genovese RL, Rantanen NW, Simpson BS: The use of ultrasonography in the diagnosis and management of injuries to the equine limb. Comp Cont Ed Pract Vet 1987; 9:945.
22. Reef VB, Martin BB, Stebbins K: Comparison of ultrasonic, gross, and histologic appearance of tendon injuries in performance horses. In Proceedings of the Annual Conference of the American Association of Equine Practitioners, 1989, p 279.
23. Genovese RL, Rantanen NW, Hauser ML, Simpson BS: Diagnostic ultrasonography of equine limbs. Vet Clin North Am Equine Pract 1986; 2:145.
24. Genovese RL, Rantanen NW, Simpson BS, et al: Clinical experience with quantitative analysis of superficial digital flexor tendon injuries in thoroughbred and standardbred horses. Vet Clin North Am Equine Pract 1990; 6:129.
25. Reef VB, Martin BB, Elser A: Types of tendon and ligament injuries detected with diagnostic ultrasound: Description and follow-up. In Proceedings of the Annual Convention of the American Association of Equine Practitioners, 1988, p 245.
26. Balasubramaniam P: Mechanism of collagen breakdown by local infiltration of steroids. In Hirohata K, Mizuno K, Matsubara T (eds): Trends in Research and Treatment of Joint Diseases. Tokyo, Springer-Verlag, 1992, p 51.
27. Garmer L: Osseous metaplasia: A complication of local corticosteroid therapy in the horse. Nord Vet Med 1965; 17:516.
28. Alexander SA, Donoff RB: The glycosaminoglycans of open wounds. J Surg Res 1980; 29:422.
29. Amiel D et al: Hyaluronate in flexor tendon repair. J Hand Surg 1989; 14A:837.
30. Spurlock GH, Spurlock SL, Parker GA: Evaluation of Hylartin V therapy for induced tendinitis in the horse. Equine Vet Sci 1989; 9:242.
31. Foland JW, Trotter GW, Powers BE, et al: Effect of sodium hyaluronate in collagenase-induced superficial digital flexor tendinitis in horses. Am J Vet Res 1992; 53:2371.
32. St. Onge R, Weiss C, Denlinger JL, et al: A preliminary assessment of the Na-hyaluronate injection into "no man's land" for primary flexor tendon repair. Clin Orthop 1980; 146:269.
33. Thomas SC, Jones LC, Hungerford DS: Hyaluronic acid and its effect on postoperative adhesions in the rabbit flexor tendon. Clin Orthop 1986; 206:281.
34. Smith RKW: A case of superficial digital tendinitis: Ultrasonographic examination and treatment with intralesional polysulphated glycosaminoglycans. Equine Vet Ed 1992; 4:280.
35. Keg PR: Experimentelle Untersuchung zur Beurteilung der Wirksamkeit von Ultraschall bei der Tendinitis des Pferdes. Pferdeheilkunde 1989; 5:285.
36. Morcos MB, Aswad A: Histological studies of the effects of ultrasonic therapy on surgically split flexor tendons. Equine Vet J 1978; 10:267.
37. Lang DC: Ultrasonic treatment of musculoskeletal conditions in the horse, dog, and cat. Vet Rec 1980; 106:427.
38. Henninger RW, Bramlage LR, Bailey M, et al: Effects of tendon splitting on experimentally induced acute equine tendinitis. Vet Comp Orthop Ther 1992; 5:1.
39. Knudsen O: Percutaneous tendon splitting: Method and results. Equine Vet J 1976; 8:101.
40. Webbon PM: The racing performance of horses with tendon lesions treated by percutaneous tendon splitting. Equine Vet J 1979; 11:246.
41. Bramlage LR: Superior check desmotomy as a treatment for superficial digital flexor tendinitis: Initial report. In Proceedings of the Annual Convention of the American Association of Equine Practitioners, 1986, p 365.
42. Bramlage LR, Rantanen NW, Genovese RL, et al: Long-term effects of surgical treatment of superficial digital flexor tendinitis by superior check desmotomy. In Proceedings of the Annual Convention of the American Association of Equine Practitioners, 1988, p 655.
43. Henninger R, Bramlage L, Schneider R: Short-term effects of superior check ligament desmotomy and percutaneous tendon spliting as a treatment for acute tendinitis. In Proceedings of the Annual Convention of the American Association of Equine Practitioners, 1990, p 539.
44. Nilsson GN, Björck G: Surgical treatment of chronic tendinitis in the horse. J Am Vet Med Assoc 1969; 155:920.
45. Wilson DA, Baker GJ, Pijanowski GJ, et al: Composition and morphologic features of the interosseous muscle in standardbreds and thoroughbreds. Amer J Vet Res 1991; 52:133.
46. Gerring EL, Webbon PM: Fetlock annular ligament desmotomy: A report of 24 cases. Equine Vet J 1984; 16:113.
47. Verschooten F, Picavet T-M: Desmitis of the fetlock annular ligament in the horse. Equine Vet J 1986; 18:138.
48. Dik KJ, Van Den Belt AJM, Ket PR: Ultrasonographic evaluation of fetlock annular ligament constriction in the horse. Equine Vet J 1991; 23:285.
49. Adams OR: Lameness in Horses. Philadelphia, Lea & Febiger, 1974, p 356.
50. Rothwell AG: Quadriceps hematoma: A prospective clinical study. Clin Orthop 1982; 171:97.
51. Järvinen M: Healing of a crush injury in a rat striated muscle. Acta Pathol Microbiol Scand 1976; 142:47.
52. Garrett W, Tidball J: Myotendinous junction structure, function, and failure. In Wo SL-Y, Buckwalter JA (eds): Injury and Repair of the Musculoskeletal Soft Tissues. Park Ridge, Ill., American Academy of Orthopedic Surgeons, 1988, p 171.
53. Armstrong RB, Ogilvie RW, Schwane JA: Exercise-induced injury to rat skeletal muscle. J Appl Physiol 1983; 54:80.
54. Schwane JA, Johnson SR, Vandenakker CB, et al: Delayed-onset muscular soreness and plasma CPK and LDH activities after downhill running. Med Sci Sports Exerc 1983; 15:51.
55. Abraham WM: Factors in delayed muscle soreness. Med Sci Sports Exerc 1977; 9:11.
56. Bishop R: Fibrotic myopathy of the gracilis muscle of a horse. Vet Med Small Anim Clin 1972; 67:270.
57. Dyson S: Calcanean tendinitis. Equine Vet J 1992; 4:277.
58. Clayton HM: Cinematographic analysis of the gait of lame horses: V. Fibrotic myopathy. J Equine Vet Sci 1988; 8:297.
59. Turner AS, Trotter GW: Fibrotic myopathy in the horse. J Am Vet Med Assoc 1984; 184:335.
60. Stashak TS: Lameness. In Stashak TS (ed): Adam's Lameness in Horses. Philadelphia, Lea & Febiger, 1987, p 730.
61. Irwin DHG, Howell DW: Fibrotic myopathy, haematomas, and scar tissue in the gaskin area of the thoroughbred. J S Afr Vet Assoc 1981; 52:65.
62. Bramlage LR, Reed SM, Embertson RM: Semitendinosis tenotomy

for treatment of fibrotic myopathy in the horse. J Am Vet Med Assoc 1985; 186:565.

63. Frost HM: The pathomechanics of osteoporosis. Clin Orthop 1985; 200:198.

64. Carter DR: The relationship between in vivo strain and cortical bone remodelling. CRC Crit Rev Biomech Eng 1981; 8:1.

65. Carter DR: Mechanical loading histories and cortical bone remodelling. Calcif Tissue Int Suppl 1984; 36:19.

66. Carter DR, Caler WE: Uniaxial fatigue of human cortical bone: The influence of tissue physical characteristics. J Biomech 1981; 14:461.

67. Copeland RW: Incidence, location and principles of treatment of stress fractures of the third metacarpal bone. In Proceedings of the Annual Convention of the American Association of Equine Practitioners, 1979, p 159.

68. Mackey VS, Trout DR, Meagher DM, et al: Stress fractures of the humerus, radius, and tibia in horses. Vet Radiol 1987; 28:26.

69. Frost HM: The pathomechanics of osteoporosis. Clin Orthop 1985; 200:198.

70. McCarthy RN, Jeffcott LB: Effects of treadmill exercise on cortical bone in the third metacarpus of young horses. Res Vet Sci 1992; 52:28.

71. Pratt GW: An in vivo model of ultrasonically evaluating bone strength. In Proceedings of the Annual Convention of the American Association of Equine Practitioners, 1980, p 295.

72. Nunamaker DM, Butterweck DM, Provost MT: Fatigue fractures in thoroughbred racehorses. Relationship with age, peak bone strain, and training. J Orthop Res 1990; 8:604.

73. Nunamaker DM, Butterweck DM, Provost MT: Some geometric properties of the third metacarpal bone: A comparison between the standardbred and the thoroughbred racehorse. J Biomech 1989; 22:129.

74. Nunamaker DM, Butterweck DM, Black J: In vitro comparison of thoroughbred and standardbred racehorses with regard to local fatigue failure of the third metacarpal bone. Am J Vet Res 1991; 52:97.

75. Ascenzi A, Bonucci E: The ultimate tensile strength of single osteons. Acta Anat 1964; 58:160.

76. Ascenzi A, Bonucci E: The tensile properties of single osteons. Anat Rec 1967; 158:375.

77. Ascenzi A, Bonucci E: The compressive properties of single osteons. Anat Rec 1968; 161:377.

78. Ascenzi A, Bonucci E: The shearing properties of single osteons. Anat Rec 1972; 172:499.

79. Curry JD: Differences in the tensile strengths of bone of different histological types. J Anat 1959; 98:87.

80. Carter DR, Spengler DM: Mechanical properties and composition of cortical bone. Clin Orthop 1978; 135:192.

81. Martin RB, Burr DB: Structure, Function and Adaptation of Compact Bone. New York, Raven Press, 1989.

82. Reilly DT, Burnstein AH: The mechanical properties of cortical bone. J Bone Joint Surg 1974; 56A:1001.

83. Reilly DT, Burnstein AH: The elastic and ultimate properties of compact bone tissue. J Biomech 1975; 8:393.

84. Walmsley R, Smith JW: Variation in bone structure and the value of Young's modulus (abstract). J Anat (Lond) 1957; 91:603.

85. Norwood GL: The bucked-skin complex in thoroughbreds. In Proceedings of the Annual Conference of the American Association of Equine Practitioners, 1978, p 319.

86. Lloyd KCK, Koblik P, Ragle C, et al: Incomplete palmar fracture of the proximal extremity of the third metacarpal bone in horses: Ten cases (1981–1986). J Am Vet Med Assoc 1988; 192:798.

87. Ross MW, Ford TS, Orsini PG: Incomplete longitudinal fracture of the proximal palmar cortex of the third metacarpal bone in horses. Vet Surg 1988; 17:82.

88. Pleasant RS, Baker GJ, Muhlbauer MC, et al: Stress reactions and stress fractures of the proximal palmar aspect of the third metacarpal bone in horses: 58 cases (1980–1990). J Am Vet Med Assoc 1992; 201:1918.

89. Wright IM, Platt D, Houlton JEF, et al: Management of intracortical fractures of the palmaroproximal third metacarpal bone in a horse by surgical forage. Equine Vet J 1990; 22:142.

90. Haynes PF, Walters JW, McClure JR, et al: Incomplete tibial fractures in three horses. J Am Vet Med Assoc 1980;177:1143.

91. Hasegawa M, Kaneko M, Oikawa M, et al: Pathological studies on distal third tibial fractures of the plantar side in racehorses. Bull Equine Res Inst 1988; 25:6.

92. Johnson PJ, Allhands RV, Baker GJ, et al: Incomplete linear tibial fractures in two horses. J Am Vet Med Assoc 1988; 192:522.

93. Pilsworth RC, Webbon PM: The use of radionuclide bone scanning in the diagnosis of tibial "stress" fractures in the horse: A review of five cases. Equine Vet J 1988; (suppl 6):60.

94. Stover SM, Johnson BJ, Daft BM, et al: An association between complete and incomplete stress fractures of the humerus in racehorses. Equine Vet J 1992; 24:260.

95. Jaffe HL: Metabolic, Degenerative and Inflammatory Diseases of Bones and Joints. Philadelphia, Lea & Febiger, 1972.

96. Tyler JA: Cartilage degradation. In Hall B, Newman S (eds): Cartilage: Molecular Aspects. Boca Raton, Fla, CRC Press, 1991, p 213.

97. McIlwraith CW, Vachon A: Review of pathogenesis and treatment of degenerative joint disease. Equine Vet J 1988; (suppl 6):3.

98. Videman T, Eronen I, Candolin T: ^{3}H-proline incorporation and hydroxyproline concentration in articular cartilage during the development of osteoarthritis caused by immobilization: A study in vivo in rabbits. Biochem J 1981; 200:435.

99. Caterson B, Lowther DA: Changes in the metabolism of the proteoglycans from sheep articular cartilage in response to mechanical stress. Biochem Biophys Acta 1978; 540:412.

100. Radin EL, Paul IL: A consolidated concept of joint lubrication. J Bone Joint Surg 1972; 54A:607.

101. Sato H, Takahashi T, Ide H, et al: Antioxidant activity of synovial fluid, hyaluronic acid, and two components of hyaluronic acid. Arthritis Rheum 1988; 31:63.

102. Aviad AD, Arthur RM, Brencick VA, et al: Synacid vs Hylartin V in equine joint disease. J Equine Vet Sci 1988; 8:112.

103. Phillips MW: Clinical trial comparison of intraarticular sodium hyaluronate products in the horse. J Equine Vet Sci 1989; 9:39.

104. McIlwraith CW: Traumatic arthritis and its treatment in the athletic horse. The Equine Athlete 1989; 2:1.

105. Yovich JV, Trotter GW, McIlwraith CW: Pharmacologic properties of polysulfated glycosaminoglycan (Adequan) and its application to treatment of equine degenerative joint disease. In Proceedings of the Annual Convention of the American Association of Equine Practitioners, 1987, p 707.

106. Hamm D, Goldman L, Jones EW: Polysulfated glycosaminoglycan: A new intraarticular treatment for equine lameness. Vet Med Small Anim Clin 1984; 79:811.

107. Yovich JV, Trotter GW, McIlwraith CW, et al: Effects of polysulfated glycosaminoglycan on chemical and physical defects in equine articular cartilage. Am J Vet Res 1987; 48:1407.

108. Trotter GW, Yovich JV, McIlwraith CW, et al: Effects of intramuscular polysulfated glycosaminoglycan on chemical and physical defects in equine articular cartilage. Can J Vet Res 1989; 53:224.

109. Hamm D, Jones EW: Intraarticular (IA) and intramuscular (IM) treatment of noninfectious equine arthritis (DJD) with polysulfated glycosaminoglycans (PSGAG). Equine Vet Sci 1988; 8:456.

110. Gustafson SB, McIlwraith CW: Intraarticular infection following intraarticular injection of medication: Diagnosis, possible etiologic factors and prevention. In Proceedings of the Annual Convention of the American Association of Equine Practitioners, 1988, p 283.

111. Pelletier J-P, Martel-Pelletier J: In vitro effects of tiaprofenic acid, sodium salicylate and hydrocortisone on human osteoarthritic cartilage degradation and synovial collagenase synthesis. Drugs 1988; (suppl 35):42.

112. Pelletier J-P, Martel-Pelletier J: Effects of steroids on neutral metalloproteinase activity in human rheumatoid and osteoarthritic cartilage. Adv Inflamm Res 1988; 12:81.

113. Behrens F, Shepard N, Mitchell N: Alteration of rabbit articular cartilage by intraarticular injections of glucocorticoids. J Bone Joint Surg 1975; 57A:70.

114. Glade MJ, Krook L, Schryver HF: Morphologic and biochemical changes in cartilage and foals treated with dexamethasone. Cornell Vet 1983; 73:170.

115. Silderberg M, Silderberg R, Hasler M: Fine structure of articular

cartilage in mice receiving cortisone acetate. Arch Pathol Lab Med 1986; 82:569.

116. Chunekamrai S, Krook LP, Lust G, et al: Changes in articular cartilage after intraarticular injections of methylprednisolone acetate in horses. Am J Vet Res 1989; 50:1733.

117. McKay A, Milne FJ: Observations on the intraarticular use of corticosteroids in the racing thoroughbred. J Am Vet Am Assoc 1976;168:1039.

118. Owen R: Intraarticular corticosteroid therapy in the horse. J Am Vet Med Assoc 1980; 177:710.

119. Swanstrom OG, Dawson HA: Intraarticular betamethasone and depomedrol: A comparative study. *In* Proceedings of the Annual Convention of the American Association of Equine Practitioners, 1974, p 249.

120. Fox RB, Fox WK: DMSO prevents hydroxyl radical mediated depolymerisation of hyaluronic acid. Ann NY Acad Sci 1983; 411:14.

121. Welch RD, Watkins JP, De Bowes RM, et al: Effects of intraarticular administration of dimethylsulfoxide on chemically induced synovitis in immature horses. Am J Vet Res 1991; 52:934.

122. Palmer S: Prevalence of carpal fractures in thoroughbred and standardbred racehorses. J Am Vet Med Assoc 1986; 188:1171.

123. McIlwraith CW: Tearing of the medial palmar intercarpal ligament in the equine midcarpal joint. Equine Vet J 1992; 24:367.

124. Kannegieter NJ: Intracarpal ligament damage as a cause of lameness in the horse. *In* Proceedings of the 12th Bain-Fallon Lectures of the Australian Equine Veterinary Association, 1990, p 175.

125. Kannegieter NJ, Burbridge HM: Correlation between radiographic and arthroscopic findings in the equine carpus. Aust Vet J 1990; 67:132.

126. Selway SJ: Intercarpal ligament impingement: A primary cause of joint pathology in the intercarpal joint. *In* Proceedings of the Annual Convention of the American Association of Equine Practitioners, 1991, p 779.

127. Park DR, Morgan JP, O'Brien T: Chip fractures in the carpus of the horse: A radiographic study of their incidence and location. J Am Vet Med Assoc 1970; 157:1305.

128. McIlwraith CW, Yovich JV, Martin GS: Arthroscopic surgery for the treatment of osteochondral chip fractures of the equine carpus. J Am Vet Med Assoc 1987; 191:531.

129. Bramlage LR, Schneider RK, Gabel AA: A clinical perspective on lameness originating in the carpus. *In* Proceedings of the Annual Conference of the American Association of Equine Practitioners, 1991, p 771.

130. Colahan P, Turner TA, Poulos P, et al: Mechanical functions and sources of injury in the fetlock and carpus. *In* Proceedings of the Annual Conference of the American Association of Equine Practitioners, 1987, p 689.

131. French DA, Barber SM, Leach DH, Doige CE: The effect of the healing of articular cartilage defects in the equine carpus. Vet Surg 1989; 18:312.

132. O'Brien TR: Radiographic diagnosis of the "hidden" lesions of the third carpal bone. *In* Proceedings of the Annual Conference of the American Association of Equine Practitioners, 1977, p 343.

133. O'Brien TR, DeHaan CE, Arthur RM: Third carpal bone lesions of the racing thoroughbred. *In* Proceedings of the Annual Conference of the American Association of Equine Practitioners, 1985, p 515.

134. DeHaan CE, O'Brien TR, Koblik PD: A radiographic investigation of third carpal bone injury in 42 racing thoroughbreds. Vet Radiol 1987; 28:88.

135. Young DR, Richardson DW, Markel MD, et al: Mechanical and morphometric analysis of the third carpal bone of thoroughbreds. Am J Vet Res 1991; 52:402.

136. Pool RR, Meagher DM: Pathologic findings and pathogenesis of racetrack injuries. Vet Clin North Am Equine Pract 1990; 6:1.

137. Schneider RK, Bramlage LR, Gabel AA, et al: Incidence, location and classification of 371 third carpal bone fractures in 313 horses. *In* Proceedings of the Annual Conference of the American Association of Equine Practitioners, 1988, p 662.

138. Ross MW, Richardson DW, Beroza GA: Subchondral lucency of the third carpal bone in standardbred racehorses: 13 cases (1982–1988). J Am Vet Med Assoc 1989; 195:789.

139. Stephens PR, Richardson DW, Spencer PA: Slab fractures of the third carpal bone in standardbreds and thoroughbreds: 155 cases (1977–1984). J Am Vet Med Assoc 1988; 193:353.

140. Martin GS, Haynes PF, McClure JR: Effect of third carpal slab fracture and repair on racing performance in thoroughbred horses: 31 cases (1977–1984). J Am Vet Med Assoc 1988; 193:107.

141. Nickels FA, Grant BD, Lincoln SD: Villonodular synovitis of the equine metacarpophalangeal joint. J Am Vet Med Assoc 1976; 168:1043.

142. White NA, Sullins KE, Spurlock SL, et al: Diagnosis and treatment of metacarpophalangeal synovial pad proliferation in the horse. Vet Surg 1988; 17:46.

143. Speirs VC: Assessment of the economic value of orthopedic surgery in thoroughbred racehorses. Vet Clin North Am Large Anim Pract 1983; 5:391.

144. Yovich JV, McIlwraith CW: Arthroscopic surgery for osteochondral fractures of the proximal phalanx of the metacarpophalangeal and metatarsophalangeal (fetlock) joints in horses. J Am Vet Med Assoc 1986; 188:273.

145. Raker CW: Calcification of the equine metacarpophalangeal joint following removal of chip fractures. Arch Am Coll Vet Surg 1985; 4:66.

146. Rooney JR: Biomechanics of Lameness in Horses. Baltimore, Williams & Wilkins, 1969.

147. Yovich JV, McIlwraith CW, Stashak TS: Osteochrondritis dissecans of the saggital ridge of the third metacarpal and metatarsal bones in horses. J Am Vet Med Assoc 1985; 186:1186.

148. Rick MC, O'Brien TR, Pool RR, et al: Condylar fractures of the third metacarpal and third metatarsal bone in 75 horses: Radiographic features, treatments, and outcome. J Am Vet Med Assoc 1983; 183:287.

149. Krook L, Maylin G: Fractures in thoroughbred racehorses. Cornell Vet 1988; (suppl 78):36.

150. Spurlock GH, Gabel AA: Apical fractures of the proximal sesamoid bones in 109 standardbred horses. J Am Vet Med Assoc 1983; 183:76.

151. Martin GS, McIlwraith CW, Turner AS, et al: Long-term results and complications of proximal interphalangeal arthrodesis in horses. J Am Vet Med Assoc 1984; 184:1136.

152. Schneider JE, Carnine BL, Guffy MM: Arthrodesis of the proximal metacarpophalangeal joint in the horse: A surgical treatment for high ringbone. J Am Vet Med Assoc 1978; 173:1364.

153. Gabel AA: Treatment and prognosis for cunean tendon bursitis-tarsitis of standardbred horses. J Am Vet Med Assoc 1979; 175:1085.

154. Moyer W, Brokken TD, Raker CW: Bone spavin in thoroughbred racehorses. *In* Proceedings of the Annual Convention of the American Association of Equine Practitioners, 1983, p 81.

155. Adams OR: Surgical arthrodesis for treatment of bone spavin. J Am Vet Med Assoc 1970; 157:1480.

156. Edwards GB: Surgical arthrodesis for the treatment of bone spavin in 20 horses. Equine Vet J 1982; 14:117.

157. Sonnichsen HV, Svalastoga E: Surgical treatment of bone spavin in the horse. Equine Pract 1985; 7:6.

158. Bohanon TC, Schneider RK, Wesbrode SE: Fusion of the distal intertarsal and tarsometatarsal joints in the horse using intraarticular sodium monoiodoacetate. Equine Vet J 1991; 23:289.

159. McIlwraith CW, Foland JW, Trotter GW: Arthroscopic surgery for the treatment of equine femoropatellar osteochondritis dissecans. *In* Proceedings of the Annual Convention of the American Association of Equine Practitioners, 1991, p 767.

160. McIlwraith CW, Foerner JJ, Davis DM: Osteochondritis dissecans of the equine tarsocrural joint: Results of treatment with arthroscopic surgery. Equine Vet J 1991; 23:155.

161. Foerner JJ, Phillips TN, MacHarg MA: Osteochondritis of the distal saggital ridge of the metacarpus and metatarsus. *In* Proceedings of the Annual Conference of the American Association of Equine Practitioners, 1990, p 533.

162. Svalastoga E, Smith M: Navicular disease in the horse: The subchondral bone pressure. Nord Vet Med 1983; 35:31.

163. Pleasant RS, Baker GJ, Foreman JH, et al: Intraosseous pressure and pathologic changes in horses with navicular disease. Am J Vet Res 1993; 54:7.

164. Turner TA: Shoeing principles for the management of navicular disease in horses. J Am Vet Med Assoc 1986; 189:298.

165. Ostblom LC, Lund C, Melsen F: Navicular bone disease: Results of treatment using egg-bar shoeing technique. Equine Vet J 1984; 16:203.
166. Ostblom L, Lund C, Melsen F: Histological study of navicular bone disease. Equine Vet J 1982; 14:199.
167. Colles CM, Hickman J: The arterial supply of the navicular bone and its variation in navicular disease. Equine Vet J 1977; 9:150.
168. Colles CM: A preliminary report on the use of warfarin in the treatment of navicular disease. Equine Vet J 1979; 11:187.
169. Colles CM: Navicular disease and its treatment. In Practice 1982; 4:29.
170. Rose RJ, Allen JR, Hodgson DR, et al: Studies on isoxuprine hydrochloride for the treatment of navicular disease. Equine Vet J 1983; 15:238.
171. Turner AS, Tucker CM: The evaluation of isoxuprine hydrochloride for the treatment of navicular disease: A double blind trial. Equine Vet J 1989; 21:338.
172. Cochran SL: The treatment of distal interphalangeal joint synovitis in sport horses. In Proceedings of the Annual Conference of the American Association of Equine Practitioners, 1990, p 281.
173. Dyson SJ: Lameness due to pain associated with the distal interphalangeal joint: 45 cases. Equine Vet J 1991; 23:128.
174. Hertsch B, Beerheus U: Der Wendeschmerz als Symptom bei der Lahmheitsuntersuchung des Pferdes—pathomorphologische, roentgenologisch und klinische Untersuchungen. Pferdeheilkunde 1988; 4:15.
175. Rendano VT, Grant B: The equine third phalanx: Its radiographic appearance. Am J Vet Radiol Soc 1978; 19:125.
176. Stashak TS: Lameness. In Stashak TS (ed): Adam's Lameness in Horses. Philadelphia, Lea & Febiger, 1987, p 486.
177. Moyer W, Sigafoos R: Preliminary experiences and uses of composite hoof wall repair. In Proceedings of the Annual Conference of the American Association of Equine Practitioners, 1991, p 681.
178. Grant BD, Balch O, Ratzlaff M, et al: The application and use of compressible plastic horseshoes—Seattle shoes. Equine Pract 1989; 11:18.
179. Jeffcott LB: Back problems in the horse: A look at past, present and future progress. Equine Vet J 1979; 11:129.
180. Jeffcott LB: Diagnosis of back problems in the horse. Comp Cont Ed Pract Vet 1981; 3:S134.
181. Jeffcott LB, Hickman J: The treatment of horses with chronic back pain by resecting the summits of the impinging dorsal spinous processes. Equine Vet J 1975; 7:115.
182. Pettersson H, Strömberg B, Myrin I: Das thorakolumbale interspinale syndrom (TLI) des reitpferdes—retrospektiver vergleich konservativ und chirurgisch behandelter fälle. Pferdeheilkunde 1987; 3:313.
183. Steckel RR, Kraus-Hansen AE, Fackelman GE, et al: Scintigraphic diagnosis of thoracolumbar spinal disease in horses: A review of 50 cases. In Proceedings of the Annual Conference of the American Association of Equine Practitioners, 1991, p 583.
184. Martin BB, Klide AM: Acupuncture for the treatment of chronic back pain in 200 horses. In Proceedings of the Annual Conference of the American Association of Equine Practitioners, 1991, p 593.
185. Jeffcott LB, Dalin G, Ekman S, et al: Sacroiliac lesions as a cause of chronic poor performance in competitive horses. Equine Vet J 1985; 17:111.
186. Dalin G, Magnusson L-E, Thafvelin BC: Retrospective study of hindquarter asymmetry in standardbred trotters and its correlation with performance. Equine Vet J 1985; 17:292.
187. Jeffcott LB, Kold SE: Clinical and radiological aspects of stifle bone cysts in the horse. Equine Vet J 1982; 14:40.
188. Foerner JJ, McIlwraith CW: Orthopedic surgery in the racehorse. Vet Clin North Am Equine Pract 1990; 6:147.
189. White NA, McIlwraith CW, Allen D: Curettage of subchondral bone cysts in the medial femoral condyles in horses. Equine Vet J 1988; 20(suppl 6):120.
190. Lewis RD: A retrospective study of diagnostic and surgical arthroscopy of the equine femorotibial joint. In Proceedings of the Annual Conference of the American Association of Equine Practitioners, 1987, p 887.
191. Kold SE, Hickman J: Use of an autogenous cancellous bone graft in the treatment of subchondral bone cysts in the medial femoral condyle of the horse. Equine Vet J 1983; 15:312.
192. Kold SE, Hickman J: Results of treatment of subchondral bone cysts in the medial condyle of the equine femur with an autogenous cancellous bone graft. Equine Vet J 1984; 16:414.
193. Gibson KE, McIlwraith CW, Park RD, Norrdin RW: Production of patellar lesions by medial patellar desmotomy in normal horses. Vet Surg 1989; 18:466.
194. McIlwraith CW: Osteochondral fragmentation of the distal aspect of the patella in horses. Equine Vet J 1990; 22:157.

16

Transport Stress

D. P. LEADON

The horse industry abounds with anecdotes (e.g., "a good big 'un will always beat a good little 'un") and numerous other unsubstantiated, but not necessarily inaccurate, assumptions. It often has been assumed that transporting horses by road, sea, or air was inherently stressful, but stress arising during transport has not been a subject that has attracted much interest in the past. Appreciating the problems inherent in transport requires "hands on" experience. This can be difficult to obtain because transport companies are highly specialized and have little room in a competitive commercial environment for well-intentioned amateurs. As a result, many people (including a significant proportion of those intimately involved with the horse industry for many years) have a very limited understanding of the horse transport industry.

An understanding of this industry and its inherent problems is essential. National and international trade and competition (including the Breeders Cup, the Japan Cup, the Hong Kong and Magic Millions invitational races, and other "group" status races, with the Olympic Games and World Equestrian Games and numerous similar sporting events) involving athletic horses is ever-increasing.

This chapter outlines the evolution of the horse transport industry and describes some of its current practices. Potential sources of stress within the transport environment are then identified, and methods of quantifying the severity of these stressors are discussed. The transport of horses necessitates their being limited to a restricted space. This confinement brings with it inherent problems in ensuring effective heat dissipation and ventilation, which, if not dealt with properly, can result in the rapid development of so-called shipping fever or pleuritis and pneumonia in susceptible horses. Appropriate management and veterinary care prior to, during, and after transport can help to reduce the incidence and severity of shipping fever, and a series of recommendations to horse owners and veterinarians therefore forms the conclusion of this contribution.

History of the Transport of Performance Horses

ROAD

Land transport of the horse may have had its origins in the eighteenth century. There are various reports of the carriage of horses in custom-built horseboxes. During the reign of Queen Anne in England (1702–1714), a horse may have been carried in this way, either for a bet or to travel it to a race meeting without tiring it,[1] and this development was accelerated by the transport of the subsequent winner of the English St. Leger, Elis, by road in 1836. This horse was transported several hundred miles from his home stabling to the racecourse faster than he could have traveled by being led or ridden, which was the usual custom. Massive gambles were won as a result of this innovation.[2]

AIR

The first known shipment of a racehorse by air is thought to have occurred on a biplane in the 1920s.[3] The first recorded Irish cargo flight which carried horses departed from Shannon for New York in 1947.[2]

Size of the Present-Day Horse Transport Industry

ROAD

There are limited statistics that reflect the traveling activities of the competition horse industry. In excess of 250 events that represent the elite sector of the equestrian disciplines, held under the auspices of the Federation Equestre Internationale (FEI), are held in Europe each year. It was estimated[4] that, on average, some 100 horses were entered in these events in Germany alone. This involved in excess of 250,000 movements of horses for these purposes in 1979. These estimates can reflect the overall growth of these activities as well as the increase in transport. It is now estimated that over 1.5 million horse movements occur in Germany in the course of all equestrian events (Haring, personal communication). The racing industry in Ireland and the United Kingdom documents over 7500 thoroughbred horses in training. These horses take part, on average, in five races per year, which represents over 35,000 movements in this sector of activity in these islands (Redmond, personal communication).

AIR

The true size of involvement of the air transport industry in the shipment of horses is also impossible to quantify with certainty, but very many horses are transported by air. In the period of the massive increase in investment that occurred in the bloodstock industry in the 1980s, the activities of one Irish-based cargo airline, Aer Turas, were devoted almost entirely to the transport of more than 8000 horses by air annually (Dowling, personal communication). These 8000 horses were composed in the main of horses traveling between the so-called tripartite countries of Ireland, the United Kingdom, and France. Currently, major international carriers, such as KLM and Lufthansa, are carrying somewhere between 5000 and 10,000 horses each year. Market forces greatly influence these totals, as may be evidenced by the profound decrease in the importation of horses by air from Europe into Australia from a total number in excess of 800 in the mid-1980s to less than 100 in 1991 (Wallace, personal communication).

Current Methods of Transport of Athletic Horses

ROAD

Athletic horses may be carried in either trailers (floats) or modified vans or lorries. Trailers, or "floats," are usually designed to carry two or three horses in Europe, but similar trailers can carry six, nine, or even more horses in the United States, for example. Heavy goods vehicle chassis lorries are often combined with purpose-built coachwork to provide individual stall accommodations for valuable athletic horses in Europe (Fig. 16–1). These vehicles may vary considerably in appearance, internal volume, and layout. They are usually designed to carry four, six, or nine horses. There is accommodation for grooms to travel with these horses, usually in the ratio of one groom for up to nine horses. The individual access that is afforded by the vehicle design permits the provision of food and water for these horses while the vehicle is moving. Food, in the form of hay and water, is usually provided to horses in transit under this system, at least every 6 to 8 hours. Journey durations can vary from a few hours to several days. The usual practice within this sector of the horse transport industry is for overnight rest in stables to be provided after every 24 hours of transport.

AIR

Air transport of horses utilizes either a jet-stall system, in which horses travel in a fully enclosed "air stable," or an open-stall system (Fig. 16–2), in which there is a lesser degree of enclosure. The open stall system is usually utilized when the entire airplane (which would be a freighter type in configuration) or a considerable section of it has been chartered by a horse transport agency. The numbers of horses that are carried in open-stall systems is determined by the type of airplane in which they are carried and the sizes of the horses to be transported. Three horses can be accommodated across the width of a narrow-bodied aeroplane, e.g., a Boeing 707 or Douglas DC8, in triple stalls. This number can be extended to four horses, provided they are relatively narrow in conformation, in quad stalls. Wide-bodied jets, e.g., a Boeing 747 or Douglas DC10, can accommodate up to seven horses across their width.

Jet stalls can carry up to three horses, separated by partitions. There is a groom entry door and space for

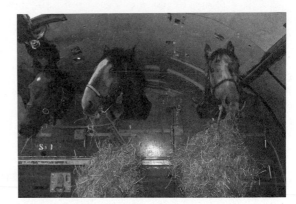

Figure 16-2. Horses in an open-stall system in a narrow-bodied aircraft.

these personnel at the front of the stall. A prototype insect-proof jet stall, for the proposed transport of horses through areas of the world in which insect-borne equine diseases are endemic, is currently being evaluated. Jet stalls are also used in charter arrangements by airlines, but they also can be used in so-called combi systems, in which passengers are carried in the front of the aircraft with freight and the horses in the jet stalls carried in the rear. Passengers are separated from the freight section by a partition.

The normal practice of the horse air transport industry is that the ideal ratio of personnel-to-animal ratio should be one groom for every three horses on the airplane. However, this ideal personnel-to-horses ratio is not always attainable because of the restricted numbers of seats available on some aircraft. Horses are usually offered hay ad libitum while the airplane is in flight, and water is usually offered every 6 to 8 hours or at landing/refueling stops.

A minority of bloodstock shipping agencies arrange for an experienced equine clinician to travel with valuable horses and/or on long-haul flights. This practice has much to recommend it. Treatment of clinical entities as and when they occur will always minimize the severity of the problems with which many clinicians are confronted when sick or traumatized horses arrive at their final destination. Provision of veterinary care is infinitely easier in aircraft using an open-stall system. Jet-stall systems are too restrictive to allow anything other than the most cursory of clinical examinations. Jet-stall systems are popular with airlines because they fit in well with modern palletized freight loading and unloading practices, thus minimizing aircraft turnaround times at airports and because they provide a rigid structure from which horses cannot escape. Jet stalls are also becoming increasing popular with horse owners who wish to move their horses rapidly around the world without having to wait for specialized horse charters to be organized. Jet-stall movements are probably now more popular than charter arrangements. As is so often the case, commercial pressures are ultimately to the detriment of welfare.

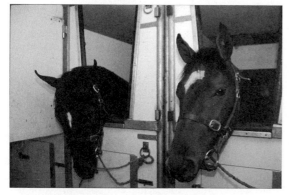

Figure 16-1. Horses in a European motor vehicle.

It is usually only in the case of charter shipments of horses that provision of clinical care during transport is a viable financial proposition.

Is the Transport of Horses Stressful for These Animals?

POTENTIAL STRESSORS WITHIN THE TRANSPORT ENVIRONMENT

Confinement, movement, noise, lack of previous exposure/experience, and the presence of exhaust or other gases, coupled with changes in air temperature, relative humidity, and the numbers of microorganisms within the inhaled air, are all potential sources of stress in the transport environment. Changes in air temperature, relative humidity, and the numbers of microorganisms within the inhaled air have been described[5] in the course of the air transport of horses.

Air temperature and relative humidity will be higher in the aircraft when it is stationary during loading or unloading and during stops for refueling than when it is airborne. The air within the aircraft while it is at altitude flows from the front to the rear of the cargo space. This air is much cooler and drier than that which is present on the earth's surface. There is therefore a temperature and relative humidity gradient from the front to the rear of the aircraft. This gradient tends to be maintained even when the aircraft is on the ground during loading and unloading or refueling stops. This occurs because the ground power units and air-conditioning systems used by stationary aircraft also promote a front to rear airflow. This variation in temperature and relative humidity reflects the inability of the flight deck crew to provide a uniform environment for horses in transit on fully loaded aircraft. This may be of clinical significance in that variations in environmental conditions can be an additional stressor that horses succumbing to shipping fever should be spared, if possible. This is the reason for the recommendation that wet- and dry-bulb thermometers should be placed within the cargo hold and monitored on an hourly basis throughout all medium- and long-haul flights.[5]

The confinement of horses within their stalls will lead to contamination of the environment with microorganisms. Bacterial numbers within the inhaled air can be maintained at levels (while the aircraft is in flight) that are comparable with those normally found in stables. Highly significant increases in bacterial numbers can occur while the aircraft is stationary. These accumulations of bacteria and other microorganisms will be inhaled and must be cleared from the respiratory system. Reduction in microorganism contamination of the environment is a gradual process that is achieved by the higher net airflows that occur during flight.[5]

The practice of tying horses by their head collars in transport results in an abnormal "head held high" posture for protracted periods. This practice may favor the spread of the normal nasopharyngeal flora into the deeper respiratory tract and facilitate the development of respiratory disease.[6] The challenge to the respiratory system will be increased where both the number of microorganisms and the relative humidity are increased, as occurs in stationary aircraft. Thereafter, mucociliary clearance of inhaled particles may be reduced as a result of the desiccating effects of exposure to dry air and low relative humidity.

These factors have therefore the potential to act as stressors of the respiratory system. Similar changes in temperature with net increases in relative humidity and contamination by microorganisms occurs in the road transport of horses (Leadon, in preparation). It is reasonable to conclude that the environment provided within aircraft and road vehicles for the transport of horses is stressful.

METHODS OF ASSESSMENT OF STRESS

Stress is a term that is easily understood, but it is an entity that is notoriously difficult to define.[7] Stress is perhaps more easily identified in its effects than by definition. The ultimate result of extreme stress is death. A literature search has failed to reveal any reliable mortality statistics for the road transport of athletic horses. This may be because fatality can often, but not always, be prevented in the road transport of athletic horses by stopping the vehicle and unloading, if necessary.

There are occasional reports of mortality resulting from frenzy in horses transported by air. The outcome of these accidents in terms of injury rather than death may be determined by the experience of the grooms on board, the presence of an experienced and properly equipped equine clinician, and the availability of suitable tranquilizers and other forms of restraint (e.g., so-called cow collars). Mortality, then, would appear to be an insufficiently sensitive indicator of transport stress in horses.

Stress has been defined as occurring when an animal is required to make an abnormal or extreme adjustment in its behavior or physiology in order to cope with adverse effects of the environment or management.[8] This definition is useful because it takes into account the multifactorial nature of the environmental stresses that may occur during transport, as has been described above.

Stress in horses also has been divided into so-called psychological stress, which is usually quantified in terms of heart rate, ACTH, cortisol, and/or beta-endorphin responses, and physical/physiologic stress, which can reflect trauma and/or disease. It is important to note that different stressors invoke differing responses in different animals and that these responses will vary with age, physiologic status, and previous experiences.[9]

MANIFESTATIONS OF STRESS

Behavior and Orientation in Relation to the Direction of Movement During Road Transport. It has been suggested[10,11] that rear facing of horses in two-horse trailers and in horse lorries[12] may result in more relaxed behavior than forward facing. However, in a study of 16 same-sex pairs of yearling horses naive to transport, it was noted[13] that rear-facing horses had fewer impacts against the trailer sides, fewer total impacts, and lower losses of balance and that they tended to have lower heart rates during the first 15 seconds of travel. However, the investigators concluded that orientation had no major effects on physiology; despite this, body orientation during transport may be an important stressor for some, although not all, horses.

Changes in Laboratory Measurements in Horses Transported by Road. It has been reported[14] that road transportation over distances of 130 to 200 km resulted in significant elevations in serum creatinine and creatine kinase (CK) in 12 clinically normal Sanfrantelli horses. Similar changes were recorded after journeys of 130 to 350 km in 16 untrained horses of various breeds[15] in aspartate amino transferase (AST), lactate dehydrogenase (LDH), alanine aminotransferase (AAT), and serum alkaline phosphatase (SAP). Increases in the activities of serum CK, AST, and LDH also have been described as a result of long journeys of unspecified length[16] and on short journeys of 70 minutes and 50 km duration.[17] Changes in AST, LDH, and creatinine also have been recorded in asses,[18] but changes in the activities of serum enzymes were not evident in ponies transported by road.[12] Significant decreases in the concentrations of the free amino acids methionine, taurine, and 3-methylhistidine have been noted in association with transport,[19] and although blood lactate and pyruvate increases may be seen, the lactate/pyruvate ratio may decrease.[20] Decreases in the serum concentrations of potassium, magnesium, and calcium also may occur.[21] Road transport has been associated with significant increases in cortisol and T_4 in a group of 20 horses that ranged in age from 4 to 7 years.[22] Elevations in the concentrations of cortisol and glucose in the peripheral circulation also have occurred in transported ponies.[12] However, 7 adult 3-day-event horses did not demonstrate elevations beyond the normal range in plasma cortisol and free fatty acids when transported over a distance of 2000 km in a 24-hour period.[23] Furthermore, transportation of acclimatized adult horses for 1 hour in a trailer did not result in any change in beta-endorphin levels.[24]

These reported changes in laboratory measurements in horses that are transported by road are probably not of clinical significance.

Changes in Laboratory Measurements in Horses Transported by Air. Significant postflight elevations in mean neutrophil counts and fibrinogen levels, which may reflect otherwise inapparent responses to confinement and transport and perhaps, too, the initial signs of subclinical and otherwise undetected respiratory disease, have been reported in apparently normal horses after long-haul flights. Total white blood cell counts (WBC), neutrophil counts ($>5.8 \times 10^9$ per liter), and fibrinogen values (>3.2 g/liter using the modified Clauss method) are higher in horses with shipping fever than those observed in normal horses from the second day after long-distance transport by air.[5]

Effects on Respiratory and Enteric Health Status. Stress as a result of transport may be a predisposing factor in the development of respiratory[5,25,26] and enteric disease.[27] Predisposition to respiratory disease after transport may be due to a marked increase in the numbers[28] and, in viral-infected horses, the activity[29] of pulmonary alveolar macrophages. Depression of cellular immunity may be related to increased cortisol levels.[28] However, road transport of seven healthy thoroughbred horses over 1160 km for 36 hours did not affect selected pulmonary alveolar macrophage functions.[30]

Effects on Subsequent Performance. Transport in trailers has been found to have relatively little effect on performance, as measured in time trials in eight quarter and thoroughbred horses transported for 8.1 km during 15 minutes or for 194 km over a 2- to 2.5-hour time period.[31] The effects of air transport are extremely difficult to quantify. However, it has been noted that racehorses that are transported long distances by air tend to have minor elevations in CK and AST on arrival. Those racehorses which have been successful in their target race on arrival after long-distance air transport have tended to lose less body weight (<10 kg) in transit than those which have raced badly (>20 kg) (Leadon, unpublished data).

Management and Veterinary Care of Horses in Transit

PRIOR TO TRANSPORT

The horse transport industry does not usually make provision for the veterinary care of horses in transit. However, veterinarians are occasionally given the opportunity to provide this care for individual horses or groups of horses of high value. Where this care or just general advice is sought, a number of measures are appropriate. The health status of horses should be checked prior to and on the day of transport with special reference to the identification of subclinical respiratory disease. This measure is advisable because it can help to identify horses that would be more likely to succumb to shipping fever than their healthy counterparts. Appropriate therapy can then be initiated and the response to this therapy can be identified prior to departure. Clinical judgment on maintenance of therapy during transport, if appropriate, can then be exercised. The shipment of horses with existing clinical respiratory disease is contraindicated unless warranted by a need for emergency hospitalization due to other considerations such as limb fracture, etc. Unnecessary medication, such as the administration of so-called prophylactic antimicrobial therapy without evidence of respiratory disease and the unjustified use of sedatives, should be avoided.

Special dietary provisions are not required for horses being transported short distances. It is the usual practice of the horse transport industry to provide horses with a light laxative diet, e.g., a series of bran mashes, prior to medium- or long-haul journeys. Care should be used in the administration of laxatives such as liquid paraffin prior to these longer journeys. Excessive fluid loss through the feces is clearly contraindicated where dehydration in transit can occur easily.

Efforts should be made to preserve the best attainable standard of air hygiene for horses in transit. Moldy hay should not be provided. Even good-quality hay should be well shaken or passed through a vacuum-driven particle remover to minimize the workload of the horses mucociliary clearance mechanisms in the confined transport environment.

DURING TRANSPORT

Figure 16–3 illustrates the factors involved in the development of shipping fever. Hay should be provided on an ad libitum basis throughout the journey, and water should be offered every 6 to 8 hours. Delays in transport should be avoided, and on road journeys, overnight rest away from the vehicle should be provided to enable horses to lower their heads and facilitate mucociliary clearance.

Clinicians who accept responsibility for the health care of horses in transit by accompanying them on a journey must make adequate preparations to enable them to fulfill this responsibility. Road transport vehicles can be diverted to the nearest veterinary clinic if the need should arise, but the available facilities may not always be either sufficient or appropriate to the needs of athletic horses. It is therefore advisable for clinicians to carry adequate veterinary supplies when accompanying horses transported by road or by air. Provision should be made to deal with the occurrence of frenzy on repeated occasions among the horses included in the shipment. Supplies for the repair of injury and treatment of respiratory disease and colic are also essential. Although there is a popular perspective that a gun should be used in emergency situations at altitude, few airline captains will endorse the use of a free bullet within the airframe at any time. The advent of modern, potent equine tranquilizers, analgesics, and anesthetics has, in my experience, obviated the requirement for the use of a gun.

The clinician must be aware of the fact that as well as having a responsibility for the horses, there is also, particularly at altitude, a responsibility for the welfare and safety of all the personnel on board. Heroic attempts at manual restraint of the occasional cases of frenzy that occur in horses in transit by lay staff devoted to their horses should be discouraged, even if the administration of a tranquilizer may result in the disqualification of the horse concerned in subsequent competition.

AFTER TRANSPORT

Cases of shipping fever do occur after short journeys, but they are not as common as those after longer journeys. Clinical evaluation should be carried out for all horses after medium- or long-haul journeys. Horses should be bright and alert, and they should take a drink and exhibit interest in palatable feed soon after arrival. Depression and inappetence with the presence of a soft cough, shallow frequent respirations, and a febrile response are classical signs of shipping fever.[32] However, the febrile response can be variable, and 53 percent of horses with shipping fever may not manifest a febrile response until 2 or sometimes even 3 days after arrival (Leadon, unpublished data). It is therefore advisable to record rectal temperature morning and evening for at least 3 days after arrival following long journeys.[7] Veterinary advice must be sought at once by horse owners if a febrile response is detected after transport.

TREATMENT OF SHIPPING FEVER

Prompt, appropriate treatment will result in a full recovery in many cases of shipping fever. However, this condition is always potentially life-threatening, and fatalities do occur. Hematology and blood biochemistry can be useful diagnostic and prognostic aids in cases of

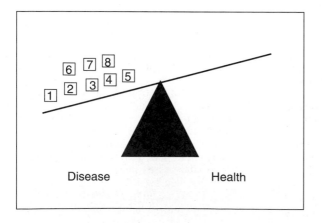

Figure 16-3. Schematic illustration of some of the factors that are involved in the development of shipping fever. 1 = preexisting respiratory disease; 2 = surges in T° and RH %; 3 = increasing nos. CFU in air; 4 = immunocompromise; 5 = dehydration; 6 = delays; 7 = prolonged exposure; 8 = other unknown factors.

pleuropneumonia. Thoracocentesis[32] is indicated where there is marked pleural effusion. The resultant drainage will provide effective and immediate relief when combined with anti-inflammatory and antimicrobial therapy. Thoracic drains (Argyle, Sherwood Medical Industries, Tullamore, Ireland) placed under local anesthesia (after ultrasonographic examination or percussion between the seventh and eighth intercostal spaces on the left side or the sixth and seventh spaces on the right, 8 to 10 cm above the point of the elbow) may be left in situ for up to 72 hours. A condom can be attached to the thoracic drain to act as a one-way valve. Some form of one-way valve is essential if the chest drain is to remain indwelling for a period of days, and it is sensible to attach a valve prior to placement of the chest drain. Some clinicians prefer to repeatedly drain the chest, if necessary, rather than to leave a chest drain in place for several days. Both approaches appear to be well tolerated in most cases. Thoracocentesis also enables cytology, biochemistry, and microbial culture to be carried out on the resultant chest cavity fluid. Aerobic infections are common, and concurrent anaerobic infections also occur. Scintillation of pleural fluid on ultrasonographic examination may reflect gas production as a result of anaerobic involvement (Marr, personal communication). Gram-positive and gram-negative organisms often can be recovered, since these organisms appear to spread to the lower respiratory tract as a result of the restricted head movement that is inevitable during transport.[6] It is therefore reasonable for clinicians to initiate a regimen of beta-lactamase and aminoglycoside antimicrobial therapy (while awaiting culture and sensitivity results). Simultaneous anti-inflammatory therapy can be very helpful, and metronidazole should be incorporated into the therapeutic regimen where anaerobic involvement is suspected or confirmed. The possibility of predisposing viral infection or complicating *Mycoplasma* infection[33] should not be overlooked. Ultrasonographic examination[34] combined with clinical pathology data can enable an objective prognosis to be formed and monitored.

THE POST-TRANSPORT RECOVERY PERIOD

Objective monitoring of the posttransport recovery period is a difficult task. There is considerable individual variation among horses in terms of responses to transport. Although it may be thought that laboratory based assessments are the most useful criteria for monitoring recovery from a journey, this is not the case in practice. Research and experimental studies in which horses are transported from their place of origin and return to it after journeys of variable duration permit use of standardized methods of laboratory evaluation. In the real world, laboratory tests carried out prior to departure are often not comparable with those available on arrival at some far distant final destination.

The subjective judgment of experienced personnel who are familiar with the horses in their care is often the best method of evaluating recovery after a journey in normal, healthy horses. However, horses should, if possible, be weighed prior to transport. The measurement and recording of body weight gain after the initial loss that is associated with transport is a useful adjunct to monitoring recovery in both healthy horses and (when combined with rectal temperature, clinical examination, laboratory data, and ultrasonography) in those which have been affected by shipping fever.

Acknowledgments

The author wishes to acknowledge the financial support of the International League for the Protection of Horses and the assistance of the International Equestrian Federation, that have enabled him to conduct a series of studies on transport stress. These studies and associated research form the basis of this contribution.

References

1. Creiger S: Land Transportation of the Horse. Live Animal Trade and Transport Magazine, November 1989, p 43.
2. Leadon FR: The Horse Transport Industry. Irish Field (Supplement), 1973, p 20.
3. Anon: Instone Air Line. Live Animal Trade and Transport Magazine, November 1989, p 39.
4. Hinriksen JK, Korner H: Problems in transport of horses. In Proceedings of the 30th Annual Meeting of the Equine Association of Animal Production, 1979, p 1.
5. Leadon DP, Daykin J, Backhouse W, et al: Environmental, haematological and blood biochemical changes in equine transit stress. In Proceedings of the Annual Conference of the American Association of Equine Practitioners, 1990, p 485.
6. Rackyleft DJ, Love DN: Influence of head posture on the respiratory tract health of horses. Aust Equine Vet 1989; 8:123.
7. Leadon DP, Frank C, Atock A: Recommendations to Horse Owners and their Representatives on the Transport of Horses. Lausanne, Switzerland, Federation Equestre Internationale, 1990.
8. Fraser D, Ritchie JSD, Fraser AF: The term "stress" in a veterinary context. Br Vet J 1975; 131:653.
9. Moberg G: Animal Stress. Baltimore, Md, American Physiological Society, 1985.
10. Tellington W, Tellington-Jones L: Endurance and Competitive Trail Riding. New York, Doubleday, 1979.
11. Creiger S: Reducing equine hauling stress: A review. J Equine Vet Sci 1982; 2:187.
12. Abbott EM: Research undertaken. Annual Report of the Animal Health Trust, Newmarket, Suffolk, 1979.
13. Clark DK, Dellmeier GR, Friend TH: Effect of the orientation of horses during transportation on behavior and physiology. Reviewed by S Creiger. Live Animal Trade and Transport Magazine, September 1991, p 34.
14. Caola G, Ferlazzo A, Panzera M: Livelli sierici di creatinina fosfochinasi in cavalli, dopo trasporto. Clin Vet 1984; 107:46.
15. Ferlazzo A, Caola G, Omero E, et al: Modificazioni sieroenzimatiche nel cavallo sedentario dopo trasporto. Arch Vet Ital 1984; 35:27.
16. Petazzi F, Ceci L: Modificazioni Seriche E Sieroenzimatiche In Cavalli Sottoposti A Strazzo Da Trasporto. Medicina 1981; 325.
17. Von B, Schmidt K-H: Untersuchungen uber das verhalten der serumenzyme aspartat-aminotransferase, creatin-kinase, lactat dehydragenase, alkalische phosphatase und des serumbilirubins bei warmblutpferden unter dem einfluss von transport, turnierteilnahme, longieren und tageszeit. Berl Munch Tierartztl Wochenschr 1980; 93:244.
18. Ferlazzo A, Panzera M, Balbo SM, et al: Su alcuni parametri ematochimici in Equus asinus L. - Influenzadello stress da trasporto. Clin Vet 1983; 106:238.
19. Omero A, Caola G, Panzera M, et al: Modificazioni dei livelli di metionina, taurina e 3-metilistidina nel quadro degli amminoacidi liberi del siero nel cavallo, dopo trasporto su strada. Clin Vet 1982; 105:197.

20. Ferlazzo A, Panzera M, Caola G, et al: Comportamento della lattacidemia e della piruvicemia nel cavallo sanfrantello dopo esercizio fisico di tipo fascio e posturale. Acta Med Vet 1982; 28:543.
21. Gaola G, Ferlazzo A, Omera A: Gli elettroliti sierici nel cavallo sanfrantello dopo esercizio fisico. Arch Vet Ital 1983; 34:122.
22. Petazzi F, Zarilli A, Ceci L: Comportamento delT3, T4 e del cortisolo in cavalli adulti sottoposti a stress da transporto. Obiettivi Doc Vet 1983; 4:55.
23. Senniksen HV, Jorgenssen K: Untersuchungen zum transportstress beim Pferd. Pferdeheilkunde 1988; 4:35.
24. McCarthy R, Jeffcott LB, Clarke I, et al: Evaluation of stress in horses. Aust Equine Vet 1990; 9:34.
25. Hayes MH: Horses on Board Ship: A Guide to Their Management. London, Hurst and Blackett, 1902.
26. Raphael CF, Beech J: Pleuritis secondary to pneumonia and/or lung abscess in 90 horses. J Am Vet Med Assoc 1982; 18:808.
27. Owen RH, Fullerton J, Barnum DA: Effects of transportation, surgery and antibiotic therapy in ponies infected with *Salmonella*. Am J Vet Res 1983; 44:46.
28. Bayly WM, Liggitt HD, Huston LJ, et al: Stress and its effect on equine pulmonary mucosal defenses. *In* Proceedings of the Annual Conference of the American Association of Equine Practitioners, 1986, p 253.
29. Anderson NV, DeBowes RM, Nyrop KA, et al: Mononuclear phagocytes of transport-stressed horses with viral respiratory tract infection. Am J Vet Res 1985; 46:2272.
30. Crisman MV, Hodgson DR, Bayly WM, et al: Effects of transport on constituents of broncho-alveolar lavage fluid from horses. Cornell Vet 1992; 82:233.
31. Slade LM: Trailer transportation and racing performance. *In* Proceedings of the 9th Equine Nutrition and Physiology Symposium, 1986, p 511.
32. Byars TD, Becht JL: Pleuropneumonia. Respiratory Disease: Medicine and Surgery. Vet Clin North Am Equine Prac 1991; 7:63.
33. Hoffman AM, Baird JD, Kloeze JH, et al: *Mycoplasma felis* pleuritis in two show-jumper horses. Cornell Vet 1992; 82:155.
34. Reef VB: Outcome and return to performance in horses with pleuropneumonia evaluated ultrasonographically. *In* Proceedings of the 8th ACVIM Forum, 1990, p 573.

Training Regimens: Physiologic Adaptations to Training

D. R. HODGSON AND R. J. ROSE

The major objectives of training are to prepare a horse for the rigors of athletic competition, to decrease the risk of injury, and to increase the work capacity. By nature, horses are gifted athletes that are also capable of undergoing substantial adaptations in response to training. Investigations examining the adaptability of the musculoskeletal, cardiorespiratory, hemolymphatic, and thermoregulatory systems have been undertaken. Some of the findings will be summarized in this section, whereas others may be found in the other sections of this chapter. Most of the measurements discussed have been used only in experimental laboratories. However, it is likely that some of the variables will be used in the future to provide objective indices of fitness and the success of training.

Muscular Responses to Exercise

ENZYMES IN MUSCLE

Aerobic Enzymes. Muscle is a remarkably plastic tissue that is remodeled when exposed to the stresses of training. In general, although by no means universally, training results in an increase in mitochondrial density, with resulting increases in the activities of enzymes in the tricarboxylic and lipid metabolic pathways, both of which contribute to increased oxidative capacity of skeletal muscle.[1-9] Endurance training produces the greatest increase in the activities of aerobic enzymes, and in the first few months of training, overall increases of more than 100 percent over pretraining values are reported.[8,10] These changes also may be associated with an increase in the number of oxidative muscle fibers within the working muscle.[1-13] Additionally, there is an increase in the density of capillaries surrounding muscle fibers, in particular the more oxidative slow-twitch (type I) and fast-twitch high-oxidative (type IIA) fibers, in response to training.[14]

Although the metabolic advantages of increases in oxidative capacity in skeletal muscle will be greatest in animals required to undertake more prolonged exercise, e.g., steeplechasing, 3-day eventing, or endurance rides, there are positive effects in animals participating in more intense activities, there being a prolongation of work capacity.

The mechanism by which the increase in oxidative capacity exerts its effects is by more efficient utilization of substrates by the metabolic pathways within the skeletal muscle. This occurs as a result of a more rapid translocation into the mitochondria of the ADP produced during muscular contraction. Since an increased ratio of ADP/ATP within the cytosol of working muscle is one of the stimuli for an elevation in glycolytic (anaerobic) energy production, the increase in oxidative capacity serves to keep this ratio low via the rapid mitochondrial uptake of ADP. A decrease in the ADP/ATP ratio reduces the stimulus for glycolysis and increases the contribution of fat to total energy production. The capacity for greater utilization of fatty acids by muscle during submaximal exercise results in a sparing of glycogen within the working muscle. This glycogen-sparing effect assists

in delaying the onset of fatigue during endurance events because there is a direct relationship between exhaustion of the intramuscular glycogen store and the onset of fatigue.[15,16]

The lower intracellular ADP/ATP ratio is also likely to have important effects during exercise at higher intensities. A beneficial effect would be provided by the augmented aerobic capacity, since this allows a greater proportion of energy to be produced by the aerobic pathways early in the exercise. Thus the production of lactate and hydrogen ions will be delayed, reducing the potential of these by-products to adversely affect the contractile apparatus, a factor that contributes to fatigue. This increase in oxidative capacity is reflected by increases in values for the metabolic variables such as V_{LA4} in response to a standardized exercise test.[17-19]

Glycolytic Enzymes. Equine skeletal muscle possesses an intrinsically high glycolytic capacity, which is reflected by high activities of the glycolytic enzymes. Such is the magnitude of the activities of the glycolytic enzymes that when compared on the basis of protein concentration, the glycolytic activity is more than tenfold greater than for the aerobic enzymes. However, there are few changes in the activities of glycolytic enzymes in response to most routine training programs.[4-6,10,20-22] In some cases, modest decreases in the activity of lactate dehydrogenase in response to training have been reported.[2,4,8,10,17,23] These findings of few, if any, changes in the activity of the glycolytic enzymes are similar to those reported for several other mammalian species.

In contrast, when training involving short-term, intense bursts of exercise is undertaken, it results in an increase in the activities of several glycolytic enzymes.[7,24] This also parallels the findings in humans and rats, where intense training has been shown to result in an increase in the glycolytic potential.

Enzymes Associated with Purine Nucleotide Metabolism. There are few reports on the effects of training on the activities of enzymes directly associated with purine nucleotide metabolism. Analogous to the situation for glycolytic activity, the intrinsic activities of creatine kinase (CK) and AMP deaminase are high in equine skeletal muscle. The greater the capacity for speed of an animal, the higher are the enzyme activities.[25,26] Training has been reported to result in limited increases in the activities of CK[21,27] and AMP deaminase.[26] The purpose of these increases has not been determined, but it has been suggested that the increase in AMP deaminase activity may be responsible for ensuring a rapid stimulation of glycolysis during the most intense forms of exercise.[26]

CAPILLARITY

The number of capillaries surrounding muscle fibers has been shown to increase in response to training.[14] The purpose of this increased capillarity appears not to be related to an increase in the supply of blood to the working muscle per se but to prolonging the transit time for blood through the capillary bed of the muscle. This increased transit time improves the potential for exchange of substrates to and metabolic by-products from the muscle fibers. During prolonged exercise, these effects allow greater uptake by muscle of glucose and free fatty acids, which are ideal fuels for the metabolic pathways, whereas during intense exercise, there is an increased capability for the offloading of oxygen and glucose and the removal of carbon dioxide, lactate, and hydrogen ions from the contracting muscles.

ALTERATIONS IN FIBER TYPES

The question as to whether the proportions of different fiber types change in response to age or training is not resolved. The proportion of type I fibers in the skeletal muscles of several breeds of horse has been shown to increase in response to advancing age (from juvenile to adult) and training.[8,10] In contrast, there is a growing body of evidence that indicates that conventional race training of adult horses induces few transformations in fiber type proportions,[5,20] although fast-twitch fibers, in particular type IIB fibers, have been demonstrated to undergo substantial increases in oxidative capacity.[28]

GLYCOGEN CONCENTRATION

The concentration of glycogen in equine skeletal muscle, usually in the range of 500 to 650 mmol glucosyl units per kilogram (dry weight), is about 50 percent higher than that reported in humans.[29] In general, training results in a moderate increase in the intramuscular glycogen store,[20,22] particularly if an adequate plane of nutrition is maintained.

Repletion of glycogen following prolonged exercise is relatively slow in the horse, taking, at times, up to 48 hours for complete replenishment.[15,16] Assuming that the diet contains sufficient calories, there is apparently little effect of nutrition on the rate of glycogen repletion.[30,31] Similarly, supplementation with glucose, either orally or intravenously, does not affect the rate of replenishment. In humans, a combination of prior training, a bout of exercise to induce glycogen depletion, and subsequent consumption of a high-carbohydrate diet result in what has been referred to as a "supercompensation" in the muscle glycogen store. To date, this effect has not been reproduced in horses. However, feeding of diets high in fat have been suggested to result in an increase in the resting concentration of muscle glycogen.[32,33] The mechanism for this increase in muscle glycogen reserve has not been established.

BUFFERING CAPACITY

Horses possess a large intramuscular buffering capacity that assists in offsetting the deleterious effects of proton accumulation during intense exercise. The importance of these systems are such that the capacity to perform high-intensity exercise is thought to be linked to the concentration of buffers within muscle.[34] Hydrolysis of phosphocreatine provides buffering in response to energy production in the myofibrils and is referred to as *dy*-

namic buffering. *Physiochemical buffering* refers to the static buffering systems within skeletal muscle provided by proteins, dipeptides, and inorganic phosphate in the myofibers. Of the physicochemical buffers, carnosine provides a large proportion of the buffering capacity of equine skeletal muscle.[35,36] A relatively tight correlation between buffering capacity and the capacity for high-intensity exercise has been demonstrated by Harris and colleagues.[37]

Training appears to exert a variable but beneficial response on muscle buffering capacity. McCutcheon and colleagues[38] demonstrated a relatively large increase in buffering capacity in response to moderate-intensity training, whereas other groups have demonstrated more modest increases.[39,40] The advantage of a training-induced increase in buffering capacity is to allow the horse to tolerate a higher proton (H^+) load in working skeletal muscle during exercise, thereby postponing the onset of fatigue.

Hematologic Responses to Training

HEMOGRAM

Erythrocytes are a vital conduit for the transport of oxygen from the lungs to the working muscle. Persson and colleagues[41] and Lykkeboe and colleagues[42] have reported increases in the total red cell pool following training in racehorses. This would provide its greatest advantage, in terms of improved oxygen transport, during intense exercise, when maximal splenic emptying has occurred. The advantage of expansion of the red cell mass is supported by the study of Persson,[43] who demonstrated a relationship between the total red cell volume and racing speed over 1000 m in standardbred trotters.

Training has been shown to result in moderate increases in the resting hematocrit, hemoglobin concentration, and red cell count.[44-46] The significance of these increases is not clear, since they may only reflect the variations in these variables encountered in response to repeated sampling.[47] As outlined in Chapter 5, changes in the horse's temperament in response to training also may influence these responses. In general, as horses progress through training, they become a little more excitable when handled, particularly when procedures such as venipuncture are being performed. This apparent short-lived anxiety may result in increases in the variables described above, making their physiologic significance open to question. The white blood cell pool, however, undergoes few, if any, changes in response to routine race training.

When compared with other types of racehorses, endurance horses frequently have lower values for resting hematocrit and other red cell indices.[48] This may be the result of an increase in the plasma volume in response to training,[49] although changes in hematologic variables did not occur in one group of horses undergoing routine training for endurance competition.[50] Leukocyte indices are not significantly affected by endurance training.[50]

PLASMA BIOCHEMISTRY

Plasma biochemical values are often integral to the diagnosis of disease syndromes in horses. For example, elevations in the plasma activities of the enzymes CK and aspartate amino transferase are common in association with myopathies, whereas increased activity of gamma glutamyl transferase has been linked to hepatic dysfunction. Despite the utility of these markers for certain diseases, minimal changes are reported when many commonly measured plasma biochemical variables are assayed throughout a routine training program.[50]

BLOOD/PLASMA VOLUME

Training has been reported to result in an increase in the plasma volume.[49] In one report, a 29 percent increase in plasma volume occurred within 2 weeks of the commencement of low-intensity training.[49] The majority of this increase occurred within 1 week of training commencing. This rapid increase in plasma volume coupled with fixed hemoglobin concentration in blood indicates that there was also an increase in the oxygen-carrying capacity of the blood. This is likely to contribute to the increase in maximum oxygen uptake $\dot{V}_{O_2max}$ that occurs early in response to training.[51] An expansion of the plasma volume is also likely to contribute to improved capacity for thermoregulation, since it would allow increased blood flow to the skin while maintaining blood flow to working muscle during exercise.

Changes in Cardiorespiratory Variables in Response to Training

HEART RATE

A reduction in heart rate during submaximal exercise has been reported in horses in response to conventional and treadmill training.[52,53] Thomas and colleagues[54] suggest that this reduction is about 10 beats/min for any submaximal speed of exercise. However, this finding is not common to all studies, with a number of reports describing no change in the heart rate response to submaximal exercise following training.[51,55–57] Maximal heart rate does not appear to be affected by the state of training.[57]

Recovery of heart rate following exercise has been suggested to be correlated with the level of fitness in racehorses. The recovery of heart rate in the first 5 minutes following galloping in thoroughbreds was reported to be a useful indicator of fitness. Heart rate recovery became more rapid as fitness improved.[52,58] In contrast, several other studies have failed to show a similar response to training.[55,56,59]

Heart rate recovery following endurance exercise is likely to be a valuable tool in the assessment of training effects. From studies conducted by Rose and colleagues[60,61] at competitive endurance rides, it is apparent the fittest horses suffering the fewest metabolic derangements (e.g., dehydration) at the compulsory rest stops

have the most consistent drop in heart rate during the rest period. This is supported by another study where poorly performing endurance horses had higher postexercise heart rates than the better-performed horses.[62]

STROKE VOLUME AND CARDIAC OUTPUT

Training has variable effects on stroke volume during exercise. In a study involving training at low speeds, there was a small but significant increase in stroke volume in response to submaximal exercise following the training.[54] In another study, Evans and Rose[57] demonstrated an increase in stroke volume and cardiac output during maximal exercise following training. These findings are in contrast to those involving submaximal exercise, since Bayly and colleagues[63] and Thornton and colleagues[53] did not demonstrate any changes in stroke volume in response to training.

MAXIMAL OXYGEN UPTAKE ($\dot{V}_{O_2max}$)

Increases in $\dot{V}_{O_2max}$ have been reported following training, with the most substantial increases occurring in the first few weeks of training.[51] Increases in $\dot{V}_{O_2max}$ from around 130 to 160 ml/kg/min (23 percent increase) have been reported following training in thoroughbred horses.[57] This increase is associated with an elevated plasma volume, arteriovenous oxygen difference, and stroke volume.[51]

Metabolic Responses to Training

LACTATE PRODUCTION AND METABOLISM

As outlined in Chapter 4, lactate is a product of muscular metabolism and accumulates in muscle and blood at higher intensities of exercise. One of the effects of training is to increase the exercise intensity at which lactate begins to accumulate within the circulation. This is referred to as the *onset of blood lactate accumulation* (OBLA), and the derived variable V_{LA4} is the speed at which a blood lactate concentration of 4 mmol/liter is achieved. This is the blood lactate concentration above which lactate is known to increase rapidly in the blood. Thornton and colleagues[53] measured the OBLA in standardbred horses and found that it related to the animals' endurance capacity during treadmill exercise. An intensive 5-week training period resulted in an increase in the V_{LA4} from 7 to almost 8 m/s. The advantage of this effect would be to increase the speed at which the deleterious effects of proton accumulation occurs during high-intensity exercise.

Application of Indices of Fitness to Horses in Training

RESTING MEASUREMENTS

As described in Chapter 11, a number of measurements have been described which may give some insight into a horse's athletic potential. These include conformational indices, estimates of heart size and blood volume, and determinations of the proportions of fibers within the muscles of locomotion. In contrast, there are few measurements which when performed in the resting horse provide information regarding the animal's fitness, despite attempts to link the two. For example, over the past 20 years, a number of equine practitioners have placed great emphasis on the relationship between values for resting red cell indices and a horse's fitness.[44] Doubtless the red cell pool is a key factor in the transport of oxygen from the lungs to the tissues, and therefore, a sufficient red cell mass and hemoglobin concentration within the blood are necessary to ensure optimal performance. However, except in the presence of anemia or other disease conditions which can be detected using hematologic or plasma biochemical analyses, there is little scientific evidence that resting hematology provides an indication of fitness in an individual horse. There is also no indication of a decrease in resting heart rate in response to training, unlike the situation in the human athlete.

EXERCISE MEASUREMENTS

Unquestionably the best indication of fitness for racing is the ability of a horse to withstand the rigors of competition and perform successfully. Since racing is stressful, often pushing a horse to near its physiologic limits, attempts have been made to define the fitness of a horse in response to exercise without necessarily exposing it to the burden of racing.

Performing exercise tests on the track for the assessment of fitness usually consists of various measurements taken during or after a standardized bout of exercise. In their elementary form, tests on the racetrack involve assessment of performance capacity and fitness by determination of the time taken for the horse to complete the competition distance. Naturally, the faster the time and the more rapid the recovery of the horse following the test, the more likely the horse is to be fit for competition. However, since this type of test requires exercise at maximal intensities, which increases the chance of injury, alternative testing schemes involving less intense exercise have been developed.

Submaximal tests involving speeds around three-quarters pace in thoroughbreds (about 800 m/min) and maximal speed tests involving distances less than those required in racing are most likely to provide the most useful information. Measurements which are relatively easily performed in association with track tests include heart rate measured using a digitally displaying heart rate meter, hematologic variables (e.g., blood volume), and blood lactate values following exercise.[64] Total blood volume may be measured soon after intense exercise using Evans blue dye (see Chap. 5). Persson[65] suggests that this variable provides an indication of performance capacity of standardbred horses.

Assessment of the relationship between work effort and heart rate in horses during exercise has been reported. Stroke volume does not change greatly with in-

creasing exercise speed,[66] and therefore, heart rate provides a guide to cardiac output in response to exercise. Usually there is a linear increase in heart rate with increasing exercise speed up to the point at which the maximal heart rate (HR_{max}) is reached. The HR_{max} is identified when there is no further increase in heart rate despite an increase in running speed. The HR_{max} does not change with training state,[57] although the speed at which HR_{max} is reached increases with increasing fitness. Persson[65] demonstrated a relationship between heart rate and the aerobic capacity of horses and suggested that the speed required to generate a heart rate of 200 beats/min (V_{200}) (see Chap. 7) provides a useful indication of aerobic capacity. By monitoring the speed at which V_{200} is achieved during training, it is possible to derive an objective assessment of how a horse is adapting to training. As an alternative to determination of V_{200}, and possibly more appropriately, a speed that represents 80 of 90 percent of HR_{max} may be used. The reasons for selecting this percentage of the HR_{max} are related to the finding that not all horses have the same HR_{max}, and therefore, a horse with an HR_{max} of 215 beats/min working at V_{200} will be exercising at a higher relative intensity than a horse with an HR_{max} of 240 beats/min. If it is assumed that HR_{max} does not increase with training, an increase in the speed at which the prescribed percentage of HR_{max} is achieved will be reflective of an increase in fitness. However, because heart rates at submaximal intensities may fluctuate considerably, depending on the extent of excitement, care should be taken when interpreting changes in heart rate.

As mentioned earlier, determination of the rate of recovery of heart rate following exercise has proven valuable, particularly when attempting to assess fitness in endurance horses[60,61] (see Chap. 7). In contrast, measurements of heart rate recovery appear to have less utility in the assessment of fitness in standardbred and thoroughbred racehorses, although a significant correlation with race performance has been reported.[67]

Much useful information can be obtained on the fitness of horses in response to standardized exercise tests on a high-speed treadmill. As described in Chapter 12, we use an incremental treadmill test comprising a 3-minute warmup at 4 m/s, followed by 90 seconds at 6 m/s, and then 1-minute steps at 8, 10, 11, 12 and 13 m/s on a treadmill set at a 10 percent slope. We find that only the most athletically gifted thoroughbred and standardbred racehorses will complete all steps, and endurance horses frequently will not continue at speeds greater than 10 m/s. We have found that the number of steps completed and the total run time provide an index of fitness and performance capacity, particularly in racehorses. Cardiovascular and respiratory variables are measured during the last 5 to 10 seconds of each exercise step. Measurements of blood lactate concentrations are made at the ends of steps involving speeds greater than 6 m/s. At speeds lower than this, excitement can result in substantial variability in values, thereby limiting their usefulness. Since plasma or blood lactate values do not reach steady state at the conclusion of each of the steps at higher intensities, it is important that tests should involve steps of the same duration and intensity when comparisons are being made.

Knowledge that training results in an increase in the speed of exercise at which a given quantity of lactate accumulates in the blood can be incorporated into training programs in one of two ways. The first is to measure the concentration of lactate in blood in response to a standardized exercise test. Alternatively, the standardized test described previously can be performed on a treadmill. We have found that the blood lactate concentration at the conclusion of the 10-m/s step provides a useful basis for the assessment of fitness. Fitter and more athletically capable horses have the lowest values after this step.

Conclusions

The horse is a naturally gifted athlete that also possesses great capacity to respond to the repeated stresses imposed by training. While there is now a substantial body of information about the adaptations occurring with training, there is still a need for more data relating to specific competitive events. One of the major problems in training horses is the objective assessment of fitness. The more widespread use of treadmills may permit changes in fitness to be assessed more critically in the future.

References

1. Essén-Gustavsson B, Lindholm A, Thornton J: Histochemical properties of muscle fiber types and enzyme activities in skeletal muscles of standardbred trotters of different ages. Equine Vet J 1980; 12:175.
2. Lindholm A, Essén-Gustavsson B, McMiken D, et al: Muscle histochemistry and biochemistry of thoroughbred horses during growth and training. In Snow DH, Persson SGB, Rose RJ (eds): Equine Exercise Physiology. Cambridge, Granta Editions, 1983, p 211.
3. Straub R, Dettwiler M, Hoppeler H, et al: The use of morphometry and enzyme activity measurements in skeletal muscles for the assessment of the working capacity of horses. In Snow DH, Persson SGB, Rose RJ (eds): Equine Exercise Physiology. Cambridge, Granta Editions, 1983, p 193.
4. Essén-Gustavsson B, Lindholm A: Muscle fiber characteristics of active and inactive standardbred horses. Equine Vet J 1985; 17:434.
5. Hodgson DR, Rose RJ, Dimauro J, et al: Effects of training on muscle composition in horses. Am J Vet Res 1986; 47:12.
6. Hodgson DR, Rose RJ: Effects of a nine-month endurance training programme on muscle composition in the horse. Vet Rec 1987; 121:271.
7. Lovell DK, Rose RJ: Changes in skeletal muscle composition in response to interval and high intensity training. In Persson SGB, Lindholm A, Jeffcott LB (eds): Equine Exercise Physiology 3. Davis, Calif, ICEEP Publications, 1991, p 215.
8. Roneus M, Lindholm A, Âsheim A: Muscle characteristics in thoroughbreds of different ages and sexes. Equine Vet J 1991; 23:207.
9. Snow DH, Guy PS: The effects of training and detraining on the activity of a number of enzymes in the horse skeletal muscle. Arch Int Physiol Biochem 1979; 87:87.
10. Roneus M: Muscle characteristics in standardbred trotters of different ages and sexes. Equine Vet J (in press).
11. Lindholm A, Piehl K: Fibre composition, enzyme activity and concentration of metabolites and electrolytes in muscles of standardbred horses. Acta Vet Scand 1974; 15:287.
12. Henckel P: Training and growth induced changes in the middle gluteus muscle of young standardbred trotters. Equine Vet J 1983; 15:134.
13. Gottlieb JR, Essén-Gustavsson B, Lindholm A, et al: Effects of a draught loaded interval training programme on skeletal muscle in the horse. J Appl Physiol 1989; 67:570.
14. Henckel P: A histochemical assessment of the capillary blood supply of the middle gluteal muscle of thoroughbred horses. In Snow DH, Persson SGB, Rose RJ (eds): Equine Exercise Physiology. Cambridge, Granta Editions, 1983, p 225.
15. Snow DH, Baxter P, Rose RJ: Muscle fiber composition and glycogen depletion in horses competing in an endurance ride. Vet Rec 1981; 108:374.
16. Hodgson DR, Rose RJ, Allen J: Muscle glycogen depletion and repletion patterns in horses performing various distances of endurance exercise. In Snow DH, Persson SGB, Rose RJ (eds): Equine Exercise Physiology. Cambridge, Granta Editions, 1983, p 229.
17. Roneus M, Essén-Gustavsson B, Lindholm A, et al: A field study of circulatory response and muscle characteristics in young thoroughbreds. In Gillespie JR, Robinson NE (eds): Equine Exercise Physiology 2. Davis, Calif, ICEEP Publications, 1987, p 376.
18. Straub R, Hoppeler H, Dettwiler M, et al: Beurtechung der trainierbarkeit und der momentanen leistungskapazitart mit hilfe von Muskeluntersuchungen beim pferd. Schweiz Arch Tierheilk 1982; 124:529.
19. Wilson RG, Thornton JR, Inglis S, et al: Skeletal muscle adaptation in racehorses following high intensity interval training. In Gillespie JR, Robinson NE (eds): Equine Exercise Physiology 2. Davis, Calif, ICEEP Publications, 1987, p 367.
20. Foreman JH, Bayly WM, Allen JR, et al: Muscle responses of thoroughbreds to conventional race training and detraining. Am J Vet Res 1990; 51:909.
21. Cutmore CM, Snow DH, Newsholme EA: Activities of key enzymes of aerobic and anaerobic metabolism in middle gluteal muscle from trained and untrained horses. Equine Vet J 1985; 17:354.
22. Nimmo MA, Snow DH, Munro CD: Effects of nandrolone phenylpropionate in the horse: 3. Skeletal muscle composition in the exercising animal. Equine Vet J 1982; 14:229.
23. Essén-Gustavsson B, Lindholm A, McMiken D, et al: Skeletal muscle characteristics of young standardbreds in relation to growth and early training. In Snow DH, Persson SGB, Rose RJ (eds): Equine Exercise Physiology. Cambridge, Granta Editions, 1983, p 200.
24. Guy PS, Snow DH: The effects of training and detraining on LDH isoenzymes in horse skeletal muscle. Biochem Biophy Res Commun 1977; 25:863.
25. Snow DH, Harris RC: Thoroughbreds and greyhounds: Biochemical adaptions in creatures of nature and man. In Gilles R (ed): Circulation, Respiration and Metabolism. Berlin, Springer-Verlag, 1985, p 227.
26. Cutmore CM, Snow DH, Newsholme EA: Effects of training on enzyme activities involved in purine nucleotide metabolism. Equine Vet J 1986; 18:72.
27. Guy PS, Snow DH: The effect of training and detraining on muscle composition in the horse. J Physiol (Lond) 1977; 269:33.
28. Valberg S, Essén-Gustavsson B, Skoglund Wallberg H: Oxidative capacity of skeletal muscle fiber types in racehorses: Histochemical versus biochemical analysis. Equine Vet J 1988; 20:291.
29. Lindholm A, Bjerneld H, Saltin B: Glycogen depletion patterns in muscle fibres of trotting horses. Acta Physiol Scand 1974; 90:475.
30. Topliff DR, Potter GD, Dutson JL, et al: Diet manipulation and muscle glycogen in the equine. In Proceeding of the 8th Equine Nutrition and Physiology Symposium, 1983, p 119.
31. Topliff DR, Potter GD, Kreider JL, et al: Diet manipulation, muscle glycogen metabolism and anaerobic work performance in the equine. In Proceedings of the 9th Equine Nutrition and Physiology Symposium, 1985, p 224.
32. Harkins JD, Morris GS, Tulley RT, et al: Effects of added dietary

fat on racing performance in thoroughbred horses J Equine Vet Sci 1992; 12:123.

33. Scott BD, Potter GD, Greene LW, et al: Efficacy of fat-supplemented diet on muscle glycogen concentration in exercising thoroughbred horses maintained in varying body conditions. J Equine Vet Sci 1992; 12:109.

34. Parkhouse WS, McKenzie DC, Hochochka PW, et al: The relationship between carnosine levels, buffering capacity, fiber type and anaerobic capacity in elite athletes. *In* Knuttgen HG, Vogel JA, Poortmans J (eds): Biochemistry of Exercise. Ill, Champaign, Ill. Human Kinetics Publishers, 1983, p 590.

35. Sewell DA, Harris RC, Marlin DJ, et al: Estimation of the carnosine content of different fibre types in the middle gluteal muscle of the thoroughbred horse. J Physiol (Lond) 1992; 455:447.

36. Marlin DJ, Harris RC, Gash SP, et al: Carnosine content of the middle gluteal muscle in thoroughbred horses with relation to age, sex and training. Comp Biochem Physiol [A] 1989; 93:629.

37. Harris RC, Marlin DJ, Dunnett M, et al: Muscle buffering capacity and dipeptide content in the thoroughbred horse, greyhound dog and man. Comp Biochem Physiol [A] 1990; 97:249.

38. McCutcheon LJ, Kelso TB, Bertocci LA, et al: Buffering and aerobic capacity in equine muscle: Variation and effect of training. *In* Gillespie JR, Robinson NE (eds): Equine Exercise Physiology 2. Davis, Calif, ICEEP Publications, 1987, p 348.

39. Fox G, Henckel P, Juel C, et al: Skeletal muscle buffer capacity changes in standardbred horses: Effect of growth and training. *In* Gillespie JR, Robinson NE (eds): Equine Exercise Physiology 2. Davis, Calif, ICEEP Publications, 1987, p 341.

40. Sinha AK, Ray SP, Rose RJ: Effect of training intensity and detraining on adaptations in different skeletal muscles. *In* Persson SGB, Lindholm A, Jeffcott LB (eds): Equine Exercise Physiology 3. Davis, Calif, ICEEP Publications, 1991, p 223.

41. Persson SGB, Larsson M, Lindholm A: Effects of training on adreno-cortical function and red-cell volume in trotters. Zentralbl Vet Med [A] 1980; 27:261.

42. Lykkeboe G, Schougaard H, Johansen K: Training and exercise change in respiratory properties of blood in race horses. Respir Physiol 1977; 29:315.

43. Persson SGB: Evaluation of exercise tolerance and fitness in the performance horse. *In* Snow DH, Persson SGB, Rose RJ (eds): Equine Exercise Physiology. Cambridge, Granta Editions, 1983, p 441.

44. Sykes PE: Hematology as an aid in equine track practice. *In* Proceedings of the 12th Annual Convention of the American Association of Equine Practiners, 1966, p 159.

45. Allen BV, Powell DG: Effects of training and time of day of blood sampling on the variation of some common hematological parameters in normal thoroughbred racehorses. *In* Snow DH, Persson SGB, Rose RJ (eds): Equine Exercise Physiology. Cambridge, Granta Editions, 1983, p 328.

46. Stewart GA, Clarkson GT, Steel JD: Hematology of the racehorse and factors affecting interpretation of the blood count. *In* Proceedings of the Annual Convention of the American Association of Equine Practitioners, 1970, p 17.

47. Persson SGB: The circulatory significance of the splenic red cell pool. *In* Proceedings of the 1st International Symposium on Equine Hematology, 1975, p 303.

48. Rose RJ, Allen JR: Hematologic responses to exercise and training. Vet Clin North Am Equine Pract 1985; 1:461.

49. McKeever KH, Schurg WA, Jarrett SH, et al: Exercise training-induced hypervolemia in the horse. Med Sci Sports Exerc 1987; 19:21.

50. Rose RJ, Hodgson DR: Hematological and biochemical parameters in endurance horses during training. Equine Vet J 1982; 14:144.

51. Knight PK, Sinha AK, Rose RJ: Effects of training intensity on maximum oxygen uptake. *In* Persson SGB, Lindholm A, Jeffcott LB (eds): Equine Exercise Physiology 3. Davis, Calif, ICEEP Publications, 1991, p 77.

52. Foreman JH, Bayly WM, Grant BD, et al: Standardized exercise test and daily heart rate responses of thoroughbreds undergoing conventional race training and detraining. Am J Vet Res 1990; 51:914.

53. Thornton J, Essén-Gustavsson B, Lindholm A, et al: Effects of training and detraining on oxygen uptake, cardiac output, blood gas tensions, pH and lactate concentrations during and after exercise in the horse. *In* Snow DH, Persson SGB, Rose RJ (eds): Equine Exercise Physiology. Cambridge, Granta Editions, 1983, p 470.

54. Thomas DP, Fregin GF, Gerber NH, et al: Effects of training on cardiorespiratory function in the horse. Am J Physiol 1983; 245:R160.

55. Milne DW, Gabel AA, Muir WW, et al: Effects of training on heart rate, cardiac output, and lactic acid in standardbred horses, using a standardized exercise test. J Equine Med Surg 1977; 1:131.

56. Rose RJ, Allen JR, Hodgson DR, et al: Responses to submaximal treadmmil exercise and training in the horse: Changes in hematology, arterial blood gas and acid-base measurements, plasma biochemical values and heart rate. Vet Rec 1983; 113:612.

57. Evans DL, Rose RJ: Cardiovascular and respiratory responses to submaximal exercise training in the thoroughbred horse. Pflügers Arch 1988; 411:316.

58. Stewart GA: Drugs, performance and responses to exercise in the racehorse: 1. Physiological observations on the cardiac and respiratory responses. Aust Vet J 1972; 48:537.

59. Skarda RT, Muir WW, Milne DW, et al: Effects of training on resting and postexercise ECG in standardbred horses, using a standardized exercise test. Am J Vet Res 1976; 37:1485.

60. Rose RJ, Purdue RA, Hensley W: Plasma biochemistry alterations in horses during an endurance ride. Equine Vet J 1977; 9:122.

61. Rose RJ: An evaluation of heart rate and respiratory rate recovery for assessment of fitness during endurance rides. *In* Snow DH, Persson SGB, Rose RJ (eds): Equine Exercise Physiology. Cambridge, Granta Editions, 1983, p 505.

62. Cardinet GH, Fowler ME, Tyler WS: Heart rates and respiratory rates for evaluating performance in horses during endurance trail ride competition. J Am Vet Med Assoc 1963; 143:1303.

63. Bayly WM, Gabel AA, Barr SA: Cardiovascular effects of submaximal aerobic training on a treadmill in standardbred horses, using a standardized exercise test. Am J Vet Res 1983; 44. 544.

64. Thornton JR: Exercise testing. Vet Clin North Am Equine Pract 1985; 1:573.

65. Persson S: On blood volume and working capacity in horses. Acta Vet Scand 1967; (suppl 19):1.

66. Evans DL, Rose RJ: Cardiovascular and respiratory responses in thoroughbred horses during treadmill exercise. J Exp Biol 1988; 134:397.

67. Marsland WP: Heart rate response to submaximal exercise in the standardbred horse. J Appl Physiol 1968; 24:98.

17B

Training Regimens: Overview

D. L. EVANS

Regular exercise results in many physiologic responses that enable horses to perform athletic activity more easily and with less risk of injury. Studies of the effects of exercise training in horses have demonstrated adaptation of the cardiovascular system, blood, muscle, tendons and ligaments, bone, and thermoregulatory mechanisms. The aim of training is to provoke adaptation of relevant body systems to enable the horse to perform specific athletic tasks.

The physiologic and psychological demands of competitive events such as the 3-day event, show jumping, dressage, endurance rides, and commercial horse racing over distances of 400 m (1/4 mile) to 3200 m (2 miles) or more are extremely different. Therefore, training should be specific to the event so as to train the appropriate structures and physiologic systems. However, in all these events, training has the common aim of producing horses that are fit, healthy, and keen to compete. Readers are referred to other chapters for details of the specific adaptations that occur in various body systems of horses after physical training.

Physical training has traditionally been partitioned into aerobic and anaerobic training and divided into endurance, sprint, and strength training. The relative importance of each of these types of training depends on the duration and intensity of the event. Classification of training into these types is arbitrary, and there is overlap. For example, sprint training probably improves endurance capacity, and anaerobic training may increase maximal aerobic capacity.

Although there have been numerous studies describing physiologic responses to training in horses, few studies have compared responses to training at different intensities and durations or responses to interval training and continuous training. In addition, there has only been one report of measurement of anaerobic capacity in horses.[1] It is therefore difficult to be prescriptive for many aspects of horse training.

Energy Demands of Specific Events

An appreciation of the energy demand of the athletic event is important for the design of appropriate training programs (see Chap. 4). The relative contributions of aerobic and anaerobic pathways to the regeneration of ATP during exercise depend on both the intensity and the duration of exercise. Trot and slow canter exercise on level terrain can be regarded as purely aerobic. This means that the transport of oxygen can support almost all the energy demand of the exercise. There is very little contribution of either the creatine phosphate or lactate anaerobic pathways, and the exercise may be continued for hours. Exercise at such intensities is called *endurance exercise*. At the other extreme, sprint exercise over 200 to 500 m (1 to 2.5 furlongs) which lasts less than about 30 to 40 seconds relies principally on anaerobic energy production.

Most quarter horse, standardbred, and thoroughbred horse races last between 20 and 200 seconds. Energy supply in all these events is a combination of anaerobic and aerobic, with the brief events predominantly anaerobic and the longer races (2000 to 3200 m) principally aerobic. The relative contributions of aerobic and anaerobic mechanisms of ATP regeneration in events that require top speed for 20 to 200 seconds have been described, although estimates of the relative contributions differ markedly.[2-4] However, it is generally agreed that a sprint of 20 to 24 seconds' duration depends almost entirely on anaerobic ATP supply or resynthesis.

A race over 1000 to 1200 m (5 to 6 furlongs) has been described as being dependent on approximately one-third aerobic and two-thirds anaerobic mechanisms for energy supply.[3] The anaerobic mechanisms are attributed to both glycolysis (about two-thirds) and the creatinine phosphate and ATP stores (one-third). These events also have been estimated to be only 5 to 15 percent aerobic.[2,4] Events over 2000 m (10 furlongs) were thought to be from 25 to almost 90 percent dependent on aerobic pathways.[3,4]

However, recent measurements of the anaerobic capacity of thoroughbred racehorses indicate that the contribution of aerobic ATP resynthesis in events lasting 60 to 120 seconds has probably been underestimated. Anaerobic capacity in thoroughbred racehorses is approximately 30 ml O_2 equivalent per kg bodyweight,[1] and anaerobic energy sources probably contribute less than 30 percent of the total energy output in all standardbred and thoroughbred races.[1] The relative contributions of aerobic and anaerobic energy supply in horse races of different durations are described in Chapter 4. The contribution of aerobic ATP resynthesis is greater in horses than in humans exercising maximally for similar durations. This may be due to the much faster rate of increase in oxygen consumption at the commencement of exercise in horses.[5]

This partitioning of energy supply for events of different durations explains why horses can maintain top speed for only about 600 to 800 m. Anaerobic energy supply is limited, and the severe acidosis in muscle during high-intensity exercise can result in depletion of ATP concentrations in muscle coincident with fatigue and decreased speed.[6]

Training Intensity

Endurance training, or slow-speed long-distance training, involves prolonged exercise at low intensities. Such exercise at speeds of about 4 to 8 m/s usually results in heart rates of less than about 160 beats/min and no accumulation of lactate in blood. Heart rate meters have been used by some trainers to ensure that the training intensity is not excessive. The main limits to endurance training in horses are time available and hot, humid environments. Deaths of horses at endurance rides illustrate that they will willingly exercise for periods that result in extreme dehydration and electrolyte imbalance.

Horses may exercise for 5 minutes to several hours per day at the trot and/or slow canter, depending on fitness, environmental conditions, time available, the aim of the training, and the ambition of the trainer. Fit standardbred racehorses often trot or slow canter for 30 to 40 minutes on "slow" days. Fit thoroughbred horses might trot or canter for 5 to 10 minutes over 3000 to 5000 m, and endurance horses often exercise for 1 to 2 hours.

Low-intensity training is usually employed for some period in the first weeks of all training programs. This training is designed to improve the aerobic capacity and limb strength and educate the horse. The duration of this "pretraining" varies markedly among breeds, countries, and trainers. Some thoroughbreds undergo only 4 to 5 weeks of slow training before moving on to fast exercise.

Many months of slow, long-distance training before commencement of faster exercise have been advocated.[2] The principal argument for longer periods of low-intensity training is the development of stronger limbs and the consequent reduced frequency of limb injury. Anecdotal evidence suggests that the incidence of injuries is lower in horses that have undertaken more slow training. Shin soreness, or bucked shins, is a common problem in the training of young horses, especially thoroughbreds.[7] There is a lower incidence of the disease in horses that do not undergo rapid race preparations.[8]

There is some evidence that prolonged periods of endurance training stimulate continued adaptation of skeletal muscle. The activities of two enzymes used as markers of oxidative capacity of muscle continued to increase throughout a 9-month training program in endurance horses.[9] The implications of prolonged periods of endurance training for improvements in maximal aerobic capacity have not been reported.

Preparation of racehorses for racing necessitates gradual increases in the speed of exercise. It is only at exercise intensities that are near maximal that improvements in anaerobic capacity and anaerobic power can be expected. Lactic dehydrogenase (LDH) concentration in skeletal muscle has been used as a marker of anaerobic enzyme activity. Interval training at high speeds on a treadmill resulted in an increased concentration of LDH in skeletal muscle, but conventional training does not have the same effect.[10] Likewise, training at a moderate intensity (80 percent of $\dot{V}_{O_2max}$) for 6 weeks does not result in increases in skeletal muscle (gluteus medius) LDH concentration, although such training did increase the muscle buffering capacity by 8 percent and the ratio of fast-twitch highly oxidative fibers to fast-twitch fibers (FTH/FT).[11] These adaptations to training did not occur in a group of horses trained concurrently at a lower intensity (40 percent of $\dot{V}_{O_2max}$). It is possible that changes in training strategies, such as interval training at intensities that are near maximal, could result in beneficial adaptations in muscle. Such training necessitates careful monitoring of the intensity of exercise. Exercise at suboptimal intensities will limit the rate of adaptation, and supraoptimal intensities may contribute to a state of overtraining.

The exercise intensity during initial weeks of training is probably not an important determinant of the rate of change in maximal oxygen consumption ($\dot{V}_{O_2max}$). There was no difference in the changes in $\dot{V}_{O_2max}$ with training in two groups of horses trained at 40 and 80 percent of $\dot{V}_{O_2max}$.[12] Intensity of training may therefore be an important factor in determining the degree of local adaptations in skeletal muscle, but not for increases in maximal oxygen consumption.

Heart rate meters have been suggested as a tool for monitoring the intensity of strenuous submaximal exercise. For example, an exercise speed resulting in a heart rate of 200 beats/min has been suggested as suitable for race training.[13] However, there have been no controlled studies which have confirmed this view. In addition, the blood lactate concentration at intensities that result in a heart rate of 200 beats/min varies greatly. In unfit horses, exercise at heart rates of 200 beats/min is likely to result in high blood lactate concentrations, and in fit horses, such exercise may result in relatively low blood lactate concentrations.

There are also practical difficulties in the use of heart rate meters during exercise in galloping horses. It is difficult for jockeys on thoroughbred racehorses to monitor heart rate and adjust speed accordingly. The maximal heart rate of some horses is also 210 to 215 beats/min, only 5 percent greater than 200. In addition, muscular adaptations may not be optimal unless exercise is at speeds that result in maximal heart rate.[10]

Measurement of blood lactate level after exercise may be a more suitable way of monitoring the intensity of the prior exercise, but there have been no studies which have compared the adaptations to training in horses exercising at controlled blood lactate concentrations.

Training Specificity

Training of horses should be specific to the athletic event involved whenever possible. This principle need not be followed rigidly, since there are circumstances when alternative types of exercise may be appropriate for some horses.

It has been shown that show jumping generates mean postexercise blood lactate concentrations of 9 ± 0.9 mmol/liter,[14] which are similar to the concentrations found in thoroughbred horses exercising at 12 to 14 m/s. Jumping exercise for racehorses may be a useful adjunct to the usual training routines. It may relieve boredom and may provide an alternative to high-speed exercise as a means of training the anaerobic capacity of the horse.

Another interesting alternative to high-speed exercise is the use of treadmill trotting in combination with weight lifting.[15] Weights were added to a rope that ran over a pulley, connected horizontally from behind the treadmill to a harness. While trotting at 4.8 m/s and lifting loads of 60 to 100 kg, heart rates increased to a mean of 209 beats/min, and blood lactate levels after exercise ranged from 5 to 16 mmol/liter. The relationships between oxygen consumption and both heart rate and blood lactate concentrations are similar for draught work and normal submaximal treadmill exercise.[16] This technique may be useful for increasing the training stimulus at low treadmill speeds. Addition of loads to the sulky has been used for training of trotting horses in Sweden.

Swimming is popular with some trainers, and many training centers provide a pool for horses. Horses use a trotting or pacing gait for swimming, and it has been noted that the breathing pattern was characterized by brief inspiration, prolonged expiration, and looked "painful."[17] Certainly many horses appear to have difficulty breathing when swimming. This is probably due to the pressure applied to the chest and abdomen of the horse by the water, which would necessitate more forceful muscular contractions in the chest wall and diaphragm to generate the same decreases in intrathoracic pressure. It may be that swimming is a good way of training the respiratory muscles. However, it also results in relatively high blood pressures compared with galloping.[18]

Free swimming is similar in intensity to trotting and slow cantering.[17] A training effect was found, since heart rate during swimming decreased over a 4-week period of regular swimming exercise. Heart rates ranged from 140 to 180 beats/min, and blood lactate concentrations only increased by two- to fourfold above resting values during the swimming. Horses were exercised for 5 minutes daily in the first week, and the duration was increased by 5 minutes each week thereafter. It was thought that swimming was appropriate for the development of basic physical fitness and for rehabilitation of horses with limb problems. Prolonged swimming for 1 hour did not cause excessive increases in body temperature. It was suggested that the direction of swimming in circular pools be changed regularly during prolonged swimming to avoid fatigue in the outside legs.

Tethered swimming may be an appropriate means of increasing the intensity of swimming. This technique involves securing the horse by a tail rope and encouraging the horse to greater effort.[18] This resulted in heart rates of 170 to 200 beats/min and blood lactate levels of between 1 and 10 mmol/liter in five unfit horses swimming for 5 minutes.

Interval Training

Interval training is defined as the use of multiple exercise bouts separated by rest periods. It offers the opportunity to increase the frequency of exercise and so increase the total training stimulus. No study has yet concluded that interval training is superior to conventional training where the total amount of exercise performed is the same. When conventional training and interval training of standardbreds were compared, no significant difference was found in postexercise heart rates. However, the total slow- and fast-work distances undertaken were the same in both training schedules.[19] Interval training over 10 weeks did not produce greater adaptation in quarter horses trotting on a treadmill.[20] Interval training of thoroughbreds appeared to offer some advantage in one study, but it is likely that the total amounts of work performed were much greater in the interval trained group.[21]

It has been shown that standardbred racehorses interval trained on a treadmill had improved metacarpal bone quality.[22] The training schedule consisted of 5 weeks of slow exercise of 6 to 12 km/day at 5 m/s. This was followed by a 9-week period of interval training, during the last 3 weeks of which the horses performed three to four intervals per day over 600 to 1000 m at or above speeds which resulted in maximum heart rate. Bone quality improved throughout the training period.

Interval training may increase the risk of injury.[4] It is therefore very important that the speed of the exercise be closely monitored and be at appropriate speeds and that recovery periods between bouts of exercise be adequate.

Overtraining

For most horse trainers, there is a delicate balance between attaining and maintaining peak fitness, and lameness or overtraining. Overtraining is defined as a loss of performance ability despite the maintenance of or an increase in training effort. Athletic performance decreases and horses must cease or reduce training for variable periods of time for recovery.

The physiologic basis of overtraining in human athletes is poorly understood,[23] but the heart rate and blood lactate response to exercise, body weight, and mood state are sometimes closely monitored to detect early overtraining during periods of intense exercise training. Two studies also have reported a distortion of the relationship between heart rate and speed of exercise as an indication of overtraining in horses. Heart rate is elevated at a set speed,[24] or the treadmill velocity at a heart rate of 200 beats/min may be decreased.[25] Regular measurement of heart rate during a standardized submaximal exercise test may assist the management of horses during periods of intense training. An increase in total red cell volume also has been reported in overtrained trotters.[25]

Disturbances to immune function also have been reported in horses during strenuous exercise training.[26] The implications of these observations for performance or the incidence or severity of disease in horses during strenuous training are unknown.

Detraining

Detraining refers to the sudden cessation of training. Many horses have their training preparations interrupted by ill-health or injury. There have been few studies of the effects of detraining, and the results are confusing.

In standardbreds, mean treadmill speed at a heart rate of 200 beats/min was not significantly different from values obtained after 5 weeks of intense training.[27] The same study found that there was no consistent change in V_{LA4} (treadmill velocity at which blood lactate is 4 mmol/liter) with detraining. It is possible that the weekly exercise tests in this detraining study maintained fitness.

Two weeks of detraining reduced $\dot{V}_{O_2max}$ to values near those before training,[13] and the value continued to decrease over a 6-week period (Fig. 17B–1). In the same horses, buffering capacity significantly decreased over a 6-week period,[11] reversing the adaptation that occurred with prior training (Fig. 17B–2). Three weeks of detraining resulted in a 12 percent decrease in $\dot{V}_{O_2max}$ in 10 thor-

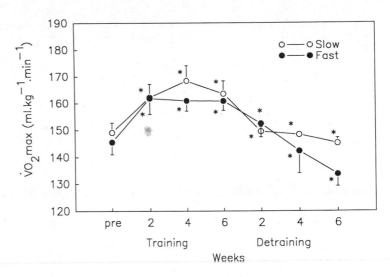

*Figure 17B-1. Maximum oxygen uptake ($\dot{V}_{O_2max}$) for horses during training and detraining. Fast group was trained at 80 percent of $\dot{V}_{O_2max}$; slow group at 40 percent of $\dot{V}_{O_2max}$ (mean ± SEM). *Significant difference from pretraining value (p < 0.01). (From Effects of training intensity on maximum oxygen uptake. In Persson SGB, Lindholm A, Jeffcott LB (eds): Equine Exercise Physiology 3, Davis: ICEEP Publications, 191, p. 77, with permission.)*

oughbreds.[28] These results suggest that there is rapid loss of some training adaptations with enforced rest. Further studies are required before any general recommendations can be made concerning the effects and time course of losses of adaptations to detraining.

Training and Rehabilitation from Injury

The effect of exercise on the healing of articular cartilage defects in the equine carpus was examined in 12 horses.[29] It was concluded that a 13-week period of graduated exercise (walking, trotting, and later cantering) after surgical creation of a cartilage defect was not detrimental to the rate of repair.

Training also increases the strength of the suspensory ligaments.[30] The mean absolute load necessary to

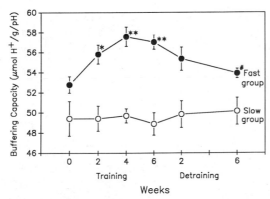

*Figure 17B-2. Muscle buffering capacity in gluteus medius muscle during training and detraining (mean ± SEM). *p < 0.05; **p < 0.01 significantly different from before training; #p < 0.05 significantly different from end of training (week 6). (From Skeletal muscle adaption to different training intensities and to detraining in different hindlimb muscles in thoroughbred horses. In Persson SGB, Lindholm A, Jeffcott LB (eds): Equine Exercise Physiology 3, Davis: ICEEP Publications, 1991, p. 223, with permission.)*

cause failure of the suspensory apparati with compression testing was higher in tissue from trained horses. In untrained horses, the site of rupture was through the suspensory ligament, whereas in the trained horses, the site of rupture in most cases was through the proximal sesamoid bones. Restoration of strength in the suspensory ligaments should employ a graduated period of exercise training.

Postexercise Recovery

There are no special strategies for recovery from prolonged exercise except provision of water, electrolytes, and a high-energy diet. Prolonged hosing with cool water may assist the cooling-down process if exercise has been conducted in a hot environment. Low-energy diets such as hay may contribute to delayed glycogen resynthesis in the 2- to 3-day period after exercise.[31]

The recovery process after intense exercise is influenced by the use of a "warm-down" period of exercise. Both walking and trotting for 20 to 70 minutes after exercise increase the rate at which blood and muscle lactate concentrations decrease after exercise. Ten minutes of activity had little effect, but by 40 minutes postexercise, blood lactate concentrations were about 4 to 10 mmol/liter lower with continuous trotting and 2 to 5 mmol/liter lower if the horses walked during recovery. These results probably reflect increased use of lactate as a substrate for aerobic metabolism supporting the postexercise activity.[32] There may be no important implications of a more rapid rate of decline in postexercise blood lactate for the recovery process other than a possible training effect of such exercise.

Conclusions

The expense and time-consuming nature of research projects examining aspects of training in horses have precluded rapid gains in knowledge in this area. There are many devotees of "scientific" horse training methods, but it is difficult to assess quantitatively the relative success of different training programs. However, a knowledge of the general principles of training should assist any trainer of the equine athlete to achieve optimal results.

Acknowledgments

The helpful suggestions offered by Michael Eaton and Alan Davie are very much appreciated.

References

1. Eaton MD, Rose RJ, Evans DL, et al. The asssment of anaerobic capacity of thoroughbred horses using maximal accumulated oxygen deficit. Aust Equine Vet 1992; 10:86.
2. Ivers T: The Fit Racehorse. Cincinnati, Esprit Racing Team, Ltd., 1983.
3. McMiken DF: An energetic basis of equine performance. Equine Vet J 1983; 15:123.
4. Bayly WM: Training programs. Vet Clin North Am Equine Pract 1985; 1:597.
5. Evans DL, Rose RJ: Dynamics of cardiorespiratory function in standardbred horses during constant load exercise. J Comp Physiol [B] 1988; 157:791.
6. Harris RC, Marlin DJ, Snow DH: Metabolic response to maximal exercise of 800 m and 2000 m in the thoroughbred horse. J Appl Physiol 1987; 63:12.
7. Nunamaker DM, Butterweck DM, Provost MT: Fatigue fractures in thoroughbred racehorses: Relationships with age, peak bone strain and training. J Orthop Res 1990; 8:604.
8. Buckingham SHW, Jeffcott LB: Shin soreness: A survey of thoroughbred trainers and racetrack veterinarians. Aust Equine Vet 1990; 8:148.
9. Hodgson DR, Rose RJ: Effects of a nine-month endurance training program on skeletal muscle composition in the horse. Vet Rec 1987; 121:271.
10. Lovell DK, Rose RJ: Changes in skeletal muscle composition in response to interval and high intensity training. In Persson SGB, Lindholm A, Jeffcott LB (eds): Equine Exercise Physiology 3. Davis, Calif, ICEEP Publications, 1991, p 215.
11. Sinha AK, Ray SP, Rose RJ: Skeletal muscle adaptations to different training intensities and to detraining in different hindlimb muscles in thoroughbred horses. In Persson SGB, Lindholm A, Jeffcott LB (eds): Equine Exercise Physiology 3. Davis, Calif, ICEEP Publications, 1991, p 223.
12. Knight PK, Sinha AK, Rose RJ: Effects of training intensity on maximum oxygen uptake. In Persson SGB, Lindholm A, Jeffcott LB (eds): Equine Exercise Physiology 3. Davis, Calif, ICEEP Publications, 1991, p 77.
13. Gysin J, Isler R, Straub R: Evaluation of performance capacity and definition of training intensity using heart rate and blood lactate measurements. Pferdeheilkunde 1987; 3:193.
14. Art T, Amory H, Desmecht D, et al: The effect of show jumping on heart rate, blood lactate and other plasma biochemical values. Equine Vet J 1990; (suppl 9):78.
15. Gottlieb M, Essén-Gustavsson B, Lindholm A, et al: Cardiorespiratory and muscle metabolic responses to draught work on a treadmill in standardbred horses. In Gillespie JR, Robinson NE

16. Gottlieb-Vedi M, Essén-Gustavsson B, Persson SGB: Draught load and speed compared by submaximal exercise tests on a treadmill. In Persson SGB, Lindholm A, Jeffcott LB (eds): Equine Exercise Physiology 3. Davis, Calif, ICEEP Publications, 1991, p 92.
17. Murakami M, Imahara T, Inui T, et al: Swimming exercises in horses. Exp Rep Equine Health Lab 1976; 13:27.
18. Thomas DP, Fregin GF, Gerber NH, et al: Cardiorespiratory adjustments to tethered-swimming in the horse. Pflugers Arch 1980; 385:65.
19. Gabel AA, Milne DW, Muir WW, et al: Some physiological responses of standardbred horses to a submaximal exercise test following conventional and interval training. In Snow DH, Persson SGB, Rose RJ (eds): Equine Exercise Physiology. Cambridge, Granta Editions, 1983, p 497.
20. Rodiek AV, Lawrence LM, Russell MA: Cardiovascular effects of intermittent or continuous treadmill conditioning in horses. J Equine Vet Sci 1987; 7:14.
21. Harkins JD, Kammerling SG, Bagwell CA, et al: A comparative study of interval and conventional training in thoroughbred racehorses. Equine Vet J 1990; (suppl 9):14.
22. McCarthy RN, Jeffcott LB: Monitoring the effects of treadmill exercise on bone by non-invasive means during a progressive fitness programme. Equine Vet J 1988; (suppl 6):88.
23. Fry RW, Morton AR, Keast D: Overtraining in athletes: An update. Sports Med 1991; 12:32.
24. Erickson BK, Erickson HH, Sexton WL, et al: Performance evaluation and detection of injury during exercise training in the quarter horse using a heart rate computer. In Gillespie JR, Robinson NE (eds): Equine Exercise Physiology 2. Davis, Calif, ICEEP Publications, 1987, p 92.
25. Persson SGB, Larsson M, Lindholm A: Effects of training on adrenocortical function and red-cell volume in trotters. Zentralbl Vet Med [A] 1980; 27:261.
26. Buschmann H, Baumann M: Alterations of cellular immune response during intensive training of event horses. J Vet Med [B] 1990; 38:90.
27. Thornton J, Essén-Gustavsson B, Lindholm A, et al: Effects of training and detraining on oxygen uptake, cardiac output, blood gas tensions, pH and lactate concentrations during and after exercise in the horse. In Snow DH, Persson SGB, Rose RJ (eds): Equine Exercise Physiology. Cambridge, Granta Editions, 1983, p 470.
28. Art T, Lekeux P: Training-induced modifications in cardiorespiratory and ventilatory measurements in thoroughbred horses. Equine Vet J 1993; 25:532.
29. French DA, Barber SM, Leach DH, et al: The effect of exercise on the healing of articular cartilage defects in the equine carpus. Vet Surg 1989; 18:312.
30. Bramlage LR, Bukowiecki CW, Gabel AA: The effect of training on the suspensory apparatus of the horse. In Proceedings of the 35th Annual Convention of the American Association of Equine Practitioners, 1990, p 245.
31. Snow DH, Harris RC, Harman JC, et al: Glycogen repletion following different diets. In Gillespie JR, Robinson NE (eds): Equine Exercise Physiology 2. Davis, Calif, ICEEP Publications, 1987, p 701.
32. Marlin DJ, Harris RC, Harman JC, et al: Influence of post-exercise activity on rates of muscle and blood lactate disappearance in the thoroughbred horse. In Gillespie JR, Robinson NE (eds): Equine Exercise Physiology 2. Davis, Calif, ICEEP Publications, 1987, p 321.

17C

Training Thoroughbred Racehorses

D. L. EVANS

In the past, many trainers of thoroughbred racehorses have been successful without a formal knowledge of the science of exercise or training. However, as in most fields of endeavor, modification of traditional techniques and application of new findings will frequently reap greater rewards. Many trainers are now using the science of equine exercise as an aid to training. This section presents some of the new research findings that are relevant to the training of thoroughbred racehorses. I will also present some personal opinions.

Training thoroughbred racehorses is probably more difficult than training endurance horses or quarter horses. The metabolic demands of thoroughbred racing over distances of 1000 to 3200 m (5 to 16 furlongs) are quite different. In addition, there have been no published studies which apportion the contribution of anaerobic and aerobic ATP supply in such events. A report of the measurement of the anaerobic capacity in thoroughbred racehorses[1] suggests that thoroughbred racing is a much more aerobic activity than previously believed.[2,3] The contribution of aerobic ATP resynthesis is probably greater than 60 percent in all thoroughbred racehorses, with about 90 percent of the energy demands in a 2-mile race likely to be supplied by oxygen-dependent metabolism. The physiology of thoroughbred training is probably similar to strategies used for training human athletes to compete over track distances of 800 to 1600 m.

Thoroughbred trainers must therefore train horses so that demands are placed on the aerobic and anaerobic energy pathways to increase both endurance and speed. A comparison of training methods for thoroughbreds in different countries illustrates that there are many ways of achieving these objectives.[4]

Phases of Training

It is convenient to divide training into three phases:

- *Phase 1:* Endurance training at speeds less than 600 m/min
- *Phase 2:* Combined aerobic and anaerobic training at 70 to 80 percent of maximal speed (750 to 850 m/min)
- *Phase 3:* Anaerobic training for development of speed and acceleration

PHASE 1: ENDURANCE TRAINING

Endurance exercise at the start of any thoroughbred training program is vital for the racing future of the horse. It involves exercise at slow speeds (trot and canter at speeds up to 600 m/min) over long distances. The distances used vary greatly among trainers.

Such exercise rapidly increases maximal oxygen consumption. Within 2 to 6 weeks, 10 to 23 percent increases in maximal oxygen consumption have been reported.[5,6] However, it is likely that prolonged endurance training over many months will result in gradual improvement in the maximal aerobic capacity of the horse, as in humans. The oxidative potential of muscle in-

creased over a 9-month period of training in endurance horses.[7]

The other important role of the initial weeks of endurance training is the development of strength in bone and soft tissue in the limbs. Recent studies have shown that these structures adapt to the training stimulus. A substantial adaptive remodeling response to conventional North American race training in 2-year-old thoroughbreds has been demonstrated in the proximal sesamoid bones.[8] Treadmill training in young thoroughbreds also improves the bone quality of the third metacarpal bone[9] and strength of the suspensory ligaments.[10] However, little is known about the durations or intensities of exercise that promote optimal adaptive responses in bone or soft tissues.

It is likely that the greatest adaptation will occur if the "overload" principle is followed. This principle is relevant to the adaptation of many body systems in horses in training. It refers to the necessity for a gradual increase in the training stimulus every 2 to 3 weeks. This period gives time for adaptation to the current training demands before increasing the stress of the training to induce further adaptations. Many of the problems found in thoroughbred training, such as bucked shins[11] and periodic inappetence,[12] are probably related to rapid increases in the intensity of training so that there has been insufficient time for adaptation.

Endurance exercise training of thoroughbreds can be conducted in many ways besides the traditional use of a jockey. Treadmill exercise at the trot and canter, jogging horses behind trucks or beside horses in carts, and swimming have been used successfully. It is important not to rely exclusively on exercise without using a jockey, especially in young horses, since this period of training is as important for development of the horse's behaviour as it is for the physical adaptations to training.

A 14-week period of treadmill training has demonstrated the effects of training on third metacarpus bone quality in 13- to 14-month-old thoroughbred horses.[9] The treadmill training program used in this study is summarized in Table 17C–1. The training did not produce any clinical signs of bucked shins but did result in several important adaptive responses in the cortices of the metacarpal bones of the young horses com-

Table 17C-1. *Treadmill Exercise Program Used to Train Six Thoroughbred Horses Aged 13 to 14 Months*[9]

Weeks of training	Training exercise
1–2	Trot 2 to 4 km/day at 4 m/s (5 %)
3–7	Trot 800 m at 4 m/s, then canter 1.0 to 1.6 km at 8 to 12.5 m/s, then trot 1.0 to 1.2 km at 4 m/s (5 %)
8–9	Trot 2 to 4 km/day at 4 m/s (5 %)
10–14	Gallop 1.2 to 1.6 km/day at speeds up to 14.5 m/s (0 %)

Note: Treadmill angle is indicated in parentheses.

Source: From McCarthy RN, Jeffcott LB: Effects of treadmill exercise on cortical bone in the third metacarpus of young horses. Res Vet Sci 52:28, 1992, with permission.

pared with unexercised controls. These included an increased amount of subcortical bone, increased bone mineral content, and increased bone stiffness. Ultrasound speed through the metacarpal bones of the trained group also increased. It was concluded that a period of graduated treadmill training in young horses resulted in adaptations of the cortex of the third metacarpal bone that provide a structure more capable of resisting exercise-induced injury. Further studies are needed to examine the implications of these responses for injury-free racing in 2-year-old thoroughbreds.

Swimming should be used sparingly in endurance training of thoroughbreds. It does promote cardiovascular fitness[13] but probably does not develop limb strength or gait coordination. Frequent use of swimming also breaks one of the major rules of training, that is, specificity. *Specificity* refers to the need for training to mimic the gait that is employed in competition so that structural changes in the limb are appropriate to the stresses of competitive events.

Typical slow-speed training in Australia involves only 4 to 5 weeks of training at a trot and canter over 3 to 5 km (2 to 3 miles) per day before moving on to faster exercise at greater than 20 seconds per furlong.[12] Thoroughbred trainers in England tend to employ greater durations of slow exercise over a period of 3 months or more, especially in 2-year-old horses. My impression is that English 2-year-olds have a lower incidence of bucked shins than Australian or North American horses. Rapid preparation of 2-year-olds in Australia has been identified as an important contributing factor in the incidence of bucked shins.[11]

It is not possible to make specific recommendations about the duration of the trotting and cantering endurance training of thoroughbreds. Thoroughbreds can canter about 10,000 meters at about 500 m/min in one bout 6 days per week after a suitable 3- to 5-month prior training and adaptation period.[14] More prolonged endurance training also has been recommended.[2] There is obviously a balance to be struck between the likely adaptive advantages and the financial cost of prolonged training periods. If conditions are hot and humid, it is appropriate to break up the endurance training into 10- to 15-minute sessions if relatively high-speed cantering is being used. This will obviate the risk of exhaustion due to hyperthermia.

Slow-speed training has been subdivided into a slow, long-distance training phase and a phase at slightly faster speeds termed *cardiovascular fitness work* for improvement of the oxygen transport system.[2] This division is entirely arbitrary, since no differences have been demonstrated in the degree or rate of change in cardiovascular fitness during training at different speeds of submaximal exercise.

One study illustrated no differences in the degree or rate of change in $\dot{V}_{O_2max}$ of horses trained at 40 and 80 percent of $\dot{V}_{O_2max}$.[6] However, the recommendation that a prolonged period of exercise at speeds up to about half pace with gradual increases in the stress of training every few weeks[2] is likely to be physiologically appropriate.

PHASE 2: COMBINED AEROBIC AND ANAEROBIC TRAINING

The overload principle dictates that the training speed should gradually approach racing speed. Training at about 70 to 80 percent of racing speed results in accumulation of lactate in the muscle and blood of the horse. This indicates that anaerobic glycolysis has been employed by some muscle cells to support the need for ATP supply. Exercise at speeds that produce high blood lactate concentrations, such as 15 to 20 mmol/liter, which approximate those found after racing, cannot be maintained for prolonged periods or be repeated daily. The inevitable consequence of attempts to do so will be lameness and/or a state of overtraining, reflected in weight loss, inappetence, loss of interest in racing, and poor performance.

However, training at 70 to 85 percent of racing speed (about 14 to 16 seconds per furlong) is an important component of thoroughbred training, since it stimulates muscle adaptations that reflect improved capacity for anaerobic ATP resynthesis. Such adaptations include increased percentage of type II fibers, increased buffering capacity, and increased concentrations of enzymes involved in anaerobic metabolism.[15,16] There seem to be large variations among trainers and countries in the techniques and relative importance of this type of training.

After a period of 4 to 5 weeks of training at a trot and canter over 2 to 3 miles/day ("pretraining"), thoroughbred trainers in Australia usually alternate between fast and slow mornings. On slow days, horses are exercised on average 5500 m at speeds between 4 and 7 m/s (trot and slow canter). On fast days, horses exercise at speeds between 12 and 16 m/s over 1000 to 2000 m after a warmup of 1000 m.[12]

Conventional training in North America reportedly employs "breeze" work at about 75 percent of maximal speed every 7 to 10 days interspersed with walking, jogging, and swimming.[14] A conventional racetrack program in the United States also has been described as gallops at near-maximal speed for 600, 800, or 1000 m every fifth day. On intervening days, horses were walked, trotted, and cantered over a total distance of about 5 km.[17]

A detailed description of a typical 9-week conventional thoroughbred training program in United States has been published.[18] Horses trotted 2400 m each day in week 1 and 4000 m each day in week 2. After 2 weeks of training at the slow speed, horses were introduced to additional 1200-m gallops at about 400 to 500 m/min. The distance of the gallops was increased to 3200 m in the sixth week. Fast gallops, or breezes, at 900 to 950 m/min were then given every 5 days over distances of 600 to 1000 m. These gallops were followed by rest days and then 3 days of the trot and gallop exercise in a 5-day rotation. The percentages of maximal heart rate achieved in the trotting, gallops, and breezes were approximately 50 to 60, 70 to 90, and 90 to 100 percent, respectively.

In England, training of the aerobic and anaerobic

systems includes regular multiple exercise bouts on hills, combined with exercise on level ground over 800 to 1600 m at about 14 to 15 seconds per 200 m. For example, 6 days of training could include 10 canters up an 800-m incline at about 20 seconds per 200 m and two workouts over 1200 m at the higher speeds. Horses canter up hills one to three times a day at speeds that usually generate postexercise blood lactate concentrations of 3 to 15 mmol/liter. These concentrations are similar to those found after single bouts of 1200-m exercise at 14 to 15 seconds per 200 m on level ground.

Two main intensities of exercise on flat sand tracks have been described for training thoroughbred horses in Germany.[19] In addition to slow work at speeds less than 11 m/s for less than 3 minutes, horses also work at faster speeds which generate high blood lactate concentrations. At a mean speed of 13 m/s for 100 seconds, average maximal postexercise blood lactate concentration was 16.3 mmol/liter.

Traditional training of thoroughbreds may not fully exploit the potential of combined aerobic and anaerobic training at strenuous submaximal speeds. Interval training of thoroughbred horses on an inclined treadmill (5 percent) at speeds of 10 to 12 m/s (about 17 to 20 seconds per furlong) resulted in increased lactate dehydrogenase concentrations in the skeletal muscle. This adaptation is not seen in traditional training programs.[16]

Strategies for increasing the volume of training which stimulate anaerobic glycolysis without causing fatigue and overtraining include increased training distance or frequency and use of exercise on hills or treadmills inclined at 5 to 10 percent.

Many horses in Australia are exercised at 70 to 80 percent of top speed for distances much less than race distance, although some trainers frequently use exercise at about 15 seconds per 200 m over distances anticipated during racing. My experience is that thoroughbreds can successfully perform exercise at that speed over 1000 m at least once daily 5 days per week in addition to daily treadmill exercise. Treadmill exercise can consist of 1600 m of trotting and slow cantering, 3-minute rest periods, and then fast canter exercise over 1200 to 1600 m. Such fast canters usually result in postexercise blood lactate concentrations of about 4 mmol/liter.

Increased training frequency can employ training at appropriate speeds on more days per week than usual or interval training. *Interval training* refers to the use of multiple workouts on the same day separated by short rest periods.[20] Interval training has been advocated as a way of increasing fitness,[2] but there have been few investigations of the possible advantages of interval training compared with continuous training.

Interval training on a treadmill does result in increased fitness, as measured by the heart rate response to exercise.[21] Recent evidence also suggests that interval training may increase the anaerobic capacity of thoroughbreds. This conclusion was based on a finding of higher rates of lactate production and increased plasma lactate clearance rates in the interval-trained horses.[14] However, differences in the responses to training in in-

terval-trained and conventionally trained horses in this study may have been due to differences in the total amount of training performed rather than a reflection of the use of interval training. The relationships between anaerobic capacity and blood lactate responses to exercise in racehorses have not been described.

An interval training program in thoroughbreds was used to investigate skeletal muscle adaptations to training.[22] After a warmup trot and canter over 1200 m, horses performed increasing numbers of 600-m gallops at speeds of 820 to 860 m/min. One-minute rest periods were given between gallops. In weeks 1–2, 3–4, 5–6, and 7–8, horses completed 1, 2, 3, and 4 × 600-m gallops, respectively. Horses galloped 3 days per week in week 1 and 5 days per week in other weeks, with 2 rest days 3 days apart. This training program significantly increased the mean V_{LA4} (exercise speed that results in blood lactate concentration of 4 mmol/liter) derived from a racetrack exercise test from 540 to 670 m/min. In addition, the percentage of highly oxidative type II muscle fibers increased from 43 to 50 percent.[22]

The advantage of hill or treadmill exercise for strenuous submaximal training is the reduced speed of the exercise and reduced likelihood of injury. When treadmills are used for such training, the work speed can be carefully controlled, and blood lactate concentrations and/or heart rates are easy to monitor in order to regulate the intensity of exercise.

Swimming is not appropriate for improving the anaerobic endurance of horses, since heart rates during swimming are generally less than 180 beats/min.[23] Moreover, swimming is not specific to competitive exercise and therefore may not stimulate adaptation in muscles recruited during running.

PHASE 3: ANAEROBIC TRAINING

Thoroughbred horse racing over any distance employs some exercise at top speed and usually necessitates rapid acceleration at some stage of the race. It is therefore important that this aspect of training not be ignored. Traditionally, there has been very little training of thoroughbreds specifically for speed and acceleration. Most top-speed exercise is given at the completion of work at submaximal speeds. For example, horses often exercise over 600 to 1600 m at 14 to 16 seconds per 200 m and then gallop over another 200 to 600 m at 95 to 100 percent of top speed.

Specific speed and acceleration training could employ frequent exercise at top speeds over 1 to 2 furlongs. Interval-training techniques would be appropriate. Sprints shorter than 40 to 45 seconds' duration are probably necessary to improve anaerobic capacity.[22] The number of brief-duration, high-speed intervals should be increased gradually every 2 to 3 weeks, with intensive training days probably limited to twice weekly. Other training days through the week can be of the slow or moderate training intensities described above. Some race fit and nearly fit thoroughbreds in England are maintained on a 3-day rotation twice weekly. Horses are given phase 1, 2, and 3 exercise on successive days. A similar regimen does not result in progressive depletion of muscle glycogen reserves.[24]

However, frequent use of high-speed interval training over 600 m or more is probably inappropriate. In eight thoroughbreds that performed four 600-m exercise bouts at near-maximal speeds with 5-minute rest periods between exercise sessions, muscle glycogen concentrations were reduced by approximately 50 percent.[25] Therefore, it would be unwise to employ frequent interval training at 95 to 100 percent of top speed over distances of 800 to 1200 m (4 to 6 furlongs). Such training may lead to overtraining and the possible disintegration of 3 to 5 months of adaptation to prior training.

Maintenance of fitness does not require intensive and frequent training. The frequency of training can be reduced when horses are racing every 2 weeks. Several days of recovery are necessary for full restoration of muscle glycogen stores.[26]

Conclusions

The difficult task for the trainer of the race fit horse is to balance the demands of racing, postrace recovery, maintenance of fitness, and mental attitude of the horse. It is unlikely that scientific formulas will ever be devised to give trainers exact recipes for management of the fit racehorse from week to week and race to race. The experience of the individual trainer and recognition of the individual attitudes, attributes, and needs of each horse in the stable then become even more important.

Acknowledgments

The helpful suggestions offered by Michael Eaton and Alan Davie are very much appreciated.

References

1. Eaton MD, Rose RJ, Evans DL, et al: The assessment of anaerobic capacity of thoroughbred horses using maximal accumulated oxygen deficit. Aust Equine Vet 1992; 10:86.
2. Ivers T: The Fit Racehorse. Cincinnati, Esprit Racing Team, Ltd., 1983.
3. Bayly WM: Training programs. Vet Clin North Am Equine Prac 1985; 1:597.
4. Staaden R: Winning Trainers Their Road to the Top. Perth, Australia, Headway International Publishing, 1991.
5. Evans DL, Rose RJ: Cardiovascular and respiratory responses to submaximal exercise training in the thoroughbred horse. Pflugers Arch 1988; 411:316.
6. Knight PK, Sinha AK, Rose RJ: Effects of training intensity on maximum oxygen uptake. In Persson SGB, Lindholm A, Jeffcott LB (eds): Equine Exercise Physiology 3. Davis, Calif, ICEEP Publications, 1991, p 77.
7. Hodgson DR, Rose RJ: Effects of a nine-month endurance training program on skeletal muscle composition in the horse. Vet Rec 1987; 121:271.
8. Nunamaker DM, Butterweck DM, Provost MT: Fatigue fractures in thoroughbred racehorses: Relationships with age, peak bone strain and training. J Orthop Res 1990; 8:604.
9. McCarthy RN, Jeffcott LB: Effects of treadmill exercise on cortical bone in the third metacarpus of young horses. Res Vet Sci 1992; 52:28.
10. Bramlage LR, Bukowiecki CW, Gabel AA: The effect of training on the suspensory apparatus of the horse. In Proceedings of the 35th Annual Convention of the American Association of Equine Practitioners, 1990, p 245.
11. Buckingham SHW, Jeffcott LB: Shin soreness: A survey of thoroughbred trainers and racetrack veterinarians. Aust Equine Vet 1990; 8:148.
12. Southwood LL, Evans DL, Bryden WL, et al: Nutrient intake of horses at thoroughbred and standardbred stables. Aust Vet J 1993; 70:164.
13. Thomas DP, Fregin GF, Gerber NH, et al: Cardiorespiratory adjustments to tethered swimming in the horse. Pflugers Arch 1980; 385:65.
14. Harkins JD, Kammerling SG, Bagwell CA, et al: A comparative study of interval and conventional training in thoroughbred racehorses. Equine Vet J 1990; (suppl 9):14.
15. Sinha AK, Ray SP, Rose RJ: Skeletal muscle adaptations to different training intensities and to detraining in different hindlimb muscles in thoroughbred horses. In Persson SGB, Lindholm A, Jeffcott LB (eds): Equine Exercise Physiology 3. Davis, Calif, ICEEP Publications, 1991, p 223.
16. Lovell DK, Rose RJ: Changes in skeletal muscle composition in response to interval and high intensity training. In Persson SGB, Lindholm A, Jeffcott LB (eds): Equine Exercise Physiology 3. Davis, Calif, ICEEP Publications, 1991, p 215.
17. McCutcheon LJ, Kelso TB, Bertocci LA, et al: Buffering and aerobic capacity in equine muscle: variation and effect of training. In Gillespie JR, Robinson NE (eds): Equine Exercise Physiology 2. Davis, Calif, ICEEP Publications, 1987, p 348.
18. Foreman JH, Bayly WM, Grant BD, et al: Standardized exercise test and daily heart rate responses of thoroughbreds undergoing conventional race training and detraining. Am J Vet Res 1990; 51:914.
19. Lindner A, Von Wittke P, Schmald M, et al: Maximal lactate concentrations in horses after exercise of different duration and intensity. J Equine Vet Sci 1992; 12:36.
20. Daniels J, Scardina N: Interval training and performance. Sports Med 1984; 1:327.
21. Harkins JD, Kammerling SG: Assessment of treadmill interval training on fitness. J Equine Vet Sci 1991; 11:237.
22. Wilson RG, Thornton JR, Inglis S, et al: Skeletal muscle adaptation in racehorses following high intensity interval training. In Gillespie JR, Robinson NE (eds): Equine Exercise Physiology 2. Davis, Calif, ICEEP Publications, 1987, p 367.
23. Murakami M, Imahara T, Inui T, et al: Swimming exercises in horses. Exp Rep Equine Health Lab 1976; 13:27.
24. Snow DH, Harris RC: Effects of daily exercise on muscle glycogen in the Thoroughbred racehorse. In Persson SGB, Lindholm A, Jeffcott LB (eds): Equine Exercise Physiology 3. Davis, Calif, ICEEP Publications, 1991, p 299.
25. Hodgson DR, Kelso TB, Bayly WM, et al: Responses to repeated high-intensity exercise: Influence on muscle metabolism. In Gillespie JR, Robinson NE (eds): Equine Exercise Physiology 2. Davis, Calif, ICEEP Publications, 1987, p 302.
26. Snow DH, Harris RC, Harman JC, et al: Glycogen repletion following different diets. In Gillespie JR, Robinson NE (eds): Equine Exercise Physiology 2. Davis, Calif, ICEEP Publications, 1987, p 701.

Training Standardbred Trotters and Pacers

D. LOVELL

Training Standardbred Racehorses

Two incidents have been indelibly stamped on my mind since my interest first turned to sports medicine and its possible implications for improvement of training methods applicable to preparing horses for racing. Both are anecdotal and have absolutely no scientific foundation, but they have very important messages.

The first occurred while I was watching the Australian movie dramatizing the life of Phar Lap, the champion racehorse. Toward the end of the movie, Harry Telford, the trainer, says to his wife in despair, "Phar Lap will win in Caliente. He'll win wherever else he races. For years I've kidded myself that I made that horse. The truth is he would have been a champion no matter who trained him. I've got 20 colts out there, all with blood lines as good as or better than his. I've trained them all exactly the same as him. Everyone's a dud. He's a freak!"

The second point relates to the chapter on the training of standardbreds by Stanley Dancer in the USTA publication *Care & Training of the Trotter & Pacer.*[1] Dancer gave an extremely detailed and intricate description of how he trained and managed the horses in his stable, which left no doubts in the readers' minds as to the importance of not overtraining horses. He then related how he traveled to New Zealand to purchase Cardigan Bay and observed in detail the methods employed to train horses in that country, which were the complete antithesis of his own. He described the concern he felt at paying so much money for a horse and then having to be able to reproduce that form under a different training and racing system. The horse's success under Dancer is history. He sums things up by stating, "A great horse is a great horse regardless of the training system you use. I think you have to use a little common sense and hit a happy medium somewhere, but aside from that, a trainer is pretty much on his own. Cardigan Bay is a perfect example of that. He was a champion while racing under two different systems."

Where are we in our quest for improvement in training techniques? Much was written and postulated in the early 1980s about how improved and scientific training methods would revolutionize race performance, but little has resulted. The definitive work undoubtedly was Tom Ivers book, *The Fit Racehorse.*[2] However, 10 years later, the "ill-equipped incompetents" Ivers refers to are still in control of the preparation of race horses, while most scientific sports medicine trainers are out of work. What has been happening?

I suggest that an aspiring training revolutionary should do two things: First, go to the racetrack, watch horses race, and make an objective observation of what has happened. Several things will become obvious:

- The 10 or 12 competitors are all trying hard to win.
- There is often very little distance between the first and last horse.
- Tactics are very important in the race. The last 400 m is usually run in fast time. As a result, it is very difficult for horses to make up ground on the leaders in this last part of the race.

- Horses are graded or assessed so that they race against other horses of similar ability.
- It is clear that racing is a competitive business, and there is more to successful performance than simply introducing a scientific conditioning program to improve the horse's performance.

Second, make a list of the top 10 trainers in your area, and then make an assessment of why you think they are successful. Again, some consistent trends emerge:

- Most successful trainers have a relatively high turnover of horses each year. This is perhaps their major secret for success. They do not persevere with horses that have little or no ability or some other problem that will prevent them from performing well. The major ingredient these trainers have for success is their ability to attract new horses from owners. Success leads to success, so owners are more willing to send horses to trainers who are producing winners.
- Successful trainers are always very good drivers, or they engage the best drivers available.
- Most successful trainers train their horses in a similar manner using techniques that are often maligned by some exercise scientists.

The important basic message is that the business of racing horses is a professional practice. Successful trainers are invariably highly qualified specialists who, in most cases, have spent many years learning their trade and developing their skills. A certain system has evolved over 200 years of horse racing that has been honed and fine-tuned again and again to develop a protocol practiced by these tradesmen. Successful trainers can prepare and present a horse for racing in a practical, cost-efficient manner, and no one has been able to demonstrate that these horses are not racing at their peak performance capability.

I believe that the major area where we have gone wrong over the last 15 years or so in trying to introduce new training techniques has been to ignore successful trainers who have so much to offer. A lot of damage has been done, and the whole field of equine exercise physiology has lost much of the initial support it had from horse people. A fresh new approach is called for.

The basis for this must surely be to first examine the obvious. Look closely at the exact techniques and methods used by trainers to prepare their horses, and make objective assessments of just what effects these actually have on the conditioning and physiology of the horse. Can the performance of an animal presented for a race, particularly one that is competing successfully, really be improved?

In training the standardbred racehorse, the definitive training manual has already been written. *The Care & Training of the Trotter & Pacer*[3] was published in 1968 and is a vital source for any student of standardbred training. Of particular relevance is the chapter on training and conditioning by Dancer.[1] Here the great trainer provides detailed and intricate programs for the preparation of a wide variety of horses for racing. Racing has changed a lot in the last 25 years, and times are considerably faster now than they were then, but the principles are the same. The improvement in race times has been due primarily to changes in track and sulky design and the evolution of a faster breed of horse brought about by the introduction of artificial insemination. Very little of the improvement can actually be credited to changes in training methods. If improvement in racetrack performance is going to be achieved, it may best be achieved by adaptations made after analysis of the strengths and weaknesses of current methods.

The present-day standardbred has been carefully selected and bred for speed and performance over many generations, and there is really not a lot of difference in the speed capabilities of the majority of horses. Most horses can pace a very fast quarter mile and so are capable of performing at competitive speeds. The successful racehorse, however, must be able to put together at least four successive quarter miles at these speeds. As well as *speed,* this requires two additional attributes, *stamina* or *endurance* and *competitiveness* or *"the will to win."* The successful racehorse must have a combination of these features, and it is the job of the horse trainer to develop these traits to produce a horse that will perform at its best on race day. All three traits are profoundly influenced by the trainer, and neglect of any area will result in suboptimal performance. The realm of the exercise sciences is related mainly to stamina. Perhaps a major contribution to failures by the "scientists" has been neglect of the other two!

[Once again, I would like to mention that genetic inheritance of the right combination of these factors is still the primary requisite for an outstanding racehorse, and no trainer will be successful with a horse that does not have them. Therefore, a trainer must be able to select from large numbers of horses if he or she is to be able to maintain a position at the top of the winning trainers' list.]

Preparing a Horse for Racing

The "art" of training horses for optimal racing performance depends on refining the factors of *speed, stamina,* and *competitiveness* in the individual and presenting the horse on race day so that none of them alone will limit performance. Arbitrarily, the three can be considered separately, but they are closely interrelated.

SPEED

Lambert,[4] referring to thoroughbreds, states, "each horse has a maximum speed at which it can run and breathe and that speed renders the horse more or less competitive. Furthermore, each horse has its own variety of structural and physiological limitations to both pace and endurance, and finally, the whole picture is made more complicated by unsoundness." He is referring to the very important fact that breathing in the horse is intimately synchronized with stride and that speed is the product of stride length and stride frequency. To increase speed, the horse has to increase stride length or frequency or both. Because of the limitations imposed by the entrainment to breathing, there is a structural and functional upper limit to each animal's speed. Superior racehorses are genetically endowed with the necessary factors to allow them to move at a faster speed than other horses.

Maximal speed is probably inherent, and little can be done to increase a horse's maximal speed. However, the trainer plays an essential role in developing this speed. The standardbred has to be able to trot or pace at high speed pulling a sulky and driver and be able to do this for much of the time while going around corners. Balancing and gearing the horse correctly are essential to allow the horse to attain maximal speed. No animal can possibly perform at its best if its legs are interfering or if the harness and gear are uncomfortable. Much of the success or otherwise of a horse's performance depends on getting all the dynamic factors correct. There are no rules, and each animal is different. The trainer must be constantly analyzing the horse's action and movement and then fine-tuning the horse's rigging. Obviously, trimming and shoeing the feet are the most crucial factor in avoiding interference, and most situations where the horse is "hanging," "going roughly," or "hiking" can be traced back to some problem in the feet. The lightest possible shoes that will protect the horse's feet and encourage the optimal flight and stride must be selected because extra weight on the horse's feet must inevitably be a factor in fatigue.

The training process also brings about radical changes in the horse's management, appearance, and body weight, all of which prepare the horse for speed. The untrained horse at pasture depends on grass and forage as the natural food. The biggest part of a pasture horse is its abdominal constituents, and this is primarily because such a high-fiber diet requires a large amount of water or fluid to allow fermentation and digestion to occur. No animal can possibly run quickly if it is anchored down by large volumes of body fluid and fiber. All the energy for performance comes from feed, so the diet must be adjusted to provide for the tremendous increase in energy requirements brought on by the increase in daily workload. Because this is brought about by changing from a high-fiber roughage diet to a grain and concentrate diet, there is a reduction in the mass of the abdominal contents. These changes are all part of the training process and require thought and attention from the trainer. The capacity for speed is increased as these changes occur.

STAMINA

If we concede that speed is not really improved by training, then stamina is a most important feature upon which to focus. A given level of work can be maintained by an individual for a finite length of time before fatigue occurs. Improving stamina implies increasing the ability to maintain that exercise intensity for longer durations or to be able to perform a higher exercise intensity for the same time. To understand what training is doing and to base training prescriptions correctly, there are certain fundamentals of physiology that must be understood and applied to training.

Progressive Loading and Training Specificity. Adaptations to training occur primarily in the musculoskeletal and cardiorespiratory systems. The changes are dynamic and continual, and the response to a workload imposed today will not be seen until some time in the future, since the body must have time to respond. The concept of progressive loading is well documented and is the means by which an increasing level of exercise is applied to continually challenge the body systems to adapt so that they are better able to perform the tasks demanded. The concept of specificity of work also has been commonly put forward, but the reasons for its importance are perhaps not as clearly understood.

All the power for locomotion and propulsion is derived from muscular contraction. Obviously, the primary muscles involved are those of the hind quarters, but all the body muscles perform some function, even if only to help in maintaining balance.

The different muscle fiber types (slow- and fast-twitch fibers) are recruited for contraction by a differential nerve supply so that for slow, steady work, only the slower, aerobic-type fibers are normally called into action. With faster or more intense exercise, more of the fast-twitch fibers are recruited, in addition to the slow-twitch fibers. Further discussion of muscle fiber types can be found in Chapter 8. When considered in relation to the muscular system, the importance of training specificity is easily appreciated. If the training load is not heavy enough, the muscle fibers recruited will not be those required during competition, so little adaptation or improvement can be expected.

Exercise Physiology and Training. Much research has now been conducted into the various training responses of equine body systems to exercise and training. Some relevant points include the following:

1. *Skeletal muscle* shows a very rapid and dramatic change in metabolic characteristics with training. The oxidative capacity of muscle has a tremendous capacity for enhancement with training. Even low-intensity, submaximal training programs have produced a very significant increase in muscle oxidative capacity. Very intense training may improve muscle glycolytic and buffering capacities.

2. *Maximal oxygen uptake* shows an initial increase with the onset of training, even at submaximal loads. The rate of increase after longer or more intense programs is not as spectacular.

The implications of these findings are that perhaps the horse, under whatever type of conditioning program, is capable of responding very rapidly to improve its ability to run fast, and all horses will give a very similar response to even relatively low workloads. The rate of change after this initial response is much slower.

3. *Exercise at speeds approaching maximum* result in a large reduction in the glycogen content of muscle. This then takes 48 to 72 hours to return to pre-exercise concentrations. Consequently, horses should have a recovery period between severe exercise bouts to allow the muscles to "fuel up" again.

4. The horse shows a tremendous *adaptive physiologic response to the onset of exercise*. The heart rate is capable of a tremendous increase from a resting rate in the low thirties to a maximal rate of approximately 220 to 240 beats/min. Since the amount of blood pumped per beat (stroke volume) remains relatively constant, there is a tremendous increase in cardiac output with exercise. The oxygen-carrying capacity of the blood is a function of the numbers of circulating red cells and increases dramatically as the packed cell volume rises from 35 to 40 percent at rest to values of 60 to 65 percent during intense exercise, the result of mobilization of a red cell reserve in the spleen. Respiratory rate increases from 10 to 21 breaths/min at rest up to values in excess of 150 breaths/min at maximal exercise. This increases the volume of air breathed in and out from 100 to 1600 to 1800 liters/min. Nature has endowed the horse with an incredible ability to perform at high speeds, a situation very different from that of the human, and it is unreasonable to expect that training methods used by human athletes should transpose to the horse.

5. *Heart rate* increases in direct relationship with the speed or workload at slower or submaximal speeds up to a certain point, after which, although the horse is capable of going much faster, the heart rate remains the same. Maximal oxygen uptake also increases in a similar pattern, and in fact, the speed at which the heart rate reaches a plateau is also the speed at which the ability of the cardiopulmonary system to supply oxygen to the muscles also reaches its maximum. Beyond this speed, energy requirements of working muscle are met by anaerobic mechanisms.

This relationship between speed and heart rate is undoubtedly the most important concept we need to be aware of if we are going to apply any sort of scientific analysis or input into training programs. The heart rate at maximum speed ($V_{HR_{max}}$) is the key training speed upon which all training programs should be based. Below this speed, the horse is not stressing its aerobic energy delivery systems to their maximum. Above this speed, anaerobic energy sources play a major role in the energy supply, and fatigue occurs quickly. At about 80 percent of $V_{HR_{max}}$, lactate, a major by-product of anaerobic metabolism, will start to accumulate in the blood. In practice, variations certainly occur, but the theory is useful when examining training programs. Many trainers have purchased heart rate meters over the years, but most have discarded them because they had no concept of how to use them. The purpose of a heart rate meter is to allow the trainer to tailor make a training program to suit an individual's $V_{HR_{max}}$. At the very least, monitoring this speed will allow the trainer to assess the horse's improvement in condition. If the training is being successful, the speed at which HR_{max} occurs will progressively increase as training progresses. This means that the aerobic capacity, or the ability of the body to perform a certain level of effort with energy supplied by the oxidative pathways, is increasing.

It is now time to introduce the concept of *total anaerobic capacity*. Production of large proportions of the energy requirement by the glycolytic pathways, as is necessary when the exercise intensity exceeds the $V_{HR_{max}}$, results in the accumulation of undesirable waste products, the principal culprit being lactate. Lactate buildup produces a dramatic fall in the pH of the muscle cell environment. This is popularly regarded, although by no means conclusively proven, to be a major cause of fatigue that limits performance. There is no question that high-intensity exercise rapidly leads to fatigue or the point at which the level of performance can no longer be maintained. Whatever the actual cause, the point is soon reached where activity at that level has to cease. Each individual has a finite capacity for supply of energy by anaerobic means during performance. Once this capacity has been reached, fatigue occurs, and performance is reduced. The correctly run race is the one where the capacity for anaerobic energy supply is reached when the horse is just past the finish post. Once again, this is an overly simplistic view, but this concept is important in understanding the tactics of racing and the principles of what we are aiming for in training horses for racing.

Tactically, if there is a certain amount of anaerobic capacity available, it must be used carefully to achieve the best result. If the horse is allowed to lead and run the race at its own pace, the situation is easy. The horse can be rated to use up its reserve at a constant rate and arrive at the finish just as the reserve expires. This rarely occurs. In most cases, three surges are necessary during a race. A sprint at the start to achieve a position, a sprint during the race to improve position, and a sprint to the finish line. If the energy reserve has been used up before the finish line, the horse will slow down and may be incapable of winning. In between these surges, the horse is eased to slow the rate of usage and, hopefully, if training has been successful, allow some degree of recovery.

The principles to aim for in training with this anaerobic capacity reserve in mind are

1. To maximize aerobic sources of energy supply so that the anaerobic energy available can be spared as much as possible.
2. To increase the amount of anaerobic power available. There is still much debate as to whether any such increase really does occur in response to training, and experimental results are inconclusive. Certainly little improvement has been detected in conventionally trained animals.
3. To increase the tolerance of the body to the waste products of glycolysis. This occurs in two ways. The ability of the body to buffer the fall in pH produced by the accumulation of lactate occurs in many ways. The main buffer is the blood bicarbonate system, and obviously, an improvement in circulation through the muscles and lungs in response to training must be beneficial. There are also local muscle buffering systems using certain amino acids, and the belief is that repetitive exposure of the muscle to lactate results in an increase in local buffering capacity. The second means of developing lactate tolerance involves an increased ability of the body to dispose of the lactate. Effects of training on this process are still open to conjecture.

Specificity and loading again must be mentioned because if the training load is not high enough to produce lactate, then no adaptive response can be expected. However, if the load is too high, fatigue will occur rapidly, and the metabolic processes will be significantly impaired. Therefore, bouts of exercise at $V_{HR_{max}}$ once again must be the aim, since this ensures that some lactate is produced and yet not at levels likely to cause rapid fatigue.

Improving stamina is therefore the collation of the body systems' responses to progressively increasing levels of repetitious workloads specific for the exercise involved that ultimately allows the individual to perform the work more efficiently.

COMPETITIVENESS

Competitiveness or "the will to win" is probably the most important of the qualities the horse needs to perform satisfactorily and is primarily an inherent characteristic that determines how good an individual is going to be. This is an intangible characteristic that is unmeasurable but essential for outstanding performance. Basically, it implies that an individual is so driven by the urge to dominate that it ignores the physiologic warning signals that the body is exceeding its capacity to absorb the by-products of maximal performance and yet still continues to perform in the face of possible breakdown.

There is also a psychological factor involved over which the trainer has a profound influence, and this is the actual freshness or state of mind of the competitor at the time of the race. This depends on the ability of the trainer to "peak" the horse for performance, and this is where the real art of training a racehorse is applied. The successful trainer seems somehow to be able to subjectively assess his or her charge and decide just how much work the horse needs to reach its peak. Overtraining is the major cause of loss of form in racehorses, and it would appear to be simply a loss of the individual's ability to perform at its best. Many attempts have been made to assess and measure physiologic values to explain a loss of form, but none has been conclusive. Those involved in the scientific training of racehorses need to be careful that they do not cause an animal to lose its competitiveness or "will to win."

Current Training Programs

The training charts outlined by Dancer[1] provide us with a basis for assessment of the workloads imposed on horses in practical training situations. The actual times now will be faster than those 25 years ago, but if it is assumed that today's times are faster primarily because of technical improvements, then the relative workloads will be similar.

In Dancer's recommendations,[1] horses were being prepared for a constant race distance of 1600 m. The 6 days per week training is broken into 4 jog days and 2 "fast" days. Initially, untrained horses are given 4 weeks of jogging only before they commence their faster work. Jogging consists of a workload of 3, 4, or 5 miles (5 to 8 km) per day at a speed of approximately 5 minutes per mile (320 m/min). Heart rates at this slow speed are extremely labile but are usually in the range of 120 to 150 beats/min. Metabolism is essentially aerobic. Fast days commence and consist of 2 days per week with three heats per day. Each heat is over a constant distance of 1 mile (1600 m), the actual race distance, and so a horse will train 6 heat miles per week. Dancer[1] aims for his untrained horses to have between 75 and 100 of these training "miles" before they race. The principle of progressive loading is applied carefully over the 12 to 16 weeks of preparation, with the miles each week becoming a little faster. Only one of these miles each week is anywhere near racing speed. When the horse is racing, the race is this fast mile. When not racing, the last heat on one of the days is the fast mile, and the other five training miles are slower.

In Dancer's examples,[1] the races were being run in times of between 2 minutes and 2 minutes and 10 seconds, and we can presume these represent maximal effort. No horses were trained at race speeds just prior to racing. On the fast training day, the horse would go in 2 minutes and 12 seconds to 2 minutes and 15 seconds, with the last 400 m in 30 seconds, or close to race speed. The other 5 miles per week were much slower. The first mile each day would be in 2 minutes and 45 seconds (580 m/min) and the other three between 2 minutes and 20 seconds (685 m/min) and 2 minutes and 30 seconds (640 m/min). All these speeds are submaximal. At 700 m/min (a mile in 2 minutes and 17 seconds), most horses are close to the speed where the heart rate becomes maximal. Dancer,[1] and by inference, many of the other North American trainers, has been "interval training" his horses all the time and at speeds just below the point at which maximal heart rate occurs. Lactate is being produced, but not at a rate that will result in a large accumulation in the bloodstream. The most significant difference between these methods and what is accepted as interval training in human athletes is the time between heats. Standardbred trainers allow 40 to 60 minutes between heats for the horse to properly "cool out."

Inadvertently, many standardbred trainers have been practicing good principles of exercise physiology all the time. These methods have evolved by trial and error over many years and have been found to be the most suitable methods for training standardbreds for racing under North American conditions. These trainers have been training by the stopwatch, not by a heart rate meter, but they have been achieving a similar result. The advent of the heart rate meter has allowed us to actually measure the relative workload. While the heart rate tends to fluctuate at slow jogging speeds, once the horse works at speeds above a 3-minute mile or around 540 m/min, the heart rate will stabilize and remain relatively constant at any given speed. At this speed, the rate will be about 180 beats/min in most horses. At speeds above this, the heart rate will climb until the maximal heart rate is reached, at which point the heart rate versus speed plateaus. Further analysis of Dancer's methods[1] will reveal that even his "fast" mile in a training week has not really been overchallenging the horse. A 2-minute and 15 second mile will be rated so that only the last 400 m is run at fast speed. The first 800 m will be run in 1 minute and 10 seconds (685 m/min), the next 400 m in 34 seconds, (705 m/min), and the final 400 meters in 31 seconds (775 m/min). The heart rates correspondingly will be submaximal for the first 800 m, at about the $V_{HR_{max}}$ speed for 400 m, and then a maximal effort (i.e., a speed greater than $V_{HR_{max}}$ for the last 400 m for the week). Exercise scientists may argue that giving the horse harder workouts will improve its fitness. Theoretically, this is correct, but how much harder? Do we increase speed, distance, or frequency? Horses, unlike human athletes, are not motivated by honor, glory, and financial rewards, so they do not have the same incentive to push themselves to near the body's limits.

Training methods in Australia and New Zealand are very different from those in the United States. The horses certainly are given more work in Australia, but racing is also different. Race distances vary from 1600 m (1 mile) to 3200 m (2 miles), with the majority of races being 1600 or 2100 m. The horse is trained for more endurance, and this is achieved mainly by increasing the "jog" miles. Most horses will jog about 10 miles on slow days. They generally have three fast work days per week but only work one period. This usually takes one of two forms: Either a 3200-m workout with the first 2400 m rated submaximally and the last 800 m in 60 to 63 seconds, with the last quarter in 30 seconds, or they work what is called "double headers," where the horse works a mile, evenly rated at around 2 minutes and 15 seconds, then stays on the track walking for 5 to 10 minutes, and then works another mile with the final 800 m at close to racing speed. Once again, the horses are rarely worked at really high speed. They are given more total distance than horses in the United States, but the faster miles each week still only total six, and most of the work is done at around $V_{HR_{max}}$. Different racing, different parts of the world, different training methods, but the basic underlying principles are really not very different. Can this be improved?

Scientific Training Programs

Much has been written about V_{200}, which is the velocity at which a horse's heart rate will stay steady at about

200 beats/min, being the ideal training speed. Similarly, the term V_{LA4}, which is the speed at which the blood lactate concentration will remain around 4 mmol/liter, has been advocated as an ideal training speed. However, exercise scientists are only talking quantitatively about the same workloads that trainers are already using. Most scientists advocate more distance, but there has been no evidence to show that this improves a horse's race performance. Professional trainers still win most of the races, and although many have tried the newer recommendations, most have reverted to their proven techniques.

Any changes to training must be reasonably simple to use, economically realistic, and seen to have benefit over the current practices. The major disadvantages of the present systems are that they are entirely subjective in their prescription. There are no rules, and nothing is measurable except for speed. Trainers determine the horse's training speed by subjective judgment. Good trainers undoubtedly have this ability as a natural instinct, and this is what sets them above their competitors. Measurable values would help the less able individuals tailor their horses' workloads and would undoubtedly make the physiologist feel better. Workloads such as V_{200} and V_{LA4} have been attempts to do this. The V_{LA4} determination is not simple, requiring multiple blood samples during a standardized exercise test. However, it is a good concept, since it determines a precise physiologic value tailored to suit each individual. The V_{200} can be measured using a heart rate meter and a standardized exercise test. Use of V_{200} has the disadvantage that it assumes that all horses have the same maximal heart rate. However, horses' maximal heart rates vary over the range 210 to 240 beats/min. A horse with a low maximal heart rate working at V_{200} will be working fairly hard. A horse with a maximal rate of 240 beats/min working at V_{200} will only be working at 80 percent capacity. A better technique is to work the horse at a percentage of maximal heart rate. This is no more difficult than determining V_{200} and physiologically is more correct.

To determine $V_{HR_{max}}$, the horse is worked four heats at submaximal speeds, and the speed and heart rate are recorded. The heats must be of long enough duration for the heart rate to stabilize at a constant value. A distance of 1000 m is suitable. Speeds for the heats should be submaximal and examples might be

Heat 1	3.00-minute mile rate, or approximately 550 m/min
Heat 2	2.45-minute mile rate (approximately 600 m/min)
Heat 3	2.30-minute mile rate (approximately 650 m/min)
Heat 4	2.20-minute mile rate (approximately 700 m/min)

The maximal heart rate for the horse also must be determined, and this is recorded during a bout of exercise at maximal speed. Heart rate versus speed is plotted, with rate on the y axis and speed on the x axis. A hori-

zontal line is drawn across the graph at the maximal heart rate value. The points are plotted for heart rate versus speed and are joined. A relatively straight line will be produced, and this line is continued upward to intersect with the heart rate maximum line (Fig. 17D–1). This point will now give the point on the x axis that is $V_{HR_{max}}$. A far simpler method involves the use of a computer-programmed linear regression calculator that will derive this at the push of a button, but not all trainers have access to these.

As the horse's fitness improves, if training is to be deemed successful, the $V_{HR_{max}}$ will increase progressively and so must be redetermined. Every 2 weeks is the minimum time, since the body must have time to respond to the loads applied. Response will be much quicker early in the training, after which the rate of improvement will slow as speeds increase, resulting in the decrease in frequency of retesting. The maximal heart rate will not change significantly and need only be determined once, but the $V_{HR_{max}}$ will increase progressively if the horse's fitness is improving.

We now have a physiologically meaningful speed that can be used to determine workload for horses in training and which can be adapted and changed easily to complement the increases in fitness as training progresses. The ways in which this speed can be used to control training are endless and depend on the whim of the trainer. The basic philosophy, however, should be that the training heats should be performed at close to this speed. In practice, nothing is ever absolute, so for safety the training speed should be calculated at just below the derived speed. A value of 90 to 95 percent of $V_{HR_{max}}$ should be calculated and horses worked at this speed.

"Interval" trainers can program whatever combinations of distance and recoveries they desire, but the speed should be constant. Any speed greater than the derived speed is going to be above $V_{HR_{max}}$, so those who wish to work the horse over a distance and then sprint home the final 400 or 800 m know the safe speed for the first part of the workout and then how fast they need to go to work at speeds above $V_{HR_{max}}$. Conventional train-

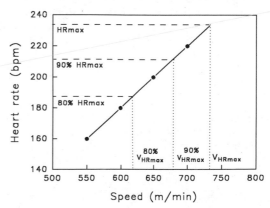

Figure 17D-1. *Calculation of percentages of maximal heart rate from measured values for heart rate at different speeds.*

ers have a speed on which to base their training miles. This speed is going to be close to the speeds already being used, but now it is simply based on measurable indices rather than the trainer's intuition.

A mention should be made of swimming as it applies to standardbred training because it is a commonly employed technique. Nothing could be less specific in training principle, but it is amazing how many horses race successfully with a swimming component in their work. Swimming does not train the glycolytic energy pathways. Heart rates obtained while swimming rarely exceed 160 to 180 beats/min and are often less in the lazier horse. While the intensity of swimming work is only moderate, most horses that swim a lot during training do so because of a lameness problem and the swimming is used to reduce the concussive effects of track work. Many of these horses have led a substantial track preparation and have been brought up to race level before the swimming becomes a major contributor to the training regimen. Swimming is used to maintain some level of exercise between races, which are in fact their fast work. Swimming does play a very useful role in conditioning. The commonly used expression that swimming is "good for the wind" is absolutely correct. Horses working on the track develop a rhythm of body and abdominal content movements that serves to help the necessary expansion and collapse of the thoracic cavity that draws air into and out of the lungs for respiration. Swimming horses have no such rhythm, and they have to rely on the respiratory groups of muscles, the intercostal and lateral chest muscles, to expand the chest cavity to draw air into their chest and the diaphragm and abdominal muscles to force air out. This is very hard work and makes these muscles perform more work than usual. How and whether this actually translates to the track are not known, but it is conceivable that some direct benefit may apply.

Suggested Training Protocol

There is no such thing as a formal training program that can be picked off the shelf and put into practice with any horse. Each animal is an individual, and what suits one might ruin another. The following is intended as a guideline only to provide a framework that must be tailored to each individual. The program outlined is for a mature horse that has raced before but has been turned out for a prolonged rest ("lay up").

PRETRAINING

Four weeks of jogging during which time the horse is reintroduced to the routine of stable life is the starting point. Diet is changed to prepare the horse for intensive training, and the body is generally toned up. Note: Unless otherwise specified, a jog = 5 minutes per mile pace.

Week 1

Monday	Jog 5000 m (3 miles) at 5 minutes per mile

Tuesday	Jog 5000 m (3 miles)
Wednesday	Jog 6000 m (4 miles)
Thursday	Jog 6000 m (4 miles)
Friday	Jog 6000 m (4 miles)
Saturday	Jog 6000 m (4 miles)
Sunday	Off

Week 2

Monday	Jog 8000 m (5 miles)
Tuesday	Jog 8000 m (5 miles)
Wednesday	Jog 8000 m (5 miles)
Thursday	Jog 8000 m (5 miles)
Friday	Jog 8000 m (5 miles)
Saturday	Jog 10,000 m (6 miles)
Sunday	Off

Week 3

Monday	Jog 10,000 m (6 miles)
Tuesday	Jog 10,000 m (6 miles)
Wednesday	Jog 10,000 m (6 miles)
Thursday	Jog 10,000 m (6 miles)
Friday	Jog 10,000 m (6 miles)
Saturday	Jog 10,000 m (6 miles)
Sunday	Off

Week 4

Monday	Jog 13,000 m (8 miles)
Tuesday	Jog 13,000 m (8 miles)
Wednesday	Jog 13,000 m (8 miles)
Thursday	Jog 13,000 m (8 miles)
Friday	Jog 13,000 m (8 miles)
Saturday	Jog 3000 m (2 miles), exercise test to derive $V_{HR_{max}}$
Sunday	Off

FOUNDATION TRAINING

The horse commences a 4-week program of interval training at a predetermined target speed. Between heats, horses are kept on the track but walked for approximately 10 minutes before the next heat. Heart rate should be monitored and a normal recovery pattern established for each horse. Any deviation from this would preclude continuing the day's session. All horses should recover to a heart rate of at least 110 beats/min while walking. Exercise testing to determine $V_{HR_{max}}$ should be repeated every 2 weeks, and the derived speed should be increasing each time.

Week 5

Monday	Jog 10,000 m (6 miles)
Tuesday	Jog 3000 m (2 miles), 2 × 1000 m at 90 percent of $V_{HR_{max}}$
Wednesday	Jog 10,000 m (6 miles)
Thursday	Jog 3000 m (2 miles), 2 × 1000 m at 90 percent of $V_{HR_{max}}$
Friday	Jog 10,000 m (6 miles)

Saturday	Jog 3000 m (2 miles), 3 × 1000 m at 90 percent of $V_{HR_{max}}$
Sunday	Off

Week 6

Monday	Jog 10,000 m (6 miles)
Tuesday	Jog 3,000 m (2 miles), 3 × 1000 m at 90 percent of $V_{HR_{max}}$
Wednesday	Jog 10,000 m (6 miles)
Thursday	Jog 3,000 m (2 miles), 3 × 1000 m at 90 percent of $V_{HR_{max}}$
Friday	Jog 3000 m (2 miles), exercise test to derive $V_{HR_{max}}$
Saturday	Jog 3000 m (2 miles), 3 × 1000 m at 90 percent of $V_{HR_{max}}$
Sunday	Off

Week 7

Monday	Jog 10,000 m (6 miles)
Tuesday	Jog 3,000 m (2 miles), 3 × 1000 m at 90 percent of $V_{HR_{max}}$
Wednesday	Jog 10,000 m (6 miles)
Thursday	Jog 3,000 m (2 miles), 3 × 1000 m at 90 percent of $V_{HR_{max}}$
Friday	Jog 10,000 m (6 miles)
Saturday	Jog 3000 m (2 miles), 3 × 1000 m at 90 percent of $V_{HR_{max}}$
Sunday	Off

Week 8

Monday	Jog 10,000 m (6 miles)
Tuesday	Jog 3000 m (2 miles), 3 × 1000 m at 90 percent of $V_{HR_{max}}$
Wednesday	Jog 10,000 m (6 miles)
Thursday	Jog 3000 m (2 miles), 3 × 1000 m at 90 percent of $V_{HR_{max}}$
Friday	Jog 3000 m (2 miles), exercise test to derive $V_{HR_{max}}$
Saturday	Jog 3000 m (2 miles), 3 × 1000 m at 90 percent of $V_{HR_{max}}$
Sunday	Off

Training to this point has been fairly similar for each individual, with the horses now having reached an almost competitive level of fitness. The program for the individual for the next 2 to 4 weeks will vary considerably. The aim is to give the horse its hardest work now to complete a solid foundation before tapering the horse for racing. It is imperative that the horse not be overtrained, and extreme care must be taken to monitor each horse to ensure it is coping with the load.

Extra heats will be introduced for most horses, and most will fit into the pattern of 3 to 5 × 1000 m every second day. Some horses may be worked heats every day. Those which are thriving and doing well should continue for a full 4 weeks. Others should stop after the second week and move into the next phase. Horses that are going to be swum should commence swimming dur-

ing this period, with the aim of being able to substitute swimming for some of the jogging and track work as the speed of the heats increases.

RACING

The horse is now prepared to race, and this involves a lightening of the overall workload to freshen the horse and introduction of some faster speeds. Again, individual requirements will vary tremendously. Time between heats may be increased for some individuals.

Week 9

Monday	Jog 6000 to 10000 m (4 to 6 miles)
Tuesday	Jog 3000 m (2 miles):
	1 × 1600 m at 90 percent of $V_{HR_{max}}$
	1 × 1600 m
	First 1200 m at 90 percent of $V_{HR_{max}}$
	Last 400 m at 110 percent of $V_{HR_{max}}$
Wednesday	Jog 6000 to 10,000 m (4 to 6 miles)
Thursday	Jog 3000 m (2 miles):
	1 × 1600 m at 90 percent of $V_{HR_{max}}$
	1 × 1600 m
	First 1200 m at 90 percent of $V_{HR_{max}}$
	Last 400 m at 110 percent of $V_{HR_{max}}$
Friday	Jog 6000 to 10000 m (4 to 6 miles)
Saturday	Jog 3000 m (2 miles):
	1 × 1600 m at 90 percent of $V_{HR_{max}}$
	1 × 1600 m
	First 1200 m at 90 percent of $V_{HR_{max}}$
	Last 400 m at 110 percent of $V_{HR_{max}}$
Sunday	Off

Week 10

Monday	Jog 6000 to 10,000 m (4 to 6 miles)
Tuesday	Jog 3000 m (2 miles):
	1 × 1600 m at 90 percent of $V_{HR_{max}}$
	First 1200 m at 90 percent of $V_{HR_{max}}$
	Last 400 m at 110 percent of $V_{HR_{max}}$
Wednesday	Jog 6000 to 10,000 m (4 to 6 miles)
Thursday	Jog 3000 m (2 miles):
	1 × 1600 m at 90 percent of $V_{HR_{max}}$
	1 × 1200 m at 90 percent of $V_{HR_{max}}$
	1 × 400 m at 110 percent of $V_{HR_{max}}$
Friday	Jog 3000 m (2 miles), exercise test to derive $V_{HR_{max}}$
Saturday	Jog 3000 m (2 miles):
	1 × 1600 m at 90 percent of $V_{HR_{max}}$
	First 800 m at 90 percent of $V_{HR_{max}}$
	Next 400 m at 110 percent of $V_{HR_{max}}$
	Last 400 m in 30 seconds.
Sunday	Off

Most horses will now be ready to present for racing. Some will need more fast quarters; others will only be worked twice a week. Jogging should be light and easy for most horses.

Conclusions

Training standardbred horses is an art, and established successful trainers are currently training effectively in terms of race performance. The use of some of the principles of exercise physiology may assist in monitoring fitness and tailoring training regimens to the needs of individual horses.

References

1. Dancer SF: Training and conditioning. In Harrison JC (ed): Care and Training of the Trotter and Pacer. Columbus, Ohio, USTA, 1968, p 186.
2. Ivers T: The Fit Racehorse. Cincinnati, Esprit Racing Team, Ltd., 1983.
3. Harrison JC: Care and Training of the Trotter and Pacer. Columbus, Ohio, USTA, 1968.
4. Lambert DH: Practical experiences in the application of sports medicine. *In* Proceedings of the Annual Convention of the American Association of Equine Practitioners, 1990, p 477.

17E

Training Endurance Horses

K. J. RIDGWAY

Principles of Conditioning Endurance Horses

Conditioning implies creating progressively adaptive changes in response to correctly applied physical and mental stresses. Key words here are *correctly applied* and the application of both *physical* and *mental* stress. It is nearly impossible to separate the subjects of conditioning and training; therefore, certain aspects of training will be interjected in this discussion.

Conditioning also implies goals, first and foremost of which needs to be concern at all times for the horse's welfare and well-being. With this principle always in mind, we can proceed with the goal of enabling the horse to withstand the three incurred stresses of performance horses—musculoskeletal, metabolic, and mental.

Ability to withstand the metabolic stress demanded of an endurance horse requires a training program that addresses the need to (1) increase the maximal oxygen uptake ($\dot{V}_{O_2max}$), (2) increase and enhance the oxidative capacity of muscle, (3) increase the efficiency of carbohydrate, fat, and protein utilization, and (4) enhance the horse's thermoregulation abilities.

The discussion of conditioning also should include selection of an appropriate horse for endurance riding. Mediocrity and great expectations make a poor marriage. It is self-defeating to waste time, money, and energy trying to develop the wrong type of horse for the job. Toward this end, one should pay attention to breed, type, conformation, and genetics so that the most appropriate horse is selected.

Selection of Endurance Horses

It is advisable to request the prospect's health care charts, especially with regard to worming, illness, and foot care. Recognize that endurance training and competition put more stress on the feet than essentially any other discipline. Good foot quality and conformation are imperative.

Of equal importance to the preceding aspects are the mental qualities of the prospective endurance horse. Look for a forward, bold-moving, alert horse. The horse should show respect for the handler but still show independence and an ability to "think" for itself. Avoid or be cautious in choosing a timid, fear-filled, or overly aggressive horse. Many endurance competitions are held on hazardous mountain trails or where wildlife, motorcycles, and trail bikes may be encountered. Horses that shy excessively can, under such circumstances, be exceedingly hazardous to *your* health.

In your search, consider the advantages of a pasture-raised horse versus a horse raised in a stall and paddock. Early physical stresses help maximize genetic potential by requiring tissue adaptation at an age when adaptation would occur in a natural environment. Such horses have encountered many obstacles and learned how to negotiate them easily. This makes conditioning progress more rapidly while also incurring less risk of injury. Additionally, horses raised in a pasture and in the company of other horses tend to be better balanced psychologically. They have learned social behavior from both their dams and from peer-group horses and tend to be more self-assured regarding their environment and relationship with other horses. They tend to be free of the vices associated with isolated box stall horses.

A candidate that is mature but has not received conditioning exercise as a young animal will require a more gradually applied stress load—allowing more time for tissue adaptation to occur. Tissue adaptation is more difficult in the case of bone because it may adapt to loading more slowly than soft tissues. For these reasons, it is more difficult to achieve the genetic athletic potential of the mature but unstressed, unconditioned horse.

Conditioning Period

It is not possible to provide hard figures regarding the precise length of time required to prepare a given horse for endurance competition. As a general statement, a 3-year-old that is ground trained and has had light exercise such as ponying or good long line exercise can be *totally* conditioned and trained for endurance riding in approximately 3 years. Much of the conditioning work actually may be accomplished while competing at a self-imposed "restricted level."

With older horses, the time can be significantly shortened by previous conditioning experience and training—if the exercise approximates the appropriate conditioning format needed for endurance performance. With horses 6 years old and older that have had some form of athletic use, it is possible to compete on a limited basis with as little as 6 months of well-executed conditioning. In all cases, the conditioning time is also dependent on any history of prior injuries and lamenesses.

There are matters that should be accomplished prior to physical conditioning. One should sit down with pen and paper and create realistic but flexible goals. The trainer must always be prepared to alter both goals and schedules to fit *current realities* of both horse and rider. Make allowances for potential layups due to injury or illness, for both horse and rider. At the same time, however, stick to your goals. Do not put off conditioning, training, and goals just to fit personal whims.

Consider your goals with regard to training and competition. Be sure to schedule such things as deworming, shoeing, immunizations, and dental care so that they do not interfere with the conditioning or competition schedule.

Records

Your next consideration should be to create a "training log," a simple form that can be used consistently and adhered to easily. At a minimum, the log should contain a record of the length of the training session, an estimate of distance traveled and time spent, and pertinent weather conditions. It is helpful to start the conditioning/training day with a written statement of your goal for that session and a comment at the end regarding results. It is also helpful if you note approximately how much time was spent at various gaits and the nature of the terrain (e.g., mountain, hard footing, deep sand, etc.). Any problems such as mental attitude, soreness, tack fit, lameness, or diseases should be noted. Such a log obviously can vary in detail but will be of value only if consistently used. Keep it simple.

Nutritional State

The feeding of endurance horses is an extremely important subject that requires diligent study. The reader is encouraged to seek out available literature on *endurance horse* nutrition. The subject is lightly broached in this section because the nutritional status of the horse is critical to the conditioning program. A properly balanced feeding program should be in place prior to commencement of conditioning and should be modified as conditioning progresses. Endurance horses expend an enormous number of calories during exercise and need high-quality roughage on a "free choice" basis, if possible. However, one should avoid feeding high levels of grains, and protein intake should be in the neighborhood of 10 to 12 percent of the ration. Calcium intake should be relatively low. Diets of strictly alfalfa (lucerne) hay as the source of roughage provide excess calcium and may lead to problems with exertional myopathies and "thumps" (properly known as *synchronous diaphragmatic flutter*). Perhaps most important of all, ensure that your endurance horse is provided with *fresh, clean water* and *"free choice"* salt. Along with achieving a good nutritional plane before starting a conditioning program, take care of the horse's worming and dental needs.

Mental Conditioning

Recall that one of your goals is to develop a bold, forward, alert, and confident horse. This starts with extensive, *gentle* ground handling and grooming to create trust and bonding. Part of this ground handling should be to develop a routine that includes a systematic body evaluation for tack rubs, wounds; painful muscles, ligaments, and tendons; condition of shoes; and overall appearance and condition. This evaluation also accustoms the horse to being handled by veterinarians during rides.

Linda Tellington Jones's "TTEAM work" provides one method of training that accelerates development of the horse's confidence in handling fear-inducing situations. The horse learns confidence when negotiating ground obstacles in hand by the use of labyrinths, mazes, and "stars" that are introduced in a nonthreatening manner. There are now many videotapes available by numerous trainers that utilize the horse's method of thinking and functioning to aid in training. The serious trainer would be well advised to explore these resources.

Dressage

The ideal riding foundation for all forms of conditioning and training stems from dressage, whether considered by that term or another. The discipline develops suppleness, flexibility, control, and rateability—vital elements in providing an important key to soundness and athletic ability. Dressage also teaches the horse sensitivity to aids and helps develop the abdominal muscles to better support the animal's back. I believe that over 80 percent of all endurance horses suffer to some extent from back problems and that many lower leg injuries stem from poor head, neck, and back carriage. It is not necessary for an endurance horse to progress to higher-level dressage work, but the ability to exercise in a long, relaxed frame, elevate the back, and travel in a collected frame (when asked) can prevent many of the back problems suffered by endurance horses.

Unfortunately, there are many dressage instructors who wish to force the horse into a collected frame or push ahead in training before the horse is ready. Seek a sensitive instructor who will progress at the pace the horse and the experience of the rider dictate.

Conditioning Different Tissue Types

Different tissues adapt at different rates. Soft tissues such as muscles, lungs, and heart characteristically condition quite rapidly. These tissues may exhibit the desired level of conditioning response in as little as 4 to 8 weeks. This often leads to the false impression that because the heart rate and respiratory recoveries are excellent, the horse is adequately conditioned. However, other tissues essential to withstanding the stress of endurance work take much longer to condition. The common denominator in tissues that achieve fitness rapidly is an extensive blood supply reflected by the presence of many capillaries (high vascularity).

As tissues become less vascular, conditioning progresses more slowly. Thus the group of tissues known as *medium-density tissues*—tendons, ligaments, joints, and hoofs—will require 6 to 12 months of proper conditioning to withstand the stress of thousands upon thousands of repetitive movements performed during an endurance event.

Bone, too, must be conditioned. This is achieved through a process of constant remodeling—removing bone from areas of lesser stress and adding bone to those areas receiving more stress. This is a process known as *Wolff's law*. A cross section of a foal's cannon is relatively circular. As the horse matures to age 2 or 3, the cannon bone becomes significantly more ovoid. In a mature horse that has received adequate stress, the bone becomes flattened and almost concave on the posterior surface, much like a leaf spring. This essential bone remodeling process is often not completed and the maximal bone density achieved until the third year of conditioning and the horse has actually been in a number of competitions.

It becomes obvious that conditioning must take place at the pace dictated by the horse's weakest link—whether that weak link is mental maturity or a limiting physical characteristic such as excess weight or a result of overstress such as tendon sheath filling or an outright injury.

Heart Rate for Measuring Fitness Level

Of all the measurements available to assess fitness and ability to continue an endurance ride, the heart rate stands paramount in both importance and informative quality. There exists a direct relationship between the heart rate and the amount of energy use occurring at any given time.

Essentially all other measurements typically used in monitoring endurance horses are reflected in heart rate and character of the pulse. For this reason, all horse people, whether in endurance or another discipline, should own and learn to properly use a stethoscope.

The first heart rate value to be determined *for each specific horse* is the *true resting heart rate*—the heart rate when the animal is resting quietly in a stall, paddock, or pasture. Typically, this rate will fall between 24 and 36 beats/min. The trainer should develop a pattern of taking a resting heart rate daily before the horse is handled. If the heart rate is elevated by 6 to 8 beats/min above normal for the horse, it provides evidence of some nature of stress. The stress may be the result of overwork on the previous day, it may relate to an injury not yet apparent (subclinical), or it may indicate that there is an impending infectious disease problem or noninfectious problem such as colic. A slightly elevated heart rate per se does not necessarily mean that the horse should not be exercised on that day, but the horse should be further examined—the legs carefully palpated, the temperature taken, and attention paid to the horse's attitude and willingness to exercise. The trainer may want to shorten the duration or decrease the intensity of the workout.

The next heart rate measurement to be recorded is a *resting rate when saddled and ready to work*. For most horses, this falls between 36 and 48 beats/min. Since the rate varies from horse to horse, it needs to be determined for each specific animal. The figure also tends to be lower in more conditioned horses, although emotions and temperament play a part. As with the true resting heart rate, elevations in the saddled and ready to work rate may indicate impending disease, lack of recovery from the preceding day's exercise, pain (tendons, ligaments, joints, muscles or internal), or psychological stress. A careful evaluation by the rider/trainer is indicated before continuing with the training schedule.

Recovery heart rates become the key to determining the level of fitness, as well as the ability to continue during conditioning or competition. Within 5 minutes of ceasing exercise, a horse fit for that particular level of exercise will exhibit recovery levels low enough to continue safely. Five minutes is an ideal time to determine level of recovery, although it can be checked at 10 minutes and still provide meaningful information. Recovery level can be determined in an even more meaningful manner by using a cardiac recovery index, subsequently explained here in detail. For a 5- or 10-minute recovery evaluation, take the heart rate immediately after dismounting and repeat after 5 minutes and again after 10 minutes.

Interpretation of Heart Rate Values

1. If the heart rate exceeds 72 beats/min within 5 to 10 minutes of ceasing exercise, the distance traveled or the speed during traveling has (at least temporarily) exceeded the horse's metabolic tolerance and level of conditioning. The horse should be rested until the heart rate drops to 64 beats/min or less. If it takes more than 15 minutes to reach this point, the trainer/rider should consider shortening the day's work and/or using less speed, i.e., decreasing the intensity of the exercise. This lack of acceptable cardiac recovery also indicates that more frequent rest periods are needed for the remainder of the day's exercise.

2. A heart rate recovery to 60 beats/min (± 4 beats/min) within 10 minutes indicates a good recovery response and adaptation to the level of applied stress.

3. If the recovery heart rate is 52 beats/min or less, it is likely that little conditioning effect will have occurred. These rates indicate that the level of exercise needs to be increased if an optimal conditioning effect is desired. This may be accomplished by increasing speed, climbing hills, or doing gymnastic exercises. A recovery to 52 beats/min or less also can be a *desired* result, e.g., at the end of a day's training workout when the rider has slowed the pace and allowed the horse to "cool down" prior to arrival at the ride's finish. A pulse of 52 beats/min or less offers proof of this adequate and desirable warmdown.

Cardiac Recovery Index (CRI)

This index provides a sophisticated measure of both recovery level and level of fitness to continue. It is based on the premise that a horse that is adequately warmed up and fit to continue exercise will exhibit a heart rate that, after trotting a specific distance, will return to a *working base rate* within approximately 30 seconds following the trot out.

A course of 80 m (250 ft) is measured. If the location is, for example, at an event's veterinary check point, the course is 40 m out and then 40 m back to the veterinary examiners. The heart rate is taken before the trot out becomes the working base rate. The horse is then briskly trotted, in hand, the 80-m distance. At the moment the trot is commenced, the time is noted; the heart rate is again determined 1 minute later. This (second) heart rate is the *recovery heart rate*. It takes most horses 25 to 30 seconds to cover the distance when trotted in hand. Knowing the typical number of seconds for a given horse to trot the 80 m in hand allows the trainer to simply trot the horse for that number of seconds and then wait the balance of the 1 minute before rechecking the heart rate. This allows the rider to use the CRI at any point on a training track without physically measuring the 80-m distance.

Interpretation of the CRI

With 10 or fewer minutes of rest after exercise, a fit horse should be able to pass the CRI test. When tested, the fit horse will exhibit a recovery rate that is equal to or lower than the working base rate. The CRI is most easily interpreted when the horse's working base rate is between 64 and 80 beats/min. At these levels, a recovery heart rate increased by 4 beats/min above the working base rate indicates that the horse has not recovered adequately. The test should be repeated after an additional 5 minutes of rest. A 4 beat/min increase has significance if the working base rate is over 64 beats/min.

If the horse has had 10 minutes of rest prior to testing, a recovery heart rate that is 8 beats/min greater than the working base rate is of more concern, especially if the base rate is over 64 beats/min. This lack of recovery is indicative that the horse has likely received too much stress, and measures need to be taken to reduce stress or cease the workout.

A horse that does not pass this test within 30 minutes of rest should not continue to exercise but should be carefully monitored—metabolic problems may ensue. Not only should the horse pass the test within this time frame, but it should, if the test is repeated, exhibit a progressively decreasing working base rate (taken before commencement of the trot out). The CRI is especially beneficial in determining *progressive recovery* by repeating the CRI tests at appropriate intervals of time. Progressive recovery provides superior evidence of both fitness and ability to continue safely, enabling delineation of the status of horses that may have subclinical metabolic problems.

Using a Measured "Reference Course"

As conditioning progresses and the horse exercises at a given heart rate, the horse will cover a measured course in progressively less time. Speed over the course can be calculated by dividing distance by elapsed time. Conversely, if the horse covers the course in the same time as in the beginning stages of conditioning, it will be able to do so at a lower heart rate. Remember that a lower heart rate indicates less oxygen consumption and less work output. Additional value accrues from using a measured course—the trainer/rider learns to recognize the horse's speed at different gaits and can better pace the horse in competition.

To be of the greatest value in recognizing conditioning progress, the course is best ridden with an onboard heart rate monitor so that a steady heart rate can be maintained. A fitness peak will be reached wherein no further improvement takes place with additional conditioning. The trainer then must seek to maintain this peak without overdoing conditioning work.

For endurance horses, a training course of 1.5 to 5 km (1 to 3 miles) is ideal. It is helpful to physically mark or mentally note some known distance reference points along the course. The course should be ridden after the horse is well warmed up and should be used for training approximately three times a week in the early conditioning phases and about once a week when the horse is more fit.

Overconditioning

If, in fact, with continued conditioning work the time to complete the course at a specific heart rate increases, it may be evidence that the horse is overconditioned and a state known as *overtraining* is occurring. In endurance riding, overtraining and overusing the horse in competition by riding too many miles or failing to allow adequate recovery time between competitions is as common, if not more common, than underconditioning.

Signs that a horse is reaching this point include weight loss despite large food intake or poor appetite, dull or dry hair coat, or a dull appearance to the eye. The horse may perform adequately but seem to lack "bottom" (the eagerness or drive to continue). Such a horse also may take longer to recover, have slower work times, and be prone to colic and nervous disorders.

Interestingly, a horse suffering from overtraining may continue to exhibit low heart rates during exercise as a result of excessive parasympathetic nerve stimulation, resulting in increased vagal nerve tone. Vagal nerve stimulation has a direct effect on the heart, preventing the heart rate from increasing appropriately in response to stress. Therefore, low heart rates are not proof that overtraining and/or overuse has not occurred. Conversely, however, consistently higher than previous exercising heart rates and slower returns to resting heart rates are consistent with overtraining and are more easily observed.

Turnout is indicated, and close monitoring is important if overtraining is truly occurring. An extended rest of several weeks is indicated to reverse this overtraining, overuse syndrome.

Aerobic Foundation

A good aerobic foundation is the basis of all conditioning regardless of the riding discipline involved. Let us define *aerobic metabolism* as the ability to utilize oxygen to burn the fuels provided by food breakdown. The carbohydrates, fats, and proteins in the forms of glycogen, volatile fatty acids, and free fatty acids provide the energy for work output. Aerobic metabolism provides the bulk of energy needed to accomplish work performed in endurance riding. In contrast to aerobic metabolism is *anaerobic metabolism,* which, by utilizing an alternate cycle of metabolism known as the *pyruvate cycle,* can burn fuel in the muscles in the absence of any available oxygen (see Chap. 4). Anaerobic metabolism provides the majority of energy for an intense work output over a very short time span of approximately 20 to 40 seconds.

When discussing aerobic versus anaerobic metabolism, it is important to realize that all exercise requires both aerobic and anaerobic metabolism. The relative contribution of each of the metabolic types depends on the speed or intensity of the exercise. This is to say that there is no magic point or heart rate at which the body suddenly switches from aerobic to anaerobic metabolism. Rather, it is a transition process starting with nearly complete aerobic metabolism and progressing with exercise intensity increases to the predomination of anaerobic metabolism.

What is known is that with conditioning, the ability to take in more oxygen and enhance oxygen utilization is greater. Thus, after conditioning, horses can exercise at higher intensities with less anaerobic contribution. Aerobic capacity is greater and the horse's speed is faster before blood lactate increases to above 4 mmol/liter, which has been described as the *anaerobic threshold*. Simply expressed, more blood will be pumped, more oxygen is carried to nourish tissues, and capacity for work output is prolonged—therefore, efficiency is greater, also resulting in less heat production.

Slow, Long-Distance Exercise

An aerobic foundation is accomplished by slow, long-distance exercise (SLD). This consists of walking interspersed with trotting and slow canters. The endurance horse performs perhaps 95 percent of exercise using aerobic energy delivery systems. To perform aerobic exercise, the horse depends on a well-developed base of slow-twitch (type I) muscle fibers. These muscle fibers are resistant to fatigue and have a greater oxidative capacity and a rich blood supply (see Chap. 8).

SLD exercise plays a principal role in enhancing the blood supply and oxygenation of these muscle fibers by increasing capillarity. SLD exercise also provides the appropriate stresses to commence (but not complete) the process of strengthening ligaments, tendons, and joints.

The procedure for building an aerobic base consists of 30- to 60-minute training sessions three to four times a week. A pace of 10 to 13 km/h (6 to 8 miles/h)—an easy working trot—is interspersed with 2 to 3 minutes of walking after approximately 10 minutes of trotting. Initially, heart rates during the working trot for an unconditioned horse are likely to be in the range of 120 to 150 beats/min. When aerobic conditioning is achieved, these rates will usually fall to a range of 70 to 110 beats/min.

These paces, barring any problems, are continued for the first month of training. In the second month, a 16-km (10-mile) workout is added. Ten-mile workouts are incrementally added once per week for 2 weeks, then two 10-mile workouts are added per week for 2 weeks, and finally, the conditioning program is increased to three 10-mile workouts per week by the third or fourth month. Incrementally adding stress is the key to any conditioning program. It is important to note the added increments in your conditioning log.

By the end of the second month of conditioning, you may want to add a fourth day to the conditioning regimen—using a hard day of exercise followed by an easy day. Three aerobic workouts per week are a minimum number when trying to improve fitness. Conversely, one should probably not exceed five workouts per week.

It is especially important to remember to *progress with conditioning at the rate of the horse's weakest link*. This weak link may be conformation, body weight, injury

(including excess filling or strain), or mental resistance to the work. One should palpate, examine and evaluate for pain and sensitivity both before and after every workout.

It is desirable during this aerobic base formation to intersperse trail work with ring work. Ring work, utilizing dressage movements, will lead to responsiveness and teaches the horse to round and strengthen its back. These goals are more easily accomplished in a better-controlled arena environment than under trail conditions.

Remember, the goals at this time are to promote the safety of both the horse and the rider, to safeguard long-range soundness, to keep the horse mentally alert and eager, and to prevent boredom and sourness. It must be cautioned that extensive continuation of SLD exercise can actually be detrimental to horses that also must be able to sprint effectively. This includes winning endurance horses and cutting, stock work, polo, racing, open jumpers, and higher-level event horses.

Speed Training

This phase of conditioning, popularized in Sweden by trainers of human runners and known as *fartlek,* comes into play by approximately the third month of conditioning. It encompasses sudden, rapid, relatively short bursts of speed interspersed throughout the exercise bout to stimulate tissues not yet addressed by slower exercise and increases the horse's metabolic capabilities. Speed training increases the aerobic capacity beyond the level achieved with the foundation (SLD) training and stimulates adaptation-evoking stresses on the medium tissues such as tendons, ligaments, joints, and hoofs, as well as having some conditioning effects on the hard tissues (bone). These speed-burst stresses are carefully added for only a few minutes at a time.

Speed training increases the capillarity of the muscles and skin. Increased capillarity means providing more available oxygen and enhancing cellular respiration. The increase in blood flow to the skin becomes very important in dissipating the immense heat buildup associated with endurance exercise. Enhanced ability to dissipate body heat is perhaps the single biggest deciding factor between being able to win, place second, complete, or not complete an event.

Horses appear to enjoy speed training and find it both fun and exciting. Because speed training can induce significant excitement in the horse and result in a lack of rider control, however, caution is advised in utilizing this regimen until the horse has adequate training and is easily rated and controlled.

The stresses of *fartlek* should be incrementally added to the program. Start with speed training only once in a training session. After a week or two, add two sessions of speed bursts to a training routine. After 2 or 3 weeks at this level, three *fartlek* sessions per workout lasting 1 to 2 minutes per speed burst are a satisfactory goal.

Along with speed training, longer periods of faster trotting are indicated at this training level. In order to maintain heart rates that produce an ongoing conditioning effect, a trainer will need to increase speed of the trot from, perhaps, 10 km/h (6 miles/h) to 13 km/h (8 miles/h) or even to 16 km/h (10 miles/h).

For this and subsequent phases of conditioning, use of an onboard heart rate monitor should be considered. A monitor enables the trainer to be far more accurate in applying appropriate stress and evaluating the horse's progress. This is not to say that evaluation of physiologic systems and progress cannot be accomplished without the use of such a monitor, but it is definitely less precise. By the same note, a heart rate monitor improperly used and without the data being recorded is nothing more than an expensive toy.

Speed training should not be initiated until the horse is well "legged up." In an unconditioned horse, speed training can create tendon, ligament, and joint sprain. The aerobic foundation previously discussed should provide an adequate base for *fartlek*.

A usable program consists of a bout of 8 to 11 km (5 to 7 miles) of training performed as a mix of working trot interspersed with 1- to 3-minute bursts of extended trot or canter. The duration and intensity of the speed phase depend on the level of fitness already achieved. If errors are to be made, err on the lower side of speed and shortened distance. Heart rates as evidenced on the onboard monitor may initially range from 160 to 200 beats/min. Do not maintain rates above 170 to 175 beats/min for more than a minute in this phase of conditioning. Once adequately conditioned, a horse's heart rates during speed training will likely range from 145 to 175 beats/min.

Interval Training

The processes involved in interval training entail exercising the horse at near-maximal speed (or near-maximal heart rates) for a given distance (or a given time) and then allowing a partial recovery by walking or jogging for a specified time (or to a specific heart rate). This procedure is then repeated for a specific number of times. Each act of repeating the process is referred to as a *repetition*.

Short, intense exercise bouts that achieve (with onboard monitors) heart rates in excess of 180 beats/min produce strength and maximize both the aerobic capacity and the anaerobic capabilities. This conditioning phase provides the "icing on the cake." It is, however, not accomplished without risk of injury to the horse. If your goal is simply completion and not necessarily competing with the front runners, this phase of conditioning is not imperative.

Interval training develops strength in tendons, ligaments, and joints, as well as strengthening hooves and increasing bone density. Muscle fibers, especially fast-twitch (type II) fibers, are brought to peak; thus maximal speed and anaerobic capabilities are achieved and aerobic capacity is maximized.

The adage that speed, not distance, injures horses holds true when doing interval training. Additionally, exercise-induced pulmonary hemorrhage can occur. Before addressing interval training, precautions for improving the level of safety should be considered.

The horse should be very well conditioned through the use of SLD and speed training before undertaking interval training. In most cases for endurance horses, interval training should not be undertaken until the second or preferably third year of training. By contrast, race horses are introduced to interval training as young as 1 or 2 years of age. On days that interval training is to be used, the horse should be carefully evaluated immediately prior to commencing the day's workout.

An enormous heat load is produced during interval training, and therefore, care should be taken in using interval training during days of high temperature—and especially if the high ambient temperature is combined with high humidity. As a guideline, if the temperature (in degrees Fahrenheit) is added to the percentage of relative humidity and the resulting number is in excess of 160, it is *not* advisable to do more than two repetitions of interval exercise.

Because of risk of injury to muscles, tendons, ligaments, joints, and feet, the terrain used for interval training should be as close to ideal as possible. Footing should be reasonably firm, resilient, and not rocky. Deep footing, such as sand, should be avoided. Hills with a gradient of 3 to 10 degrees can be utilized to produce the needed stress without speed. This will still create the stress needed for maximal strength development of muscles, tendons, and ligaments. High rates of speed greatly increase concussion and possible damage. On the positive side, however, these same concussive stresses are useful in strengthening bone. Problems from increased concussion can be minimized if terrain gradients are used in the early stages of interval training and a flat track and increased speed are used later.

A thorough and adequate warmup is helpful in minimizing injury. For this reason, intervals should not be done until near the end of the day's workout. By the same token, a warm-down after interval training should be thorough and followed by careful palpation of all limbs.

Regarding repetitions, it is safest to start with one interval (a gallop followed by walk/jog to partial recovery). No repetitions should be used during the first week. Repetitions should be performed no more frequently than twice a week and on days that are maximally spaced. In the second week, incorporate one interval, and follow the walk/jog phase with another repetition. Interval training should be included in the schedule only once a week at this time (the second week). During the third week, add one session of interval training with the initial interval plus two repetitions. Be very cautious if, beginning with the fourth week, a third repetition is added to the initial gallop/jog combination. Many horses cannot handle a total of three such repetitions. Once repetitions are in place, it is not usually necessary, nor advisable, to do interval training more than once a week.

Interval-Training Formats

Format 1. Perform a maximal gallop for a measured distance—usually 1.6 km (1 mile). Then allow a partial recovery by briskly walking or slowly jogging the horse for 400 m (1/4 mile). Then perform the appropriate number of repetitions. This procedure can be used if an onboard heart rate monitor is not available.

Format 2. Perform a maximal gallop for a measured time (usually 2 minutes), followed by a brisk walk or slow trot for 2 minutes. Follow this with the appropriate number of repetitions. This format, like the first format, is useful when a heart rate monitor is not available.

Format 3. Select a target heart rate in the "anaerobic" range, (e.g., 200 beats/min). Govern the horse's pace to maintain the selected heart rate for a specified time, e.g., 2 minutes. The gallop is then followed by a brisk walk or slow trot until the targeted partial recovery rate of, for example, 90 or 100 beats/min is met. This is then followed by the appropriate number of repetitions.

Format 3 does require the use of an onboard heart rate monitor but is highly advantageous in assessing the physiologic state of the horse during the intervals and whether the horse can handle the desired number of repetitions. If the horse has to slow down considerably to maintain peak heart rate, or if recovery time to the target recovery rate lengthens, fatigue is setting in and the horse is not yet capable of handling further repetitions. It should be evident that format 3 provides a greater margin of safety.

This bears repeating: The importance of following a thorough cool-down with a visual examination and hands-on palpation of all four legs cannot be overemphasized. The same examination should be repeated prior to the next workout.

Natural Gait Selection

Each horse has a speed at which it will physiologically choose to change gaits as speed increases or decreases. When changing gaits because of speed increase, the heart rate will actually drop when the horse makes its upward transition. This indicates that less effort is required even though the speed is the same or even greater. As speed is again increased, the heart rate will again rise and then fall as the transition to a canter occurs. (This transition phenomenon is, however, not noted in the transition from rapid canter to full gallop.)

This phenomenon is explained by heart rate and oxygen consumption. As the horse becomes more conditioned, it is capable of traveling faster in a given gait while still maintaining a slower heart rate. This then allows the rider to ask the horse for a faster or more extended gait requiring less energy burn and thus delaying the onset of fatigue.

With an onboard heart rate monitor, the rider can, by asking for upward transition to trot or canter *before* the point where extra oxygen consumption is required, maintain the same or even higher rate of speed. Energy conservation has been maximized while maintaining or increasing the pace.

Utilizing Gait Extension

The trainer must recognize the difference between gait extension and simply traveling faster at a given gait. Extension implies longer stride rather than increased frequency of stride. Extension requires more muscular effort and will therefore hasten the onset of fatigue—especially in the less fit horse.

However, if wisely used, gait extensions do have benefit both in conditioning and in competition—whereby distance can be traversed rapidly with an economy of energy expenditure. Gait extension in conditioning also adds incremental stress to further develop the medium-density tissues, fast-twitch muscle fibers, and bone density. The increased heart rate, carefully monitored, increases the conditioning effect.

However, excessive use of extended gaits increases risk of injury. As fatigue sets in, fine neuromuscular coordination is lost, the foot is not properly placed, muscles prematurely contract, and injury to muscles, tendons, ligaments, joints, and bone can follow. Endurance horses are particularly prone to suspensory ligament sprains, many of which occur from overutilization of the extended trot.

Allowing or encouraging the horse to periodically switch to the next higher gait is helpful. In early phases of training, major gait extension should not be maintained for more than 1 to 2 minutes. In many fully conditioned horses, the extension may be maintained for 10 to 20 minutes, although breaks from extension approximately every 5 minutes should be encouraged. This is to say that an extended trot should be broken by periods of cantering or walking. This allows different muscle groups to come into play and diminishes the workload of muscles most used in performing the extension.

Maintaining Performance Level

Horses that have reached the desired level of fitness do not have to be exercised daily to maintain the attained level. If they are in a heavy competition cycle—competing every weekend or every 2 weeks—significant conditioning between events can lead to metabolic problems and overtraining-induced lameness. Additionally, horses on heavy competition schedules often have trouble maintaining weight. Light riding once or twice a week interspersed with pasture turnout, ponying, or longeing (or a combination of these) will maintain fitness.

The ability to maintain a fitness level can be assessed using the previously described measured reference course and by good heart rate monitoring. Attention should be paid to visual and palpation examinations in conjunction with all workouts and competitions.

Return to Performance after Layoff or Injury

Injuries are, unfortunately, a part of life with all athletic horses. However, a significant level of fitness is maintained, even with a 3- to 4-week period of forced rest. Such layoff periods can be prescribed for injuries if it is recognized that only a small decrease in fitness will occur.

The trainer must, however, be aware that the horse will lose performance "sharpness," particularly where fine-tuned neuromuscular coordination is critical. This is more important in the case of event horses, jumpers, and dressage horses but also should be recognized as having some importance in endurance horses. Time should be allowed to restore that sharp edge of performance before competing again. This may entail only 1 or 2 weeks to fine-tune the performance level after a 3-week layup.

After longer layups, such as 3 or 4 months, most endurance horses can be brought back to the previous level of fitness in 6 to 8 weeks. It is, however, cautioned that each horse must be viewed as an individual and reconditioned at a rate compatible with the strengthening of that animal's weakest link.

Conclusions

Start the lengthy process of conditioning with the selection of a good prospect. Recognize that there is a considerable time and effort commitment that must be made—choose your prospect carefully. Pay attention to the horse's past health record, its conformation, and whether it is of appropriate type for endurance performance. Give yourself the best possible chance for success by paying close attention to worming, dental needs, proper nutrition, housing, tack fit, shoeing, and riding skills.

Set realistic goals that are reasonable but also flexible. Maintain a training record. Lay out a measured test course to periodically check the horse's progress and level of condition. Use heart rates, recovery heart rates, and the cardiac recovery index to monitor health and conditioning progress. Create a habit of examining the horse before and after every workout.

Develop an adequate aerobic foundation by using a combination of ring and trail work. Use dressage work to maximize suppleness and flexibility, remembering always to condition and train with the goal of strengthening the horse's weakest link.

If success is to be attained, a horse must do in training what is expected in performance. Nothing but slow, long-distance exercise will create an athlete that is capable of nothing but slow, long-distance exercise. Training progression should include speed training and, finally, for peak performance, interval training. Be conservative in adding each stress increment associated with speed training and especially so when adding repetitions in interval training.

Frequently review your goals and be willing to modify "deadlines" as necessary. Most important of all, do not lose sight of the goals of enjoying the horse and the sport. Pay *much more* consideration than just lip service to the welfare of the animal. Without happy, sound, and fit horses, there is no sport.

Training the Event Horse

S. J. DYSON

An event horse has to perform three basic disciplines: dressage, cross-country, and show jumping. A top-class horse must show at least moderate ability in dressage and show jumping and excellent ability in cross-country. In a 3-day event, the weighting of the three phases is approximately 2:1:5 (dressage, show jumping, and cross-country). The speed and endurance day of a 3-day event (three-star; see below) comprises two roads and tracks phases of approximately 4000 and 12,000 m, respectively, performed at 220 m/min, between which is the steeplechase phase (2760 or 3105 m at 690 m/min). The cross-country (phase D) which follows covers approximately 5700 to 6840 m, the optimal speed being 570 m/min. Thus a 3-day event horse must have both stamina and speed and must be inherently sound, since there are three horse inspections and two examinations during the course of the event, at any of which the horse may be eliminated if unsound. This section describes the selection and training of a potential 3-day event horse; the principles apply equally to preparation for a 1-day event. The main levels of competition are novice (preliminary), intermediate (one- and two-star 3-day event), and advanced (three- and four-star 3-day event). Obviously, the ability of the horse, quality of the training, and capability of the rider will determine the level reached.

Selection of Raw Material

TYPE AND CONFORMATION

The prerequisites of an event horse are speed, stamina, and soundness. Traditionally, the thoroughbred horse has excelled. Athough thoroughbred cross horses have excelled at lower levels of competition, generally they have lacked the speed and stamina required for advanced and championship level 3-day events, although there are a few notable exceptions, most particularly at the 1992 Olympics. Pure warmblood horses have generally been too slow despite good dressage and jumping ability. Experience has shown that thoroughbred horses are easier to get fit, usually requiring less work and therefore reducing wear and tear. They are probably better able to cope with conditions of high temperature and humidity. Selective breeding programs for show jumpers and dressage horses have unquestionably been successful, notably in Germany, Holland, Denmark, Sweden, and France. As yet there have only been limited attempts to breed event horses, and it is probably too early to say how successful these have been, although unquestionably there are some stallions that have sired a number of good horses. If progress is to be made, there must be more selection of both mares and stallions.

During the speed and endurance phase, the horses have to carry a minimum of 75 kg (rider with or without tack and additional weight); to carry more than this is potentially a disadvantage, especially for a small horse. The optimal size is probably 155 cm (15.3 hands) to 163 cm (16.2 hands); bigger horses tend to be less maneuverable during the cross-country phase and to be plagued by unsoundness problems.

There are only limited studies which objectively relate conformation to soundness, none of which relate specifically to event horses. Consistent soundness is of paramount importance to an event horse. There is a high incidence of superficial digital flexor tendinitis, suspensory ligament desmitis, degenerative joint disease of the metacarpophalangeal (fetlock) joints, and foot-related problems in event horses. The event horse has to cover many miles in training and in competition and may compete over uneven terrain, sometimes including stony roads and tracks. It has repeatedly to jump drop fences. Therefore, I believe that selection for good conformation (and hence potential soundness) is important.

The feet should have good horn quality, with reasonably thick, concave soles. The front feet should be set on directly beneath the central limb axes and should be of adequate size relative to body size. The pastern-foot angle should be straight; avoid either excessively upright pasterns, which may be associated with an increased risk of fetlock problems, or very sloping pasterns, which place excessive strain on the suspensory apparatus. The carpi (knees) should be straight, with the metacarpi (cannon bones) set on directly beneath. If the cannon bones are set on laterally (to the outside) relative to the carpi, this will predispose to the development of "splints." An excessively straight hock angle and/or hyperextension of the hind fetlocks should be avoided because this conformation has been associated with a high incidence of suspensory ligament problems. The tubera sacrale (the bony prominences which make the "jumpers bump") should be level; a steep angle between the tubera sacrale and tubera ischii may reflect potential good jumping ability. An excessively long back should be avoided because this may predispose to back muscle problems. Although not relating specifically to soundness, many good event horses have had a very prominent wither. Ideally, an event horse should have a well set on neck of reasonable length. This will help the horse to move with a correct outline for dressage and avoid the criticism of "neck too short."

ACTION

An event horse does not have to move as well as a dressage horse, and unquestionably, a significant proportion of horses who move exceptionally well in front are inclined to be a little careless in front when jumping and not "pick up" properly. Many thoroughbreds have a rather straight hindlimb conformation and have difficulty in truly engaging the hindlimb. A potentially good horse must have natural hindlimb impulsion and engagement helping natural self-carriage. This should help the horse to show variations within pace, i.e., working, medium, and extended paces.

It is not vital that an event horse moves completely straight. However, it is important that it does not interfere, resulting in self-inflicted trauma. The horse should be observed moving in hand on a hard surface, viewed from the front and from behind, watching limb flight and foot placement and the position of the limb during weight bearing. Avoid a horse that appears to place excessive torque on a joint during weight bearing. Hindlimb flight sometimes changes when the horse is ridden, so action also should be assessed when ridden.

JUMPING ABILITY

An event horse does not need the scope of a show jumper but *must* be reasonably careful when required to jump. There have been good event horses which have been careless show jumpers, but two or three fences down can be extremely influential. The event horse must be quick and clever, show reasonable scope, and have a bold attitude. It must show willingness to jump small ditches and to go into water. Scope, carefulness, and boldness are all reasonably innate, although by careful training, all aspects can be improved. It can be difficult to assess these factors in a horse unaccustomed to jumping; therefore, it is easier to make an accurate judgment on a horse which has had a basic introduction to jumping. When first introduced to water, some horses may be very hesitant and nappy, but generally this should not be repeated if the horse is reliably going to jump boldly into water. The good event horse jumps quickly and cleanly from bank to bank of a ditch. The attitude toward ditch jumping can usually be assessed at a small ditch.

MENTAL ATTITUDE

Both the dressage and show-jumping phases require a degree of calmness, whereas cross-country requires boldness and enthusiasm. There are many good event horses which have been difficult horses: difficult to handle in the stable or difficult to mount or inclined to be nappy. These strong "character" traits, if harnessed, can be to the horse's advantage. The "fizzy" temperament can be much more difficult to cope with, especially if manifest in both dressage and show-jumping phases. Mental attitude can be changed to some extent, but this often requires tact, patience, and flexibility of approach.

Training to Compete at Novice Level

At novice level, the horse is required to perform a simple dressage test, including movements in medium walk, working trot, and working canter; to show direct transitions from trot to halt and halt to trot; and to demonstrate lengthened strides in trot. The maximum height of show jumps is 1.15 m (3 ft, 9 in). The cross-country course comprises approximately 22 fences, maximum height 1.08 m (3 ft, 6 in), to be ridden at an optimal speed of 520 m/min. The course length is approximately 2000 to 2500 m and thus has an approximate duration of 4 minutes.

FLAT TRAINING (DRESSAGE)

Flat work is the training basis not only for dressage but also for show jumping and cross-country. The more balanced, supple, maneuverable, and controlled the horse is on the flat, the better will be its jumping performance. Progressive flat work will develop strength and fitness of specific muscle groups and may thereby enhance jumping performance. The aims of training at this level are to establish a horse that accepts the bit and goes freely forward and straight, responding to the leg aids. The horse must learn to accept the leg. Balance, cadence, suppleness, and obedience must be established. Through repetition and reward, the horse learns to understand the aids and in doing so develops muscular strength, coordination, and fitness. With progressive work in the correct way, there should be gradual enlargement of the muscles of the top line, thoracolumbar region, and hindquarters.

Although in the dressage test the horse has to perform circles in trot of 20-m diameter, it should be borne in mind that turns off and onto the center line of the dressage arena are effectively part of a 10-m circle, so the horse must be sufficiently well balanced to perform 10-m circles in trot. The horse will be competing in an arena 20 × 40 m, and it must therefore develop confidence in working within such confines.

Nonetheless, it may be helpful when first teaching and developing medium paces to work in much larger areas. The horse will compete on a grass surface and must be accustomed to working on grass, remembering that conditions may be far from ideal—either hard and slippery or poached and holding. Although there are many potential benefits of riding regularly on all-weather surfaces, the horse's musculoskeletal system must be attuned also to working on firmer surfaces. The horse also must be sufficiently obedient to work straight through uneven or muddy ground and not try to avoid it. Mental attitude must not be ignored; the horse must learn to become obedient without losing natural animation. The several discipline demands of horse trials make it unlikely that the horse will become bored. Nonetheless, the value of hacking out must not be underrated, remembering that basic training can continue. In order to cope with the difference between working at home and in the competition environment, it is preferable that the horse should be working above the level at which it is competing. Thus, ideally, the horse should be capable of performing leg yielding, shoulder in, countercanter, and both medium trot and canter. At intermediate level, the horse will be expected to perform rein backs, and it should learn this movement at novice stage.

It is of great benefit, from the mental point of view, if the horse performs in pure dressage competitions before facing the demands of three different disciplines. The horse should continue to compete in pure dressage once its horse trials career is underway so that the horse does not always anticipate that a cross-country will follow. Horses also can become "arena crafty," knowing that in competition they will not be disciplined; pure dressage competitions thus become a valuable schooling ground in these circumstances. This applies throughout the horse's trials career.

JUMPING

Although some jumping ability is innate, the horse requires training to learn how to judge the height of a fence, when to take off, and how to adjust stride length on the approach to and between fences. The training program must help to instill confidence and carefulness and will through repetitive exercises develop neuromuscular coordination, muscular strength, and the agility to adjust stride length. The horse must learn to jump both from trot and from a regular canter rhythm, and although it must learn to respect the rider, it must not be dominated by the rider. It must be able to think and act for itself. This is all achieved through gymnastic exercises and jumping small individual fences and fences at related distances. The horse must be capable and thoroughly used to jumping at least the competition height of fences and preferably 8 cm (3 in) higher. Experience at pure show jumping competitions is invaluable.

The horse must develop confidence and trust in the rider and boldness to tackle all sorts of cross-country fences, especially drop fences, ditches, steps, jumping into dark from light, corners, and angled fences. The horse must learn to jump from a quicker speed than for show jumping but must not unduly sacrifice accuracy and carefulness. First, the horse must develop accuracy and judgment of height of fences and takeoff point by the same techniques for show jumping. It must be taught to jump straight and "hold a line." Second, the horse must be introduced slowly to small cross-country obstacles, jumping first in show jumping style. Only later, when the horse has developed confidence and technique, should a faster approach be used. It also must be remembered that it is speed between fences that is far more important with respect to matching the optimal time rather than the speed in the immediate approach to a fence. At all costs, the horse's confidence must not be spoilt; fences should be selected carefully and not attempted until the horse is ready to do so. Do not tackle a coffin without first gaining the horse's confidence over a similar ditch; there will always be another day. Choose an easy water jump with a wide, light approach and a good sound bottom for the first entry into water; have another horse to give a lead and to instill confidence.

FITNESS

There are three priniciples aspects of fitness: fitness of the cardiovascular system, the respiratory system, and the musculoskeletal system. The horse must be sufficiently fit that the work of warming up for and performing the dressage and show-jumping phases and completing the cross-country does not unduly tire it. A tired horse is much more likely either to make enforced errors or to injure itself. Tendon and ligament injuries are principally fatigue injuries.

For novice 1-day horse trials, the work required to prepare the horse adequately for the three phases, interspersed with hacking, is probably sufficient to get the horse adequately fit, especially if the hacking involves some hill work. Nonetheless, some horses need to learn

to gallop and will require additional training to do so, preferably working alongside a more experienced horse. Cantering with a group of horses provides an exciting environment and may encourage the horse to breathe deeply.

The preceding statements assume that the horse is working for 1 to 1½ hours daily, most of the time working at trot and canter. Therefore, the overall work program combines flat work, jumping, and hacking exercise, preferably with daily turnout. This is important both for the horse's mental attitude and so that the horse is moving about as much as possible. If turnout facilities are limited, walking on a horse walker is also beneficial.

It is important also that the horse should learn to balance itself cantering up and down hill, and if the local terrain is flat, some effort must be made to find suitable ground. This work also will benefit the horse from an overall fitness point of view. Fitness will be discussed in much greater detail in the section entitled Preparation for the First 3-Day Event.

Training to Compete at Intermediate Level and the First 3-Day Event

Progression from novice to intermediate level is a significant jump. The majority of horses have the ability to compete at novice level, but additional scope and speed are required to compete successfully at intermediate level. The horse's mental attitude may have changed; some horses become more excitable, having been over cross-country courses multiple times, and this, combined with increased fitness, can provide difficulties, especially in the dressage arena. A solid foundation of training is therefore of great value. To perform an intermediate-level dressage test, the horse will require greater self-carriage in order to show greater variations within a pace (a distinct difference between working and medium trot and canter) and to perform lateral work.

FLAT WORK AND JUMPING

Regular flat-work training must proceed to instill further obedience and to develop further muscular strength and coordination and self-carriage. Some horses are rather limited in their natural paces, so special work must be done to develop the horse's stride so that a clear difference can be shown between working and medium paces. Working over trot poles, flat on the ground or slightly raised, set either in straight lines or around the perimeter of a circle, can be very helpful to increase lift and length of the stride in trot.

The horse must develop the ability to jump bigger fences, both show jumping (1.20 m, or 3 ft, 11 in) and cross-country (1.15 m, or 3 ft, 9 in). A premium should be placed on straight, accurate jumping. The horse must have learned to "hold a line" to cope successfully both with combination fences and corner and arrowhead fences. This discipline can be taught over small fences, but the horse also must jump larger fences to develop further muscular strength and coordination. Continued gymnastic exercises are invaluable. The horse will need to be bolder and have great confidence in its rider to cope with larger, "trappier" cross-country fences. The horse will have to learn to go cross-country at a faster speed than previously (570 m/min). This does not necessarily mean jumping the fences themselves from a faster speed, but it does mean learning to accelerate quickly away from a fence and being in sufficient control that the horse can easily be slowed down a little just a short distance from a fence.

In preparation for the first 3-day event, the horse also must learn how to tackle steeplechase fences, the ability to jump from a regular rhythm at a faster speed. The horse will probably be galloping more quickly in this phase than previously and must learn to cruise reasonably effortlessly at this speed (640 to 660 m/min). All this must be combined with maintaining the horse's carefulness, and again, continued gymnastic exercises are very helpful as well as competing in pure show jumping competitions.

FITNESS (TRAINING)

Fitness implies being able to carry out the work required without undue fatigue. Fatigue results in buildup of muscle lactic acid and exhaustion of muscle glycogen (energy) stores and potentially predisposes to injury (e.g., lameness). In a fit horse there is increased oxidative capacity of muscle (i.e., increased ability to utilize oxygen), an increased number of capillaries (small blood vessels) around muscle fibers, an increase in the amount of enzymes in the muscle cells which metabolize free fatty acids (an important energy source), thus sparing the glycogen stored in the muscles and increasing the *anaerobic threshold* (the stage at which muscle cells start to produce lactic acid). Fast work conditions the horse to recruit the fast-twitch, low oxidative muscle fibers (i.e., cells that have a lesser demand for oxygen). In a fit horse, the cardiovascular and respiratory systems are conditioned to provide adequate nutrient and oxygen supplies to the muscle cells so that lack of supply is not a limiting factor (for further details, see Chap. 8).

Fitness (training) becomes of increasing importance at intermediate and higher levels. The general daily work will not be adequate to enable the horse to compete at either intermediate-level 1-day horse trials or 3-day events (one and two star) because of the longer distances (2400 to 3620 m at 1-day events) and faster speeds (570 m/min) required. The training program will ultimately be geared to reaching peak fitness for the 3-day event. It is important to map out a program that allows some leeway so that if the horse sustains a minor injury and misses 7 to 10 days of work, this should not unduly alter the peak level of fitness. Nonetheless, it should be borne in mind that once a horse has achieved a level of fitness, this level will be maintained for 1 to 2 weeks despite box rest.

If, for example, the horse has been kept in regular work, flat work, and jumping between two event seasons, then the aims of the fitness program are to increase the horse's ability to work for longer periods at faster speeds without placing undue stress on the musculoskeletal, cardiovascular, and respiratory systems. It is difficult to dictate a precise program suitable for all horses and all conditions because there are a number of variable factors, including the type of horse (pure thoroughbreds are often far easier to condition and generally innately gallop better and more easily than thoroughbred crosses) and the local terrain (most importantly the availability of hills makes a great deal of difference). The work surfaces also have some influence; regular work on a soft all-weather menage or on an indoor arena surface is usually more demanding than working on grass.

The musculoskeletal system has to be conditioned so that the musculotendinous units do not become unduly fatigued. Likewise, the cardiovascular and respiratory systems need to be conditioned so that the horse is working as economically as possible. The result of conditioning is that the horse can work either at a set speed over a set distance with progressively shorter recovery periods to resting heart and respiratory rates or can work at faster speeds and/or over a long distance without undue prolongation of the recovery time. Cardiovascular conditioning should be undertaken so that horses can maintain heart rates of at least 200 beats/min (a typical heart rate at speeds equal to or greater than 500 m/min) for prolonged periods (10 to 12 minutes).

There is little doubt that this progressive increase in fitness can be done most economically by hill work in terms of minimizing undue stress placed on the musculoskeletal system and in terms of actual distance covered and time expended. Both slow hill work (walking and trotting) and fast hill work (variable speed and distance canters) should be used. In order to reach the same level of fitness, a horse worked predominantly on flat terrain will have to exercise over longer distances (and for longer periods of time). The horse may have to compete either on soft or hard ground, and it is my opinion that to minimize risk of injuries, it is appropriate to train the horse on a variety of surfaces, e.g., trot work on roads and canter work on grass (if not excessively hard) or on a variety of all-weather surfaces.

The concept of interval training can be adapted to suit the type of horse and the terrain available for canter work. This technique involves the repetition of work sessions, with short recovery periods between each session, so that the horse progresses toward baseline pulse and respiratory rates but undergoes another session before reaching these levels. Generally, three repeat sessions, each of similar length, are used over similar distances, sometimes with a progressive increase in speed. For example, the horse may start with three 3-minute canters at approximately 500 m/min (heart rate of 180 to 200 beats/min) with 2- to 3-minute rest periods (heart rate declining to approximately 110 beats/min), increasing progressively to three 8-minute canters at approximately 550 to 570 m/min with 2- to 3-minute intervals. A "non-interval" training program uses much longer periods of continuous cantering (e.g., up to 12 to 14 minutes). Both types of programs can be combined. Long periods of continuous cantering can, with appropriate facilities, sometimes be done as lose schooling. The horse must learn to canter in balance and in a regular rhythm, and this can be of benefit to the horse both mentally and physically.

Exercise to increase aerobic fitness will be performed at approximately 3- to 4-day intervals to fit in with the rest of the training schedule and competitions. Once the horse has reached adequate fitness for 1-day horse trials, the trials can substitute for one intense training day.

The fitness of a horse at any particular stage in the training program can be gauged to a certain extent by the level of the pulse and respiratory rates at the termination of the third repeat, the pattern of respiration, and the rate at which the pulse and respiratory rates decline toward baseline levels. Obviously, these factors will be influenced to some extent by temperature and humidity, wind speeds, and to a much lesser extent temperament of the horse. Recovery should be close to complete within 5 to 8 minutes of finishing training, depending on the duration and speed of the exercise. Fitness of the musculoskeletal system is difficult to gauge objectively. Exercise to condition the cardiovascular and respiratory systems should result in adequate adaptations of the musculoskeletal system, provided that work surfaces are chosen carefully and the training is not done by swimming.

Some horses are difficult to work, especially those which are inherently lazy; these horses may be helped by exercising as one of a group. A typical fitness training program is outlined in Table 17F–1. It should be borne in mind that this will have to be adapted depending on the baseline level of fitness of the horse, the available terrain, and the way in which the horse adapts to the training program. Obviously, if the interval training is done up hills, then the interval between each canter session will in part be dictated by the time to descend the hill before the next ascent.

Pulse rates can be quite difficult to assess by palpating an artery of an excited, restless horse. The heart rate can be counted easily using a stethoscope, or alternatively and most easily, a heart rate monitor can be used. These are, however, quite expensive. I believe that, with experience, a good rider develops a "feel" for how fit the horse is, but more objective measurements of pulse and respiratory rate during recovery are valuable for the less experienced rider or for the "lazy" horse. Assessment of both the pulse (heart) and the respiratory rate is valuable, rather than either one in isolation. With experience in working horses on specific training areas, the rider will develop a feel for how quickly a horse will get fitter and for the rate of recovery after a set work period.

Table 17F-1. Outline Training Program for the Final 12 Weeks Leading up to the First 3-Day Event

	Day						
Week	1	2	3	4	5	6	7
1	Day off (DO)	School and hack	Jump and hack	Hack and canter 3 × 3 min	School and hack	School and hack	Hack and canter 3 × 3 min
2	DO	School and hack	Jump and hack	3 × 4 min (500 m/min)	School and hack	School and hack	3 × 4 min
3	DO	School and hack	Jump and hack	3 × 4 min	School and hack	School and hack	Competition or 3 × 4 min
4	DO	School and hack	Jump and hack	3 × 5 min	School and hack	School and hack	3 × 5 min
5	DO	School and hack	Jump and hack	3 × 5 min	School and hack	School and hack	Competition
6	DO	School and hack	Jump and hack	3 × 5 min	School and hack	School and hack	3 × 5 min
7	DO	School and hack	Jump and hack	3 × 5 min (550 m/min)	School and hack	School and hack	Competition
8	DO	School and hack	Jump and hack	3 × 6 min	School and hack	School and hack	3 × 6 min (570 m/min)
9	DO	School and hack	Jump and hack	4 × 6 min	School and hack	School and hack	Competition
10	DO	School and hack	Jump and hack	3 × 7 min (550 m/min and one repeat at 650 m/min)	School and hack	School and hack	Competition
11	DO	School and hack	Jump and hack	3 × 7 min	School and hack	School and hack	School/jump
12	Canter and gallop	School and hack	School, first inspection	Dressage	Dressage	Speed and endurance	Show jumping

Note: It is assumed that the horse was being schooled and hacked for up to 1.5 hours daily by week 1.
Hacking includes several long periods (minimum 10 minutes) of trotting. Obviously, the schedule must be flexible to fit in with competitions, availability of dressage and jumping trainers, and the way in which the horse is adapting to the fitness program.

When preparing the horse for competitions, it is quite important to know something about the terrain at which key competitions are to be held. If these are over hilly terrain, it is quite important that the horse has done at least some of the fitness work over similar conditions. Going uphill places more demands on the cardiovascular and respiratory systems. The musculoskeletal system must be trained so that the horse can balance itself, most especially downhill, without undue fatigue.

At intermediate-level (one- and two-star) 3-day events, the horse will be required to carry a minimum of 75 kg (165 lb) during the speed and endurance phase. For many riders this is no problem; the combined weight of rider without or with the saddle will reach this weight. The horse will be accustomed to working with this weight. A problem may arise with small female riders who may have to carry up to an additional 24 kg of "dead weight." Should the conditioning work be done with or without this extra weight? Logically, it would seem probable that the horse will be likely to tire more rapidly if suddenly expected to carry an extra 20 kg or more. However, in my experience, provided that the extra weight is evenly distributed, well packed, and the horse accepts it and it does not affect its way of moving or jumping, there are only limited benefits to doing the training work with the extra weight as opposed to without. The key to success is the way in which the weight is distributed. I have used a saddle with approximately 6 kg of lead in the lining, two flasks containing lead (6 to 8 kg) attached to the front of the saddle, and additional lead in a weight cloth. Thus a large proportion of the weight is not "hanging down" on the dorsal midline, which is inevitable if a traditional weight cloth is used. Some of the routine training exercise is done with the weighted saddle, and the horse is jumped a couple of times with the full load of extra weight.

With a properly planned fitness program, the loss of 7 to 10 days of work in preparation for a 3-day event should be immaterial in terms of fitness. Swimming is a possible substitute for a limited amount of canter work but has limitations; it stresses the cardiovascular and respiratory systems quite well, but swimming uses different muscles and therefore is inadequate for conditioning the musculoskeletal system properly.

Prevention of Veterinary Problems

MUSCULOSKELETAL PROBLEMS

During the training program and in daily work it is important to try to prevent potential veterinary problems, most especially those related to the musculoskeletal system. The horse must be trimmed and shod regularly, correct balance of the foot being of paramount importance, if necessary, every 4 weeks. More problems will arise if feet start to overgrow the shoes slightly (e.g., corns, hoof cracks) than if the shoes are regularly reset even if the hoof walls are brittle. Various feed supplements (e.g., those containing methionine and biotin) may help to improve hoof wall quality in some horses.

Pads tend to result in deterioration of hoof quality beneath the pad and premature loosening of the shoe. I am opposed to long-term use of pads, but I believe that there is a place for pads at a 3-day event, if the roads and tracks phase is stony or rough, to try to prevent foot bruising. Considerable controversy surrounds the use of studs. Studs used only in the outside branch of the shoe will result in imbalance of the foot and abnormal load bearing and twisting. Therefore, provided that the horse does not have a tendency to interfere, I advocate the use of studs in both the inside and outside branches of the shoe. The greatest benefit for studs is in the dressage and show-jumping phases of a competition. Studs should be avoided under all circumstances for the roads and tracks phase.

The horse should have new shoes for a 3-day event, preferably fitted approximately 7 days prior to the first inspection. This allows sufficient time to deal with any problems, if, for example, the horse was inadvertently "pricked." Nonetheless, the shoes will still have a deep fullering line which will facilitate grip. If the horse is usually shod long and wide at the heels, it may be prudent to fit the shoe a little more tightly, because loss of a shoe during the speed and endurance phase may have devastating short-term consequences.

Leg protection will not prevent strains (over stretch injuries) of tendons and ligaments, but *some* boot and leg protector and bandage combinations can help to minimize results of direct trauma to the limbs—minimize the result of the horse hitting a fixed fence or striking into itself. I strongly advocate the use of boots and/or bandages and overreach boots for all training, jumping schooling, and competitions. Brushing boots or tendon boots must be substantial to absorb concussion and withstand a heavy, sharp blow, conform to the horse's limb, and be of appropriate length. If the boots are too long or too tight, the horse's action may be interfered with, and damage may be done to the skin, subcutaneous tissues, and/or the superficial digital flexor tendon. Most overreaches occur during cross-country schooling or at competitions and can result in a laceration and severe bruising of a heel bulb with associated lameness. The risks of severe bruising are reduced by appropriate protection. Traditional rubber overreach boots sometimes "turn up." "Petal" boots are less likely to turn up but are noisy and trap mud; the fastenings sometimes rub. Neoprene boots with Velcro fastenings are also less likely to turn up, do not rub, and provide more protection from trauma.

It is essential to monitor the limbs very carefully on a daily basis; it is vital to know how the limbs look and feel, how they vary with exercise, and how they vary with changes in the environmental temperature. Early warning signs of impending tendon and ligament damage such as focal heat, slight swelling, enlargement of a vein, and pain must be recognized. Failure to notice these signs and to take appropriate action may result in disaster. Remember that the absence of lameness does not preclude the existence of significant tendon or ligament damage. Soft-tissue swellings may disappear rapidly with cold treatment, bandaging, and box rest, but this does not necessarily imply that any underlying problem has resolved.

Professional advice should be sought whenever in doubt. The appropriate use of diagnostic ultrasonography by an experienced veterinarian can be invaluable for deciding whether there is or is not significant underlying damage. Tendon and ligament problems are of far higher incidence and greater importance to an event horse compared with a show jumper or dressage horse and can terminate a horse's career.

Try to avoid the practice of standing the horse in bandages when not in work; it is important to know how the horse's limbs look and feel without bandages. Similarly, after an event or fast work, be aware that routine use of cooling agents, cold poultices, and bandages can mask clinical signs. Be aware that signs of tendon injury may be delayed for several days after an event, most especially if the limbs have been bandaged. Also important in the prevention of injury is the selection of appropriate work surfaces. Remember that if a horse is going to compete on hard ground, it must do some conditioning work on hard ground. It is important that any work program progressively increase in intensity and that the horse is always fit enough for the expected level of competition. The horse always must be appropriately warmed up; human athletes are very aware of the risks of injury associated with inadequate warmup. Likewise, the horse must be limbered up progressively.

The event horse frequently works under saddle, and it is important that the saddle fits appropriately. If numnahs or saddle pads are used, these should remain still under the saddle and should be kept clean and in a good state of repair. Problems with saddle sores are all avoidable with proper management. Some horses seem prone to develop muscular soreness in the thoracolumbar region. This often reflects an incorrect way of working. Such horses must be encouraged to work with engagement of the hindlimbs and in a "round" outline, in balance. These horses may benefit from both lunge work and loose cantering.

RESPIRATORY PROBLEMS

Be aware that if a horse is going to perform optimally, not only should the musculoskeletal system be trained appropriately, but it also must have an optimally functioning respiratory system. Low-grade chronic obstructive pulmonary disease can significantly compromise performance and effectively slow the horse down. It is my opinion that all event horses competing at this level should be kept as far as possible under dust-free management conditions, i.e., bedded on good-quality wood shavings or paper and fed soaked hay or horsehage both at home and in transit and when staying away at competitions. A previously symptom-free horse can have acute-onset clinical signs of respiratory distress if bedded on straw for only one night at a competition.

GENERAL HEALTH

It is important not to overstress a horse that is slightly below par, and therefore, careful attention must always be paid to the horse's attitude and appetite. Daily monitoring of rectal temperature at a similar time can provide a useful indicator of anything that might be wrong. It also may be worthwhile to perform hematologic estimations (complete blood count) at 1- to 2-month intervals so that the "normal" for that particular horse is established. If problems arise, a comparison can then be made with the horse's baseline figures. It is difficult to interpret the significance of, for example, a low-normal hematocrit without comparison with baseline figures for the particular horse.

DIET AND ELECTROLYTES

Whenever the horse is competing away from home, attention must always be paid to the diet. Avoid sudden changes of concentrates or forage. The horse's diet must as far as practically possible remain unchanged.

If the horse is going to compete under hot conditions, it will be inclined to sweat a lot and lose electrolytes; supplementation is therefore important. I think that it is probably best and safest to offer electrolyte supplementation (other than just salt, sodium chloride) in the water, giving the horse free choice of normal or electrolyte-supplemented water.

RHABDOMYOLYSIS

There is a significant incidence of exertional rhabdomyolysis ("tying up") in event horses, usually occurring during competitions, especially 3-day events. Clinical signs usually develop in the speed and endurance day, either during the steeplechase (phase B) or the second roads and tracks phase (phase C) or in the compulsory 10-minute "halt" between phases C and D (cross-country). It is important to carefully assess the moving horse both when it enters the 10-minute box and approximately 5 minutes later because it is often then that the first signs of stiffness become apparent. Less commonly, a horse "ties up" at the end of cross-country, usually in association with hot, humid weather conditions. The reason(s) for "tying up" are poorly understood. If it does occur, consideration should be given on future occasions to an extended warmup phase prior to the start of phase A. It appears that some horses may be unable to absorb and/or utilize some dietary electrolytes and that such horses may benefit from appropriate dietary supplementation with sodium chloride, potassium chloride, and/or calcium carbonate. Determination of fractional excretion clearance ratios of specific electrolytes (sodium, potassium, chloride, calcium, and phosphate) while the horse is in full work on its normal ration is helpful in some cases. Dietary supplementation is then based more objectively on these results.

Training to Compete at Advanced Level and Up to Championship (Four-Star) 3-Day Events

FLAT WORK

At advanced level, the horse must be well established in lateral work (shoulder in and half-pass) and countercanter, be able to perform simple changes and rein back, and to show clear differences between working, medium, and extended paces. Bear in mind that a pure dressage horse is not asked, in a competition situation, to perform half-passes and extended paces until it is also supposed to be working in collection. Movements are easier to perform from collection, and therefore, it is reasonable to expect the event horse at this level to be working toward collection. It also must be recognized that most event horses do not have the same natural engagement of the hindlimbs, self-carriage, and paces of a dressage horse. They are expected to perform obediently and calmly when very fit, in a tense atmosphere, with many potential distractions. Once again, the importance of firm training foundations is emphasized. The young advanced horse must be taught new movements and continue to develop strength and neuromuscular coordination to perform these new movements and to improve balance and self-carriage. The older, established advanced horse must work to maintain suppleness and improve on weaknesses.

JUMPING

The size of fences in both show jumping (1.25 m, or 4 ft, 1 in) and cross-country (1.20 m, or 3 ft, 11 in) is higher than at intermediate level, and the horse must be used to jumping at this height or preferably higher. Grid work remains important to maintain suppleness and agility. Pure show-jumping competitions are invaluable and should be regarded as an important part of training for this phase when accuracy and carefulness are so important. Controlled boldness is essential in cross-country; this comes both from natural bravery and also from avoiding frights in the training and competitions up to this level. Jumping big cross-country fences in training is not important, but maintaining the horse's confidence for jumping combination fences, ditch fences, and drop fences is important. This can be achieved by schooling over fences smaller than those encountered in competition.

FITNESS

Fitness becomes of supreme importance because of the faster speeds and longer distances at advanced 1-day horse trials (600 m/min, 3250 to 4000 m) and 3-day events (570 m/min, 5700 to 6840 m at a three-star competition). Nonetheless, it must be borne in mind that the speed for 1-day horse trials is faster than that for 3-day events. Speed predisposes to injury; remember, usually the goal ultimately is to be successful at a 3-day event rather than at a 1-day event. Horses that have been trained to competition level several times usually are much easier to train than a horse that has never previously been trained to peak fitness. Frequently, the first 3-day event, if completed successfully, transforms a horse; it becomes keener, bolder, and often gallops better.

Long breaks (more than 2 months) out of training, unless enforced through injury, are undesirable. Although horses maintain some fitness when turned out in a field for a prolonged period, additional work is beneficial, especially for the musculoskeletal systems. Human athletes do not take long breaks from training, although they may modify their training programs. This is of particular importance for older horses which may have had some problems associated with the musculoskeletal system. Therefore, although it may be appropriate and beneficial to allow the horse 6 to 8 weeks turnout at the end of an autumn (fall) season, longer periods should be avoided.

The fitness program leading up to a three-star (or four-star) 3-day event must build up to either more repeat work sessions in an interval training period (e.g., four repeats) and/or longer work sessions at faster speeds (Table 17F–2). It should be remembered that the steeplechase phase at three- and four-star 3-day events has an optimal speed of 690 m/min. Thus over distances of 2760 or 3105 m (three star) or 3105 or 3450 m (four star), the total duration of effort ranges from 4 to 5 minutes.

If the horse is competing at championship (four-star) level, it may have to perform under very different environmental conditions from those to which it is accustomed. There is no doubt that conditions of high temperature and high humidity are especially dangerous, with a very real risk of compromise of the horse's normal thermoregulatory system and subsequent heat stress. Under these circumstances, it is of vital importance that the horse be monitored carefully throughout the speed and endurance phase. The horse must not be unduly pressed when it is showing genuine signs of fatigue, and the speed must be moderated accordingly. The horse must be cooled as effectively as possible during the compulsory 10-minute halt between phases C and D and at the end of phase D. This means moving air (a breeze or an air current created by fans), together with moving the horse to promote evaporation and liberal amounts of iced cold water being sponged over the horse and scraped off. There is little danger of cooling the horse too rapidly. In hot conditions, it is not unusual for the horse to finish with a rectal temperature of 41°C (106°F), but this should decrease rapidly to 39°C (102°F) within 30 to 40 minutes.

At present, we have little data available concerning the optimal preparation for competing under conditions of high temperature and humidity or at significantly higher altitude levels (e.g., sea level versus 1500 m above sea level). Obviously, the horse should be as fit as possible, and it should be taught to drink during the competition. We do not know if acclimatization is beneficial and if there is an optimal acclimatization period. We do not know how the competition should be modified if combined temperature and humidity levels are dangerously high; whether the length of one or more phases should be reduced and/or the speed.

The Problem Horse

Several problems other than overt lameness or illness may arise and include lethargy, difficulty in getting the horse fit, premature fatigue, and poor performance. Any of these problems need to be looked at from a broad

Table 17F-2. *Outline Training Program for the Final 8 Weeks Leading up to a Three- or Four-Star 3-Day Event (also see Table 17F–1)*

Week	Day 1	2	3	4	5	6	7
1	Day off (DO)	Dressage, hack	Jump, hack	Hack and canter, 3 × 6 min (500 m/min)	Hack	Dressage, hack	Hack and canter, 3 × 6 min
2	DO			3 × 6 min			3 × 6 min
3	DO	Dressage competition		3 × 7 min (550 m/min)			Competition
4	DO		Show-jumping competition	3 × 8 min			Competition
5	DO			3 × 8 min			3 × 8 min
6	DO			3 × 8 min (570 m/min)			Competition
7	DO			3 × 8 min			3 × 8 min (last 2 min 640 m/min)
8	Dressage		First inspection	Dressage	Dressage	Speed and endurance	Show jumping

viewpoint, which must include assessment of the horse as a whole (especially musculoskeletal, cardiovascular, and respiratory systems), the training program and expected level of fitness, the diet of the horse, and the ability of both the horse and the rider. Not all performance-related problems have a medical basis.

Faced with a horse with lethargy, with difficulty in getting fit, or with premature fatigue, clinical appraisal obviously should include a routine clinical examination plus evaluation of routine hematology (complete blood count). An endoscopic examination of the upper respiratory tract should be performed to rule out functional abnormalities of the upper airway or an undue amount of mucus in the trachea, reflecting lower airway inflammation. Presuming that the resting heart rate and rhythm are normal and that there are no significant murmurs, it might be worth recording an electrocardiogram tracing during exercise if facilities are available. For further details, see Chapter 14 on evaluation of poor performance.

If the horse is performing poorly, as much as possible should be found out. Has the horse had a recent fall? Has the horse recently moved up a grade? How is the poor performance manifest—stiffness, unwillingness or difficulty in performing certain movements, unexpected refusals at jumps, not jumping straight, or anything else? Such problems may reflect a training difficulty, lack of ability by the horse and/or rider, lack of confidence, or a pain-related problem. Subtle reduction in stride length or reduced hindlimb impulsion may well reflect a low-grade bilateral forelimb or hindlimb lameness. Low-grade back pain for whatever reason may compromise performance. If there are no obvious abnormalities of the musculoskeletal system, it may be worthwhile treating the horse with an oral analgesic drug (e.g., phenylbutazone, flunixin meglumine, or ketoprofen) to try to establish whether there is a pain-related problem. The horse must be treated at a high enough dose for a long enough time (e.g., phenylbutazone 2 g twice daily for 7 to 10 days) if a meaningful result is to be achieved. Nonetheless, it must be recognized that not all pain-related problems are improved by the use of analgesics; some fascial or muscle pain only responds to local rather than systemic therapy. The potentially beneficial role of some forms of physiotherapy should not be underestimated.

Conclusions

There are few aspects of training that have been investigated scientifically in event horses. Training an event horse is an art to which a little science can currently be applied. Within the scope of this book, it is not possible to cover comprehensively all aspects of training, but it is hoped that this section provides a foundation from which to build, bearing in mind that all horses are individuals. We must continue to learn both from advances in applied science and from the horses themselves.

Acknowledgments

I would like to thank Lars Sederholm for his constructive cricitism of the manuscript and the many riders, trainers, and veterinarians with whom I have shared discussions over the last several years.

17G

Training Show Jumpers

H. M. CLAYTON

The Sport of Show Jumping

The first officially organized jumping competitions were included in the program for the Royal Dublin Society's show in 1864. There were three competitions; the first was a high jump of gorse and three rails, the second was a wide jump of hurdles, and the third was a stone wall. The dimensions of the jumps are no longer known, but a wooden fence used in a qualifying competition was 1.35 m high. Over the following years, show-jumping competitions rapidly gained popularity in England and continental Europe, and the first international jumping trials were included in the World Exhibition in Paris in 1900.

In the early years of the twentieth century, Italians dominated the international jumping scene largely due to the outstanding performances of Federico Caprilli, the first proponent of the forward seat, which was demonstrated at the International Horse Show in Turin in 1901. Despite some initial opposition, the forward seat was later adopted by all cavalry schools. Riding a horse called Melopo, Caprilli established a high jump record of 2.08 m and a long jump record of 7.40 m in 1902. In the same year, the German riders performed so abysmally that the emperor forbade their participation in international competitions.

When the Olympic games were revived in 1896 in Athens, the intent was to include equestrian events. However, the logistics of transportation and organization proved insuperable, and it was not until the 1912 Stockholm Olympics that dressage, show jumping, and eventing were included. Since 1956, women have been accepted as team members, and show jumping is now one of the few sports in which men and women compete as equals.

The first Olympic show-jumping course consisted of 15 fences, some of which were combinations and some of which were jumped twice for a total of 29 jumping efforts. The maximum dimensions were 1.40 m high and 4 m wide. Today, the maximum dimensions under the rules of the International Equestrian Federation (FEI) are 1.70 m high (except in puissance, power, and skill or a high jump record) 2.00 m wide for a spread fence (except a triple bar, for which the limit is 2.20 m), and 4.50 m wide for the water jump (except when trying to establish a record).[1]

Conformation

A horse's conformation undoubtedly affects its jumping ability, but data correlating specific conformational attributes to success in jumping competitions are limited. Typically, good jumpers are tall at the withers[2] with a long, straight shoulder. The ratio between the chest girth and wither height tends to be relatively low in good show jumpers, as does the ratio between cannon circumference and wither height.[2] Anecdotal evidence suggests that good jumpers have long forearm and leg segments so that the knees and hocks are close to the ground. When the horse is viewed from behind, width through the hip and gaskin is desirable.

Biomechanics

Biomechanics applies the laws of mechanics to living systems. In jumping horses, mechanical laws govern the trajectory of the center of gravity and the rotation of the horse's body during the airborne phase. Mechanical considerations are also involved in the stride adjustments that precede the takeoff and follow the landing.

Horses usually approach and move away from a fence in a canter. In this gait, the sequence of limb placements in each stride is trailing hindlimb (TrH), followed by the leading hindlimb (LdH) and trailing front limb (TrF), which make impact almost simultaneously, and finally, the leading front limb (LdF). After the LdF leaves the ground, there is usually a short suspension before the next impact of the TrH. When a horse is cantering on a left lead, the TrH is the right hindlimb, the LdH is the left hindlimb, the TrF is the right front limb, and the LdF is the left front limb. On a right lead, the sequence is reversed.

The stride in which the horse jumps the fence is called the *jump stride* (JS). It is characterized by a long suspension between liftoff of the LdH and impact of the TrF, during which the horse is airborne over the fence. The airborne phase is called the *jump suspension;* the hindlimb stance phases preceding the jump suspension constitute the *takeoff,* and the front limb stance phases following the jump suspension are referred to as the *landing.* The strides preceding (*approach strides)* and following (*move-off strides)* the jump stride are named from the jump outwards (Figure 17G–1). Starting three full strides before the jump, they are known as approach stride 3 (A3), approach stride 2 (A2), approach stride 1 (A1), and jump stride (JS), move-off stride 1 (M1), move-off stride 2 (M2), and move-off stride 3 (M3).[3] The strides A1 and M1 are highly modified canter strides; A1 initiates the upward movement of the forehand prior to takeoff, while M1 reestablishes the horse's balance after landing. The horizontal velocity, stride length, and stride rate for strides A2, A1, JS, and M1 are shown in Table 17G–1.

APPROACH

The horse approaches the fence in a canter at a suitable speed in accordance with its strength and level of technical skill. Generally, a more experienced jumper can cope with a faster approach through being stronger and having better control of its motor skills. If the takeoff speed is too fast, the horse may not be able to generate enough force sufficiently rapidly to clear the fence in good form. Consequently, the horse either hits the fence or clears it by making a compensatory action such as rolling a shoulder or twisting in the air.

The stride length is adjusted during the approach so that the takeoff occurs at an appropriate distance from the base of the fence. In a study of four Grand Prix horses jumping vertical and square oxer fences with a height and width of 1.10 to 1.40 m, no significant difference was found for the limb displacements from the base of the fence in strides A2, A1, JS, or M1.[4] Therefore,

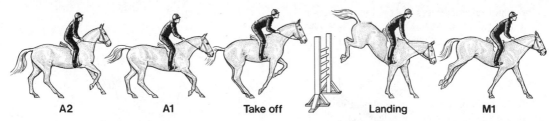

Figure 17G-1. Outline drawing of horse and rider during the approach, jump, and move-off (A2, approach stride 2; A1, approach stride 1; JS, jump stride; M1, move-off stride 1).

the takeoff distance was the same regardless of fence height or width, within the range tested, and any adjustments in stride were made prior to stride A2. The limb placed closest to the fence on the take off side is usually the LdF in stride A1.[4] One study found a correlation between fewer penalties during a competitive round and the tendency to place the LdF closest to the base of the fence on the takeoff side.[5]

During the approach strides up to and including A2, the horse canters in a collected frame. The head and neck are elevated, the nose is ahead of the poll (see Fig. 17G-1), and the TrH and LdF make impact almost synchronously.[6]

Compared with the preceding strides, A1 is a short, quick stride (see Table 17G-1),[6] in which the horse's motion is often described as "patting the ground." Stride A1 has a four-beat rhythm due to dissociation of the diagonal limb pair, with the LdH making impact before the TrF. The head and neck stretch forward and down as the horse lowers its center of gravity prior to initiation of the upward movement (see Fig. 17G-1). The front limbs are thrust forward in a strutting action, hitting the ground at a more acute angle than usual,[6] which allows them to decelerate the forward movement of the body.[7] Consequently, there is a significant reduction in horizontal velocity during stride A1 (see Table 17G-1). The front limbs also provide a large vertical force that starts the upward movement of the forehand. Since the TrF exerts a higher peak vertical force[7] and has a longer stance duration than the LdF,[6] it makes a greater contribution to the upward impulse. A short suspension follows liftoff of the LdF,[6,7] and then the hindlimbs hit the ground to initiate the takeoff.

TAKEOFF

During the takeoff, impact of the TrH may precede that of the LdH, but often the two hindlimbs are placed almost synchronously.[6,8] Initially, the hindlimbs decelerate the forward movement, but then a large horizontal accelerative force is applied in the later part of the takeoff.[7] The hindlimb stance duration is longer during takeoff than in a normal stride, which allows the generation of a large impulse.[6] Since the center of gravity lies ahead of the line of action of the force exerted by the hindlimbs against the ground, this force imparts angular momentum that causes the horse's body to rotate forward around the center of gravity during the jump suspension. As a consequence of the angular momentum, the horse takes off from the hindlimbs and lands on the forelimbs.

Some important mechanical characteristics of the jump, including the path of the center of gravity and the angular momentum, are established during the takeoff and cannot be changed until the horse makes contact with the ground or some other object. Sometimes horses bank a fence (push off the top of a solid fence) or make adjustments such as dropping the hindlimbs between the rails of an oxer in an attempt to compensate for a takeoff that is mechanically inappropriate.

JUMP SUSPENSION

During the jump suspension, horses use different styles or techniques. Jumping ability is optimized by adopting a technique that minimizes the height discrepancy between the top of the fence and the horse's center of gravity. When the horse bascules (flexes the vertebral column), it lowers the position of the center of gravity within its trunk. Elevation of the limbs as they pass over the fence minimizes the height to which the center of gravity must be raised for all the body parts to clear the fence. In the front limbs, elevation of the lower limb is accomplished by swinging the point of the shoulder forward and upward, which pulls the elbow forward. With the upper limbs in this position, the horse able to flex

Table 17G-1. Mean Values for Velocity, Stride Length, and Stride Rate in Four Horses Jumping a Vertical Fence 1.55 m High

	Approach stride 2	Approach stride 1	Jump stride	Move-off stride 1
Velocity (m/s)	7.3	6.3	5.9	6.5
Stride length (m)	4.1	2.4	4.9	3.3
Stride rate (strides per second)	1.8	2.6	1.2	1.9

the elbow and raise its knees. As the hindquarters pass over the fence the lumbosacral joint extends to elevate the hindquarters, while extension of the hip joint raises the lower limbs.

LANDING

The TrF makes impact first with an almost vertical orientation, quickly followed by the LdF, which has a more acute angulation to the ground.[6] Both front limbs experience high peak vertical forces as they absorb the concussion of landing. The TrF, which has a very short stance duration at landing, provides some horizontal propulsion to assist in moving the horse away from the jump, while the LdF reverses the direction of rotation of the trunk around the center of gravity. The trunk continues its downward trajectory as it passes over the front limbs.

MOVE-OFF

In the short suspension that follows landing, the hindquarters swing underneath the trunk. The TrH is placed further from the fence than the TrF but closer than the LdF.[4,5] In contrast to the fairly predictable position of the TrH, that of the LdH is quite variable. Sometimes it lands adjacent to the TrH; other times the two hindlimbs are widely separated. The LdH placement seems to depend on the horse's balance during the landing and move-off. Stride M1 covers a short distance, but the stride rate is approximately the same as that of stride A2 (see Table 17G–1). It has a distinct four-beat rhythm due to dissociation of the diagonal limbs with the LdH preceding the TrF.[6] In the subsequent move-off strides, the horse reestablishes a normal stride pattern.

Physiologic Demands of Show Jumping

The majority of show-jumping competitions require a minimum speed in the range of 325 to 400 m/min, although the average speed during a round may be considerably faster when time is a deciding factor. Heart rate recordings have shown that the exercise intensity is greater than would be expected from the average speed due to the fact that large amounts of energy are expended in overcoming the body's inertia during takeoff and landing.

The warmup for a show jumping competition involves a moderate exercise intensity at an average heart rate of 96 beats/min,[9] but with peak values as high as 173 beats/min.[10] The heart rate peaks each time the horse jumps a practice fence, and there appears to be a direct correlation between heart rate and fence height, which may be related to a faster speed of approach to the larger fences.[10] While the horse waits at the in gate, the heart rate is in the range of 71 to 93 beats/min. During a competitive round, the heart rate rises steadily as the horse progresses around the course,[9,11] as shown in Figure 17G–2, reaching peak values as high as 205 beats/min. The fact that the heart rates are so high confirms that show jumping is a strenuous sport despite the

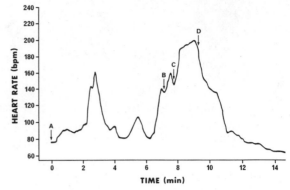

Figure 17G-2. *Heart rate of a horse from the start of the warmup until after the warm-down following a competitive jumping round. (A) Start of warmup. (B) Horse enters course. (C) Start of the round. (D) End of the round and start of recovery. (From Art T, Amory H, Desmecht D et al: Effect of show jumping on heart rate, blood lactate and other biochemical values. Equine Vet J. 1990; (suppl 9): 78, with permission)*

relatively slow average speed. It has been suggested that the energy expended by a show jumper is equivalent to galloping the same distance at a speed of 600 m/min.[9]

The onset of blood lactate accumulation occurs at heart rates in excess of 150 to 160 beats/min,[12] so it is not surprising that show jumping is associated with a marked elevation in blood lactate.[9,11,13] Significant alterations also have been recorded in the packed cell volume, which rises as high as 60 percent from a resting value of around 35 percent, and the red blood cell count, which has been shown to increase to 9.49×10^6 from a resting value of 5.8×10^6 due to the ejection of red blood cells from the spleen.[10]

A rise in plasma cortisol from a resting value of 67.6 mmol/liter to 118.7 mmol/liter has been found after a show-jumping competition.[9] Cortisol levels reflect adrenal activity and physiologic stress, and during exercise, the extent of the rise is related to the duration and/or intensity of the workout. The cortisol increase in show jumpers is less than in thoroughbred racing (high intensity) or endurance racing (long duration). During competitions, experienced jumpers have significantly smaller increases in plasma cortisol than inexperienced jumpers, suggesting that horses become conditioned to the psychological stress of the show environment.[3]

Show jumping is associated with reductions in plasma Ca^{2+}, Cl^-, and HCO_3^-, an increase in Na^+, and no change in K^+ concentrations.[3,11] Total plasma protein increases, and this finding, together with the increased plasma Na^+, is indicative of a reduction in plasma volume due to a net movement of fluid out of the extracellular compartment. There is a metabolic acidosis due to the increased HCO_3^-, and this is associated with the substantial increase in lactic acid. Marked increases in the activities of lactate dehydrogenase, creatine kinase, and aspartate aminotransferase have been found, but not in gamma glutamyl transferase following jumping competition.[3,11]

Overall, the physiologic response to show jumping suggests that the relatively slow average speed belies the intense effort required to jump fences every 5 seconds or so. Anaerobic metabolism makes a significant contribution to the energy supply, as shown by the accumulation of lactate.

Training on the Flat

Course designers rely heavily on technical problems to sort out a field of high-class show jumpers rather than depending on the size of the fences alóne. Consequently, show jumpers must be well schooled on the flat so that the horse is ridable and obedient between fences and is able to cope with the adjustments in stride length and the tight turns that are required in competition. The well-trained show jumper turns, moves laterally, and adjusts the stride length immediately in response to the rider's aids. Practice of these skills improves the horse's motor control and teaches it to move efficiently and economically, thereby saving energy and delaying the onset of fatigue due to lactate accumulation.

In classic dressage training, the horse works through six steps of rhythm, suppleness, contact, straightness, impulsion, and collection, and this progression is also applicable to flat training for show jumpers. The horse should move in a round frame supple in the jaw with direct flexion at the poll, the vertebral column flexed. When the horse works in this frame, it develops the muscles along the top line, allows engagement of the hindquarters, and facilitates the development of collection. Lateral bending of the vertebral column and lateral flexion at the poll are equally important. The horse is taught to yield laterally both to the rein (shoulder yielding) and to the leg (leg yielding), which improves ridability and adjustability between fences. The more classical exercises of shoulder in, shoulder out, haunches in (travers), and haunches out (renvers) are particularly beneficial for lateral suppleness. Turns and circles are performed in true flexion and in counterflexion to improve lateral suppleness and control.

From the start of the training program, the horse must learn to respond promptly and calmly to the aids to go forward, come back, and move laterally; instant obedience becomes increasingly important as the horse progresses through the levels of competition, and it is best to establish this type of discipline at an early stage. Frequent transitions help to keep the horse's attention focused, and when they are performed correctly, transitions between and within the gaits engage the hindquar-

ters. Consequently, the forehand becomes lighter, and this facilitates the rider's control.

The importance of being able to adjust the horse's stride length cannot be overemphasized; many of the problems on a course involve related distances between fences that require the ability to shorten or lengthen the stride in order to arrive at an appropriate takeoff distance. Furthermore, because horses breathe in rhythm with the stride when cantering and galloping, the most energetically efficient way of changing speed is to lengthen and shorten the stride while maintaining a constant rhythm or stride rate. Each time the rhythm changes, extra energy is expended in breathing until the new rhythm is established.

The ability to turn quickly becomes increasingly important at the higher levels of competition. Turning skills are enhanced by teaching the horse to sit on the hindquarters during tight turns.

It takes a long time to develop the technical skills required to be competitive in high-level show jumping. The best results are achieved through a combination of schooling exercises, together with appropriate strength training and suppling to reduce the risk of breakdown. Adaptations in the ligaments and tendons occur very slowly, and the technical training should not be rushed lest musculoskeletal injuries occur due to inadequate conditioning.

Training Over Fences

As in training on the flat, there are different systems of training over fences. This section will give only an outline of the objectives and a reasonable order of progression, with the methods of achieving these objectives being left to the discretion of the experienced trainer. The best results are always obtained by modifying the exercises and the rate of progression in accordance with the individual horse's talents and deficiencies. Schooling over fences proceeds hand-in-glove with schooling on the flat, and the exercises used to improve jumping skills at any stage of training are limited by the horse's flatwork ability. Strength training exercises should be integrated into the program to strengthen appropriate muscle groups and reduce the risk of injury.

Training over fences aims to improve the horse's technical jumping skills but inherent ability also plays an important role. In one study, a group of horses was classified as poor, intermediate, or good jumpers at the start of a 9-month training program. When the same horses were reevaluated after completing the training program over fences, it was found that the classifications had not changed.[2] In other words, inherent ability had more influence on the horse's final skill than training.

The work over fences may include jumping on the lunge, free jumping in a jumping lane, and ridden exercises. At an early stage in the training program, the horse should learn to walk, trot, and canter over rails on the ground to improve coordination and develop a greater awareness of limb position. When the horse is able to trot rhythmically over five rails [1.2 to 1.5 m (4 to 5 ft) apart], it is an easy step to include a small cross-pole after the trot rails.

The progressive development of jumping skills involves negotiating single fences at a trot and later at a canter, jumping two fences at an easy related distance, and jumping small grids that incorporate bounce, one, two, and three stride distances. Ground lines may be used to encourage the horse to take off at a suitable distance from the base of the fence so that there is room to elevate the front legs. Placing poles on the takeoff and landing sides help to ensure that the peak of the jumping arc is centered on the middle of the fence. The position of the placing poles relative to the base of the fence depends on the way the horse jumps and the problems that need to be corrected.

Gymnastic jumping grids are invaluable for teaching the horse to jump in good form and for correcting faults in technique. The profile of the fences (vertical, ramped oxer, square oxer, etc.) and the distances between them are adjusted in accordance with the training objectives. Ideally, the horse learns to adjust its stride length and to take off at an appropriate trajectory to clear the fence without overjumping it. After a lesson has been mastered technically, multiple repetitions can be used to build muscular strength in a highly sport-specific manner.

Fences set at related distances are used to teach the horse to adjust stride length. In the early stages, the horse is asked to add a stride in a line by shortening the stride length. Later the horse is asked to take out a stride by increasing the stride length, taking care that the horse does not flatten the arc when jumping from a longer stride.

In the early stages of training, horses should jump frequently to facilitate the learning of technical skills and to promote musculoskeletal adaptations in response to the unique orientation of the stresses on the limbs. Since the tissues adapt slowly over a period of many months, it is wise to restrict the jumping activities to small fences for at least 3 to 6 months. During this time, a variety of fence types can be introduced, including verticals and oxers, solid fences, narrow fences, and small ditches. The objective is for the horse to approach the fences straight, in a good rhythm, and with a confident but relaxed attitude. Over the fence, the horse should lower its head and neck, round its back, and raise the lower limbs as high as necessary to clear the jump in good form but without overjumping. The horse should move away from the fence with a relaxed, rhythmic stride, prepared to shorten or lengthen as necessary.

As the training over fences progresses, new skills are introduced, including bending lines, jumping on an angle, and coping with difficult distances in combinations. The horse should master normal, short, and long strides in a two-stride distance and then in a one-stride distance. By maintaining the same approach speed, the horse is encouraged to adjust between the fences rather than changing the takeoff or landing distances. Gradually, the size of the fences is increased, but progress is slow in accordance with the rate of musculoskeletal adaptation.

Conditioning the Show Jumper

The successful show jumper combines a unique blend of power, precision, and speed. The airborne time over each fence is only about half a second, and most of the time in the ring is spent cantering or galloping between fences. However, each jump involves brief periods of rapid energy expenditure at takeoff and landing which call for powerful contractions in specific muscle groups. These intense muscular efforts are repeated every 5 seconds or so.

In designing a conditioning program for show jumpers, three areas are addressed: cardiovascular fitness, muscular strength, and suppleness. Cardiovascular conditioning improves the aerobic capacity while maintaining sufficient anaerobic power for the energy-intensive aspects of the competition, strength training enhances muscular power in the appropriate muscle groups, and suppling exercises improve the horse's athleticism and reduce the risk of injury.

CARDIOVASCULAR CONDITIONING

Cardiovascular conditioning improves the ability of the cardiovascular, respiratory, and muscular systems to produce energy by the appropriate metabolic pathways for the sport. In show jumping, the proportions of the total energy requirement supplied by aerobic and anaerobic metabolism depend on the fitness of the horse, the size and number of fences, the length of the track, and the horse's speed on course. A relatively long Derby course relies more heavily on aerobic metabolism than a speed competition over a short, twisting course, when the faster speed and shorter recovery time between fences place a greater demand on anaerobic metabolism.

In a horse that has recently started work under saddle, cardiovascular conditioning begins with a period of slow, long-distance work in which the frequency of exercise is every second day, the duration is short (10 to 15 minutes), and the exercise intensity is low (walking, trotting). An incremental increase in either the duration or intensity (speed) of the work is applied on a weekly basis. Gentle gradients are introduced in the later stages of the slow, long-distance program, with the horse working up, down, and across the slope.

The objective of the slow, long-distance phase is to get the horse fit enough to exercise for about 50 minutes average speed of 6 to 8 km/h (4 to 5 miles/h), *(45)* including 2- to 3-minute periods of cantering. It takes 6 to 12 months to complete the slow, long-distance phase, depending on the age, breed, and history of the horse. As a general rule, the younger the horse, the slower is the rate of progression. On completion of the slow, long-distance phase, there is a gradual transition to an interval training format in which cardiovascular workouts are performed three times a week, and progressively more of the conditioning is done at a canter because this is the gait used in competition.

Initially, two 2-minute canters are performed at a speed of 350 m/min, separated by a 2-minute rest at a walk. Progressive loading involves increasing the number of repetitions to three, after which the duration is raised to 3 minutes and then 4 minutes. There is an equal increase in the rest interval to maintain a 1:1 work/rest ratio. The next step is to raise the speed of the canters to 375 m/min and then 400 m/min. At this stage, a workout consists of three 4-minute canters at 400 m/min separated by 4 minutes of walking. The heart rate during the workouts is in the range of 130 to 160 beats/min, and it should fall below 100 beats/min in the rest intervals.

Speed play is introduced into the periods of cantering at a fairly early stage to recruit the fast-twitch muscle fibers; the horse accelerates over a distance of 50 to 100 m and then decelerates to the previous cantering speed. Initially, two accelerations are included in a workout, and the number is increased by two per week until 10 short sprints are performed in each workout. During the sprints, the heart rate reaches 160 to 170 beats/min. The next step is to increase the distance of some of the sprints to 100 to 200 m. When the horse reaches this stage, it is ready to compete in novice competitions.

For horses moving up the competitive levels, the intensity of the speed play is increased by accelerating and decelerating more sharply, sprinting at faster speeds, or using a slight uphill gradient. The heart rate is maintained at 170 to 200 beats/min for periods of 20 to 60 seconds.

Show jumpers use a considerable amount of energy in overcoming inertia, and this is a major contributor to the anaerobic nature of the sport. The effects of inertia are felt every time the horse accelerates, decelerates, or turns. Taking off and landing over a jump require an intense muscular effort and are particularly expensive energetically. Therefore, an important component of the cardiovascular conditioning program is inertial drills, which include acceleration sprints and turning drills.[14]

In an acceleration sprint, the horse accelerates from a standing start, maintains the speed over a short distance, and then slows to a walk. A work/rest ratio of 1:6 is used due to the high intensity of the workouts. In the rest intervals, the horse performs suppling exercises at a relaxed trot or a walk. Progressive loading is applied by increasing first the number, then the duration, and finally, the speed (intensity) of the acceleration sprints. The use of an uphill gradient is a good method of increasing the intensity. Some horses get very excited by acceleration sprints, and if this is the case, it is preferable to use high-intensity speed play instead.

An example of an inertial drill for show jumpers is to have the horse accelerate over a distance of 50 m, decelerate, turn through 180 degrees, and then accelerate again. Using an IT format, two to four accelerations, decelerations, and turns constitute one work, and this is followed by a rest interval in which the horse performs suppling exercises at a relaxed trot. A work/rest ratio of 1:6 is appropriate for this type of exercise. Gymnastic jumping also can be regarded as a sport-specific inertial drill due to the large energy expenditure in overcoming inertia at each takeoff and landing.

STRENGTH TRAINING

Jumping is a highly specialized activity. Strength training for show jumpers is aimed at developing explosive power in the muscles that provides the force needed to elevate the horse's body mass into the air at takeoff. Elevation of the center of gravity over the fences is minimal over fences less than 1 m high, but muscular strength becomes progressively important over larger fences. Strength training should mimic the range and speed of joint motion used in the sport. Each time the horse takes off over a fence, the stifle and hock joints flex deeply and then extend powerfully to project the horse's body into the air. Strength training exercises that use a similar motion pattern include gymnastic jumping and bounding up steep gradients.

Strength training is introduced after completion of the slow, long-distance phase and is performed two or three times a week, which balances the need for sufficient muscular stimulation with enough rest. A strength training workout causes some minor (microscopic) tissue damage which is repaired on the days between workouts. If the exercises are repeated too frequently, damage accumulates, predisposing to injury or breakdown. In the annual conditioning cycle, the ideal time to improve strength is during the off season from competition.

Over a period of 6 months, it is possible to increase the strength in specific muscle groups by as much as 50 to 100 percent, which will produce a measurable improvement in performance. During the competitive season, if the horse has a heavy competition schedule, the gains in strength will be maintained without the need for specific strength training workouts. In horses that are competing lightly, a single strength training workout each week is sufficient for maintenance.

It is important that the horse work in good form throughout the strength training exercises to ensure that the appropriate muscle groups are trained. As fatigue develops, the horse compensates by using different muscles, and the exercise is then counterproductive because the wrong muscles are strengthened. The trainer must be alert to this possibility, and either correct the horse's technique or stop the exercise as soon as compensatory movements occur. In contrast to the situation in human athletes, strength training is not continued to exhaustion in horses because of the risk of injury. Instead, the workout is terminated when signs of muscular fatigue occur.

Gradients. Bounding up a steep gradient is useful for strength training in jumpers; the two hindlimbs are pulled forward beneath the trunk and then are extended forcefully as they push off against the ground in a movement that mimics takeoff. Since the joints of the hindlimbs move through a wide range of motion, this exercise also benefits suppleness. The fact that the horse takes several bounds in succession prepares the muscles for the repeated takeoffs in a combination. An IT format is used, in which bounding up the gradient is the work and descending at a walk is the rest interval. A work/rest ratio of 1:6 is appropriate.

Gymnastic Jumping. Gymnastic jumping is a highly sport-specific strength training method for show jumpers. By adjusting the height and width of the fences and the distances between them, the trainer can improve the horse's mental and physical agility as well as its muscular strength. Gymnastic jumping also strengthens the muscles responsible for snapping up the front legs after take-off, enabling the horse to raise its knees higher and faster.

The key factors in using gymnastic jumping as a strength training tool are, first, that the horse be familiar with the technical skills and, second, that sufficient repetitions be performed to stimulate muscular adaptation. For strength training, an IT format is used, with a work/rest ratio of 1:6. Jumping through the grid is the work, and returning to the start of the grid at a trot or walk is the rest interval. Suppling exercises are performed in the rest intervals. Progressive loading is accomplished by a weekly increase in the size or number of fences or in the number of repetitions performed. The use of a series of small fences (60 to 90 cm high) leading to two or three large fences at the end of the grid is good muscular preparation for jumping through combinations, and it emphasizes the development of explosive muscular power in the hindquarters.

When the horse jumps regularly, the bones, ligaments, and tendons are strengthened in a highly sport-specific manner that cannot be achieved by other types of exercise. Even experienced jumpers should be schooled over fences at least once a week to maintain the strength of these tissues.

SUPPLING EXERCISES

Suppleness is important for enabling the horse to jump in good form, for maximizing the horse's athletic ability, and for minimizing the risk of injury. A greater range of joint motion benefits the equine athlete by providing more shock absorption when the leg is on the ground, thereby reducing the incidence of injuries. It also allows the horse to apply forces against the ground over longer periods of time, producing increased velocities and accelerations. A limited range of motion is associated with an inferior ability to generate momentum and absorb impact forces.

Some aspects of suppleness are specific to jumping sports. When the horse bascules over a jump by rounding (flexing) the neck and back, it lowers the position of its center of gravity within the trunk, and this reduces the muscular effort required to clear the fence. Movements originating at the base of the neck are important in jumpers because the head and neck are used to adjust the horse's balance and to change the location of the center of gravity. Therefore, suppleness in the neck and back should receive continual attention throughout the horse's career. Other parts of the body in which suppleness is particularly important in show jumpers include the shoulder region, which determines the ability to elevate the lower limb. In the hindlimbs, the lumbosacral and hip joints are important because they are responsi-

ble for elevating the hindquarters over the apex of the fence.

Suppling exercises are performed daily. They increase the range of joint motion by reducing tension and resistance in the muscles or connective tissues (tendons, ligaments, joint capsules), and regular suppling progressively increases the range of motion of a joint or set of joints. A period of 3 months produces significant improvements in flexibility, but suppling exercises should continue to be a part of the daily routine throughout the horse's athletic career. The amount of tissue lengthening that persists after a suppling exercise ceases depends on the force used to stretch the tissues and the duration over which the force is applied.[14] High-force, short-duration stretching at low temperatures favors elastic deformation. This is a temporary change which is reversed when the force is removed. Permanent lengthening of the ligaments and tendons is maximized when a low force is applied for a longer duration to tissues that are warm. Cold tissues are also more brittle and susceptible to tearing, so the horse should be thoroughly warmed up by a period of active forward movement before starting the suppling exercises.

Suppling exercises are classified according to whether the stretching force is passive or dynamic in nature, and both types are useful and beneficial in jumping horses. Integration of the suppling exercises into the daily routine is accomplished by starting the workout with a forward-moving warmup to increase the temperature of the tissues, after which dynamic suppling exercises become an integral part of the warmup, the workout, and the warm-down. Passive suppling is performed after exercise each day while the tissues are still warm.

Dynamic Suppling. Dynamic suppling involves rapid rotation of a joint through its range of motion as a result of muscular contraction or weight bearing. Examples of dynamic suppling exercises that are a part of the normal schooling routine include turns, circles, voltes, and lateral movements (leg yielding, shoulder in/out, haunches in/out, half-pass). The beneficial effects of this type of exercise arise from the fact that the scapulae slide across the chest wall, the hindlimbs swing through a wide arc of motion, and the vertebral column undergoes flexion, bending, and rotation. Other exercises that have a dynamic suppling effect include walking and trotting over raised rails, gymnastic jumping, and bounding up steep gradients. All these exercises are associated with active flexion and extension of the joints through a wide range of motion.

Since the shoulder movements responsible for snapping up the horse's knees at takeoff are brought about by active muscular contractions, gymnastic jumping has a highly sport-specific effect in terms of both dynamic suppling and strength training. For the hindlimbs, gymnastic jumping and bounding up steep gradients fulfill the dual objectives of improving strength while enhancing suppleness in the lumbosacral and hip joints. The suppling effect comes from working the joints through a wide range of motion; the hindlimbs are pulled forward beneath the body at impact, which flexes the lumbosacral and hip joints, and then are extended fully as the horse pushes off against the ground.

Passive Suppling. Passive suppling involves a slow, controlled movement of a joint to the limit of its range of motion through the application of an external force. Because the force is applied slowly, it avoids stimulating a reflex muscular contraction that would oppose the stretch. When the limit of movement in a particular direction is reached, the stretched position is held for 20 seconds to enhance permanent elongation of the ligaments, tendons, and joint capsules. Passive suppling is used to bring about long-term increases in the range of motion in the neck, shoulders, and hips, to promote relaxation, and to reduce postexercise muscular soreness. As with all types of suppling exercises, the tissues should be warmed up before passive suppling is performed. This is best accomplished by a period of exercise under saddle or on the lunge, which means that it is more appropriate to perform passive suppling during or after, rather than before, a workout.

In show jumpers, the ranges of motion in the shoulder region and the hip joints are maximized by stretching them in all directions using a series of passive suppling exercises which have been described in detail elsewhere.[14] The horse should be in a quiet environment and standing squarely before starting. It is safer if the horse is held by an assistant rather than being tied up, and the person performing the stretches should have plenty of room to maneuver on all sides of the horse.

The front leg is pulled forward and upward to stretch the elbow and shoulder, keeping the knee slightly bent to relieve tension in the flexor tendons and suspensory ligament. In turn, the leg is moved backward, medially, and laterally, with one hand applying pressure above the horse's knee. Each stretched position is held for 20 seconds.

In the hindlimb, passive suppling concentrates on the hip joint. The hindlimb is pulled forward with the stifle and hock flexed to about 90 degrees, with the tibia vertical and the cannon bone horizontal. By applying upward pressure from below the hock, the tibia and stifle are raised and the hip joint is flexed. When the leg is stretched backward, the hock is flexed to 90 degrees, with the tibia horizontal and the cannon bone vertical. Gentle pressure is applied to the front of the stifle, pulling the femur back to extend the hip joint. In the medial stretch, the stifle and hock are moderately extended so that the hock of the stretched leg moves across in front of and slightly above the opposite hock. For the lateral stretches, the whole leg is moved laterally.

Other suppling exercises that are not strictly passive in nature because the horse is responsible for the movement involve feeding a tidbit in different positions, such as between the front legs to flex the neck and at the flank to bend the neck laterally.

Other Considerations

Show jumpers that are not completely sound pose a conditioning problem. Usually these are older horses with chronic injuries to the flexor tendons or suspensory or check ligaments or mild osteoarthritis. These horses have sufficient experience that they do not need to jump frequently to improve their technical skills, but unless they jump at least once a week, the strength of the musculoskeletal tissues is compromised. If the horse is saved for big competitions and then rested between shows, the tendons and ligaments lose strength and become vulnerable to injury. The best insurance against injury is to perform adequate strengthening exercises early in the horse's career and to maintain the strength by jumping small fences once or twice a week during the off season. Shortcuts in strength training for jumpers may lead to strains of the suspensory ligament, check ligament, or superficial flexor tendon. If a layoff is unavoidable, adequate time must be allowed during the reconditioning period for the support tissues to regain strength. These tissues adapt very slowly, but unless sufficient time is allowed, there is an increased risk of breakdown when full work is resumed.

The food intake of show jumpers should be restricted to a maximum of 1.5 percent of body weight daily to reduce the weight of water retained in the intestine by large amounts of fibrous food.[15] Concentrates are fed as needed to maintain condition and performance. When horses sweat copiously or frequently, electrolytes are added to the feed or water to ensure adequate replenishment. Plain water must be freely available so that excess electrolytes can be excreted in the urine. A good electrolyte mixture is three parts sodium chloride (common salt) to one part potassium chloride. For show jumpers, this mixture is fed at a rate of 1 to 2 tablespoons daily.

When the horse is at a show, the stable routine is adjusted as necessary to ensure that the horse is produced in top form. Specific considerations include ensuring adequate rest, providing water throughout the day, and adjusting the diet to allow for traveling and different levels of exercise. When the horse is out of the stall (warming up, waiting to compete, competing), stress is reduced by having drinking water available as required and by taking measures to warm or cool the horse according to the weather. When the weather is cool, blankets are used to conserve body heat, and the horse is kept moving to prevent chilling. When it is hot, heat buildup is reduced by standing the horse in the shade and using cool water to sponge the horse down between rounds. Since show jumpers accumulate fairly large amounts of lactate during a round, they should be warmed down with a few minutes of easy exercise after leaving the ring. This hastens lactate removal from the muscles, allows a gradual redistribution of blood flow away from the working muscles, and reduces postexercise muscular soreness. Massage and passive stretching are also beneficial for reducing muscular soreness after strenuous exercise.

References

1. Fédération Equestre Internationale: Rules for jumping events. Fédération Equestre Internationale, Paris, 1992.

2. Fabiani M: Próba wczesnej oceny zdolności koni do skoków. II Konie z Zakladów Treningowych w Kwidzynie i Bialym Borze. Prace Mat Zootech 1973; 4:39.

3. Clayton HM: Terminology for the description of equine jumping kinematics. J Equine Vet Sci 1989; 9:341.

4. Clayton HM, Barlow DA: The effect of fence height and width on the limb placements of show jumping horses. J Equine Vet Sci 1989; 9:179.

5. Deuel N, Park J-J: Kinematic analyses of jumping sequences of Olympic show jumping horses. *In* Persson SGB, Lindholm A, Jeffcott LB (eds): Equine Exercise Physiology 3. Davis, Calif, ICEEP Publications, 1991, p 158.

6. Clayton HM, Barlow DA: Stride characteristics of four Grand Prix jumping horses. *In* Persson SGB, Lindholm A, Jeffcott LB (eds): Equine Exercise Physiology 3. Davis, Calif, ICEEP Publications, 1991, p 151.

7. Merkens HW, Schamhardt HC, van Osch GJVM, et al: Ground reaction force analysis of Dutch warmblood horse at canter and jumping. *In* Persson SGB, Lindholm A, Jeffcott LB (eds): Equine Exercise Physiology 3. Davis, Calif, ICEEP Publications, 1991, p 128.

8. Leach DH, Ormrod K, Clayton HM: Stride characteristics of horses competing in Grand Prix jumping. Am J Vet Res 1984; 45:888.

9. Lekeux P, Art T, Linden A, et al: Heart rate, hematological and serum biochemical responses to show jumping. *In* Persson SGB, Lindholm A, Jeffcott LB (eds): Equine Exercise Physiology 3. Davis, Calif, ICEEP Publications, 1991, p 385.

10. Barrey E, Valette JP: Measurement of heart rate, blood lactate and hematological parameters during show jumping competitions ranging from regional to international level. *In* Proceedings of the Association of Equine Sports Medicine, 1992.

11. Art T, Amory H, Desmecht D, et al: Effect of show jumping on heart rate, blood lactate and other biochemical values. Equine Vet J 1990; (suppl 9):78.

12. Persson SGB: Evaluation of exercise tolerance and fitness in the performance horse. *In* Snow DH, Persson SGB, Rose RJ (eds): Equine Exercise Physiology. Cambridge, Granta Editions, 1983, p 441.

13. Covalesky ME, Russoniello CR, Malinowski K: Effects of show-jumping performance stress on plasma cortisol and lactate concentrations and heart rate and behavior in horses. J Equine Vet Sci 1992; 12:244.

14. Clayton HM: Conditioning Sport Horses. Saskatoon, Canada, Sport Horse Publications, 1991.

15. Meyer H: Nutrition of the equine athlete. *In* Gillespie JR, Robinson NE (eds): Equine Exercise Physiology 2. Davis, Calif, ICEEP Publications, 1987, p 644.

18

Drugs and Performance

R. A. SAMS AND K. W. HINCHCLIFF

Doping is defined as the administration or use of substances with the exclusive aim of attaining an artificial and unfair increase of performance.[1] Doping agents can be administered to performance horses with the aims of attaining standards of athletic performance in the ostensibly normal and healthy animal greater than would be attained without the agent, of restoring athletic performance in an injured animal (e.g., ameliorating the effects of lameness), and of decreasing performance, usually for illicit purposes.

A large number of agents have been administered to horses with the expectation, whether well founded or not, of altering performance. It is not unreasonable to expect that even greater numbers and varieties of compounds will be inflicted on performance horses as new drugs and new pharmacologic classes of drugs are developed. It is unimportant, for most of these compounds, to determine whether they alter performance. It suffices that adequate analytical expertise is available and demonstrably employed to detect doping agents and that the rules of racing provide potent disincentives to illicit drug use. However, the situation is less clear-cut for drugs that are used for treatment of clinical disorders in performance horses.

The use of "legitimate" drugs to treat clinical disorders in the immediate prerace period raises many ethical and regulatory issues. It is not appropriate that there be a full discussion of these issues in this chapter, but they will be examined in a cursory fashion. The primary concern should be for the welfare of the animal being administered the drug. Legitimate drug use should not be prevented where a clear and accepted medical indication exists. The question then arises as to whether an animal requiring such therapy is fit to race. *Prima facie,* it would appear that such an animal should be prevented from racing, but by doing so, animals with relatively trivial ailments (such as a dermatologic complaint requiring anti-inflammatory drug administration) could be prevented from racing, thereby forfeiting weeks and months of training and depriving the betting public of a competitor. Conversely, the administration of analgesic or anti-inflammatory drugs to a horse to permit it to overcome a serious or potentially serious condition, such as a fractured splint bone, is ethically unacceptable. One aspect of the problem is then, What are the effects on athletic performance of drugs used legitimately in racehorses? This issue is of concern to the betting public and is best exemplified by the current controversy in the United States over the use of furosemide in racehorses and can be summarized as follows: Are horses administered the drug thereby endowed with enhanced athletic capabilities?

In this chapter we address aspects of drug detection in performance horses, including a relatively nontechnical discussion of the more common analytical techniques, their advantages, and their limitations. The effects of various drugs on athletic capacity of horses are then examined. Surprisingly little information exists in this area, and we have included, where it seems appropriate, a discussion of the pharmacology of selected groups of drugs in both horses and human beings.

Analytical Methods Used to Detect Doping of Horses

The administration of drugs with the potential to affect the performance of horses in competition is generally prohibited by law or by the rules of the organization or commission with the responsibility for regulating the event. Furthermore, the presence of a drug or a drug metabolite in a test sample collected from a horse after competition is generally considered *prima facie* evidence that the prohibited drug was carried in the body of the animal during the contest.

Collection and testing of samples from horses in competition began in Europe in the early 1900s as a result of widespread rumors of drug use to affect performance. Early methods used there were based on relatively insensitive crystal or color tests that had been developed to detect drugs in plant extracts or toxicologic specimens. Testing in the United States was instituted in the mid-1930s after an investigation by the Federal Bureau of Narcotics revealed the use of heroin, cocaine, and other potent drugs to influence performance. The tests used in Europe were generally adopted by U.S. chemists. Tests with increased sensitivity and specificity were introduced later with the advent of chromatographic, immunologic, and spectroscopic methods. In addition, recent research on the identification of drug metabolites excreted in the urine of horses has permitted racing analysts to report the presence of these substances. The purpose of the first section of this chapter is to describe analytical methods currently used to detect and identify drugs and drug metabolites in test samples collected from horses in competition.

Definitions of Terms

Several terms used to describe analytical methods may have different meanings or be unfamiliar to most readers of this chapter. Therefore, the terms will be defined here so that their use in this chapter will be more clearly understood.

- *Specificity.* Specificity is the ability of a test to detect the presence of a particular drug when it is present. Thus a test with high specificity reliably detects the presence of a drug and does not give rise to significant numbers of false-positive results (i.e., a test result indicating the presence of a drug when none is present). Specificity is assessed by a variety of techniques, including studies of cross-reactivities of similar drugs in immunoassay tests.
- *Sensitivity.* The sensitivity of a method is the rate of change of some measured property of the drug (e.g., absorption of ultraviolet light) with change in concentration (or amount) of the drug. This definition of sensitivity can be expressed mathematically as follows:

$$\text{Sensitivity} = dx/dc$$

- where x is the measured property and c is the concentration of the drug.
- *Limit of detection.* The limit of detection is the lowest concentration (or amount) of a drug that can be detected. However, the statistical method used to identify this concentration varies considerably among laboratories and may lead to differences in interpretation. The limit of detection is often defined as the concentration that gives rise to a signal that is three times the background noise level.
- *Limit of quantitation.* The limit of quantitation is the lowest concentration of a drug that can be measured reliably. The limit of quantitation is often defined as that concentration which gives rise to a signal that is 10 times the background noise level. A drug in a test sample at a concentration less than the limit of quantitation but greater than the limit of detection is present at a *trace* concentration. Other uses of the term *trace concentration* are inappropriate and should be avoided.
- *Screening test.* A screening test is a preliminary test used to determine whether foreign substances may be present in the test sample. Screening tests are designed to detect a wide range of prohibited substances quickly and inexpensively so that those samples possibly containing prohibited substances can be subjected to more definitive tests. Screening tests may reveal the identity of a prohibited substance or may merely indicate the presence of some unidentified foreign substance.
- *Confirmation test.* A confirmation test is a second test based on a different chemical principle from that used to detect the presence of the drug in the screening test. The confirmatory test is used to establish the identity of a prohibited substance to a reasonable degree of certainty. Mass spectrometry is the confirmation test of choice, although other tests may be used in certain circumstances.
- *Determinative test.* A determinative test is a test used to determine the concentration of a foreign substance in a test sample. Several racing jurisdictions have adopted rules establishing a maximum plasma or urine concentration for therapeutic drugs (e.g., phenylbutazone or furosemide) or for substances present as contaminants or natural components of feeds (e.g., caffeine, salicylic acid, and arsenic). The measurement of the drug concentration in the test sample requires the use of a determinative test.
- *Prerace testing.* Prerace testing is testing where samples (usually blood) are collected from horses before they race and sufficient screening tests are completed so that racing officials can disqualify a horse from competing if a prohibited substance is detected. Conclusive identification of the detected substance is generally not necessary if no additional penalty is to be imposed on the trainer, owner, or horse. However, most laboratory practices mandate conclusive identification of the drug in the test sample either before or after reporting the findings to the racing officials. Because of the time required for confirmatory testing, complete identification

may not be feasible before the scheduled time of the race.

- *Postrace testing.* Postrace testing involves testing of samples collected from horses after completion of the race. Horses are selected for testing by rule (e.g., all winning horses) or by racing officials based on their assessment of each horse's performance (e.g., beaten favorites) in the race. Test samples are collected under the control and supervision of a regulatory veterinarian in a secure area under strict chain of custody procedures, labeled with unique identification numbers, and sealed in the presence of the trainer or designated representative of the trainer. The samples are then shipped or delivered to an official testing laboratory. After completing the tests, the laboratory reports the test results to the racing officials. Purse money is usually not paid until the laboratory has completed all testing and has reported no drug violations. In the event of a positive report by the laboratory, the racing officials will determine the identity of the horse and responsible individual (usually the trainer of the horse) from the information obtained by the regulatory veterinarian at the time of sample collection. The racing officials may then disqualify the horse, order redistribution of any purse money, and fine or suspend the license of the responsible party after conducting a hearing in an attempt to determine the facts of the alleged drugging incident.

The following sections describe in greater detail the methods used for screening test samples for prohibited substances and those used to confirm the identify of drugs detected by screening tests. The advantages and limitations of various methods will be reviewed.

Screening Tests

Screening tests are employed to determine whether prohibited substances are present in test samples. Preliminary extraction procedures are generally performed to isolate the drug from many of the endogenous substances present and to concentrate the drug in a small volume of solvent. Extractions may be performed using either liquid-liquid or solid-phase extraction techniques.

Liquid-liquid extraction is performed by (1) adjusting the pH of the test sample so that the drug or drugs of interest will not be ionized, (2) adding an immiscible organic solvent or solvent mixture (e.g., 25% isopropanol in methylene chloride), (3) mixing the two phases to facilitate partitioning of the drug into the organic phase, (4) centrifuging to separate the phases, (5) transferring the organic phase to another vessel and, (6) evaporating the organic phase to concentrate the drug. Additional steps may be added to increase the purity of the isolated drug, as shown in Figure 18–1.

Solid-phase extractions are performed using small plastic tubes containing from 200 mg to 5 g of a solid adsorbent consisting of silica gel or other solid to which specific functional groups such as hydrocarbon chains

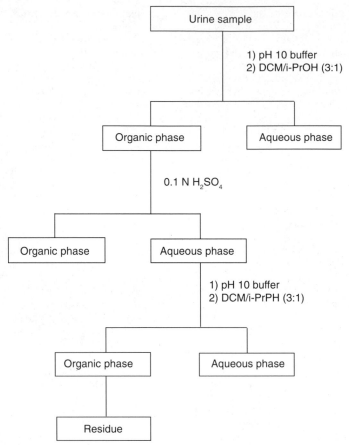

Figure 18-1. *Scheme describing the liquid/liquid extraction of basic drugs from a urine sample. (DCM = dichloromethane; i-PrOH = isopropyl alcohol)*

or ion-exchange groups have been covalently linked. The adsorbent is washed and buffered to the proper pH before the test sample is added. This step ensures that the drugs of interest will be retained on the column during subsequent wash steps that remove normal urine components. Then a portion of the test sample is poured into the extraction tube and allowed to drip from the column or is forced through at a controlled rate using vacuum or positive pressure. The adsorbent is then washed with water or organic solvents or solvent mixtures to elute unwanted sample components, washed with buffer to adjust the pH to a value that will permit elution of the drugs of interest, and then washed with eluting solvent to remove the drugs from the tube. The eluent is collected in a test tube, and the solvent is evaporated to concentrate the drug. A typical solid-phase extraction scheme for isolating a basic drug from urine is shown in Figure 18–2. Test sample extracts from liquid-liquid or solid-phase extraction procedures are then subjected to chromatographic screening tests as described in the following section.

CHROMATOGRAPHIC METHODS

Chromatographic methods have found wide application as screening tests for drugs in horse urine because of their high resolving power (i.e., their ability to separate closely related compounds), high sensitivity, and ease of use. Chromatographic methods are based on differential rates of migration of drugs in a gas or liquid phase flowing over a liquid or solid support. Various types of chromatography are generally named according to the nature of the mobile and stationary phases involved. For example, gas-liquid chromatography is a form of chromatography in which the stationary phase is a liquid and the mobile phase is a gas. A drug that interacts more strongly with the stationary phase is carried more slowly by the mobile phase than a drug that interacts less strongly with the stationary phase. Drugs may be detected while they are on the stationary phase (e.g., planar forms of chromatography such as paper and thin-layer chromatography) or as they exit from the stationary phase in the flowing mobile phase (e.g., tubular

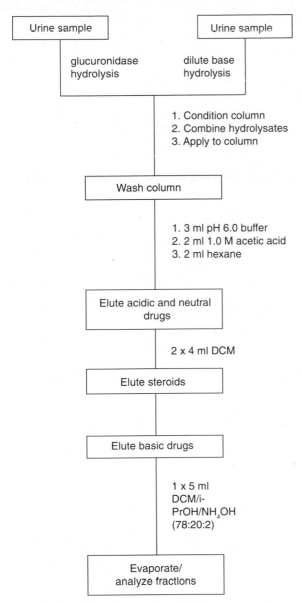

Figure 18-2. Scheme depicting the solid phase extraction of acidic, neutral, steroidal, and basic drugs from a urine sample after hydrolysis of conjugates (DCM = dichloromethane; EtOAc = ethyl acetate; i-PrOH = isopropanol).

forms of chromatography such as gas and liquid chromatography).

Thin-Layer Chromatography

Thin-layer chromatography (TLC) is a mode of chromatography performed on thin plates of glass, plastic, or metal foil covered with an adsorbent material such as silica gel, alumina, cellulose, or other material. After the plate is placed vertically in a small volume of a single solvent or a solvent mixture in a closed solvent chamber, the solvent rises up the plate by capillary action. Drugs migrate up the plate at different rates depending on the strength of their interaction with the adsorbent and the ability of the solvent to compete with the drug for binding sites on the adsorbent. The plate is removed from the solvent chamber when the solvent has risen a fixed distance (typically 4 to 10 cm), allowed to dry, and then examined under ultraviolet light and exposed to various reagents to reveal the presence of separated drugs. The distance that a drug migrates in a specified system is a characteristic of the drug and can be used for preliminary identification. However, the specificity of this approach is only moderate because several drugs or endogenous substances may have the same or similar migration distance due to the relatively low resolving power of thin-layer chromatography. Specificity may be enhanced by the use of specific visualization reagents that reveal the presence of limited numbers of substances. For example, certain specific visualization reagents reveal the presence of drugs containing the phenothiazine nucleus, whereas less specific reagents reveal the presence of all nitrogen-containing compounds.

Thin-layer chromatography was first used in racing chemistry laboratories in the 1960s, and its use was advanced by the contributions of Maylin,[2] who introduced microtechnique thin-layer chromatographic methods with increased sensitivity and decreased analysis times, and by Combie and colleagues,[3] who introduced high-performance thin-layer chromatography and new visualization reagents with increased sensitivity and specificity for many drugs. Most racing chemistry laboratories relied almost exclusively on thin-layer chromatographic screening tests from the mid-1970s to the late 1980s but have supplemented or replaced these tests with immunologic methods in order to detect certain drugs not detected in thin-layer chromatographic tests.

Advantages of thin-layer chromatography as a screening test for detecting drugs or drug metabolites in extracts of horse urine are as follows:

1. All materials for thin-layer chromatography are available from a number of vendors; consequently, material shortages are rare.
2. Costs of all materials for thin-layer chromatography are relatively low.
3. Thin-layer chromatographic methods have been extensively validated for the detection of a large number of drugs and drug metabolites in extracts of horse urine or blood.
4. Thin-layer chromatography is suitable for batch analysis.
5. The limit of detection for many drugs, particularly those which have a legitimate therapeutic use, is adequate for effective control.

However, several disadvantages of thin-layer chromatography have limited its usefulness:

1. The limit of detection for some drugs is inadequate to control their use in horses; for these drugs, a more sensitive chromatographic technique or immunoassay must be used.
2. Drugs must be extracted from the test sample before thin-layer chromatographic analyses can be performed; this additional step is costly in terms of time and personnel.
3. Thin-layer chromatographic testing is difficult to automate.
4. The use of some thin-layer chromatographic visualization reagents is restricted or prohibited due to concerns about personal health or environmental contamination; for example, certain reagents used to visualize the barbiturates contain mercury salts and may no longer be used in certain laboratories due to local restrictions.
5. Thin-layer chromatographic test results are usually determined by visual inspection of the thin-layer plate after application of various reagents; consequently, test interpretation is somewhat subjective.

Gas Chromatography

Gas chromatography (GC) is a mode of chromatography in which drugs are carried by a carrier gas through a narrow tube containing solid support particles coated with a thin film of liquid or through a thin capillary tube containing a thin film of liquid on the inner walls of the tube. Drugs dissolved in a small volume of suitable solvent are introduced into one end of the tube and are immediately heated to volatilize them so that they can be swept through the tube by the moving carrier gas. The tube is heated to maintain the volatility of the drugs. The rates of migration of the drugs through the tube are decreased by interaction with the liquid film. Thus drugs that interact strongly with the liquid film will require longer times to travel the length of the tube than drugs that interact less strongly. As the drugs exit the tube, they are carried to a detector. Different detectors used in conjunction with gas chromatography include the flamezionization detector (FID), the thermionic-specific detector (TSD), and the electron-capture detector (ECD). The time from introduction of the sample into the tube to the appearance of a chromatographic peak is the retention time of the drug. The retention time is characteristic of the drug under the specific conditions of temperature, carrier gas flow rate, dimensions of the tube, nature of the liquid phase within the tube, and other factors. The appearance of a peak at the correct retention time does not prove the presence of a drug in a sample, since several drugs or other substances may have the same or similar retention times under a given set of conditions. However, the presence of a peak at the characteristic retention time of a prohibited substance would be considered sufficient reason to conduct a confirmatory analysis of the sample extract.

The FID is an excellent and reliable detector that has become the most commonly used gas chromatographic detector. Factors contributing to its popularity include its ability to detect nearly all substances except the fixed gases, its high sensitivity and stability, its simplicity of design, and its ease of operation. Gas chromatography with FID detection has been used to screen for various drugs in biologic extracts. However, small amounts of prohibited substances may not be detected because this detector responds to nearly all compounds. Consequently, a small peak in a chromatogram containing a large number of bigger peaks may be difficult to discern.

The thermionic-specific detector ("nitrogen" detector) was developed in response to a need for a more sensitive and selective detector for nitrogenous compounds. Since most drugs with the potential to affect the performance of horses contain one or more nitrogen atoms (see Table 18–1), this detector is particularly useful as a gas chromatographic detector when screening for these classes of drugs. Several racing chemistry laboratories are currently using or are developing methods for gas chromatographic screening using this detector. Limits of detection less than 1 ng/ml are possible if conditions for drug extraction and chromatographic separation are optimized.

The electron-capture detector (ECD) was developed in the early 1960s as a very sensitive detector for detecting halogenated compounds such as DDT and other halogenated pesticides.[4] Blake and colleagues[5] prepared various halogenated derivatives of drugs (e.g., amphetamine, methylphenidate, acepromazine) (Fig. 18–3) to dramatically lower the limits of detection of the ECD for these substances. This development led to the introduc-

Table 18-1. *Examples of Drugs Containing One or More Nitrogen Atoms*

Drug class	Examples
Local anesthetics	Bupivacaine, mepivacaine, procaine
Opiates	Hydromorphone, morphine, oxymorphone
Anticholinergic drugs	Atropine, glycopyrrolate, scopolamine
Tranquilizers	Acepromazine, azaperone, promazine
Stimulants	Amphetamine, caffeine, mazindol
Bronchodilators	Albuterol, clenbuterol, terbutaline
Anti-inflammatory drugs	Flunixin, phenylbutazone
β blockers	Propranolol, sotalol, timolol
Analgesics	Detomidine, dipyrone, xylazine
Antihistamine drugs	Cimetidine, pyrilamine, tripelennamine

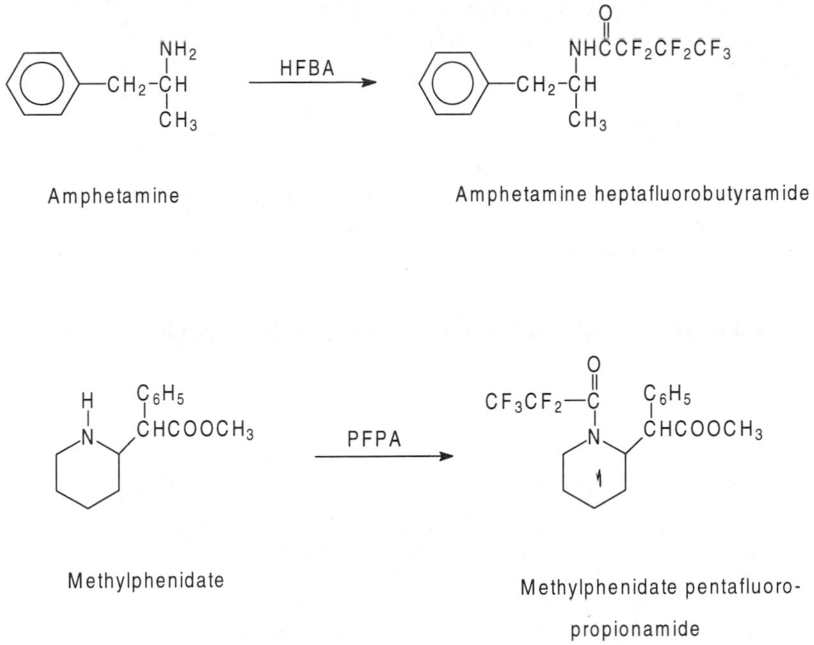

Figure 18-3. *Reaction of amphetamine with heptafluorobutyric anhydride (HFBA) and methylphenidate with pentafluoropropionic anhydride (PFPA) to form fluorinated derivatives detected with high sensitivity by the electron capture detector.*

tion of the first effective prerace testing methods for drugs in blood samples collected from horses.

Gas chromatography has the following advantages as a screening test for drugs in extracts of horse urine:

1. Low limits of detection are common with certain detectors such as the TSD and ECD.
2. Highly automated, unattended operation with automatic data recording is possible with modern instruments.
3. Very high resolution is possible with capillary columns.
4. Test results can be interpreted with a high degree of objectivity.

On the other hand, gas chromatographic screening procedures have some disadvantages:

1. Samples must be extracted before gas chromatographic analysis.
2. Polar drugs, those with high molecular masses, and unstable drugs are often not amenable to gas chromatographic analysis; for example, most peptide drugs are too polar and have such high molecular masses that they are unsuitable for gas chromatographic analysis.
3. Analyses must be performed sequentially.

High-Performance Liquid Chromatography
High-performance liquid chromatography (HPLC) is a mode of chromatography in which a liquid mobile phase is pumped through a narrow-diameter tube packed with small particles (typically 3 to 10 μm in diameter) of silica gel, alumina, or other material. In many cases, the surfaces and pores of these particles are modified by co-

valent bonding to hydrocarbon chains such as the octadecyl group or ion-exchange groups. Drugs are separated from each other and from other substances in the sample extract due to different degrees of interaction with the groups on the surfaces and in the pores of these particles. Drug molecules are carried by the mobile phase as it is pumped through the column. As the mobile phase exists the column, it flows through one or more detectors connected in series. The types of detectors most commonly used in HPLC analyses are discussed in the following sections.

ULTRAVIOLET ABSORPTION DETECTOR. The ultraviolet absorption detector measures the absorption of ultraviolet light by the drug as it flows through a small detector cell. This detector is available at a fixed wavelength (usually set at 254 nm), selectible wavelengths, continuously variable wavelengths, or as a diode-array detector. This detector is the most widely used detector for drug screening because of its high sensitivity, high reliability, and broad applicability. This detector is being used in a number of laboratories to screen for drugs in extracts of horse urine. Nonsteroidal anti-inflammatory drugs and corticosteroids are two classes of drugs that are readily detected by HPLC with ultraviolet absorption detection.

FLUORESCENCE DETECTOR. The fluorescence detector measures the fluorescence of a drug or drug derivative. This detector is generally more sensitive and more selective than the ultraviolet absorption detector. However, fluorescent derivatives often must be prepared in order to permit fluorescent detection of selected drugs due to the limited number of compounds with native fluorescence.

ELECTROCHEMICAL DETECTOR. The electrochemical detector is used to detect those substances which are electroactive at a suitable electrode such as platinum, gold, or carbon paste in response to an applied potential. This detector is very sensitive and specific but is rarely used to screen for drugs because so few drugs are detected by it. However, it can be used in series after an ultraviolet absorption detector or fluorescence detector to increase the scope of testing. Numerous HPLC methods have been reported for the very sensitive determination of various narcotic drugs such as morphine[5] and nalbuphine,[6] alkaloids such as apomorphine,[7] bronchodilators such as albuterol,[8] and catecholamines such as epinephrine,[9] norepinephrine,[10] and dopamine[10] in extracts of plasma and urine. This detector is likely to have increased use in the future as additional methods based on its use are developed.

Immunologic Methods

Immunologic methods are targeted analyses characterized by low limits of detection and high specificity. These methods are based on the complexation between an antigen and an antibody. Labeled antigen competes with unlabeled antigen in the sample for a limited number of antibody binding sites. As the concentration of antigen in the sample increases, less labeled antigen is able to bind to the antibody. After this interaction has been allowed to occur, either bound or free labeled antigen is separated and measured. The concentration of bound labeled antigen decreases as the concentration of unlabeled antigen increases. The first immunologic methods used radiolabeled antigens and nonspecific precipitation of the antigen-antibody complex to separate free from bound radiolabeled antigen.

RADIOIMMUNOASSAY

Radioimmunoassay (RIA) methods were first described in 1959 by Yalow and Berson.[12] Numerous RIA tests were commercially available in kit form by the late 1960s. One of the first RIA tests to achieve widespread use in racing chemistry was a test for fentanyl (FEN-RIA-200) marketed by IRE (Institut National des Radioelements, Fleurus, Belgium). This sensitive and specific RIA test detects fentanyl with a limit of detection of approximately 0.02 ng fentanyl and cross-reacts with some fentanyl metabolites. After Frincke and Henderson[13] identified the major metabolite of fentanyl (Fig. 18–4) in horse urine, analysts used the RIA test for fentanyl to screen horse urine samples for this metabolite and confirmed its presence in extracts of test samples after hydrolysis of the metabolite to despropionylfentanyl (see Fig. 18–4). Other RIA tests for opiates, amphetamines, and fentanyl analogues were quickly introduced into racing chemistry following the successful use of the RIA test for fentanyl. Radioimmunoassay tests are still used in racing chemistry, but they have been largely replaced by more modern immunoassays because these tests do not involve the use of radioisotopes and do not generate hazardous wastes that have become increasingly expensive to remove from the laboratory.

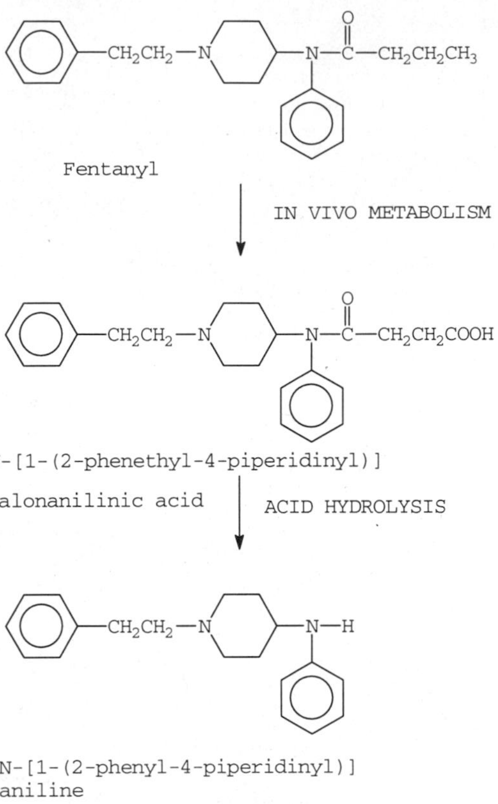

Figure 18-4. *Metabolism of fentanyl to N-[1-(2-phenethyl-4-piperidinyl)] malonanilinic acid in the horse. Acid hydrolysis of this metabolite affords N-{1-(2-phenyl-4-piperininyl}] aniline which is also known as N-despropionylfentanyl. This substance is identified by analysts to prove fentanyl administration to horses.*

ENZYME-MULTIPLIED IMMUNOASSAY TECHNIQUE

Enzyme-multiplied immunoassay technique (EMIT) tests were developed to detect drugs of abuse (e.g., benzoylecgonine and other cocaine metabolites, morphine and codeine, amphetamine and methamphetamine, phencyclidine and marihuana metabolites) in human urine samples and to provide therapeutic drug monitoring for certain drugs with low therapeutic indices (e.g., gentamicin and lidocaine) in humans. These tests are highly specific and often detect the drug at very low concentrations. Racing analysts have used EMIT assays for opiates, amphetamines, and lidocaine, among others, to screen for the presence of these prohibited substances. These tests are occasionally used in racing chemistry but have been largely supplanted by other types of immunoassay tests developed specifically for racing chemistry because of their lower cost and greater range of detectable drugs.

FLUORESCENCE POLARIZATION IMMUNOASSAY TEST

Fluorescence polarization immunoassay (FPIA) tests were developed for the same purposes as EMIT assays and have been used similarly in racing chemistry. These tests are occasionally used but are somewhat more expensive (approximately $2 to $3 per sample per drug) than tests developed specifically for use in racing chemistry. However, reagent costs typically include the cost of leasing all instrumentation necessary to perform the test. The FPIA assays are highly automated, and test results are easily interpreted even by inexperienced analysts.

ENZYME-LINKED IMMUNOSORBENT ASSAY

The first practical enzyme-linked immunosorbent assay (ELISA) tests were introduced by Engvall and Perlmann[14] and Van Weemen and Schuurs[15] as an alternative to radioimmunoassay tests. Drug labeled with an enzyme competes with drug in the test sample for a limited number of antibody binding sites. After the unbound labeled drug has been removed by washing, a substrate for the enzyme is added. The bound enzyme reacts with the substrate to produce a visible color change. The color is intense when the sample contains no drug but is less intense or colorless when the sample contains drug. These tests have the advantages of stable reagents that can be stored for long periods without loss of activity, the ability to read test results visually, automation and high throughput with the use of microtiter plates, and higher sensitivity due to the amplification of the signal by enzyme activity. ELISA tests developed specifically for use in racing chemistry were introduced by Soma and colleagues[16] and Weckman and colleagues[17] in the late 1980s. These ELISA tests were developed for the detection of fentanyl or its metabolites in horse urine and were used to replace the RIA test for fentanyl which was irregularly available from IRE. Other ELISA tests for drugs that may affect the performance of horses were rapidly introduced after the initial success and widespread acceptance of the fentanyl ELISA test. For the first time, effective tests were available specifically for drugs of interest to racing chemists. A partial list of ELISA tests specifically developed for use in racing chemistry is shown in Table 18–2.

One of the major advantages of ELISA tests is their extreme sensitivity. Limits of detection of 1 ng/ml for many substances are typical of ELISA methods, whereas limits of detection of 25 to 1000 ng/ml are typical for many substances detected by thin-layer chromatographic screening methods. Some drugs such as etorphine are administered in such small doses that the drug concentration in urine is less than the limit of detection of thin-layer chromatographic screening methods. Therefore, the use of these drugs will go undetected as long as thin-layer chromatographic methods are used exclusively. That such drugs were being used in racehorses was clearly demonstrated when ELISA tests for oxymorphone, etorphine, the fentanyl class (i.e., fentanyl and fentanyl analogues such as sufentanil and alfentanil), bumetanide, phenothiazine tranquilizers, and terbutaline were introduced, because positive results for these drugs were reported almost immediately. In some cases, use of the drugs was detected for the first time,

Table 18-2. Representative List of Drugs and Drug Classes Detected by ELISA Tests Used in Racing Chemistry Laboratories

Alfentanil
Amphetamine
Azaperone
Barbiturates
Boldenone
Bumetanide
Buprenorphine
Butorphanol
Carfentanil
Clenbuterol
Corticosteroids
Cromolyn sodium
Detomidine
Dexamethasone
Droperidol
Ethacrynic acid
Etorphine
Fentanyl
Fluphenazine
Furosemide
Glycopyrrolate
Haloperidol
Hydromorphone
Isoxsuprine
Mazindol
Methylphenidate
Methadone
Methamphetamine
Morphine
Nandrolone
Oxymorphone
Phenylbutazone
Progesterone
Promazine family
Pyrilamine
Reserpine
Sufentanil
Sulfamethazine
Triamcinolone
Tricyclic antidepressants

and widespread use of some of these drugs in racing was revealed. Oxymorphone was detected in numerous quarter horse racing samples, including several samples collected at Riodiuso Downs from horses competing in the All-American Futurity Races. These latter samples had been tested independently by two laboratories using conventional thin-layer chromatographic screening methods, and no foreign substances had been detected. Eleven samples were reported to contain etorphine and 19 were reported to contain bumetanide when ELISA tests for these drugs were first used to test urine samples collected from horses racing in Ohio in 1989.

Some of the early ELISA tests introduced into racing laboratories were plagued with problems that caused chemists to resist their use or question their utility. ELISA test reagents were sometimes unstable or plates were unevenly coated with antibodies, causing tests to perform poorly. The cross-reactivities of some of the antibodies used in early ELISA tests developed for use in racing laboratories were poorly characterized. Therefore, some ELISA tests were detecting substances (sometimes naturally occurring substances) that the tests were not designed to detect, and analysts were misled by the test results. Additionally, racing laboratories had difficulty increasing their budgets for more than a few ELISA tests because costs were approximately $100 for each 96-well microtiter plate and reagents. Thus ELISA testing for only 10 drugs or drug classes would increase the cost of testing by $10 for the ELISA test materials plus the additional costs for ELISA testing personnel. For many laboratories, such an increase would have meant more than a 100 percent increase in the cost of testing. In addition, many confirmatory assays were not sufficiently sensitive to identify drugs that had been detected by ELISA tests. Consequently, many ELISA test results could not be confirmed, thereby frustrating analysts and wasting scarce resources. Eventually, ELISA test quality and performance improved, costs decreased, and improved confirmation techniques were developed. The entry of a second commercial vendor of ELISA tests for the racing industry was instrumental in these changes. The presence of a second vendor is essential for continued test improvement and new test development.

Commercial vendors of ELISA tests for use in horse racing have produced a number of tests for the detection of therapeutic substances such as isoxsuprine, butorphanol, acepromazine, and lidocaine. The use of ELISA tests for therapeutic substances has dramatically increased the detection times for some of these substances. For example, butorphanol is readily detected by a thin-layer chromatographic screening test for approximately 1 day after a single therapeutic dose of this drug. However, the ELISA test for butorphanol may detect this drug for 7 days after the same dose. Furthermore, the use of ELISA tests has allowed detection of isoxsuprine for approximately 5 weeks and acepromazine for 6 weeks after multiple doses of these drugs. Thus large numbers of positive reports for therapeutic substances may result from the introduction of ELISA tests for these substances if veterinarians are not cautioned that increased withdrawal times are necessary. Policies and practices regarding notification of increased withdrawal times vary from one jurisdiction to another. In some jurisdictions, veterinarians are notified that new tests are being introduced and increased withdrawal times will be necessary. Grace periods and feedback from the laboratory are often provided in order to avoid unnecessary drug violations for trainers in these jurisdictions. In other jurisdictions, new ELISA tests for therapeutic substances are introduced without notice to trainers and veterinarians. In many cases, multiple positive reports have been issued by the laboratory before veterinarians have discovered an appropriate withdrawal time for the drug or have stopped using that drug to treat race horses.

The use of ELISA tests has many advantages:

1. ELISA tests are characterized by low limits of detection and high specificity.
2. ELISA tests are suitable for batch analysis; approximately 90 tests can be performed simultaneously on a 96-well microtiter plate.
3. ELISA tests can be performed with minimal instrumentation, and test results can be read visually, thereby reducing instrumentation costs.
4. ELISA tests can be automated, and test results can be determined instrumentally, thereby increasing objectivity of test interpretation.
5. Substances such as polyethyleneglycol that may interfere with chromatographic test interpretation usually do not affect performance or interpretation of ELISA tests.
6. ELISA tests are performed directly on the sample without the need for preliminary extraction.
7. The volume of sample required for ELISA testing is very small (10 to 100 μl in most cases).

On the other hand, ELISA tests suffer from some limitations:

1. ELISA tests are expensive to develop; development costs for some ELISA tests have approached $50,000 per test.
2. Some ELISA test materials are of biologic origin and are therefore subject to problems of instability and variability.
3. The limits of detection of ELISA tests for some therapeutic drugs such as butorphanol and isoxsuprine are so low that therapeutic use of these drugs in the horse is impractical if the testing laboratory uses these tests to their limits of detection.
4. Antibodies to the drug or drug class must be developed or purchased commercially; if antibodies must be developed, then considerable time may be spent modifying the hapten to make it immunogenic.

Thus ELISA tests are excellent screening tests for targeted analysis of drugs in horse urine. They possess many advantages and relatively few disadvantages compared with other screening tests. Most laboratories are now using ELISA tests in conjunction with one or more chromatographic tests to screen for drugs in horse urine.

Targeted Analysis

Screening tests such as those based on immunologic methods are used to test for specific drugs or groups of closely related drugs. Such screening tests are used for *targeted analyses,* in which the test is designed to reveal the presence of a specific drug or closely related class of drugs. These screening tests are often very sensitive and specific for the targeted drug but insensitive to the presence of other foreign substances. For example, an immunoassay test for etorphine detects the presence of this drug at urine concentrations as low as 1 ng/ml but is not known to react to the presence of any other substance. An obvious disadvantage of targeted analyses is that the laboratory will fail to detect the presence of those prohibited substances for which it is not testing. Thus the use of a prohibited substance may go undetected for years and its use become widespread.

Characteristics of targeted analyses are as follows:

1. A single drug or limited number of closely related drugs is detected.
2. Targeted analyses may have a very low limit of detection for the targeted drug.
3. The methods for targeted analyses are often expensive to develop (costs of $50,000 to develop an immunoassay screening test for a single drug are common).
4. The methods are relatively expensive to perform (costs of $1 to $2 or more for materials per drug tested are usual).
5. Nontargeted drugs are generally not detected, and their use will go undetected until a method is developed to detect them.
6. Interference from other substances usually is minimal.
7. Excretion data for the targeted drug will usually have been obtained during validation of the test procedures.

Survey Analysis

Other screening tests such as those based on chromatographic methods usually are used to screen for the presence of any foreign substance that is present at a concentration greater than the limit of detection of the method for that substance. These screening tests are used to perform *survey analyses*. Some drugs will be detected after their first use if the laboratory employs survey analyses for screening and the drug is present in the test sample at a concentration greater than the limit of detection. For example, the presence of azaperone metabolites was detected in test samples submitted to the Ohio State University Analytical Toxicology Laboratory because the laboratory was using a chromatographic test procedure that was able to detect these metabolites in extracts of the test samples. This particular test detects a large number of basic drugs and drug metabolites that are excreted as glucuronic acid conjugates in urine. The azaperone metabolites were detected by this screening test but were not identified until subjected to a confirmatory test. This particular screening test had been used for several years to test all samples submitted to the laboratory. However, no evidence for the presence of the azaperone metabolites had been found until the samples in question were tested. Thus this screening test could detect the presence of azaperone, which was probably detected on, or soon after, its first use. This probably prevented its widespread use in racing, in contrast to the situation with etorphine administration.

Characteristics of survey analyses are as follows:

1. A wide range of drugs may be detected by one test procedure.

2. The limit of detection for some drugs may be very low, but the limit of detection may vary from one drug to another within the same test.
3. The test may be very specific, and specificity may vary from one drug to another.
4. The test may reveal the presence of a foreign substance but not identify it.
5. Tests for survey analyses are generally less expensive to develop than are tests for targeted analyses.
6. Tests are relatively inexpensive to perform, particularly when the cost is expressed on a per-drug basis.
7. A new drug may be detected on its first use if it is present in the test sample at a concentration greater than the limit of detection.
8. Excretion data for all drugs and metabolites potentially detected by the test will not have been acquired during validation of the test procedure.

Confirmation Methods

Confirmation methods are employed after one or more screening tests have indicated the presence of a prohibited substance in the test sample. These tests are based on a different chemical principle from the screening test. Therefore, an immunoassay test would not be used to confirm the findings of an immunoassay screening test because there is too much risk of a false-positive finding. Chromatographic tests may be used to confirm the results of a chromatographic screening test, particularly if a different mode of chromatography is used and it can be demonstrated that the two tests are not correlated. However, gas chromatography/mass spectrometry has been the confirmation method of choice for most drugs since the late 1970s, when laboratories first acquired these instruments.

GAS CHROMATOGRAPHY/MASS SPECTROMETRY

This confirmation method involves the coupling of a gas chromatograph and a mass spectrometer via a transfer line or a glass jet separator. Separation of the drugs from each other and from other substances in the sample extract occurs in the gas chromatograph. The effluent from the gas chromatograph then exits directly into the ionization source of the mass spectrometer, where high-energy electrons collide with molecules of the drug causing them to become ionized. Collision of high-energy electrons with drug molecules causes ejection of electrons from drug molecules, leaving each with a net positive charge. Collision of the high-energy electron with the drug molecule also imparts energy to this positively charged ion, causing it to dissipate the excess energy by breakage of the weakest bonds in the molecule. The resulting ions (both the initial ion formed upon collision of the molecule with the electron and the resulting fragment ions) are focused into an analyzer where the mass-to-charge ratio and the abundance of each ion are measured. Abundances of ions are determined by their resistance to further fragmentation. Thus the most stable ions usually will be present at the highest relative abundance. For this reason, the ion corresponding to the molecular ion may be present at low abundance or may not be detectable at all.

The abundances of all ions are presented as a mass spectrum, with the most abundant ion at 100 percent relative abundance. The mass spectrum of the trimethylsilyl (TMS) derivative of morphine is shown in Figure 18–5. The TMS derivative was prepared to increase the volatility of morphine and to improve the quality of the gas chromatographic separation of morphine from other components of the sample extract. The ion at m/z 429 is termed the *molecular ion* because it corresponds to the ion produced by loss of an electron from a molecule of the di-TMS derivative of morphine; all other ions in the mass spectrum correspond to fragments of the molecular ion or other fragment ions. Fragmentation pathways producing the ions can be predicted with some degree of certainty and may aid in the identification of unknown compounds.

Mass spectra of different substances are almost always different, and mass spectra of closely related substances may be quite different, as is shown in the mass spectra of procaine and lidocaine in Figure 18–6.

The mass spectrum of each drug is characteristic, since the fragmentation pathways are determined by the strengths of the bonds and the spatial relationships between the functional groups of the molecule. Therefore, mass spectra of the same drug obtained in different laboratories are virtually identical, particularly if standardized protocols for tuning, calibration, and operation are followed. Consequently, extensive mass spectral libraries, including several available in computer-searchable software, have been created to assist in the identification of unknown substances.

Mass spectra of optical isomers are identical and those of geometric or structural isomers or homologues may be identical or so similar that identification is not possible based on comparison of mass spectra. Optical isomers cannot be differentiated unless they are first converted to derivatives containing a second chiral center (e.g., derivitization of amphetamine isomers with *N*-trifluoroacetyl-L-prolyl chloride to produce diastereoisomeric amide derivatives)[18] or separated from each other on a chiral column before entry into the mass spectrometer. Geometric and structural isomers as well as homologues often can be differentiated from each other by their gas chromatographic retention times. For example, the mass spectra of the diastereomers ephedrine and pseudoephedrine are virtually identical, but their gas chromatographic retention times differ by more than a minute on a standard 30-m capillary column, thereby permitting differentiation of these drugs.

The limit of detection of gas chromatographic/mass

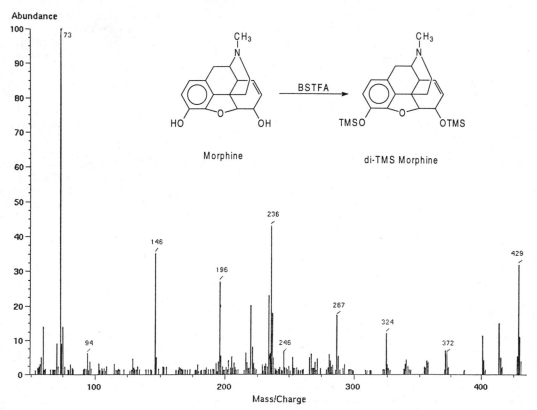

Figure 18-5. *Mass spectrum of the di-TMS ether derivative of morphine (TMS = trimethylsilyl). The ion at a mass to charge ratio (m/s) of 429 in this mass spectrum is termed the molecular ion because it results from the loss of an electron from a molecule of the derivative.*

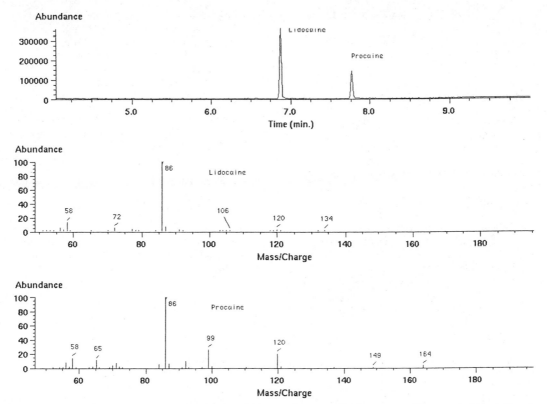

Figure 18-6. *Mass spectra of procaine (middle panel) and lidocaine (lower panel). The presence of ions at m/z 65 and 99 and greater abundance of the ion at m/z 120 in the mass spectrum of procaine differentiate it from lidocaine; m/z is the mass to charge ratio. The mass chromatogram (upper panel) demonstrates that procaine elutes nearly one minute later than lidocaine.*

spectral methods depends on various factors, including sample preparation techniques and the mode of operation of the mass spectrometer. When the mass spectrometer is used to confirm the identity of a drug detected in a targeted analysis, sample extraction and drug purification can be optimized for that drug and the mass spectrometer operating parameters adjusted to decrease the limit of detection of the instrument for the substance of interest. In this case, limits of detection approaching 1 ng/ml or less are possible. The sensitivity of the mass spectrometer can be increased, albeit with a possible loss of specificity, by monitoring only those ions which are characteristic of the compound of interest. This technique is known as *selected ion monitoring* and may decrease the limit of detection by one to two orders of magnitude.

Mass spectral limits of detection for some substances are higher than the ELISA limits of detection. Therefore, a drug may be detected but not confirmed and no positive report can be issued by the laboratory.

On the other hand, it may not be possible to optimize extraction and purification steps, and the operating parameters of the instrument cannot be adjusted to maximize sensitivity of detection if the mass spectrometer is being used to identify an unknown substance detected in a survey analysis. Under these conditions, much

higher limits of detection are likely to be encountered. Selected ion monitoring techniques obviously cannot be used to identify unknown substances because the specific ions to be monitored are unknown. Furthermore, some substances are not sufficiently volatile to pass through the gas chromatographic column and into the mass spectrometer or may decompose during this process. Furthermore, an unknown substance may give rise to a mass spectrum that is not contained in a library of spectra and which cannot be interpreted. Thus analysts may detect substances in screening tests but not be able to identify them in confirmation tests even if a mass spectrum is obtained. Analysts will often communicate the results of these tests to racing officials with the hope that some pattern of drug use can be uncovered by investigation of the trainers of the horses from which the test samples containing the unidentified substances have been collected.

Gas chromatography/mass spectrometry was first used in racing chemistry laboratories in the mid-1970s, and by 1980 its use was widespread throughout the world. Today, all racing chemistry laboratories have access to at least one mass spectrometer system, and many have access to two or more instruments. Modern gas chromatograph/mass spectrometer systems are highly automated, computer controlled, and relatively easily maintained compared with instruments available only a few years ago.

LIQUID CHROMATOGRAPHY/MASS SPECTROMETRY

This confirmation technique couples the resolving power of high-performance liquid chromatography with the high sensitivity and specificity of mass spectrometry. Owing to the difficulty of removing the liquid mobile phase before entry into the source of the mass spectrometer, development of LC/MS instruments has been slower than that of GC/MS instruments. A number of interfaces have been developed and are now commercially available. One of the more satisfactory of these interfaces is the heated nebulizer interface. This interface in conjunction with an atmospheric pressure ionization (API) system in a triple-stage quadrupole mass spectrometer developed by Sciex in Thornhill, Ontario, Canada, has permitted several drug and metabolite identifications that were previously difficult or impossible to perform. Instruments employing the heated nebulizer interface and API capability have been purchased by the three Canadian laboratories providing testing services to Agriculture Canada. Research reported by these laboratories attests to the usefulness of this system in the identification of prohibited substances in test samples collected from horses. These laboratories have reported the use of LC/MS/MS methods for the identification of detomidine[19] and xylazine metabolites,[20] reserpine,[21] and glycopyrrolate[22] in test samples collected from horses. The LC/MS or LC/MS/MS approach is of particular advantage when identifying drugs that are not amenable to gas chromatographic separation because they are charged (e.g., glycopyrrolate), have high molecular mass (e.g., reserpine), are thermally labile and decompose during GC/MS analysis (e.g., xylazine metabolites), or are difficult to separate from endogenous substances (e.g., detomidine metabolites).

Determinative Tests

Determinative tests are used to determine the concentration of various substances in test samples collected in those racing jurisdictions which control one or more substances with a quantitative limit. Several therapeutic substances such as phenylbutazone, flunixin, and furosemide are permitted in test samples in some jurisdictions, provided that the concentration is less than the maximum permitted concentration or threshold concentration for that substance. For example, phenylbutazone is permitted at threshold concentrations of 2.0, 2.2, 3.0 or 5.0 μg/ml in blood samples in various racing jurisdictions but not permitted at any concentration in other jurisdictions in the United States. Other substances such as arsenic, salicylic acid, dimethylsulfoxide (DMSO), and theophylline that are occasionally found as trace components or contaminants of feeds are permitted in test samples, provided that the concentration in the test sample is less than the threshold concentration for that substance. Various quantitative tests such as high-performance liquid chromatography (e.g., phenylbutazone,

flunixin, furosemide, salicylic acid, and theophylline), gas chromatography (DMSO), and atomic absorption spectrophotometry (e.g., arsenic) are used to determine the concentrations of these substances.

Most determinative tests involve the use of a chromatographic method such as high-performance liquid chromatography or gas chromatography, but various spectroscopic methods may be used in certain cases. A typical high-performance liquid chromatogram illustrating the determination of phenylbutazone in an extract of horse plasma is shown in Figure 18–7.

Prerace Testing

Prerace testing was first proposed in the 1960s by horse owners who wanted the protection afforded by a prerace disqualification as opposed to a postrace drug violation with loss of purse, damaged reputation, and suspension of license of the trainer. They further argued that bettors would be more assured of the integrity of racing if prerace testing were instituted.

As a result of these efforts, prerace testing began in Maryland in the early 1960s, with testing based on relatively insensitive ultraviolet absorption measurements. These methods were capable of detecting phenylbutazone, sulfonamide antibacterial drugs, and a limited number of other drugs. The scope of prerace testing was extended to include stimulants such as amphetamine, methamphetamine, and methylphenidate with the introduction of sensitive gas chromatographic screening procedures by Blake and colleagues in Ohio in the late 1960s.[5] The scope of testing was further increased to include a wide variety of acidic, basic, and neutral drugs with the introduction of microtechnique thin-layer chromatography by Maylin and colleagues in New York in the 1970s.[2] More recently, immunoassay tests were developed specifically for use in screening prerace blood samples collected from horses in Illinois for a variety of drugs, including morphine.[23] These tests demonstrated

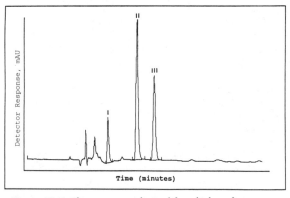

Figure 18-7. Chromatogram obtained from high performance liquid chromatographic analysis of an extract of a plasma sample containing 5 μg/ml each of phenylbutazone (III) and oxyphenbutazone (I). An internal standard (cycloprofen, II) was added to the plasma sample before extraction to increase precision and accuracy of the analysis.

the feasibility of detecting several drugs not previously detected in prerace blood samples. Despite these technical advances, however, prerace testing has been largely abandoned because of logistics problems, insufficient sensitivity of testing methods for certain drugs, and high costs of operating a field laboratory at the race track.

Postrace Testing

Postrace testing was developed in Europe in the early 1900s and was instituted in the United States at Tropical Park in 1933 after an investigation by the Federal Bureau of Narcotics revealed widespread use of cocaine, heroin, and stimulants in samples collected from horses racing in various states. Postrace testing of samples was quickly instituted in other racing states in the United States and the rest of the world. Postrace test methods in the early years were based on relatively insensitive spot tests and crystallographic methods, and few performance-modifying drugs were detected. Most reported violations involved the use of therapeutic medication administered too close to the time of sample collection. However, the introduction of more sensitive methods such as chromatographic tests and immunoassays has in the last 20 years made it possible to detect and confirm the presence of a wide variety of therapeutic and nontherapeutic drugs in test samples. Furthermore, research conducted in a number of laboratories has resulted in the conclusive identification of metabolites of several drugs (e.g., fentanyl, detomidine, xylazine, lidocaine, and azaperone).

Racing analysts formed the Association of Official Racing Chemists (AORC) in 1947. The AORC is a professional organization of racing analysts who must pass a practical examination for full membership in the organization. The organization provides an annual forum for exchange of information on the latest test methods developed by members and results of other studies. Furthermore, the association publishes quarterly reports of drugs identified in test samples so that members will be alerted to new trends in drug use and test methods. Recently, racing analysts representing the AORC have agreed on minimum criteria for identification of drugs in test samples. Several laboratories have recently been accredited by laboratory accrediting bodies in their countries, and analysts in the United States have been developing an accreditation program in conjunction with the Association of Racing Commissioners International Quality Assurance Program. Future developments in drug detection methods and efforts of racing analysts to improve the quality of testing are likely to increase the control of doping substances. The following section will review the effects of several classes of drugs on exercise performance in horses.

Investigation of Drug Effects on Athletic Performance

The capacity for elite athletic performance can be detected in part by an examination of the physiologic responses of the individual to intense or graded exertion. Similarly, the effect of drugs on athletic performance may be detectable by comparison of the physiologic responses to graded or steady-state exertion performed in the presence and absence of the drug. This type of examination in the horse has only recently become feasible with the development of high-speed treadmills and instruments for measuring respiratory and hemodynamic variables during running.

MODELS FOR EXAMINING DRUG EFFECTS DURING EXERTION

The best test of athletic performance is an actual race against peers. However, this is not a practical means by which to repeatedly assess athletic performance in an experimental situation. Although various epidemiologic studies of the effect of furosemide on athletic performance have been conducted, such studies are marred by constraints on experimental design that often prevent a clear resolution of the experimental question. The most notable example of this is the study by Sweeney and colleagues[24] that reported a significant effect of furosemide in decreasing race times in thoroughbred horses. This study is marred by the knowledge of the investigators, owners, trainers, and jockeys regarding the nature of the treatment and the inevitable selection bias that then existed as owners and trainers withdrew poorly performing animals from the study. Additionally, there was no control over administration of other medications, such as phenylbutazone, or access to feed and water after furosemide administration, or the route of furosemide administration (IM and IV). Epidemiologic studies are capable of providing important and useful information about the topic at issue, as did the report of Sweeney and colleagues,[24] but they are unable to demonstrate cause-and-effect relationships or elucidate mechanisms.

Studies of a drug in the resting horse are invaluable in providing basic pharmacokinetic and pharmacodynamic information. Exertion, however, profoundly alters the metabolic state of the horse and may result in markedly different pharmacodynamics and pharmacokinetic values than in the resting state. Information regarding drug effects and pharmacokinetics obtained in the resting horse cannot, therefore, be extrapolated directly to the exercising horse.

Earlier studies of drug effects in exercising horses were usually of a design such that the drug or placebo was administered, various measurements were made in the resting horse, the horse was exercised, and the measurements were retaken soon after the end of the run.[25] It is apparent that such studies do not provide anything but the most indirect evidence as to the effect of the drug on the variables studied during exertion. Information is obtained about the recovery phase but not about the events occurring during running.

Drug effects can be assessed during exertion, although the type of exercise test employed depends in large part on what is of interest to the investigator. An investigation of drug effects on endurance performance should be examined during a prolonged bout of submaximal exertion. Similarly, documenting likely drug effects on standardbred, quarter horse, or thoroughbred racehorses requires an exercise test of high intensity and short duration. Such high-intensity, short-duration exercise tests can take either of two forms: an incremental speed test or a brief, intense single-speed test. Incremental speed tests involve progressive, planned increases in speed and/or incline to progressively increase the workload, as illustrated by the Bruce test in human exercise physiology.[26] Such a test provides information about the responses of the individual at various exertion intensities, including the determination of the rate of maximal oxygen consumption ($\dot{V}_{O_{2max}}$) and the workload at which it occurs, and endurance time. Such tests are widely used in human exercise physiology for clinical and experimental purposes. Single-speed tests do not provide any information about the individual's response to various workloads but would appear to be a more realistic model of the stresses imposed during an actual race.[27] The exertion intensity used in such tests is often near maximal and may be determined from information gained during incremental exertion tests. Single-speed tests provide information about the changes in responses over the course of the exertion test and have the potential to be valuable in detecting subtle drug-induced effects during exertion.

The development of high-speed treadmills suitable for use with horses has greatly facilitated the collection of physiologic data during strenuous exertion in horses. Perhaps of even greater importance from an experimental point of view is the capability to accurately and precisely control the intensity and duration of separate trials. It is possible to accurately reproduce work intensities and duration from day to day, thus eliminating a major cause of experimental error in trials conducted at race tracks. The use of standardized exertion tests permits the collection of specific information that can be used for comparative purposes at later repetitions of the test or that can be compared with accumulated data from other individuals.[28]

INDICES OF ATHLETIC CAPABILITY

It may be possible to determine the likely effect of a drug on athletic capacity by examining the effect of the drug on selected physiologic responses to exertion. The best indicator of athletic capability is a competitive race among peers, but as discussed above, this is not a suitable model for experimental purposes. Various measurements have been investigated in both human and veterinary medicine as indicators of athletic capacity. The variables most often used are the maximal rate of oxygen consumption ($\dot{V}_{O_{2max}}$), running speeds and endurance time (time to volitional exhaustion), the heart rate/speed relationship, and blood lactate concentrations during running.

There is a high correlation ($r = 0.90$) between $\dot{V}_{O_{2max}}$ and running speed in humans,[29] and $\dot{V}_{O_{2max}}$ is accepted as the best measure of aerobic work capacity in humans.[30] It is generally accepted that $\dot{V}_{O_{2max}}$ in horses is similarly related to running speed and aerobic work ca-

pacity and will therefore provide a useful, and probably the most important, variable to be monitored in tests to assess the effects of drugs on performance. As important as $\dot{V}_{O_{2max}}$ in the prediction of athletic capability is the economy of running.[31] Of two athletes with identical $\dot{V}_{O_{2max}}$ values, the more economical athlete will achieve $\dot{V}_{O_{2max}}$ at a higher work rate (i.e., speed) than the less economical athlete. Overall, however, the best predictor of athletic performance is the "power," measured as the greatest workload achieved or the fastest speed achieved on the treadmill.[31]

The relationship between heart rate and speed (or work intensity) is linear over a range of work intensities below the individual's maximal work rate.[32] When a test procedure is strictly standardized, the relationship between heart rate and work intensity is precise and reproducible.[28] Examination of the heart rate/speed relationship may therefore provide another means to detect drug effects during running.

The accumulation of lactate in the blood during running provides an index of the contribution of anaerobic metabolism to energy production. Blood lactate concentrations increase as an exponential function of workload in horses, with the more rapid rise occurring in the less fit animals.[33] Determination of blood lactate concentrations during exertion is therefore a useful addition to the measurement of $\dot{V}_{O_{2max}}$, an index of aerobic metabolism, in the investigation of drug effects in the running horse.

Drug Groups

DIURETICS

Furosemide

Furosemide is the most widely used diuretic drug in performance horses in North America.[34–36] In horses, furosemide is rapidly eliminated, having alpha, beta, and gamma half-lives of 5.6, 22.3, and 158.5 minutes, respectively.[37] The elimination half-life of furosemide is longer after intramuscular administration.[38] The majority of intravenously administered furosemide is eliminated unchanged in the urine within 4 hours.[39] Furosemide inhibits chloride transport in a number of tissues, including the thick ascending limb of the loop of Henle, vascular smooth muscle, and tracheal epithelium, by binding to the chloride binding site of the $Na^+ = K^+ = 2Cl^-$ cotransporter.[40–44] Furosemide also may exert some of its pharmacologic effects by increasing prostaglandin production.[45,46]

Furosemide produces a diuresis, natriuresis, and chloruresis in horses,[47–49] through inhibition of the reabsorption of sodium and chloride in the thick ascending limb of the loop of Henle.[50] Urine production during the 4 hours after furosemide administration (1 mg/kg) to horses averages 25 ml/kg of body weight.[51] The furosemide-induced diuresis causes a reduction in plasma volume of resting horses denied access to water.[51,52] Plasma concentrations of potassium, chloride, calcium, and hydrogen decrease, while sodium concentrations are unchanged following furosemide administration to horses.[38,49,52] Furosemide-induced losses of sodium and water are associated with increased consumption of both salt and water in horses.[53] During the first hour after intravenous furosemide administration, urinary potassium excretion is approximately three times greater than that of a control period (690 versus 244 μEq/kg per hour) and represents approximately 69 percent of the extracellular fluid potassium content.[54] Therefore, furosemide-induced hypokalemia may well be a result of increased urinary losses of potassium, although there may be a redistribution of potassium within the body. Furosemide administration results in increases in venous pH, P_{CO_2}, and bicarbonate concentration.[49,54,55] Furosemide administration results in a transient decline in urine pH.[49,54]

In addition to its effect on the kidney, furosemide also affects the cardiovascular and respiratory systems. Intravenous furosemide administration to horses causes an immediate and significant decrease in right atrial pressure, pulmonary arterial pressure, pulmonary arterial wedge pressure, cardiac output, and stroke volume.[52,56] Furosemide affects systemic hemodynamics at least partly by increasing the ease with which veins distend with blood (compliance), thereby increasing their ability to contain a volume of blood (capacitance).[57,58] The vasodilatory effects of furosemide appear to be dependent on the presence of kidneys.[59]

Furosemide has bronchodilatory activity in a number of species, including horses.[60-64] In ponies with recurrent obstructive airway disease, i.e., "heaves," intravenous and nebulized furosemide increases dynamic compliance and decreases pulmonary resistance but does not affect arterial P_{O_2} or arterial P_{CO_2}.[65] Dynamic compliance and pulmonary resistance of normal ponies are not affected by furosemide.[65]

Indomethacin and other nonsteroidal anti-inflammatory drugs inhibit the diuretic, natriuretic, and chloruretic responses to furosemide.[66,67] The mechanism of this interaction is inhibition of loop prostaglandin synthesis; indomethacin does not inhibit the tubular secretion of furosemide.[67] The effect of nonsteroidal anti-inflammatory drugs on the pharmacologic effects of furosemide in horses has only been examined in running horses; flunixin meglumine and phenylbutazone inhibit the hemodynamic effects of furosemide in running horses.[56]

Furosemide modifies the hemodynamic response to exertion in both horses and ponies. Running is associated with marked changes in cardiovascular function in horses. Cardiac output increases from resting values of approximately 70 ml/kg per minute to 600 ml/kg per minute during exertion of maximal intensity. Cardiac filling pressures also increase; mean left atrial pressures exceed 70 mmHg and mean right atrial pressures exceed 40 mmHg during intense exertion.[56,68] Similarly, mean pulmonary artery pressure may exceed 80 mmHg,[69] and pulmonary artery wedge pressure increases from resting values of approximately 18 to 56 mmHg during intense exertion.[70] Administration of furosemide results in a significant attenuation of the exercise-induced increase in pulmonary arterial pressure, right atrial pressure, and

mean aortic pressure of ponies and horses.[56,69,71,72] Furosemide also attenuates the exercise-induced increase in pulmonary artery wedge pressure (an indicator of left atrial pressure) and, therefore, presumably pulmonary capillary pressure of horses.[73] The hemodynamic effects of furosemide are dose-dependent and are inhibited by prior flunixin meglumine or phenylbutazone administration.[56,74]

Furosemide is the most commonly used drug to prevent exercise-induced pulmonary hemorrhage (EIPH), despite the lack of a clear rationale for its use.[75] The pathogenesis of EIPH has not been elucidated,[76] although it has been demonstrated recently that stress failure of pulmonary capillaries occurs in horses during high-intensity exertion.[77] It is theorized that capillary rupture and subsequent hemorrhage into alveoli occur because of the high pulmonary capillary pressures generated in the horse.[78] Furosemide, by reducing pulmonary capillary pressure, may therefore reduce the incidence of pulmonary capillary wall failure, thereby reducing the severity of exercise-induced pulmonary hemorrhage.[73]

The efficacy of furosemide in reducing the incidence or severity of EIPH is questionable. Pascoe and colleagues[78] compared the repeatability of endoscopic observations of EIPH in horses with no treatment, placebo, and furosemide. The repeatability of EIPH scores, which were based on endoscopic assessment of the amount of blood in the trachea, was good for repeat observations on untreated horses ($p < 0.001$), fair to good after placebo treatment ($p < 0.01$), but poor after furosemide treatment ($p < 0.1$), suggesting an undefined effect of furosemide on the severity of EIPH.[78] Consistent with Pascoe and colleague's finding[78] that furosemide does not reduce the incidence of EIPH in previously EIPH-positive horses, there was no significant difference in the incidence of EIPH of untreated or furosemide-treated EIPH-positive horses.[79] Furthermore, 61.5 percent of 52 previously EIPH-positive horses given furosemide before a race remained EIPH-positive after the race.[24]

Furosemide may affect athletic performance. Furosemide administration improved the race times of a selected group of thoroughbred racehorses; the better horses ran faster after furosemide.[80] Furthermore, furosemide decreases the standardized race times of EIPH-negative geldings,[24] although the results of this study have been criticized.[81] However, furosemide does not reduce the time required for trained standardbred horses to run 1.6 km at maximum speed.[38,82] A retrospective analysis of track times of horses performing with and without furosemide at Louisville Downs did not reveal a statistically significant effect of furosemide.[38]

Bumetanide and Ethacrynic Acid

Bumetanide and ethacrynic acid are structurally different from furosemide, but both are potent diuretics that inhibit chloride transport in the loop of Henle, as does furosemide.[83] Ethacrynic acid given orally to adult horses induces a dose-dependent diuresis; 400 mg (PO) induces a diuresis that, assessed subjectively, is maximal

1 hour after dosing and persists for 3 hours.[84] Ethacrynic acid also increases urinary sodium excretion of ponies.[48] Bumetanide is a benzoic acid derivative with potent diuretic activity. Bumetanide is a potent diuretic when administered intravenously or intramuscularly to horses at dose rates of 10 to 20 μg/kg.[85,86] Bumetanide is a potent saluretic and kaliuretic in humans[87] and is likely to exhibit similar activity in horses, although this activity has not been demonstrated conclusively in horses.[48,88] The elimination half-life of bumetanide in horses in 6.3 minutes after intravenous administration and 11 to 27 minutes after intramuscular administration.[86]

ANABOLIC/ANDROGENIC STEROIDS

The anabolic/androgenic steroids are a group of compounds similar in structure to testosterone. Modification of the testosterone molecule has resulted in the production of compounds with reduced androgenic activity but maintained anabolic activity.[89,90] Various modifications have been made to the basic steroid structure to enhance its lipid solubility, thereby rendering it more soluble in the lipid vehicles used for parenteral injection, or to decrease its metabolism by the liver, thereby decreasing the "first-pass effect" and permitting oral administration.[91] After parenteral administration, the duration of effect of the anabolic steroid depends to a large extent on the rate with which it is released from the injection site. The rate of release is determined by the chemical nature of esters of the compound. Acetic and propionic acid esters permit rapid absorption and a short duration of action, while laureate, decanoate, and heptanoate esters slow absorption and extend the duration of action.[92]

Testosterone is the most potent anabolic steroid; however, because of its potent androgenic effects, other anabolic steroids are often preferred. The steroid hormones exert their effect by binding to intracellular protein receptors. The hormone-receptor complex then interacts with nuclear material to induce the synthesis of specific RNA and, consequently, proteins.[91] Testosterone acts in most body tissues, although the active intracellular hormone depends on the tissue.[93] Testosterone is metabolized to the more active 5α-dihydrotestosterone by 5α-reductase in reproductive tissues, whereas in muscles, which have little 5α-reductase activity, testosterone is the predominant anabolic hormone.[93] This difference in tissue sensitivity to testosterone is important in mediating the effect of the synthetic anabolic/androgenic agents. Synthetic anabolic steroids are not metabolized by 5α-reductase and therefore exert minimal androgenic activity (activity in reproductive and central nervous system) but considerable anabolic activity (activity in muscle cells).

The anabolic steroids all increase nitrogen retention and lean body weight and enhance muscular growth in animals with low levels of naturally occurring anabolic/androgenic hormones, such as females and castrated males.[94] There is little indication of a prolonged anabolic effect of low to moderate doses of anabolic/androgenic steroids in intact male animals.[94] Similar results have

been reported in studies of the use of anabolic/androgenic agents in horses.[95,96]

The effect of the anabolic/androgenic steroids on athletic performance is hotly debated in human sports medicine. Definitive answers in humans are unlikely because of the need for double-blind, randomized trials, ethical concerns over the administration of very large doses ("megadoses") of anabolic steroids to research subjects, and the difficulty in ensuring adherence to the study protocol and absence of use of other agents, such as growth hormones, estrogens, and antihypertensive medication. The literature on the effect of anabolic/androgenic steroids has been reviewed.[90,94,97] In summary, studies of anabolic steroid administration to animals have generally failed to demonstrate an effect of these compounds on muscle strength or athletic capacity. Anabolic steroids do not increase the maximal rate of oxygen consumption in laboratory animals, humans, or horses.[98]

The use of anabolic/androgenic steroids is associated with a number of adverse side effects. Virilization (masculinization) is often pronounced in females, castrated males, and prepubescent males.[91,97] Impaired reproductive function is noticeable in both fillies and stallions and is attributable to the direct effect of anabolic/androgenic hormones on the pituitary-gonadal axis.[97,99]

SYMPATHOMIMETICS

The sympathetic nervous system mediates many of the homeostatic functions vital for existence. Increased activity of the sympathetic nervous system occurs during periods of stress, whether it be psychological or induced by cold, hemorrhage, or physical activity. Most of the actions of the sympathomimetic amines—the naturally occurring catecholamines and drugs that mimic their actions—can be explained through their effect to mimic the activity of the sympathetic nervous system. Catecholamines and the sympathetic amines produce, among other effects, bronchodilation, positive inotropy and chronotropy, altered vasomotor tone (either vasodilation or vasoconstriction, depending on the vascular bed and agent), and altered carbohydrate and fat metabolism.[100] Both epinephrine and norepinephrine and the sympathetic amines isoprenaline (isoproterenol), salbutamol (albuterol), and terbutaline exert one or more of these effects in horses.[101,102] The predominant use of catecholamines or sympathetic amines in horses is in the relief of airway constriction associated with chronic obstructive pulmonary disease. Sympathomimetic agents used to effect bronchodilation in horses include clenbuterol, terbutaline, and isoproterenol.

Isoproterenol has been used to induce bronchodilation in horses. Stimulation of bronchial β_2-receptors induces bronchodilation, while stimulation of cardiac β_1-receptors effects positive inotropy and chronotropy. However, isoproterenol is equipotent as a stimulant of β_1- and β_2-adrenoreceptors, and extrapulmonary side effects, such as tachycardia, can be unavoidable and problematic.[103] Drugs with relatively greater affinity for β_2-

than for β_1-adrenoreceptors have been developed in an attempt to avoid this problem. Such drugs include clenbuterol, terbutaline, and salbutamol. Of these, only clenbuterol has been studied extensively in horses.

Clenbuterol

Clenbuterol is a β_2-adrenergic agonist with pronounced cardiopulmonary effects in horses.[104] Intravenous administration of clenbuterol to healthy horses (0.8 μg/kg) reduces nonelastic pulmonary resistance for longer than 3 hours and causes a transitory increase in heart rate and decrease in mean arterial pressure.[104] Clenbuterol also reduces the maximal change in pleural pressure during respiration in horses with chronic obstructive disease.[105] This effect is apparent after both oral and intravenous administration. Clenbuterol also has tocolytic and repartitioning effects.[105,106]

The effect of clenbuterol on various physiologic values of running horses has been reported. Clenbuterol hydrochloride (0.8 μg/kg IV) produced a significantly higher heart rate in two of four stages and 10 minutes after the end of a graded exertion test in adult horses.[107] Significant changes in P_{O_2} (increased) and P_{CO_2} (decreased) were noted but were of such small magnitude that they were unlikely to be of physiologic significance. Similar changes were not detected during more intense exertion in fit thoroughbred horses.[108] Nor did clenbuterol alter respiratory mechanics of clinically normal horses during an incremental exercise test.[109] Thus it appears that clenbuterol administration to clinically normal horses shortly before exertion does not markedly alter the physiologic responses of the horses. The effect of clenbuterol on responses to exertion of horses with chronic obstructive airway disease is not reported.

Amphetamine

Amphetamine is an indirectly acting sympathomimetic amine; its mechanism of action involves release of norepinephrine from storage sites in nerve terminals.[110] Consequently, the effects of amphetamine administration are predominantly those of α- and β_1-adrenergic stimulation, which in humans include increases in both systolic and diastolic blood pressure and a reflex reduction in heart rate.[110] The primary effect of amphetamine is in the central nervous system.[111] Central effects of amphetamine include medullary and cortical stimulation and possibly reticular activating system stimulation.[110] Stimulation of these areas results in mood elevation, euphoria, and a decreased sense of fatigue in humans.[111] Amphetamine also acts to increase the metabolic rate and hence increase oxygen consumption, and it increases the plasma free fatty acid concentration.[112] Amphetamine may be ergogenic in human beings, improving measures of acceleration, lactate accumulation, and time to exhaustion but not muscular power, speed, or maximal aerobic capacity.[111]

In resting horses, amphetamine produces an increase in the respiratory rate of 9 breaths per minute without altering the heart rate.[25,113] Amphetamine sulfate administered intravenously 30 to 60 minutes before a gallop produces an immediate postrace heart rate that is significantly less than that of controls.[25] Smetzer and colleagues[113] reported a similar observation with doses of amphetamine of 150 and 300 mg per horse. However, in another trial in which amphetamine was administered intravenously (0.55 mg/kg) 20 minutes before a submaximal exertion test, the heart rates of the treated horses were higher than those of control horses after completion of the run.[114] Cardiac arrhythmias occur during the immediate postexertion period in amphetamine-treated horses.[25,113] The dysrhythmias included second-degree atrioventricular (AV) block, sinus arrhythmia, and ventricular or AV junctional beats.[113] The dysrhythmias resolved in 3 to 5 minutes.[25] Amphetamine also increases respiratory rate, rectal temperature, and blood lactate concentration immediately after high-speed trotting or pacing.[114]

Amphetamine has been used by human athletes because of its ability to reduce fatigue and enhance athletic performance.[111,115] Apparently for the same reasons, the effect of amphetamine in horses also has been investigated. Administration of amphetamine to thoroughbred horses before each of five trials increased the speed over the corresponding control gallop; however, the overall difference was not statistically significant.[116]

Methylamphetamine

Methylamphetamine produces variable effects on heart rate after exertion; its effects appear to depend on the intensity and possibly the duration of the exertion involved.[117] Methylamphetamine improved performance in a variety of submaximal speed tests at doses of 0.1 to 0.4 mg/kg intramuscularly.[25]

Methylphenidate

Methylphenidate is structurally related to amphetamine, and its pharmacologic effects are essentially those of the amphetamine.[100] The time for cardiac deceleration after lunging was longer in horses administered methylphenidate than in untreated horses.[116] Methylphenidate increased recovery heart rate, respiratory rate, venous lactate concentration, rectal temperature, and cardiac output after a submaximal exertion test of trained standardbred horses.[114] Methylphenidate consistently increased the speed of running in four types of exertion test.[116]

Ephedrine

Ephedrine is both an α- and β-adrenergic agonist that stimulates heart rate and increases cardiac output of humans.[100] The administration of ephedrine to horses does not affect heart and respiratory rates after lunging, nor speed performance.[117]

Cocaine

Cocaine is a naturally occurring alkaloid with potent peripheral sympathomimetic activity and central nervous system stimulating effects.[118] Cocaine is also an effective local anesthetic, an effect enhanced by cocaine's induction of localized vasoconstriction and consequent delayed absorption and dissipation from the site of application. The mechanism of the peripheral effects of cocaine is unclear but may be due to inhibition of reuptake of norepinephrine at presynaptic terminals of sympathetic nerves, direct stimulation of release of catecholamines from peripheral nerves, or centrally mediated release of adrenal catecholamines.[111] Whatever the mechanism, cocaine administered intravenously to humans and horses elevates blood pressure and heart rate and may induce dysrhythmias.[118,119] The central nervous system effects of cocaine administration to humans include euphoria, a positive alteration in mood, and a decreased sense of fatigue. These effects are likely to be the result of cocaine inhibiting reuptake of dopamine in the CNS, with a resultant increase in dopamine concentration at dopamine (D_2) receptors.[111]

The effect of cocaine on exercise capacity has recently been the subject of review.[111] Briefly, cocaine may enhance athletic capacity for short-term, intense exertion but not for prolonged, submaximal activities. The effect of cocaine on athletic capacity of horses has received minimal attention. In a recent study, cocaine increased heart rate and mean arterial pressure of horses during an incremental exercise test.[119] Cocaine also reduced the anaerobic threshold in a dose-dependent fashion and resulted in cocaine-treated horses having higher blood lactate concentrations at maximal work intensities.[119] Notably, endurance time was significantly prolonged by cocaine administration.[119]

SYMPATHOLYTICS

The adrenergic receptors, via increased sympathetic nervous system activity and increased concentrations of circulating epinephrine and norepinephrine, play significant roles in mediating the physiologic and metabolic responses to exertion. Therefore, it is not surprising that β blockade modifies these responses and impairs exercise performance.[120–124] Furthermore, given that the β-adrenergic system is composed of two receptor subtypes, β_1 and β_2, which subserve different physiologic functions, it is apparent that nonselective and selective β blockade have the potential to modify different physiologic responses to exertion. The modification of the physiologic responses by both selective and nonselective β blockade during exertion has been investigated extensively in humans, in part because of the importance of β blockade and exercise in cardiac rehabilitation programs. The effects of a number of different β blockers on the physiologic responses to exertion have been examined in humans and animals.

β-Adrenergic blockade reduces exercise performance and increases the perception of fatigue.[121,123–131] Nonselective β blockade (propranolol) causes a greater reduction in exercise performance than selective (metoprolol, atenolol) β blockade.[123,124,128,132–134]

The potency of β-blocking agents has been expressed as their ability to inhibit exercise-induced tachycardia,[121] and inhibition of exercise-induced tachycardia has been used as evidence of effective β blockade. Inhibition of exercise-induced tachycardia is observed with both selective and nonselective β blockade. A significant correlation exists between plasma metoprolol concentration and inhibition of exercise-induced tachycardia, but no such relationship exists for propranolol.[121,134]

β blockade attenuates the exertion-induced increase in cardiac output,[126,130,135,136] which is not surprising given the coincident inhibition of the exertion-induced tachycardia. Selective and nonselective β blockade has similar effects.[135] However, the effect of the attenuation of exertion-induced tachycardia on cardiac output is partially offset by an increase in stroke volume,[126,135,136] although this may not occur in horses.[130] β blockade also attenuates the exertion-induced increase in mean and systolic arterial pressures,[121,134,135] reduces total peripheral resistance,[135,137] and increases central venous pressure.[126] These changes are in accordance with the echocardiographic demonstration of increased end-diastolic volume and systolic myocardial shortening during semisupine exercise following atenolol administration. Sexton and Erickson[131] also reported that propranolol (0.22 mg/kg IV) in ponies subjected to a standard incremental exertion test attenuated the elevation in pulmonary artery flow velocity (an indicator of cardiac output) and right ventricular dP/dt while augmenting the increase in mean pulmonary artery and right ventricular pressures. Propranolol did not alter the response of the mean systemic arterial pressure to exertion.[131] The increased preload, as evidenced by elevated right ventricular and central venous pressures, favors an increase in stroke volume during exertion under β blockade. The negative inotropic effects of propranolol, as assessed by dP/dt, are likely to contribute to the attenuation of cardiac output during exertion under β blockade.

The peripheral circulatory response to exertion during β blockade is unclear. In active muscles, the increased blood flow during exercise is produced by metabolite-induced vasodilation; the role of the peripheral β_2 receptors in this response is believed to be of minor importance.[138] Reductions in muscle blood flow due to local effects of the β blockade are not believed to be important in the reduction of performance capacity. Changes in skeletal muscle contractile properties with β blockade have not been observed and thus are not believed to limit performance.[139,140]

β blockade appears to reduce the rate of maximal uptake of oxygen, but the effect on $\dot{V}_{O_2}$ at submaximal work rates is variable. In the face of the attenuation of the exercise-induced increases in cardiac output by β blockade, oxygen consumption is maintained to a greater or lesser degree by an increase in the arterial-venous oxygen difference during submaximal exertion.[126,130,136] At maximal work rates, however, the increased arterial-venous oxygen difference can no longer compensate for the decreased cardiac output, and $\dot{V}_{O_2max}$ is diminished. Both selective and nonselective β blockade appears to similarly influence oxygen uptake during exertion.

β blockade modifies the metabolic responses to exertion, with nonselective blockade having a greater effect than selective β_1 blockade. β_2 receptor stimulation increases the activity of phosphorylase and hormone-sensitive triglyceride lipase, increasing the rates of glycogenolysis and lipolysis, respectively. β_2 receptor blockade therefore reduces the rates of glycogenolysis and lipolysis. These effects are manifest as a reduced blood glucose concentration (due to inhibition of hepatic glycogenolysis), decreased blood lactate concentration (due to inhibited muscle glycogenolysis), and decreased blood free fatty acid and glycerol concentrations (due to inhibited lipolysis).[130,141] The greater affinity of propranolol than metoprolol for β_2 receptors explains the differences observed in blood concentrations of glucose, lactate, and free fatty acids with exertion during selective and nonselective blockade. The inhibition of energy metabolism may explain, at least in part, the effects of β blockers in decreasing dynamic performance.

In horses, sweating is under β-adrenergic control.[142] Propranolol reduces the sweating response of isolated equine skin after stimulation with either epinephrine or terbutaline[142] and of maximally exercised horses.[124] These findings indicate that β blockade may impair the thermoregulatory responses of horses. Interestingly, propranolol increases the temperature of blood in the pulmonary artery of ponies but not that in the right atrium of horses during exertion on a treadmill.[130,131]

The effects of the β-receptor blocking drugs on the physiologic and metabolic responses to exertion are the result of impaired β-receptor–mediated responses. Both selective and nonselective β blockers modify various physiologic responses to exertion. These effects are most apparent with high-intensity exertion (at or approaching $\dot{V}_{O_2max}$). Attenuation of the exertion-induced increase in heart rate is primarily responsible for the reduction in physical performance. At submaximal workloads, the effect of β blockade on heart rate is offset by increases in stroke volume, which acts to maintain cardiac output, and the arterial-venous oxygen difference. Performance also may be reduced by inhibition of the β_2-mediated effects on energy metabolism.

SEDATIVES AND TRANQUILIZERS

The sedatives and tranquilizers used frequently in equine practice are phenothiazine derivatives (promazine, chlorpromazine, acepromazine) and the α_2-adrenergic agonists (xylazine, detomidine, and romifidine).[143] Other agents, such as chloral hydrate, reserpine, and the barbiturates, are principally of historical interest; they have a minimal role in contemporary practice.

Promazine, Acepromazine, and Chlorpromazine
The predominant mechanism of action of the phenothiazine derivatives is as dopamine antagonists in the mesolimbic-mesocortical and nigrostriatal regions of the brain.[143] The mesolimbic-mesocortical pathway is involved in behavior, while the nigrostriatal pathway is integral to the coordination of voluntary movement. The phenothiazines therefore reduce spontaneous motor activity in horses.[144] Phenothiazines also block the peripheral actions of catecholamines, an action that may account for acepromazine's hypotensive effect.[145,146] The phenothiazine derivatives have little or no analgesic activity.[147]

Promazine does not influence a number of physiologic variables of horses during a submaximal exertion test[116] but does increase the heart rate immediately after completion of a high-speed run.[25] Chlorpromazine increases the heart rate and causes penile ptosis of male horses during submaximal running on a track.[148]

As in humans, sedatives reduce athletic performance of horses.[115] Both acepromazine and promazine reduce performance in horses subjected to a short gallop or cavalleti.[116] Promazine significantly decreases speed of thoroughbred horses when administered 30 to 60 minutes before a simulated race.[25] Chlorpromazine has a pronounced effect in decreasing running speed of thoroughbred horses.[148]

α_2-Adrenergic Agonists
The α_2-adrenergic agonists exert their sedative and analgesic effects by binding to α_2 receptors in the central nervous system and suppressing axonal release of norepinephrine and dopamine.[143,149] α_2-Adrenergic receptors are found in many other tissues of the body,[149] and this is likely to account for the endocrine and cardiovascular effects of the α_2 agonists. The cardiovascular effects of the α_2 agonists are due to the combined effects of inhibition of central nervous system sympathetic tone and norepinephrine release from peripheral sympathetic nerves and an apparent reflex increase in vagal tone secondary to α_2-agonist–induced increase in systemic blood pressure.

Xylazine, detomidine, and romifidine are α_2 agonists available for use in horses.[143] Although their relative potencies vary, all three drugs are potent analgesics and sedatives in horses. Both xylazine and detomidine exert dose-dependent effects on systemic hemodynamics of conscious horses. Xylazine and detomidine cause an initial brief increase in systemic arterial pressures which is followed by a more prolonged hypotension.[150] Heart and respiratory rate and cardiac output are reduced, while cardiac filling pressures are increased by xylazine or detomidine administration to horses.[150] These drugs also decrease intracranial pressure in conscious horses,[151] cause hyperglycemia[152,153] and increase insulin secretion,[152] and transiently increase urine output.[153]

While the α_2 agonists are drugs frequently used in performance horses, the effect of α_2 agonists on athletic capacity of horses has not, to our knowledge, been reported. However, one would expect, given the profound sedative, hemodynamic, and endocrine effects of these drugs, that athletic capacity would be decreased for a period of hours after the administration of these drugs.

METHYLXANTHINES

Theophylline (and its complex with ethylenediamine, aminophylline), theobromine, and caffeine are methylxanthine alkaloids that share similar structures, pharmacologic effects, and mechanisms of action.[154] All act as stimulants of the central nervous system and heart, relax smooth muscle, induce diuresis, and increase basal metabolic rate and plasma concentrations of free fatty acids.[154] The precise mechanism of action of the methylxanthines is unclear, although three mechanisms have been suggested[154]: (1) intracellular translocation of calcium, (2) inhibition of phosphodiesterase and subsequent accumulation of intracellular cyclic nucleotides, and (3) antagonism of extracellular adenosine receptors.

Caffeine

Ingestion of caffeine by humans causes increased alertness (i.e., less drowsiness and clearer thought) but impairs coordination and task performance.[111] Increasing doses of caffeine increase CNS stimulation, resulting in, progressively, nervousness and anxiety, restlessness, insomnia, tremors, hyperesthesia, and convulsions.[111] Caffeine also affects skeletal muscle function. In vitro caffeine potentiates twitch tension, and in vivo, it increases muscle force output at low electrical frequencies (10 to 59 Hz) but does not alter the strength of maximum voluntary contractions.[111] Caffeine does not improve short-term or maximal power output in humans,[111] although it may[155] or may not[156] improve endurance performance.

Caffeine increases spontaneous locomotor activity in horses, but the effect is short-lived and apparent only after intravenous injection of the drug.[157] Caffeine (2.5 and 5.0 g per horse SC) enhances running performance, as assessed by timed runs, of thoroughbred horses.[158] It should be noted that the running speeds in these trials were likely not maximal. Heart rates during submaximal exercise and recovery are higher after caffeine administration than during drug-free trials.[158] Variable effects on performance and heart and respiratory rates were observed in two horses administered caffeine (4.0 and 16.0 mg/kg PO)[117]; insufficient data are presented to draw any conclusions.

Theophylline

Theophylline is a potent dilator of constricted airways and is often used in the treatment of recurrent obstructive pulmonary disease (heaves, COPD) in horses. Theophylline, like caffeine, has pronounced effects on other body systems, including the central nervous system, heart, and kidneys. Theophylline induces dose-dependent increases in heart rate, sweating, sensitivity to auditory and visual stimuli, urine flow, and muscle tremors in horses.[159] The suggested upper therapeutic plasma concentration of theophylline in horses is 15 μg/ml.[159]

Theophylline affects some of the physiologic responses of horses to exertion. Theophylline accentuates both the heart rate and blood lactate concentration responses of horses to incremental exertion on a treadmill.[160,161] The effect of theophylline on athletic performance in horses is unknown, although in humans, intravenous aminophylline does not increase maximal oxygen uptake, maximum work rate, or maximum minute ventilation.[162]

NONSTEROIDAL ANTI-INFLAMMATORY DRUGS

Nonsteroidal anti-inflammatory drugs (NSAIDs) act by inhibiting the activity of cyclooxygenase (prostaglandin synthetase), thereby reducing the rate at which various prostaglandin compounds, such as prostacyclin (PGI), prostaglandin $F_{2\alpha}$, prostaglandin E, and thromboxane, are formed from arachidonic acid.[163] Inhibition of prostaglandin synthesis is thought to be the principal mechanism by which the NSAIDs exert their potent anti-inflammatory, antipyretic, and analgesic activities.[163,164]

Prostaglandins are widely distributed in the body and mediate or modulate a variety of physiologic and pathophysiologic processes in many organ systems and tissues, including the hematopoietic, cardiovascular, and reproductive systems.[165] In addition to their role in inflammation, several of the prostaglandins have notable effects on the cardiovascular system. In general, prostaglandin E_2 and prostacyclin (also known as PGI_2) are vasodilatory compounds, whereas prostaglandin $F_{2\alpha}$ is a vasoconstrictor.[166] These actions, in addition to the local production of prostaglandins in vascular beds, raise the possibility that prostaglandins contribute to the regulation of various regional circulations.[167]

There is a mounting body of evidence that the prostaglandins are involved in mediating some of the cardiovascular responses to exertion. The plasma concentrations of PGE_2, 6-keto $PGF_{1\alpha}$, and $PGF_{2\alpha}$ in humans increase during running,[168,169] and exercise increases the urinary excretion rate of a metabolite of prostacyclin, 2,3-dinor-6-keto-prostaglandin $F_{1\alpha}$, but not of the metabolite of thromboxane, 2,3-dinor-thromboxane B_2.[170] Exercise on a stationary cycle induces a twofold increase in femoral venous PGE_2 concentrations over those measured at rest, indicating a net production of PGE_2 in working muscle.[171] Similarly, the plasma concentration of 6-keto-prostaglandin $F_{1\alpha}$ increased during incremental treadmill exertion in horses.[172] Clearly, in humans and horses, exertion is associated with increased production of prostaglandins and increased plasma concentrations of various prostaglandins of their stable metabolites.

The increases in prostaglandin production and/or plasma concentration during exertion indicate a physiologically important role for the prostaglandins during exertion because inhibition of prostaglandin synthesis alters the physiologic responses to exertion.[173–180] Both indomethacin and aspirin inhibit exercise-induced increases in calf muscle and forearm blood flow in humans.[177,178] Indomethacin accentuates the exercise-induced increase in systolic and diastolic arterial pressures and decreases the heart rate response to exercise.[177] Indomethacin also decreases the hyperemic response to isometric and dynamic forearm exercise in humans.[179] These actions may be due to the local effects of inhibition of prostaglandin production on systemic hemodynamics and also to the inhibition of prostaglandin-mediated systemic cardiovascular reflexes arising in active muscle.[174]

There are a number of NSAIDs used in horses,[181,182]

with phenylbutazone enjoying extensive use in performance horses.[183,184] Phenylbutazone is a potent anti-inflammatory and analgesic in horses. Consistent with the other NSAIDs, phenylbutazone's principal pharmacologic activity probably results from its inhibition of prostaglandin production.[184] There is a substantial body of evidence that phenylbutazone exerts this effect in the horse. For example, phenylbutazone inhibits thromboxane B_2 (the stable metabolite of thromboxane A_2, the biologically active compound) production in the normal horse,[185] prevents an increase in plasma concentrations of 6-keto-prostaglandin $F_{1\alpha}$ (6-keto-$PGF_{1\alpha}$, the stable metabolite of prostacyclin) in horses after endotoxin challenge,[186] and inhibits prostaglandin E_2 (PGE_2) production in an equine model of acute inflammation.[187]

The effect of NSAID administration on the physiologic and biochemical responses to exertion in horses has been examined only scantily. Phenylbutazone has not been shown to enhance the performance of racehorses. However, the administration of NSAIDs does alter the speed/blood lactate concentration relationships of horses. Administration of flunixin meglumine (1 mg/kg IM) or meclofenamic acid (2.2 mg/kg PO) before running results in lower postexercise venous lactate concentrations than occur during drug-free trials.[188] Meclofenamic acid also increases the onset of blood lactate accumulation (running speed at which a blood lactate concentration of 4 mmol/liter is produced) and decreases the extrapolated venous lactate concentration at V_{200}. Whether these effects of NSAIDs alter athletic performance is unknown.

A further factor to consider when discussing the effect of the NSAIDs on athletic performance is the ability of these drugs to decrease the pain associated with musculoskeletal disease. Traditional wisdom is that lame horses do not perform as well in athletic competition as sound horses. The administration of phenylbutazone or other NSAIDs to lame horses may therefore allow them to compete more effectively.

SODIUM BICARBONATE

Muscular work is associated with increases in the concentration of lactate and hydrogen ions in muscle cells. These changes occur as energy for muscle contraction is provided by anaerobic glycolysis, the metabolism of glucose to lactate and pyruvate. Under aerobic conditions, lactate is metabolized, and hydrogen ions are consumed through pyruvate and the citric acid cycle to carbon dioxide. However, if oxygen supply is limited or metabolic rate is high, then lactate and hydrogen ions accumulate in the muscle cells. If the buffering capacity of the cell is exceeded, the intracellular pH falls, the activity of pH-sensitive processes in the cell declines, and the cell's ability to generate power diminishes.[189] It has been suggested that sodium bicarbonate delays the onset of fatigue by providing additional buffering and thereby slowing the decline in intracellular pH. Metabolic alkalosis ... mate the release of lactate from muscle cells, ... ues and affect cellular creatine phosphate and ... id chro-

ATP concentrations, nor does it increase muscle performance.[190,191] The mechanism by which sodium bicarbonate exerts any ergogenic effect is unclear.

There have been numerous studies of the effect of sodium bicarbonate on athletic capacity in humans.[192–194] Comparison of the studies is confounded by the range of doses of sodium bicarbonate used, including doses that are now regarded as ineffective (0.2 g/kg and less), the variable time between ingestion and the exercise test, and the variety of exercise tests employed.

Sodium bicarbonate ingestion significantly decreases 400- and 800-m race times, race duration being approximately 59 and 126 seconds, respectively.[195,196] The time to exhaustion on cycle ergometers at a workload 125 percent of that producing peak aerobic power, approximately 75 seconds, and at a workload of 95 percent of maximal oxygen consumption, approximately 180 seconds, was significantly increased by sodium bicarbonate ingestion.[197,198] Sodium bicarbonate also increased the duration of the last of five exhaustive cycle rides by 42 percent[199] and decreased the time taken to complete the fourth and fifth swim sprints of 5 91.4-m sprints separated by 2 minutes,[200] indicating an ergogenic effect of sodium bicarbonate during exhaustive interval exercise. Ratings of perceived exertion, a subjective assessment of the intensity of exercise, were lesser after sodium bicarbonate ingestion.[201]

Sodium bicarbonate ingestion did not increase time to exhaustion (approximately 100 seconds) during a cycle ergometer ride at a work rate equivalent to 125 percent of that required to produce maximal oxygen consumption.[202] Furthermore, mean and peak power outputs during three 30-second Wingate anaerobic tests (separated by 6 minutes) were not affected by sodium bicarbonate ingestion.[203] Similarly, alkalosis did not affect peak power output during a cycle ergometer ride to exhaustion (approximately 20 minutes).[204]

The consensus opinion presently is that sodium bicarbonate, at doses of 0.3 or 0.4 g/kg (larger doses cause gastrointestinal discomfort and diarrhea in humans) ingested approximately 2 to 2.5 hours before an appropriate event, may be ergogenic. The ergogenic effect of sodium bicarbonate is apparent in events of maximal or near-maximal intensity lasting between 1 and 10 minutes or in repeated bouts of exhaustive exercise of less than 1-minute duration.[192,193]

Sodium bicarbonate administration to horses produces a metabolic alkalosis,[205–212] with a dose of 0.6 g/kg body weight producing a greater and longer-lasting elevation in blood pH than a dose of 0.3 g/kg. Subsequent to the oral administration of 0.6 g/kg of bicarbonate to adult horses, jugular venous blood pH is elevated for at least 12 but less than 24 hours.[205] The time to peak pH after bicarbonate administration is reported to be 8 hours after a dose of 0.6 g/kg[205] and 2.5 to 3 hours after 0.4 g/kg.[205] Increases in blood pH are associated with increases in bicarbonate concentration.

Ingestion of sodium salts may affect the concentration of various plasma constituents.[213] The effect of sodium bicarbonate ingestion on plasma constituents, other than hydrogen ion and bicarbonate, of sedentary animals or humans has received limited attention despite the fact that the quantity of sodium given is quite large.[214] Administration of sodium bicarbonate at a dose rate of 0.3 g/kg (3.9 mmol sodium per kilogram) represents a quantity of sodium equal to approximately 12 percent of extracellular sodium. Not surprisingly, then, ingestion of sodium bicarbonate (0.6 or 1 g/kg) increases serum osmolality, and the increase is largely because of an increase in serum sodium concentration.[207,213] Serum potassium concentrations decrease[206] or remain unchanged, and serum concentrations of chloride are unaffected by sodium bicarbonate.[207]

The effect of sodium bicarbonate on plasma and/or blood volume has received little attention. Serum protein concentrations of horses administered sodium bicarbonate (0.6 g/kg) are reported to be lower than those of control (water) horses,[207] suggesting that sodium bicarbonate increased plasma volume. In horses receiving the same number of moles of sodium either as sodium chloride or as sodium bicarbonate, horses receiving sodium bicarbonate had higher plasma total protein values during maximal exercise than horses given sodium chloride.[212] However, in splenectomized horses, there was no effect of oral sodium bicarbonate (1 g/kg) or sodium chloride (0.7 g/kg) administration on plasma volume (Hinchcliff and colleagues, unpublished observations).

Sodium bicarbonate alters the acid-base, plasma lactate, and muscle metabolite responses to exercise. Sodium bicarbonate also produces respiratory depression.[212] The magnitude of these changes varies with the dose of sodium bicarbonate used, the type of exercise (including duration and intensity), and the site of blood sampling (arterial, arterialized venous blood, peripheral venous, or mixed venous). However, there are some consistent changes associated with sodium bicarbonate administration.

At similar work intensities, blood pH, lactate, and bicarbonate concentrations are higher in animals or humans administered sodium bicarbonate than in the untreated state.[207,208,215] However, at exhaustion, mixed venous blood pH of horses is unaffected by sodium bicarbonate, suggesting that the higher initial pH in horses receiving bicarbonate increases the quantity of hydrogen ions buffered. Sodium bicarbonate administration increases plasma or blood lactate concentrations over those of untreated horses or humans during submaximal or exhaustive exercise.[196,198,208,211,212,214] The greater lactate concentrations in plasma or blood of sodium bicarbonate–treated individuals is the result of increased lactate efflux from skeletal muscle and is not due to increased lactate production.[191]

Similar to the use of sodium bicarbonate in human beings, studies of the effect of sodium bicarbonate on athletic capacity in horses have produced conflicting results. Greenhaff and colleagues[207] administered sodium bicarbonate (0.6 g/kg) or water (control) to 24 thoroughbred horses in a crossover trial and did not detect a significant difference in the time (approximately 69 seconds) required to complete a simulated 1000-m race. Similarly, Harkins and Kamerling[211] did not detect a sig-

nificant effect of sodium bicarbonate (0.4 g/kg) on race times of 16 thoroughbred horses. The time to exhaustion (approximately 1200 seconds) during a submaximal exercise test performed on a treadmill was not affected by sodium bicarbonate administration (0.3 g/kg).[208]

Significant effects on race times or time to exhaustion have been demonstrated by other investigators. The time for six thoroughbred horses to complete a 1600-m sprint on a racetrack was reduced by sodium bicarbonate administration (0.4 g/kg).[209] The risk of this result occurring by chance alone was less than 1 in 10 ($p <$ 0.1).[209] Standardbred horses completed a 1-mi race in 1.1 seconds less after sodium bicarbonate administration (0.3 g/kg) than after receiving water ($p < 0.1$).[210] Lloyd and colleagues[212] reported significantly longer run time in horses given sodium bicarbonate compared with an equimolar dose of sodium chloride. Hinchcliff and colleagues[216] demonstrated a significant effect of sodium bicarbonate (1 g/kg) and sodium chloride (0.7 g/kg) compared with water on time to exhaustion (approximately 500 seconds) during an incremental exercise test on a treadmill.

The effect of sodium bicarbonate on athletic capacity of horses is unclear. It appears, however, that if sodium bicarbonate is to exert an ergogenic effect, it will likely do so in events of longer than 120 seconds' duration or during events in which there are multiple exhaustive bouts of exercise with insufficient time to completely recover between bouts, such as may occur with standardbred racing in the United States. On balance, it is likely that sodium bicarbonate does not improve race times where the race lasts less than 60 seconds. One must, however, be cognizant of the fact that it is exceedingly difficult to reliably detect small improvements in race times, even though such small improvements may be very important in an actual race.[214]

Gastrointestinal discomfort is frequently reported in human beings who ingest large quantities of sodium bicarbonate (>0.4 g/kg) or insufficient water.[193] Theoretically, cardiac dysrhythmias may develop secondary to the serum electrolyte abnormalities encountered after sodium bicarbonate ingestion,[193] but sodium bicarbonate–induced dysrhythmias are not reported in the horse. The concurrent administration of furosemide and sodium bicarbonate to horses induces profound metabolic alkalosis and severe serum electrolyte abnormalities[217] and should be avoided. Fatal aspiration pneumonia has been observed in horses after the inadvertent intratracheal administration of sodium bicarbonate solution.

Conclusion

Modern screening and confirmatory methods for detecting and identifying drugs and drug metabolites are vastly improved over methods used only a few years ago. These improvements have resulted from the introduction of immunoassay methods with increased sensitivity and reliability and the development of new confirmatory techniques utilizing improved isolation techniques and gas chromatography/mass spectrometry and liqu matography/mass spectrometry. Lower limits of detection for therapeutic substances will require longer withdrawal times for these substances or abandonment of their use altogether in racing horses.

It is difficult to draw any firm conclusions about the effect of the drugs discussed above on athletic capability of the performance horse. The chief obstacle lies in the widely divergent tests of athletic capability used, undoubtedly an indicator that no single technique can be used as a means of investigating or even defining athletic capability in the horse. The high-speed treadmill has greatly facilitated the measurement of physiologic variables during exertion in the horse and has permitted the development of standardized tests. These should enable more detailed investigation of the effects of various drugs on physiologic responses to exercise in the horse.

References

1. Oseid S: Doping and athletes: Prevention and counseling. J Allergy Clin Immunol 1984; 73:735.
2. Maylin GA: Microtechniques in thin layer chromatography. *In* Proceedings of the 3rd International Conference of Racing Analysts and Veterinarians, Lexington, Ky, 1979, p 3.
3. Combie J, Blake JW, Nugent TE, et al: Furosemide, *Patella vulgata* β-glucuronidase and drug analysis: Conditions for the enhancement of the TLC detection of apomorphine, butorphanol, hydromorphone, nalbuphine, oxymorphone, and pentazocine in equine urine. Res Commun Chem Pathol Pharmacol 1982; 35:27.
4. Lovecock JE: Electron absorption detectors and techniques for use in quantitative analysis by gas chromatography. Anal Chem 1963; 35:474.
5. Blake JW, Huffman R, Noonan J, et al: GLC and the electron capture detector. Am Lab 1973; 5:63.
6. Joel SP, Osborne RJ, Slevin ML: An improved method for the simultaneous determination of morphine and its principal glucuronide metabolites. J Chromatogr 1988; 430:394.
7. Dube LM, Beaudoin N, LaLande M, et al: Determination of nalbuphine by high-performance liquid chromatography with electrochemical detection: Application to clinical samples from post-operative patients. J Chromatogr 1988; 427:113.
8. Yang R-K, Hseih JY-K, Kendler KS, et al: Rapid determination of apomorphine in brain and plasma using high-performance liquid chromatography. J Chromatogr Sci 1984; 7:191.
9. Emm T, Lesko LJ, Leslie J, et al: Determination of albuterol in human serum by reversed-phase high-performance liquid chromatography with electrochemical detection. J Chromatogr 1988; 427:188.
10. Krstulovic AM: Investigations of catecholamine metabolism using high-performance liquid chromatography: Analytical methodology and clinical applications. J Chromatogr 1982; 229:1.
11. Dutton J, Copeland LG, Playfer JR, et al: Measuring L-DOPA and dopamine in urine and plasma to monitor therapy of elderly patients with Parkinson disease treated with L-DOPA and a DOPA decarboxylase inhibitor. Clin Chem 1993; 39:629.
12. Yalow RS, Berson SA: Assay of insulin in human subjects by immunoassay. Nature 1959; 184:1648.
13. Frincke JM, Henderson GL: The major metabolite of fentanyl in the horse. Drug Metab Disp 1980; 8:425.
14. Engvall E, Perlmann P: Enzyme linked immunosorbent assay (ELISA): Quantitative assay of IgG. Immunochemistry 1971; 8:871.
15. Van Weemen B, Schuurs AHWM: Immunoassay using antigen-enzyme conjugates. FEBS Lett 1971; 15:232.
16. Soma LR, Felsburg P, Hopkins J, et al: Enzyme-linked immunoassay (ELISA) for the detection and quantitation of fentanyl: Prototype for a unique system. *In* Proceedings of the 7th International Conference of Racing Analysts and Veterinarians, 1988, p 135.
17. Weckman TJ, Tobin T, Tai H-H, et al: Detection of fentanyl and fentanyl derivatives using radioimmunoassay and enzyme-linked immunosorbent assay. *In* Proceedings of the 7th International Conference of Racing Analysts and Veterinarians, 1988, p 123.
18. Liu JH, Ku WW: Determination of enantiomeric N-trifluoroacetyl-L-prolyl chloride amphetamine derivatives by capillary gas chromatography/mass spectrometry with chiral and achiral stationary phases. Anal Chem 1981; 53:2180.
19. Chui YC, Mutlib A, Esaw B, et al: Detection of detomidine and its metabolites in equine plasma and urine. *In* Proceedings of the 9th International Conference of Racing Analysts and Veterinarians, 1992, p 85.
20. Mutlib AE, Chui YC, Young LE, et al: Characterization of xylazine metabolites produced in vivo and in vitro by LC/MS/MS and GC/MS. Drug Metab Disp 1992; 20:840.
21. Sams RA. Unpublished observations, 1992.
22. Mendonca M, Ryan M, Todi F: Glycopyrrolate: Detection and elimination in the horse. *In* Proceedings of the 9th International Conference of Racing Analysts and Veterinarians, 1992, p 327.
23. McDonald J, Gall R, Wiedenbach P, et al: Immunoassay detection of drugs in racing horses: III. Detection of morphine in equine blood and urine by a one step ELISA method. Res Commun Chem Pathol Pharmacol 1988; 59:259.
24. Sweeney CR, Soma LR, Maxson AD, et al: Effect of furosemide on the racing times of thoroughbreds. Am J Vet Res 1990; 51:772.
25. Stewart GA: Drugs, performance and responses to exeircse in the racehorse: 2. Observations on amphetamine, promazine, and thiamine. Aust Vet J 1972; 48:544.
26. McArdle WD, Katch FI, Katch VL: Exercise Physiology: Energy, Nutrition, and Human Performance, 3d ed. Philadelphia, Lea & Febiger, 1991.
27. Seeherman HJ, Morris EA: Application of a standardised treadmill exercise test for clinical evaluation of fitness in 10 thoroughbred racehorses. Equine Vet J 1990; (suppl 9):26.
28. Thornton JR: Exercise testing. Vet Clin North Am Equine Pract 1985; 1:573.
29. Shephard RJ: Tests of maximum oxygen intake: A critical review. Sports Med 1984; 1:99.
30. Åstrand PO, Rodahl K: Textbook of Work Physiology: Physiological Bases of Exercise, 2d ed. New York, McGraw-Hill, 1977, p 99.
31. Noakes TD: Implications of exercise testing for prediction of athletic performance: A contemporary perspective. Med Sci Sports Exerc 1988; 20:319.
32. Persson SGB: Evaluation of exercise tolerance and fitness in the performance horse. *In* Snow DH, Persson SGB, Rose RJ (eds): Equine Exercise Physiology. Cambridge, Granta Editions, 1983, p 111.
33. Thornton JR, Essen-Gustavsson B, Lindholm A, et al: Effects of training and detraining on oxygen uptake, cardiac output, blood gas tensions, pH and lactate concentrations during and after exercise in the horse. *In* Snow DH, Persson SGB, Rose RJ (eds): Equine Exercise Physiology. Cambridge, Granta Editions, 1983, p 470.
34. Gabel AA, Tobin T, Ray RS, et al: Furosemide in horses: A review. J Equine Med Surg 1977; 1:215.
35. Hinchcliff KW, Muir WW: Pharmacology of furosemide in the horse: A review. J Vet Intern Med 1991; 5:211.
36. Hinchcliff KW, Mitten LA: Furosemide, bumetanide, and ethacrynic acid. Vet Clin North Am Equine Pract 1993; 9:511.
37. Chay S, Woods WE, Rowse K, et al: The pharmacology of furosemide in the horse: V. Pharmacokinetics and blood levels of furosemide after intravenous administration. Drug Metab Dis 1983; 11:226.
38. Tobin T, Roberts BL, Swerczek TW, et al: The pharmacology of furosemide in the horse: III. Dose and time response relationships, effects of repeated dosing, and performance effects. J Equine Med Surg 1978; 2:216.
39. Roberts BL, Blake JW, Tobin T: The pharmacology of furosemide in the horse: II. Its detection, pharmacokinetics, and clearance from the urine. J Equine Med Surg 1978; 2:185.
40. Amedee T, Large WA, Wang Q: Characteristics of chloride currents activated by noradrenaline in rabbit ear artery cells. J Physiol (Lond) 1990; 428:501.

41. Halligan RD, Shelat H, Kahn AM: Na$^+$-independent Cl$^-$-HCO$_3^-$ exchange in sarcolemmal vesicles from vascular smooth muscle. Am J Physiol 1991; 260:C347.
42. Welsh MJ: Inhibition of chloride secretion by furosemide in canine tracheal epithelium. J Membrane Biol 1983; 71:219.
43. Martinez-Maldonado M, Cordova HR: Cellular and molecular aspects of the renal effects of diuretic agents. Kidney Int 1990; 38:632.
44. Breyer J, Jacobson HR: Molecular mechanisms of diuretic agents. Annu Rev Med 1990; 41:265.
45. Miyanoshita A, Terada M, Endou H: Furosemide directly stimulates prostaglandin E$_2$ production in the thick ascending limb of Henle's loop. J Pharmacol Exp Ther 1989; 251:1155.
46. Lundergan CF, Fitzpatrick TM, Rose JC, et al: Effect of cyclooxygenase inhibition on the pulmonary vasodilator response to furosemide. J Pharmacol Exp Ther 1988; 246:102.
47. Garner HE, Hutcheson DP, Coffman JR, et al: Urine electrolyte and diuretic responses to seven dosage levels of lasix. *In* Proceedings of the Annual Meeting of the American Association of Equine Practitioners, 1975, p 87.
48. Alexander F: The effect of ethacrynic acid, bumetanide, frusemide, spironolactone and ADH on electrolyte excretion in ponies. J Vet Pharmacol Ther 1982; 5:153.
49. Freestone JF, Carlson GP, Harrold DR, et al: Influence of furosemide treatment on fluid and electrolyte balance in horses. Am J Vet Res 1988; 49:1899.
50. Weiner IM, Mudge GH: Diuretics and other agents employed in the mobilization of edema fluid. *In* Gilman AG, Goodman LS, Rall TW, Murad F (eds): The Pharmacological Basis of Therapeutics. New York, Macmillan, 1985, p 887.
51. Muir WW, Kohn CW, Sams R: Effects of furosemide on plasma volume and extracellular fluid volume in horses. Am J Vet Res 1978; 39:1688.
52. Hinchcliff KW, McKeever KH, Muir WW: Furosemide-induced changes in plasma and blood volume in horses. J Vet Pharmacol Ther 1991; 14:411.
53. Houpt KA, Northrup N, Wheatley T, et al: Thirst and salt appetite in horses treated with furosemide. J Appl Physiol 1991; 71:2380.
54. Hinchcliff KW: Modification of the Physiologic Responses to Sustained Exertion in Horses by Phenylbutazone and Furosemide. Ph.D. dissertation, The Ohio State University, 1990.
55. Rose RJ, Gibson KT, Suann CJ: An evaluation of an oral glucose-glycine-electrolyte solution for the treatment of experimentally induced dehydration in the horse. Vet Rec 1986; 119:522.
56. Olsen SC, Coyne CP, Lowe BS, et al: Influence of furosemide on hemodynamic responses during exercise in horses. Am J Vet Res 1992; 53:742.
57. Johnston GD, Hiatt WR, Neis AS, et al: Factors modifying the early nondiuretic vascular effects of furosemide in man: The possible role of renal prostaglandins. Circ Res 1983; 53:630.
58. Dikshit K, Vyden JK, Forrester JS, et al: Renal and extrarenal hemodynamic effects of furosemide in congestive heart failure after acute myocardial infarction. N Eng J Med 1973; 288:1087.
59. Bourland WA, Day DK, Williamson HE: The role of the kidney in the early nondiuretic action of furosemide to reduce elevated left atrial pressure in the hypervolemic dog. J Pharmacol Exp Ther 1977; 202:221.
60. Robuschi M, Pieroni M, Refini M, et al: Prevention of antigen-induced early obstructive reaction by inhaled furosemide in (atopic) subjects with asthma and (actively sensitized) guinea pigs. J Allergy Clin Immunol 1990; 85:10.
61. Bianco S, Pieroni MG, Refini RM, et al: Protective effect of inhaled furosemide on allergen-induced early and late asthmatic reactions. N Engl J Med 1989; 321:1069.
62. Verdiani P, DiCarlo S, Baronti A, et al: Effect of inhaled frusemide on the early response to antigen and subsequent change in airway reactivity in atopic patients. Thorax 1990; 45:377.
63. Bianco S, Vaghi A, Robuschi M, et al: Prevention of exercise-induced bronchoconstriction by inhaled furosemide. Lancet 1988; 2:252.
64. Karlsson J, Choudry NB, Zackrisson C, et al: A comparison of the effect of inhaled diuretics on airway reflexes in humans and guinea pigs. J Appl Physiol 1992; 72:434.
65. Broadstone RV, Robinson NE, Gray PR, et al: Effects of furose-

66. Kirchner KA: Prostaglandin inhibitors alter loop segment chloride uptake during furosemide diuresis. Am J Physiol 1985; 248:F698.
67. Chennavasin P, Seiwell R, Brater DC: Pharmacokinetic-dynamic analysis of the indomethacin-furosemide interaction in man. J Pharmacol Exp Ther 1980; 215:77.
68. Jones JH, Smith BL, Birks EK, et al: Left atrial and pulmonary artery pressures in exercising horses. FASEB J 1992; 6:A2020.
69. Erickson BK, Erickson HH, Coffman JR: Pulmonary artery and aortic pressure changes during high-intensity treadmill exercise in the horse: effect of frusemide and phentolamine. Equine Vet J 1992; 24:215.
70. Manohar M: Pulmonary artery wedge pressure increases with high-intensity exercise in horses. Am J Vet Res 1993; 54:142.
71. Goetz TE, Manohar M: Pressures in the right side of the heart and esophagus (pleura) in ponies during exercise before and after furosemide administration. Am J Vet Res 1986; 47:270.
72. Manohar M: Effect of furosemide administration on systemic circulation of ponies during severe exercise. Am J Vet Res 1986; 47:1387.
73. Manohar M: Furosemide attenuates the exercise-induced rise in pulmonary artery wedge pressure in horses. Physiologist 1992; 35:231.
74. Olsen SC, Coyne CP, Lowe BS, et al: Influence of cyclooxygenase inhibitors on furosemide-induced hemodynamic effects during exercise in horses. Am J Vet Res 1992; 53:1562.
75. Sweeney CR: Exercise-induced pulmonary hemorrhage. *In* Robinson EN (ed): Current Therapy in Equine Medicine. Philadelphia, WB Saunders Co, 1987, p 603.
76. Donaldson LL: A review of the pathophysiology of exercise-induced pulmonary haemorrhage in the equine athlete. Vet Res Commun 1991; 15:211.
77. West JB, Mathieu-Costello O, Logemann RB, et al: Stress failure of pulmonary capillaries in racehorses with exercise-induced pulmonary hemorrhage (abstract). FASEB J 1992; 6:A2048.
78. Pascoe JR, McCabe AE, Franti CE, et al: Efficacy of furosemide in the treatment of exercise-induced pulmonary hemorrhage in thoroughbred racehorses. Am J Vet Res 1985; 46:2000.
79. Sweeney CR, Soma LR: Exercise-induced pulmonary hemorrhage in thoroughbred horses: Response to furosemide or hesperidin-citrus bioflavinoids. J Am Vet Med Assoc 1984; 185:195.
80. Soma LR, Laster L, Oppenlander F, et al: Effects of furosemide on the racing times of horses with exercise-induced pulmonary hemorrhage. Am J Vet Res 1985; 46:763.
81. Vulliet R: Questions experimental design in study on effects of furosemide on racing times of thoroughbreds. Am J Vet Res 1991; 51:1505.
82. Milne DW, Gabel AA, Muir WW, et al: Effects of furosemide on cardiovascular function and performance when given prior to simulated races: A double-blind study. Am J Vet Res 1980; 41:1183.
83. Lant A: Diuretics. Clinical pharmacology and therapeutic use, part I. Drugs 1985; 29:57.
84. Todi F, Fenwick J: Excretion of three diuretics, furosemide, trichlormethiazide and ethacrynic acid in the horse. *In* Johnston GH (ed): Proceedings of the 5th International Conference on Control of the Use of Drugs in Racehorses. Toronto, Canadian Section, Association of Official Racing Chemists, 1983, p 209.
85. Frey HH, Fitzek A, Wintzer HJ, et al: Use of bumetanide, a potent diuretic, to obtain urinary samples for dope testing in horses. Am J Vet Res 1976; 37:1257.
86. Delbeke FT, Debackere M, Desmet N, et al: Pharmacokinetics and diuretic effect of bumetanide following intravenous and intramuscular administration to horses. J Vet Pharmacol Ther 1986; 9:310.
87. Asbury MJ, Gatenby PBB, O'Sullivan S, et al: Bumetanide: Potent new "loop" diuretic. Br Med J 1972; 1:211.
88. Frey HH: Diuretic effect of high-ceiling diuretics in ponies (letter). J Vet Pharmacol Ther 1983; 6:157.
89. Snow DH: Anabolic steroids. Vet Clin North Am Equine Prac 1993; 9:563.
90. Lombardo JA, Hickson RC, Lamby DR: Anabolic/androgenic steroids and growth hormone. *In* Perspectives in Exercise Science. Indianapolis, Benchmark Press, 1991, p 249.

91. Wilson JD: Androgens. *In* Gilman AG, Rall TW, Nies AS, Taylor P (eds): The Pharmacological Basis of Therapeutics, 8th ed. New York, McGraw-Hill, 1990, p 1413.

92. Beroza GA: Anabolic steroids in the horse. J Am Vet Med Assoc 1981; 179:278.

93. Mooradian AD, Morley JE, Korenman SG: Biological actions of androgens. Endocr Rev 1987; 8:1.

94. Lamb DR: Anabolic steroids. *In* Williams MH (ed): Ergogenic Aids in Sports. Chicago, Ill, Human Kinetics Publishers, 1983, p 164.

95. Snow DH, Kerr MG, Nimmo MA, et al: Alterations in blood, sweat, urine, and muscle composition during prolonged exercise in the horse. Vet Rec 1982; 110:377.

96. Skelton KV, McMeniman NP, Dowsett KF: The effects of anabolic steroids on nitrogen metabolism in young horses. *In* Proceedings of the 11th Equine Nutrition and Physiology Symposium, 1989, p 114.

97. Blanchard TL: Some effects of anabolic steroids: Especially on stallions. Comp Cont Ed Pract Vet 1985; 7:s372.

98. Thornton JR, Dowsett KF, Mann R, et al: Influence of anabolic steroids on the response to training of 2 year old horses. *In* Persson SGB, Lindholm A, Jeffcott LB (eds): Equine Exercise Physiology 3. Davis, Calif, ICEEP Publications, 1991, p 503.

99. Maher JM, Squires EL, Voss JL, et al: Effect of anabolic steroids on reproductive function of young mares. J Am Vet Med Assoc 1983; 183:519.

100. Hoffman BB, Lefkowitz RJ: Catecholamines and sympathomimetic drugs. *In* Gilman AG, Rall TW, Nies AS, Taylor P (eds): The Pharmacological Basis of Therapeutics, 8th ed. New York, McGraw-Hill, 1990, p 187.

101. Snow DH: Metabolic and physiological effects of adrenoceptor agonists and antagonists in the horse. Res Vet Sci 1979; 27:372.

102. Anderson MG, Aitken MM: Biochemical and physiological effects of catecholamine administration in the horse. Res Vet Sci 1977; 22:357.

103. Adams HR: New perspectives in cardiopulmonary therapeutics: Receptor-selective adrenergic drugs. J Am Vet Med Assoc 1984; 185:966.

104. Shapland JE, Garner HE, Hatfield DG: Cardiopulmonary effects of clenbuterol in the horse. J Vet Pharmacol Ther 1981; 4:43.

105. Sasse HHL: Clinical aspects of current beta-agonist use in veterinary medicine. *In* Hanrahan JP (ed): Beta-Agonists and Their Effects on Animal Growth and Carcass Quality. Essex, Mass, Elsevier Applied Publishing, 1987, p 60.

106. Zeman RJ, Ludeman R, Easton TG, et al: Slow to fast alterations in skeletal muscle fibers caused by clenbuterol, a beta-2-receptor agonist. Am J Physiol 1988; 254:E726.

107. Rose RJ, Allen JR, Brock KA, et al: Effects of clenbuterol hydrochloride on certain respiratory and cardiovascular parameters in horses performing treadmill exercise. Res Vet Sci 1983; 35:301.

108. Rose RJ, Evans DL: Cardiorespiratory effects on clenbuterol in fit thoroughbred horses during a maximal exercise test. *In* Gillespie JR, Robinson NE (eds): Equine Exercise Physiology 2. Davis, Calif, ICEEP Publications, 1987, p 117.

109. Slocombe RF, Covelli G, Bayly WM: Respiratory mechanics of horses during stepwise treadmill exercise tests, and the effect of clenbuterol pretreatment on them. Aust Vet J 1992; 69:221.

110. Weiner N: Norepinephrine, epinephrine, and the sympathomimetic drugs. *In* Gilman AG, Goodman LS, Rall TW, Murad F (eds): The Pharmacological Basis of Therapeutics. New York, Macmillan, 1985, p 145.

111. Conlee RK: Amphetamine, caffeine and cocaine. *In* Lamd DR, Williams MH (eds): Perspectives in Exercise Science and Sports Medicine, Vol 4: Ergogenics: Enhancement of Athletic Performance. Ann Arbor, Mich, Brown-Benchmark, 1991, p 285.

112. Chandler JV, Blair SN: The effect of amphetamines on selected physiological components related to athletic success. Med Sci Sports Exerc 1980; 12:65.

113. Smetzer DL, Senta T, Hensel JD: Cardiovascular effects of amphetamine in the horse. Can J Comp Med 1972; 36:185.

114. Gabel AA, Milne DW, Ray RS, et al: A double-blind study of the effects of amphetamine and methylphenidate on physiological parameters in standardbred horses performing submaximal exercise tests. *In* Snow DH, Persson SDG, Rose RJ (eds): Equine Exercise Physiology. Cambridge, Granta Editions, 1983, p 521.

115. Lombardo JA: Stimulants. *In* Strauss RH (ed): Drugs and Performance in Sports. Philadelphia, WB Saunders Co, 1987, p 69.

116. Sanford J, Aitken MM: Effects of some drugs on the physiological changes during exercise in the horse. Equine Vet J 1975; 7:198.

117. Aitken MM, Sanford J, Mackenzie G: Factors influencing deceleration of the heart and respiratory rates after exercise in the horse. Equine Vet J 1973; 5:8.

118. Ritchie JM, Greene NM: Local anesthetics. *In* Gilman AG, Rall TW, Nies AS, Taylor P (eds): The Pharmacological Basis of Therapeutics, 8th ed. New York, McGraw-Hill, 1990, p 311.

119. McKeever KH, Hinchcliff KW, Gerken DF, et al: Effects of cocaine on incremental treadmill exercise in horses. J Appl Physiol (in press).

120. Cain SM: Exercise O_2 debts of dogs at ground level and at altitude with and without β-block. J Appl Physiol 1971; 30:838.

121. Anderson SD, Bye PTP, Perry CP, et al: Limitation of work performance in normal adult males in the presence of beta-adrenergic blockade. Aust NZ J Med 1979; 9:515.

122. Bengtsson C: Impairment of physical performance after treatment with beta blockers and alpha blockers. Br Med J 1984; 288:671.

123. Kaiser P: Running performance as a function of the dose-response relationship to β-adrenoceptor blockade. Int J Sports Med 1982; 3:29.

124. Snow DH, Summers RJ, Guy PS: The actions of the β-adrenoreceptor blocking agents propranolol and metoprolol in the maximally exercised horse. Res Vet Sci 1979; 27:22.

125. Schnabel A, Kindermann W, Salas-fraire O, et al: Effects of β-adrenergic blockade on supramaximal exercise capacity. Int J Sports Med 1983; 4:278.

126. Epstein SE, Robinson BF, Kahler RL, et al: Effects of beta-adrenergic blockade on the cardiac response to maximal and submaximal exercise in man. J Clin Invest 1965; 44:1745.

127. Hughson RL, MacFarlance BJ: Effect of propranolol on the anaerobic threshold and maximum exercise performance in normal man. Can J Physiol Pharmacol 1981; 59:567.

128. Anderson RL, Wilmore JH, Joyner MJ, et al: Effects of cardioselective and nonselective beta-adrenergic blockade on the performance of highly trained runners. Am J Cardiol 1985; 55:149d.

129. Tesch PA, Kaiser P: Effects of beta-adrenergic blockade on O_2 uptake during submaximal and maximal exercise. J Appl Physiol 1983; 54:901.

130. Plummer C, Knight PK, Ray SP, et al: Cardiorespiratory and metabolic effects of propranolol during maximal exercise. *In* Persson SGB, Lindholm A, Jeffcott LB (eds): Equine Exercise Physiology 3. Davis, Calif, ICEEP Publications, 1991, p 465.

131. Sexton WL, Erickson HH: Effects of propranolol on cardiopulmonary function in the pony during submaximal exercise. Equine Vet J 1986; 18:485.

132. Lundborg P, Astrom H, Bengtsson C, et al: Effect of β-adrenoceptor blockade on exercise performance and metabolism. Clin Sci 1981; 61:299.

133. Kaiser P: Physical performance and muscle metabolism during β-adrenergic blockade in man. Acta Physiol Scand 1984; 536:1.

134. Sklar J, Johnston GD, Overlie P, et al: The effects of a cardioselective (metoprolol) and a nonselective (propranolol) beta-adrenergic blocker on the response to dynamic exercise in normal men. Circulation 1982; 65:894.

135. Joyner MJ, Freund BJ, Jilka SM, et al: Effects of β-blockade on exercise capacity of trained and untrained men: A hemodynamic comparison. J Appl Physiol 1986; 60:1429.

136. Cronin RFP: Hemodynamic and metabolic effects of beta-adrenergic blockade in exercising dogs. J Appl Physiol 1967; 22:211.

137. Schroder G, Werko L: Hemodynamic studies and clinical experience with nethalide, a beta-adrenergic blocking agent. Am J Cardiol 1965; 15:58.

138. Fellenius E: Muscle fatigue and β-blockers: A review. Int J Sports Med 1983; 4:1.

139. Alway SE, Hughson RL, Green HJ, et al: Contractile properties of the human triceps surae following prolonged exercise and β-blockade. Clin Physiol 1987; 7:151.

140. Hughson RL, Green HJ, Alway SE, et al: The effects of β-blockade on electrically stimulated contraction in fatigued human triceps surae muscle. Clin Physiol 1987; 7:133.

141. Opie LH: Effect of beta-adrenergic blockade on biochemical and metabolic responses to exercise. Am J Cardiol 1985; 55:95d.

142. Bijman J, Quinton PM: Predominantly β-adrenergic control of equine sweating. Am J Physiol 1984; 246:R349.

143. Dyke TM: Sedatives, tranquilizers, and stimulants. Vet Clin North Am Equine Pract 1993; 9:621.

144. Ballard S, Shults T, Kownacki AA, et al: The pharmacokinetics, pharmacological responses and behavioral effects of acepromazine in the horse. J Vet Pharmacol Ther 1982; 5:21.

145. Muir WW, Skarda RT, Sheehan W: Hemodynamic and respiratory effects of a xylazine-acetylpromazine drug combination in horses. Am J Vet Res 1979; 40:1518.

146. Parry BW, Anderson GA, Gay CC: Hypotension in the horse induced by acepromazine maleate. Aust Vet J 1982; 59:148.

147. Booth NH: Psychotropic agents. *In* Booth NH, McDonald LE (eds): Veterinary Pharmacology and Therapeutics. Ames, Iowa, Iowa State University Press, 1988, p 363.

148. Fujii S, Yoshida S, Kusanagi C, et al: Pharmacological studies on doping drugs for race horses: IV. Chlorpromazine and phenobarbital. Jpn J Vet Sci 1975; 37:133.

149. Daunt DA, Maze M: α_2-Adrenergic agonist receptors, sites, and mechanism of action. *In* Short CE, Poznak AV (eds): Animal Pain. New York, Churchill Livingstone, 1992, p 165.

150. Wagner AE, Muir WW, Hinchcliff KW: The cardiovascular effects of xylazine and detomidine in horses. Am J Vet Res 1991; 52:651.

151. Moore RM, Trim CM: Effect of xylazine on cerebrospinal fluid pressure in conscious horses. Am J Vet Res 1992; 53:1558.

152. Thurmon JC, Neff-Davis C, Davis LE, et al: Xylazine hydrochloride-induced hyperglycemia and hyperinsulinemia in thoroughbred horses. J Vet Pharmacol Ther 1982; 5:241.

153. Thurmon JC, Steffey EP, Zinkl JG, et al: Xylazine causes transient dose-related hyperglycemia and increased urine volumes in mares. Am J Vet Res 1984; 45:224.

154. Rall TW: Drugs used in the treatment of asthma. *In* Gilman AG, Rall TW, Nies AS, Taylor P (eds): The Pharmacological Basis of Therapeutics, 8th ed. New York, McGraw-Hill, 1990, p 618.

155. Casal DC, Leon AS: Failure of caffeine to affect substrate utilization during prolonged running. Med Sci Sports Exerc 1985; 17:174.

156. Graham TE, Spriet LL: Performance and metabolic responses to a high caffeine dose during prolonged exercise. J Appl Physiol 1991; 71:2292.

157. Greene EW, Woods WE, Tobin T: Pharmacology, pharmacokinetics and behavioral effects of caffeine in horses. Am J Vet Res 1983; 44:57.

158. Fujii S, Yoshida S, Kusanagi C, et al: Pharmacological studies on doping drugs for race horses: II. Caffeine. Jpn J Vet Sci 1972; 34:141.

159. Errecalde JO, Button C, Mulders MSG: Some dynamic and toxic effects of theophylline in horses. J Vet Pharmacol Ther 1985; 8:320.

160. Kallings P, Persson S: Effects of theophylline and nonsteroidal anti-inflammatory drugs on pulse and blood lactate responses to exercise in horses: A preliminary report. *In* Snow DH, Persson SGB, Rose RJ (eds): Equine Exercise Physiology. Cambridge, Granta Editions, 1983, p 538.

161. Ingvast-larsson C, Kallings P, Persson S, et al: Pharmacokinetics and cardiorespiratory effects of oral theophylline in exercised horses. J Vet Pharmacol Ther 1989; 12:189.

162. Elliot CG, Nietrzeba RM, Adams TD, et al: Effect of intravenous aminophylline upon the incremental exercise performance of healthy men. Respiration 1985; 47:260.

163. Insel PA: Analgesic-antipyretics and antiinflammatory agents. *In* Gilman AG, Rall TW, Nies AS, Taylor P (eds): The Pharmacological Basis of Therapeutics, 8th ed. New York, McGraw-Hill, 1990, p 638.

164. Malmberg AB, Yaksh TL: Hyperalgesia mediated by spinal glutamate or substance P receptor blocked by spinal cyclooxygenase inhbition. Science 1992; 257:1276.

165. Campbell WB: Lipid-derived autacoids: eicosanoids and platelet activating factor. *In* Gilman AG, Rall TW, Nies AS, Taylor P (eds): The Pharmacological Basis of Therapeutics, 8th ed. New York, McGraw-Hill, 1990, p 600.

166. Aiken JW: Prostaglandins. J Cardiovasc Pharmacol 1985; 6:S413.

167. Oates JA, Fitzgerald GA, Branch RA, et al: Clinical implications of prostaglandins and thromboxane A_2 formation. N Engl J Med 1988; 319:761.

168. Demers LM, Harrison TS, Halbert DR, et al: Effect of prolonged exercise on plasma prostaglandin levels. Prostaglandin Med 1981; 6:413.

169. Ritter JM, Blair IA, Barrow SE, et al: Release of prostacyclin in vivo and its role in man. Lancet 1983; 317.

170. Wennmalm A, Fitzgerald GA: Excretion of prostacyclin and thromboxane A_2 metabolites during leg exercise in humans. Am J Physiol 1988; 255:H15.

171. Nowak J, Wennmalm A: Influence of indomethacin and of prostaglandin E_1 on total and regional blood flow in man. Acta Physiol Scand 1978; 102:484.

172. Birks EK, Giri SN, Li C, et al: Effects of exercise on plasma concentrations of prostaglandins and thromboxane B_2. *In* Persson SGB, Lindholm A, Jeffcott LB (eds): Equine Exercise Physiology 3. Davis, Calif, ICEEP Publications, 1991, p 374.

173. Morganroth ML, Young EW, Sparks HV: Prostaglandin and histaminergic mediation of prolonged vasodilation after exercise. Am J Physiol 1977; 233:H27.

174. Stebbins CL, Longhurst JC: Bradykinin-induced chemoreflexes from skeletal muscle: Implications for the exercise reflex. J Appl Physiol 1985; 59:56.

175. Pivarnik J, Kayrouz T, Senay LC: Plasma volume and protein content in progressive exercise: Influence of cyclooxygenase inhibitors. Med Sci Sports Exerc 1985; 17:153.

176. Staessen J, Cattaert A, Fagard R, et al: Hemodynamic and humoral effects of prostaglandin inhibition in exercising humans. J Appl Physiol 1984; 56:39.

177. Cowley AJ, Stainer K, Rowley JM, et al: Effect of aspirin and indomethacin on exercise-induced changes in blood pressure and limb blood flow in normal volunteers. Cardiovasc Res 1985; 19:177.

178. Cowley AJ, Stainer K, Rowley JM, et al: The effect of aspirin on peripheral haemodynamic changes following submaximal exercise in normal volunteers. Cardiovasc Res 1984; 18:511.

179. Kilbom A, Wennmalm A: Endogenous prostaglandins as local regulators of blood flow in man: Effect of indomethacin on reactive and functional hyperaemia. J Physiol 1976; 257:109.

180. Zambraski EJ, Dodelson D, Guidotti SM, et al: Renal prostaglandin E_2 and F_2 alpha synthesis during exercise: Effects of indomethacin and sulindac. Med Sci Sports Exerc 1986; 18:678.

181. Lees P, Higgins AJ: Clinical pharmacology and therapeutic uses of nonsteroidal anti-inflammatory drugs in the horse. Equine Vet J 1985; 17:83.

182. Kallings P: Nonsteroidal antiinflammatory drugs. Vet Clin North Am Equine Pract (in press).

183. Tobin T, Kamerling S, Nugent TE: Drugs and equine performance: A review. *In* Snow DH, Persson SGB, Rose RJ (eds): Equine Exercise Physiology. Cambridge, Granta Editions, 1983, p 510.

184. Tobin T, Chay S, Kamerling S, et al: Phenylbutazone in the horse: A review. J Vet Pharmacol Ther 1986; 9:1.

185. Hardee MM, Moore JN: Effects of flunixin meglumine, phenylbutazone and a selective thromboxane synthetase inhibitor (UK-38,485) on thromboxane and prostacyclin production in healthy horses. Res Vet Sci 1986; 40:152.

186. Moore JN, Hardee MM, Hardee GE: Modulation of arachidonic acid metabolism in endotoxic horses: Comparison of flunixin meglumine, phenylbutazone, and a selective thromboxane synthetase inhibitor. Am J Vet Res 1986; 47:110.

187. Higgins AJ, Lees P: Phenylbutazone inhibition of prostaglandin E_2 production in equine acute inflammatory exudate. Vet Rec 1983; 113:622.

188. Johansson IM, Kallings P, Hammarlund-Udenaes M: Studies of meclofenamic acid and two metabolites in horses: Pharmacokinetics and effects on exercise tolerance. J Vet Pharmacol Ther 1991; 14:235.

189. Kirkendall DT: Mechanisms of peripheral fatigue. Med Sci Sports Exerc 1990; 22:444.

190. Spriet LL, Lindinger MI, Heigenhauser GJF, et al: Effects of alkalosis on skeletal muscle metabolism and performance during exercise. Am J Physiol 1986; 251:R833.

191. Lindinger MI, Heigenhauser GJF, Spriet LL: Effects of alkalosis on muscle ions at rest and with intense exercise. Can J Physiol Pharmacol 1990; 68:820.

192. Linderman J, Fahey TD: Sodium bicarbonate ingestion and exercise performance: An update. Sports Med 1991; 11:71.

193. Williams MH: Bicarbonate loading. *In* Sports Science Exchange. Sports Nutrition Gatorade Sports Science Institute, 1992, p 36.

194. Heigenhauser G, Jones N: Bicarbonate loading. *In* Lamb DR, Williams M (eds): Ergogenics: Enhancement of Performance in Exercise and Sport. Dubuque, Iowa, Brown and Benchmark, 1991, p 183.

195. Goldfinch J, McNaughton L, Davies P: Induced metabolic alkalosis and its effects on 400-m racing time. Eur J Appl Physiol 1988; 57:45.

196. Wilkes D, Gledhill N, Smyth R: Effect of acute induced metabolic alkalosis on 800-m racing time. Med Sci Sports Exerc 1983; 15:277.

197. Bouissou P, Defer G, Guezennec CY, et al: Metabolic and blood catecholamine responses to exercise during alkalosis. Med Sci Sports Exerc 1988; 20:228.

198. Iwaoka K, Okagawa S, Mutoh Y, et al: Effects of bicarbonate ingestion on the respiratory compensation threshold and maximal exercise performance. Jpn J Physiol 1989; 39:255.

199. Costill DL, Verstappen F, Kuipers H, et al: Acid-base balance during repeated bouts of exercise: Influence of HCO_3. Int J Sports Med 1984; 5:228.

200. Gao J, Costill DL, Horswill CA, et al: Sodium bicarbonate ingestion improves performance in interval swimming. Eur J Appl Physiol 1988; 58:171.

201. Robertson RJ, Falkel JE, Drash AL, et al: Effect of blood pH on peripheral and central signals of perceived exertion. Med Sci Sports Exerc 1986; 18:114.

202. Katz A, Costill DL, King DS, et al: Maximal exercise tolerance after induced alkalosis. Int J Sports Med 1984; 5:107.

203. Parry-Billings M, MacLaren DPM: The effect of sodium bicarbonate and sodium citrate ingestion on anaerobic power during intermittent exercise. Eur J Appl Physiol 1986; 55:524.

204. Kowalchuk JM, Heigenhauser GJF, Jones NL: Effect of pH on metabolic and cardiorespiratory responses during progressive exercise. J Appl Physiol 1984; 57:1558.

205. Greenhaff PL, Snow DH, Harris RC, et al: Bicarbonate loading in the thoroughbred: Dose, method of administration and acid-base changes. Equine Vet J 1990; (suppl 9):83.

206. Hinchcliff KW, McKeever KH, Muir WW, et al: Effect of oral sodium loading on acid:base responses to horses to intense exercise. *In* Proceedings of the 13th Equine Nutrition and Physiology Symposium, 1993, p 121.

207. Greenhaff PL, Hanak J, Harris RC, et al: Metabolic alkalosis and exercise performance in the thoroughbred horse. *In* Persson SGB, Lindholm A, Jeffcott LB (eds): Equine Exercise Physiology 3. Davis, Calif, ICEEP Publications, 1991, p 353.

208. Lawrence LM, Miller PA, Bechtel PJ, et al: The effect of sodium bicarbonate ingestion on blood parameters in exercising horses. *In* Gillespie JR, Robinson NE (eds): Equine Exercise Physiology 2. Davis, Calif, ICEEP Publications, 1987, p 448.

209. Kelso TB, Hodgson DR, Witt EH, et al: Bicarbonate administration and muscle metabolism during high intensity exercise. *In* Gillespie JR, Robinson NE (eds): Equine Exercise Physiology 2. Davis, Calif, ICEEP Publications, 1987, p 438.

210. Lawrence L, Kline K, Miller-Graber P, et al: Effect of sodium bicarbonate on racing standardbreds. J Anim Sci 1990; 68:673.

211. Hardkins JD, Kamerling SG: Effects of induced alkalosis on performance in thoroughbreds during a 1600-m race. Equine Vet J 1992; 24:94.

212. Lloyd DR, Evans DL, Hodgson DR, et al: Effects of sodium bicarbonate on cardiorespiratory measurements and exercise capacity in thoroughbred horses. Equine Vet J 1993; 25:128.

213. Ross EJ, Christie SBM: Hypernatremia. Medicine 1969; 48:441.

214. Rose RJ, Lloyd DR: More than just a milkshake. Equine Vet J 1992; 24:75.

215. Greenhaff PL, Harris RC, Snow DH, et al: The influence of metabolic alkalosis upon exercise metabolism in the thoroughbred horse. Eur J Appl Physiol 1991; 63:129.

216. Hinchcliff KW, McKeever KH, Muir WW, et al: Effect of oral sodium bicarbonate on indices of athletic performance in horses. *In* Proceedings of the 72nd Conference of Research Workers in Animal Disease, 1991, p 30.

217. Freestone JF, Carlson GP, Harrold DR, et al: Furosemide and sodium bicarbonate–induced alkalosis in the horse and response to oral KCl or NaCl therapy. Am J Vet Res 1989; 50:1334.

Index

Note: Page numbers in *italics* refer to illustrations; page numbers followed by t refer to tables.

ISBN 0-7216-3759-0

90038

9 780721 637594